Exercise and Sport Sciences Reviews

Volume 22, 1994

EXERCISE AND SPORT SCIENCES REVIEWS

Volume 22, 1994

Editor

JOHN O. HOLLOSZY, M.D.

Professor of Medicine
Department of Internal Medicine
Washington University School of Medicine
St. Louis, Missouri

American College of Sports Medicine Series

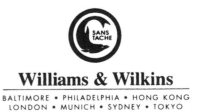

Williams & Wilkins

BALTIMORE • PHILADELPHIA • HONG KONG
LONDON • MUNICH • SYDNEY • TOKYO

A WAVERLY COMPANY

Editor: Timothy H. Grayson
Associate Editor: Carole E. Pippin
Copy Editor: Shelley Potler
Designer: Norman W. Och
Illustration Planner: Lorraine Wrzosek
Production Coordinator: Trudy Rutherford

RC
1200
.E94
V 22
July 1999

Copyright © 1994
American College of Sports Medicine

Printed in the United States of America
(ISBN 0-683-00036-5)

94 95 96 97
1 2 3 4 5 6 7 8 9 10

Preface

Exercise and Sport Sciences Reviews, an annual publication sponsored by the American College of Sports Medicine, reviews current research concerning behavioral, biochemical, biomechanical, clinical, physiological, and rehabilitational topics involving exercise science. The Editorial Board for this series currently consists of 15 recognized authorities who have assumed responsibility for one of the following general topics: athletic medicine, biochemistry, biomechanics, environmental physiology, epidemiology, exercise physiology, gerontology, growth and development, metabolism, molecular biology, motor control, physical fitness, psychology, rehabilitation, and sociology. The organization of the Editorial Board should help foster the commitment of the American College of Sports Medicine to publish timely reviews in areas of broad interest to clinicians, educators, exercise scientists, and students. The goal for this Editorial Board is to provide reviews in each of these 15 areas whenever sufficient new information becomes available on topics that are likely to be of interest to the readership of *Exercise and Sport Sciences Reviews.* Further, the Editor selects additional topics to be developed into chapters based on current interest, timeliness, and importance to the above audience. The contributors for each volume are selected by the Editorial Board members and the Editor.

John O. Holloszy, M.D.
Editor

Contributors

Paul J. Arciero, Ph.D.
Department of Medicine
Division of Endocrinology
Metabolism and Nutrition
University of Vermont
Burlington, Vermont

Neil Armstrong, Ph.D.
School of Education
Physical Education Association Research Centre
University of Exeter
Exeter, United Kingdom

Steven N. Blair, P.E.D.
Director of Epidemiology
The Cooper Institute for Aerobics Research
12330 Preston Road
Dallas, Texas

Ingrid K. M. Brenner, M.Sc.
School of Physical and Health Education
Queen's University
Kingston, Ontario, Canada

Gregory D. Cartee, Ph.D.
Biodynamics Laboratory
University of Wisconsin/Madison
Madison, Wisconsin

Wojtek J. Chodzko-Zajko, Ph.D.
School of PERD
163 MACC Annex
Kent State University
Kent, Ohio

J. Larry Durstine, Ph.D.
Department of Exercise Science
University of South Carolina
Columbia, South Carolina

Michael I. Goran, Ph.D.
Department of Medicine
Division of Endocrinology
Metabolism and Nutrition
University of Vermont
Burlington, Vermont

William L. Haskell, Ph.D.
Stanford Center for Research in Disease Prevention
Stanford University
Palo Alto, California

Charles S. Houston, M.D.
77 Ledge Road
Burlington, Vermont

Andrew S. Jackson, P.E.D., F.A.C.S.M.
Department of Health and Human Performance
University of Houston
Houston, Texas

Ira Jacobs, Dr. Med.Sc.
Environmental Physiology Section
Defence and Civil Institute of Environmental Medicine
North York, Ontario, Canada

William E. Kraus, M.D.
Department of Medicine
Duke University Medical Center
Box 3327
Durham, North Carolina

Andrea M. Kriska, Ph.D.
Department of Epidemiology
Graduate School of Public Health
University of Pittsburgh
Pittsburgh, Pennsylvania

Robert M. Malina, Ph.D., F.A.C.S.M.
Department of Kinesiology and Health Education
University of Texas
Austin, Texas

Lucie Martineau, Ph.D.
Environmental Physiology Section
Defence and Civil Institute of Environmental Medicine
North York, Ontario, Canada

Kathleen A. Moore, M.S.
Department of Psychology
c/o School of PERD
163 MACC Annex
Kent State University
Kent, Ohio

Michelle F. Mottola, Ph.D.
Faculty of Kinesiology
Thames Hall
University of Western Ontario
London, Ontario, Canada

Mark A. Pereira, M.S.
Department of Epidemiology
Graduate School of Public Health
University of Pittsburgh
Pittsburgh, Pennsylvania

Eric T. Poehlman, Ph.D.
Division of Gerontology
Department of Medicine
University of Maryland
Baltimore, Maryland

Doris A. Taylor, Ph.D.
Duke University Medical Center
Box 3327
Durham, North Carolina

Carol E. Torgan, Ph.D.
Duke University Medical Center
Box 3327
Durham, North Carolina

Richard W. Tsika, Ph.D.
University of Illinois at Urbana-Champaign
Department of Physiology and Biophysics
524 Burrill Hall
Urbana, Illinois

Andre L. Vallerand, Ph.D.
Environmental Physiology Section
Defence and Civil Institute of Environmental Medicine
North York, Ontario, Canada

Anton J. van den Bogert, Ph.D.
Faculty of Physical Education
University of Calgary
2500 University Drive N.W.
Calgary, Alberta, Canada

Joanne R. Welsman, Ph.D.
School of Education
Physical Education Association Research Centre
University of Exeter
Exeter, United Kingdom

Larry A. Wolfe, Ph.D., F.A.C.S.M.
School of Physical and Health Education
Queen's University
Kingston, Ontario, Canada

Kevin E. Yarasheski, Ph.D.
Metabolism Division
Washington University School of Medicine
St. Louis, Missouri

Contents

1
High Adventure: The Romance between Medicine and Mountaineering

CHARLES S. HOUSTON, M.D.

We are the pilgrims, master; we shall go
Always a little further; it may be
Beyond that last blue mountain barred with snow.
>   —James Elroy Flecker

My theme is searching, seeking, looking for something. As my professor of medicine, Robert Loeb, liked to say "Seek and ye shall find—maybe. But seek not and you won't find a damn thing." Scientists are always searching for answers, for truth, for solutions. Usually others have gone before us—so we *re*-search. Scientists are true pilgrims, going always a little further, looking for final answers.

Mountaineers too are searchers, whether for an elusive summit or the even more elusive self. "Whom have we conquered?" said one great climber. "None but ourselves." In science, as in climbing, there is always something more beyond that last blue mountain. And in life: "There are other Anapurnas in the lives of men," wrote Maurice Herzog.

Fortunately not every one is a wanderer; most of us are content to follow beaten paths, accepting conventional wisdom, risking little, and doing the world's work.

This essay describes the *romance between mountaineering and science*, commingling bits of the history of medicine and of exploration—not all of medicine, but that part we call altitude physiology. And not all exploration, but only mountaineering. Both are quests, both have rich victories and tragic defeats. Both attract men and women to push the envelope of the possible.

Along the way I will challenge some beliefs accepted as fact by our forebears but called fables today. I'll describe the dragons they saw and muse about the "dragons" of today.

Two thousand years ago, Chinese poets and artists rapturously described the beauty, the peace, the majesty of mountains. A few pilgrims climbed them.

Emperor Xuandi (91–49 BC) of the Han dynasty described Five Sacred Mountains, each of which had some special attribute. They were said to be the abodes of celestial beings to whom sacrifices were made by emperors, prayers said by the people, and poems written by scholars. The ancient

1

Greeks also revered mountains; their gods lived on magnificent Olympus, and it was not to be violated.

The ancient Chinese had a system of medical science quite alien to that of Hippocrates and Aristotle; much of it has persisted for 2500 years. Western science does not comprehend acupuncture and tai chi, so we tend to scoff at them, but they are used by—and seem to benefit—millions of people as they have for thousands of years. Traditional Chinese medicine is not based on what we call "scientific principles," yet it competes successfully in today's marketplace.

Did Chinese healers seek "truth" in science? Did they try to determine why their herbal medicines or acupuncture worked? Yes, but not as we do, not with rigor and the myriad measurements we can make today. Their evaluation was more pragmatic: if a treatment or a herbal mixture worked, they used it and did not ask why.

On high hills the Chinese found a spiritual peace many of us seek. Today our mountaineers compete on incredibly difficult routes to the highest summits. Why? What for? Old Chinese culture was sophisticated and elaborate, and their values of life, success, and achievement were worlds apart from ours.

Sometimes our predecessors saw danger in mountains. In Emperor Wudi's time (156–86 BC), General Du Qin urged that no envoys be sent to Kashmir because the mountains along the way were too perilous. South of the Karakoram ranges, he reported:

> travellers have to climb over Mount Greater Headache, Mount Lesser Headache, and the Fever Hills . . . they must support each other by ropes . . .

These obstacles lay athwart one branch of the ancient Silk Road, the most heavily traveled road in the world. The most dangerous portion was 120 km long, from Kezbak Pass across the 3600-meter Mustgah Pass to Kashgar. Over this road silk, tea, pottery, coinage, and skills of well drilling and paper making flowed westward, while wool and cotton, jewelry, and glass went eastward from Europe.

Other Chinese were pilgrims and also traveled far. Fa-Hsien (334–420 AD) and his companions wandered most of Asia for 15 years seeking enlightenment in hundreds of Buddhist monasteries. After crossing the Safeid Koh, on the way to the Kohat pass, Too-Kin wrote the first description of high-altitude pulmonary edema:

> Fa-Hsien and the two others proceeding southwards, crossed the Little Snowy Mountains. On them the snow lies accumulated both winter and summer. On the north side of the mountains, in the shade, they

suddenly encountered a cold wind which made them shiver and unable to speak. Hwuy-King could not go any farther. A white froth came from his mouth and he said to Fa-Hsien, "I cannot live any longer. Do you immediately go away, that we do not all die here"; and with these words he died.

Too-Kin also described snow blindness and other mountaineering perils:

> The snow reflects a white light so strong that the traveller has to shut his eyes and cannot see anything. Only after he has made sacrifices to the King of the Dragons will his eyesight be restored.
> The lakes in the Congling mountains are inhabited by poisonous dragons that breathe out poisonous clouds when enraged, causing downpours, blizzards and sandstorms from which no one can possibly escape alive. Congling is called "Snowy Mountains" by the natives.

Another early Buddhist missionary, Xuan Zang (602–664 AD), was also an outstanding mountaineer. In his masterpiece of geography and travel, *Travels to the Western Regions,* he described crossing passes and climbing mountains in the Tien Shan, Kun Lun, and Karakoram ranges. His highest climb was Lingshan (6000 m)—making him the first high-altitude climber. He wrote:

> The journey is arduous and dangerous and the wind dreary and cold. Travellers are often attacked by fierce dragons so that they should neither wear red garments nor carry gourds with them, nor shout loudly. Even the slightest violation of these rules will invite disaster.

The dragon theme recurs for many centuries and in many countries. Earlier generations in China had seen dragons as benevolent, so sacred that only high nobility could show dragon themes on their clothing. Next dragons were thought malevolent. In Europe many centuries later, reputable scientists took notarized statements from people who had been attacked by an extraordinary variety of dragons. Several distinguished scientists published beautiful illustrations of these monsters. What did they see? Where are these dragons today?

So far as we know neither Fa-Hsien nor other early explorer-mountaineers sought to understand the cause of the illness that afflicted them on mountains. In the sixteenth century, when some of Mirza Muhammad Haider's men and thousands of his horses died of mountain sickness on the high steppes of Central Asia, he tossed it off as "damgiri"—due to poisonous emanations from plants or minerals. In the same period Father Jose Acosta astutely blamed "thinne aire" for the acute mountain sickness he experienced on the stairs over high Pariacaca pass in the Andes. His contemporary Father Alonzo Ovalde agreed:

> When we come to ascend the highest point of the mountain, we feel an aire so piercing and subtile that it is with much difficulty we can breathe, which obliges us to fetch our breath quick and strong and to open our mouths wider than ordinary, applying to them likewise our handkerchiefs to protect our mouth and break the extreme coldness of the air and to make it more proportinable to the temperature which the heart requires, not to be suffocated; this I have experienced every time I have passed this mighty mountain.

A century later, among the Himalayas, Gruber repeated Acosta's "subtile aire" theory, but added:

> In summer certain poisonous weeds grow there which exude such a bad smell and dangerous odor that one cannot stay up there without losing one's life.

Such medical myths (we could liken them to dragons) persisted for many centuries as travelers blamed vapors from certain plants or minerals, and in fact one name—*soroche*—means antimony.

Then came a momentous experiment. Until the start of the seventeenth century, Aristotle's beliefs had been generally interpreted to fit the Church dogma that a vacuum, being nothing, could not exist, although "If God wished to create a vacuum he certainly could." Two great philosopher-scientists, Galileo and Descartes, disagreed. The former suspected there could be a vacuum, but waffled over details, while Rene Descartes flatly denied the possibility. The argument spread: Giovanni Baliani and Jean Rey and Rafael Magiotti became belivers. Jesuit Emmanuel Maignan, an unsung genius of that period, seems to have prompted the demonstration around 1640 by Gaspar Berti, which initiated the great advances.

Berti was a modest mathematician who left no records, and Father Maignan, one of the keenest minds of the century, wrote a long letter describing how Berti erected a tall leaden pipe against the wall of his house and arranged a series of taps or stop-cocks so that the pipe could be filled from a small tank at the top and then sealed. The lower end of the pipe was open and immersed in a cask of water.

> When the tap was opened, the water flowed out of the pipe into the cask . . . When it was closed, not all of it flowed out and it soon stood

quite still . . . when the tap R was opened . . . behold! the water rushed in with a loud noise, filling the space previously abandoned by the water.

Berti had demonstrated that a vacuum existed above the column of water (18 cubits, or about 396 inches high), and Magiotti and Baliani were satisfied that the water was held up by the weight of the air, as Beeckman had predicted years earlier. Exactly who developed from Berti's tall, water-filled lead pipe the simple mercury barometer is disputed, but Evangelista Torricelli has been given credit, and we measure atmospheric pressure in units named torr in his honor.

Within a few years came another great step forward: Florin Perier climbed a small mountain, the Puy du Dome, in southern France, carrying the Torricellian barometer and proved Acosta and Ovalde right: air was indeed thinner—less heavy—the higher one went. The Galilean-Aristotelian concepts of weight, pressure, and fluidity fell easily into the idea of impalpable air.

In Bavaria, Otto von Guericke made a simple vacuum pump and gave a dramatic demonstration of the weight of the atmosphere. By evacuating two copper hemispheres fitted snugly to each other, he showed that atmospheric pressure held them together so strongly that teams of horses could not separate them until the vacuum within was released.

Robert Boyle built his own pump, and with the Fellows of the Royal Society in London placed different substances and animals in a bell jar, which was then evacuated to see what happened when atmospheric pressure was decreased. Robert Hooke sat in a wooden barrel of his design as some of the air was pumped out, "taking him up" to about 4000 feet in the first decompression chamber ascent. Boyle's many correspondents took barometers to distant places and confirmed Perier's observations on the Puy do Dome.

Then we find a scientific "dragon": the myth of phlogiston advanced in 1669 by Johann Becher. He postulated that all substances were made of three kinds of "earth"' vitrifiable, mercurial, and combustible (not unlike the concepts that prevailed 2000 years earlier). When a substance was burned, the combustible portion was released. Georg Stahl soon named this portion "phlogiston," and some attributed to phlogiston a negative weight to explain inconvenient observations! Others thought that it was a "principle" rather than a substance. The phlogiston theory stimulated many experiments and survived for more than a century, even after oxygen was isolated and shown to be essential for life and combustion.

Not for still another century would lack of oxygen be proven the major cause of mountain sickness. Did the Chinese have an inkling of this? Were they curious? What did these pilgrims, these seekers, experience or find on their mountain journeys—besides dragons?

Chinese traders sought profit. Chinese poets sought beauty, while Fa-Hsien sought enlightenment. Alexander the Great and Haider were grabbing empires. The mummified man recently found on an alpine glacier was seeking something 2000 years ago—was he a hunter, prospector, or could he have been a daring explorer? Were there any others?

There were a few. King Peter of Arragon was described by a contemporary cleric as:

> a man of splendidly stout heart, a valiant knight, and learned in the arts of war . . . he was a man of great courage and did many feats of daring.

Sometime around 1275, the king decided to climb Pic Canigou, a small mountain in the Pyrenees, for no better reason than "to make the experiment and to ascertain what there was on top of it." He and his companions had a rough time:

> They began to hear very horrible and terrible thunder claps; in addition to this flashes of lightening began to appear and storms of hail to fall . . . all these so terrified them that they threw themselves on the ground and lay there, as it were, lifeless in their fear.

But, after soothing and feeding his companions, the King went on and

> with great labor made the ascent alone and when he was on the top of the mountain he found a lake there; and when he threw a stone into the lake, a horrible dragon of enormous size came out of it and began to fly around and to darken the sky with his breath.

Here is the dragon theme in Europe, 800 years after Fa-Hsien, and 500 years before Scheuchzer collected eyewitness accounts in the Alps.

When Domp Julian of Beaupre, perhaps the second true mountaineer, climbed formidable Mont Aiguille in 1492, he found the top to be

> covered with a beautiful meadow which it would take forty men to mow; there is also a beautiful herd of chamois which will never be able to get away.

But no dragons. This was an extraordinary climb, up a steep 800-foot face, first driving wooden pegs into a vertical crack and then creeping along narrow ledges; it was so difficult that no one repated it for four hundred years. At the time of the second ascent, the meadow and the chamois had disappeared.

Soon after this, a famous genius, Leonardo Da Vinci, went even higher, onto a mountain which

> has its base at so great a height as this, which lifts itself above almost all the clouds; and snow falls seldom there, but only hail when the clouds are highest.

There has been great argument over which mountain it was: he called it Monboso (most likely Monte Rosa), and he probably reached the Col d'Olen at 10,000 feet, where Mosso much later built a laboratory.

Another early mountaineer, Seigneur de Villamont, was more daring and more specific when in June 1588 he climbed Roche Melon which was said to be

> the highest mountaine of all the Alpes, saving one of those that part Italy and Germany. Some told me it was fourteen miles high; it is covered with a very Microcosm of clowdes . . . As the day broke, we continued the stiff ascent, which we found more difficult than it had been at first, with the result that I wanted to turn back . . . until, having got more than three leagues high, I had to fasten irons to my hands and feet in order to climb, and also for fear of falling down the precipices, which threatened us with a horrible death.

These "irons" may have been those described a few years earlier by Josias Simmler, a Swiss inn-keeper, who published a guidebook detailing the clothing and equipment needed for Alpine travel, and how to avoid avalanches and frostbite. He included one dragon picture! Much of his remarkable book *De Alpibus Commentarius* is still fresh and relevant today.

Villamont seems to have climbed what is only a small mountain simply from curiosity. Acosta, Ovalde, and others in the Society of Jesus needed to cross high mountain passes to reach the natives high in the Andes whom they wished to convert. Their contemporary, physician Conrad Gesner, found spiritual and physical refreshment on mountains. His companion, Professor Marti, saw written on a boulder on a summit an ancient Greek inscription:

> Love of mountains is best.

Gesner and Marti seem to have been among the few who climbed for pleasure in those days; what little mountain travel was done was utilitarian.

Meanwhile in China, Xu Xiake, born in 1586, was a great explorer and writer. His book *The Travels of Xu Xiake* describes similar use of ropes and crampons, and a rudimentary ax with which he cut steps on steep snow and ice during many of his climbs.

The first of what we would call "direct aid" climbing had been done almost two thousand years earlier, when Alexander the Great was seeking to conquer the world. His army assaulted the Sogdian (or Ariamazes) Rock, a mighty fort on a thousand-foot pinnacle. The 30,000 defenders scoffed at Alexander's demand for their surrender. According to Arrian, the King was furious, so at night, in winter:

> There were some 300 men who in previous sieges had had experience in rock-climbing. These now assembled. They had provided themselves with small iron tent-pegs, which they proposed to drive into the snow, where it was frozen hard, or into any bit of bare earth they might come across, and they attached to the pegs strong flaxen lines . . . then driving their pegs either into bare ground or into such patches of snow as seemed most likely to hold under the strain, they hauled themselves up, wherever each could find a way. About thirty lost their lives during the ascent—falling in various places into the snow, their bodies were never recovered—but the rest reached the summit just as dawn was breaking.[a]

The awestruck defenders immediately surrendered. We don't know of a similar exploit until 1492, when Domp Julian drove his wooden pegs into the cliffs of Mont Aiguille; he was seeking only to obey the orders of his king.

There are many accounts of men who climbed for practical reasons, including Moses, warriors like Philip of Macedon, philosopher-scientist Empedocles, Marco Polo, and travelers on the ancient trade routes. Hannibal and Caesar crossed passes to conquer other lands. Perier climbed a hill to see whether barometric pressure fell as altitude increased. Conrad Gesner, in his book *On the Admiration of Mountains* published the same year as Simmler's, wrote:

> I have determined for the future, so long as the life divinely granted to me shall continue, each year to ascend a few mountains, or at least one . . . partly for the sake of bodily exercise and the delight of the spirit.

---

[a]Curtius Rufus Quintus has a slightly different version: he wrote that the soldiers drove their 'wedges' into cracks between the rocks; be claimed the rock was 30 furlongs (6000 feet) high.

At the time it was so firmly believed that the body of Pontius Pilate lay in the small lake on the summit of Pilatus, that the death penalty was paid by those who disturbed the waters. Thirty years after Gesner's climb, in 1585, Johann Muller, Pastor of Lucerne, climbed Pilatus with a group of brave citizens and threw stones into the small dark lake from which evil dragons and all sorts of natural disasters had been said to emerge. Nothing happened. In his encyclopedia of natural history, Gesner included descriptions of some 250 species of dragons that were said to roam the mountains.

Mountaineering as a sport really began only in the mid seventeen hundreds, when two British gentlemen of leisure described the magnificence of the highest mountain in Europe. Their book and lectures brought both the adventuresome and the scientists to the remote village of Chamonix beneath beautiful Mont Blanc. Others like generalist Marc Bourrit and Johann Jakob Scheuchzer had already been there to catalog the flora and fauna, including dragons and other fearsome creatures that were reliably reported to roam the peaks and valleys. Few of these visitors actually climbed.

The science of mountain medicine was also born in Chamonix with the visit of Horace Benedict de Saussure, who made the second ascent of Mont Blanc (4350 m) in 1787. Impressed by his sensations on the summit, he recorded his pulse, respirations, temperature, and symptoms on that and other mountains, and wrote perceptively:

> I was out of breath by the rarity of the air; however by resting a moment every thirty or forty paces, but without sitting down, so far recovered my breath, as to be able in about forty minutes to get to the edge of the avalanche which had fallen the previous night, and which we had heard from our tent. There we all stopped for some minutes in hope that after having rested our lungs and legs we should be able to get over the avalanche pretty quick and without resting to take breath, but in that we deceived ourselves, the sort of weariness which proceeds from the rarity of the air is absolutely insurmountable; when it is at its height, the most eminent peril will not make you move a step faster.
>
> Since the air (on the summit of Mont Blanc) had hardly more than half of its usual density, compensation had to be made for the lack of density by the frequency of inspirations . . . That is the cause of the fatigue that one experiences at great heights. For while the respiration is accelerating, so also is the circulation.

De Saussure did not quite take the next step. Ten years earlier, Priestley and Lavoisier had isolated oxygen and proven that it was the "vital spirit" that John Mayow much earlier had shown was necessary for life. Not for a hundred years would bits of knowledge be put together proving that lack of oxygen due to decreased atmospheric pressure was the cause of mountain sickness.

After De Saussure, many travelers described the symptoms experienced when they went higher than 3000 m. From 1797 to 1802, Alexander von Humboldt traveled extensively in South America and climbed to 5700 m on Chimborazo, an altitude record not matched for thirty years. He wrote:

> We all became by degrees much distressed; a constant desire to vomit, together with vertigo, were the most prominent symptoms, and proved far more trying than the difficulty of breathing which we likewise suffered from.
>
> The distress, the weakness, and the desire to vomit certainly came as much from the lack of oxygen in these regions as from the rarity of the air.

Humboldt seems to have been the first to propose that lack of oxygen was the cause, but later, confusingly, he refers to the "lessened quantity of oxygen in the same volume of air." He also read an article by Dr Berard purporting to show that atmospheric pressure held joints together and suggesting that the fatigue experienced at altitude was due to loosening of the coxofemoral joint. Humboldt picked up this idea which soon became popular:

> It would be better to examine the probability of the effect of a lessened air pressure upon weariness when the legs are moving in regions where the atmosphere is greatly reduced . . . the leg, attached to the body, is supported when it moves, only by the pressure of the atmospheric air.

Lack of oxygen was ignored in a small book published in 1853 by Professor Stanhope Speer. After summarizing physiological observations made by many contemporary climbers on high mountains, mostly relating to the pulse rate, Speer nearly got it right when he wrote:

> These symptoms (of mountain sickness) may be referred to a threefold source, viz., a gradually increasing congestion of the deeper portions of the circulatory apparatus, increased velocity of the blood, and loss of equilibrium between the pressure of the external air and that of the gases existing within the intestines . . . the causes of mountain sickness are themselves the result of a change from a given atmospheric pressure and temperature, to one in which both are greatly and suddenly diminished.

In fairness, remember that oxygenation of blood was not proven until Paul Bert did so fifty years later, although Aristotle, and much later Lower, had already commented that dark venous blood changed color when exposed to air. Mayow had even placed freshly drawn arterial blood under his bell jar and watched bubbles appear as he pumped out the air.

Though not much came of it. Junod began to study mountain sickness by repeating Robert Hooke's experiment: he placed a man in a large sphere which he "took up" to an altitude of about 1250 m by evacuating the air—just as Hooke had done two hundred years earlier! Junod went on to treat a great range of afflictions by "decompressing" the lower half of the body; this was as profitable as Liebig's row of chambers in which one or two persons could relax while being "taken up" to altitude for an hour or two.

Bouguer remained for three weeks on the summit of Pichincha in the Andes and felt no symptoms after the first few days. He and a few other travelers commented that natives who lived at altitude did not suffer as much as did the sea-level residents, early indications of acclimatization.

In 1700, Johann Jakob Scheuchzer was a distinguished professor of physics in Zurich, who often vacationed in the Alps, where he developed a theory describing the formation of glaciers and collected plants. He was attracted to studying dragons by carvings of them on some public buildings and especially because of a "dragon stone" in a museum in Lucerne. A dragon stone, or bezoar, can be cut out of a dragon's head while the dragon is asleep, lulled with soporific herbs. Scheuchzer's curiosity and credibility were stirred by the anesthesia required to operate on the sleeping dragon! He obtained notarized statements from men of good reputation who had seen or even been attacked by dragons in the Swiss Alps, and believed completely in dragons in 1726, when he published two large illustrated folios. But in 1745 he dismissed the dragon stories as fables. We don't know whether he tried to obtain a bezoar, which had such magical properties as antidote for poisons.

A century before this, Father Alonzo Ovalde, a Jesuit, had been shown dragon stones during his travels in the Andes, where he suffered from altitude in 1649. He brought home a large bezoar, which he was told came, not from a dragon, but from guanacos (chamois, wild goats like those in Europe). Bezoars were used to treat many infirmities and poisonings including bites from venomous serpents and poisonous plants. He reported that:

> The virtue of these bezoar-stones is very well known and experienced; people of quality take them, not only in time of sickness, but also in health, to preserve it; the way of using them is to put them whole into the vessel which holds wine or water, or into the glass out of which one drinks and the longer they stay in, the more virtue they communicate . . . it would have more virtue to grate a little of the stone to powder, and drink it; whatsoever way it is taken it comforts the heart, purifies the blood, and the using of it is looked upon as a preservative against all infirmities.

Another distinguished naturalist, Ulisse Aldrovandi, also published a beautifully illustrated set of folios with many dragons, but I saw no bezoar stones in his books.

Medical science has had its own dragons—strongly held beliefs that endured for centuries. One that relates to medicine, Galen's description of the circulation of the blood, suppressed contrary evidence for a thousand years until Servetus proved him wrong and was burned at the stake for this heresy. Aristotle was certain that a vacuum was impossible, and Galileo waffled about it (he was already suspect to the Church) until Baliani and Berti demonstrated that a vacuum could be created.

Belief in the philosopher's stone survived for many centuries: it could cure many varieties of illness and transform base minerals to precious ones. Spontaneous generation of life required careful experiments to disprove. Belief in phlogiston rivaled oxygen for almost a century. These misbeliefs are some of the "dragons" of science; there were—and still are—many others.

Except as incidental, studies of altitude illness languished for more than fifty years after De Saussure, during which 57 ascents of Mont Blanc were made, two by women. Then in 1851 a London physician, Albert Smith, described his own ascent so vividly that hundreds took up the sport, beginning the Golden Age of Alpine climbing. Though Smith's symptoms suggest that he had developed high-altitude cerebral edema near the summit, he seems to have had no interest in altitude physiology. But others, like Friedrich von Tschudi, exploring the Andes in 1838–1842, had described their mountain sickness vividly.

My panting mule slackened his pace, and seemed unwilling to mount a rather steep ascent which we had now arrived at. To relieve him I dismounted, and began walking at a rapid pace. But I soon felt the influence of the rarefied air, and I experienced an oppressive sensation which I had never known before. I stood still for a few moments to recover myself, and then tried to advance. My heart throbbed audibly; my breathing was short and interrupted. A world's weight seemed to lie upon my chest; my lips swelled and burst; the capillaries of my eyes gave way, and blood flowed from them. In a few moments my senses began to leave me. I could neither see, hear, nor feel distinctly. A grey mist floated before my eyes, and I felt myself involved in that struggle between life and death which, a short time before, I fancied I could discern on the face of nature. Had all the riches of earth, or the glories of heaven, awaited me a few hundred feet higher, I could not have stretched out my hand toward them. In that half senseless state I lay stretched on the ground until I felt sufficiently recovered to remount my mule.

It is interesting that many of the early mountaineers—even into the nineteenth century—described bleeding from the nose, lips, and eyes, which is rare today. And they often do not mention the headache, which is such a common symptom.

After Smith's adventures, in the next 35 years every Alpine summit was reached, and as skill increased, a new climb passed through stages, described by Mummery as "an impossible peak, the most difficult climb in the Alps, and finally an easy day for a lady." Climbers began to visit the high Andes and Himalaya.

Mountain sickness was frequently described, based on little study but many theories. Conrad Meyer-Ahrens, a leading Zurich physician, in 1854 covered all bases:

> Mountain sickness is due to (a) decrease in the absolute quantity of oxygen, (b) rapidity of evaporation, (c) intensity of light, (d) expansion of intestinal gases and (e) weakening of the coxo-femoral articulation.

This "weakening" or dislocation of the coxo-femoral articulation was favored by others too. The distinguished physicist John Tyndall, a delightful writer and astute observer, wrote of his ascent of Mont Blanc in 1857:

> I counted the number of paces which we were able to accomplish without resting, and found that at the end of every twenty, sometimes at the end of fifteen, we were compelled to pause. At each pause my heart throbbed audibly, as I leaned upon my staff, and the subsidence of this action was always the signal for further advance. My breathing was quick but light and unimpeded. I endeavored to ascertain whether the hip joint, on account of the diminished atmospheric pressure, became loosened, so as to throw the weight of the leg upon the surrounding ligaments, but could not be certain of it.

Some distinguished scientists argued that diminished atmospheric pressure caused the fluids of the body to expand. An American surgeon blamed earth's magnetism. For several centuries emanations from plants (rhubarb, marigolds, heather) or minerals (antimony, lead) had been blamed for what was called *damgiri, puna, mareo, or soroche*.

Then came a great man. After studying law, Paul Bert took his degree in medicine and studied respiration under Claude Bernard. He met a Paris physician, Denis Jourdannet, a wealthy patron of the arts and sciences, who had traveled in Mexico. They became friends and fellow-workers. Jourdannet provided equipment for Bert's innovative studies: the decompression chambers and the gas analysis equipment. Bert extracted gases from the blood of animals exposed to decreased pressures, and defined a portion of the familiar oxyhemoglobin dissociation curve.

Describing his observations in Mexico and his work with Bert, Jourdannet wrote:

> Anoxemia is the counterpart of anemia . . . An ascent above 3000 m is equivalent to a barometric disoxygenation of the blood as a bleeding is to a corpuscular disoxygenation.

Jourdannet subsidized Bert's magnificent book *La Pression Barometrique,* an extraordinary encyclopedia of all that was then known—or believed—about altitude sickness.[b] Bert and Jourdannet showed beyond reasonable doubt, that lack of oxygen was the main, if not the only cause of the symptoms experienced on high mountains. Bert did not climb, and Jourdannet was a traveler rather than a mountaineer. But one of their contemporaries was both doctor and climber.

Angelo Mosso was already an experienced mountaineer and physiologist when he was attracted by the writings of German poet-doctor Albrecht Haller:

> Even though the air be reduced to half its weight, it may still be breathed without difficulty as I experienced on the mountains.

Mosso challenged Haller and Bert with his studies in a decompression chamber and, beginning in 1893, in a laboratory built for him by Queen Margherita of Italy on Monte Rosa at 5470 m. His observations convinced him that the decrease of carbon dioxide in the blood that resulted from overbreathing at altitude was more influential than lack of oxygen as a cause of mountain sickness. He coined the work "acapnia" and thought he could relieve—or prevent—symptoms by adding a small amount of carbon dioxide to the air as his subjects were "taken up" in his chamber. His book *Life of Man on the High Alps* is rich in laboratory observations and mountain experiences.

Other scientists were also turning to high summits. Joseph Vallot was studying mountain flora and geology when he was attracted to Mont Blanc. First he sought to determine whether or not mountain sickness was caused by a decrease in body temperature, which was then a popular theory. In

---

[b]This work, ignored at the time, was translated in 1942 by Charles and Mary Hitchcock and is indispensable to mountain physiology.

1887, he spent three nights on the summit of Mont Blanc in a tent and was so impressed that he decided to build a laboratory in which to pursue more research.

He went about it carefully, arriving in Chamonix with 19 cases containing three duplicate sets of instruments, one to be read in the valley, one half-way up the mountain, and one in a small building he had arranged to have built in a safe spot somewhat below the summit. After he had made many meteorological measurements and had proved that body temperature was not affected by altitude, his building was abandoned. A new one was erected in 1898; it has been rebuilt and enlarged and is an active research laboratory today.

Soon after the first Vallot shelter was completed, a distinguished astronomer, Jules Janssen, spent a few days there and decided to build his own observatory on the summit for spectroscopic analysis of the air, which was ideally clear; after much difficulty his shelter was completed in August 1891. Believing that exertion was a major cause of the mountain sickness he suffered, he later had himself pulled up the mountain on a sled and felt none of the unpleasant symptoms that affected the 42 men who dragged him.

One member of Janssen's party, Dr. Egli-Sinclair, had to depart, and a young Chamonix doctor, Etienne Henri Jacottet, took his place. Jacottet climbed up too rapidly, soon became ill, and died. An autopsy by Dr Wizard read in part:

> Poumon: couleur violet, gonfle, fonce, congestion bilaterale, oedeme considerable muqueeuse bronchique injectee fortement. Le liquide de la coupe est ecumeneux. Congestion egale partout. Foie, rate, reins normaux. Pas de'oedeme des jambes.

This is a good description of the pathology of high-altitude pulmonary edema. Jacottet's vivid letter to his brother, writtten in his last hours, have made him the first martyr to high-altitude science. Another member of the group, Dr. Imfeld, suffered a severe stroke shortly after descent.

Dr. Hugo Kronecker was consultant for the railroad being built up to the shoulder of a beautiful Swiss peak, the Jungfrau. To decide whether passengers on the train would feel ill from the altitude, he had seven men and women carried in chairs up to 3600 m; like Janssen, they did not have mountain sickness. Kronecker believed that diminished atmospheric pressure dilated the blood vessels, straining the heart, and he described six cases that probably were not heart failure but high-altitude pulmonary edema.

In 1870, Nathan Zuntz moved from country practice to a university professorship and soon the rapid increase in mountain tourism and some deaths during high balloon flights led him into altitude research. Zuntz became another pioneer through his interest in metabolism and respiratory physiology, both in his decompression chamber and during mountain expeditions to the Alps, Pikes Peak, and the Canary islands. With colleague Adolph Loewy and assistants Mueller and Gaspari he wrote another of the classics in physiology: *Hohenklima und Bergwanderung.*

These were the beginnings of a great surge of interest in altitude physiology. Soon leading scientists were making expeditions to mountains all over the world. Zuntz invited Barcroft, Douglas, and Durig to join an expedition to the peak of Teneriffe (12,200 ft) in 1909, specifically to look at Mosso's acapnia theory. Two years later came the first scientific expedition to Pikes Peak (14,100 ft), originating when young Yandel Henderson invited Haldane to come to America to study high altitude!

At the time, John Scott Haldane had been studying caisson illness—a problem for workers building dams or tunnels and working under increased pressure. He was also interested in carbon monoxide poisoning—a prominent cause of oxygen lack. Like Paul Bert he took up problems of decreased atmospheric pressure as well and became a major player in altitude studies for two decades. He, Douglas, and Schneider accepted Henderson's invitation, and the party spent 6 weeks on the summit of Pikes Peak. Mabel Fitzgerald, refused a place in this male party, rode a horse throughout the Colorado Rockies and analyzed the hemoglobin content of blood and alveolar gases of hundreds of miners living at altitude, landmark research that has not been surpassed.

Haldane's data on Pike's Peak convinced him that the alveolar cells could actually secrete oxygen, thus making the oxygen pressure in the pulmonary artery higher than that in the alveolus.

Joseph Barcroft, an imaginative physiologist interested in mountaineering, disagreed. He spent 10 days at sea level in a sealed room where the oxygen was gradually decreased. Using a large needle, recently described by Stadie, Barcroft drew arterial blood and collected alveolar air samples. He found that his arterial blood contained less oxygen than his alveolar air; Haldane's theory was disproven.

In 1923, Barcroft organized a party to study acclimatization in the Andes, at Cerro de Pasco and Morococha. Their observations are included in two charming and stimulating books about mountain medicine: Barcroft's *The Respiratory Functions of the Blood: Lessons from High Altitude* and, in 1934, *The Architecture of Physiological Function*. Studies there confirmed his finding that alveolar air contained more oxygen than arterial blood.

Apparently these men did not know of the first comprehensive clinical description of altitude illnesses, written in 1913 by Thomas Ravenhill, doctor for a mining company at 15,000 feet in the Andes. Like case reports by Zuntz and Kronecker, Ravenhill's article lay undiscovered in an obscure journal for many years.

As for mountaineers, it had long been believed that to spend a night above 20,000 feet would be fatal, and the rate of climb was painfully slow.

But Dr. and Mrs. Bullock Workman said they slept reasonably well during many weeks above 20,000 feet, and in 1905 Dr. Tom Longstaff, very well acclimatized, climbed from 17,600 to 23,360 feet in 10 1/2 hours. In 1906, Longstaff published his doctoral thesis, titled *Mountain Sickness and its Probable Cause,* in which he tends to agree with Mosso that acapnia contributes to the signs and symptoms of altitude illness. Since then men and women have survived many nights much higher, even on top of Everest. Another "dragon" had perished!

By the end of the nineteenth century, an attempt on Everest seemed possible, as Tibet became more amenable. The summit even seemed attainable as climbers pushed their ceiling higher and higher. In 1892, a distinguished surgeon-mountaineer, Clifford Dent, predicted the summit would be reached; unfortunately he was somewhat mistaken about the cause of altitude illness:

> A far more important factor (than abdominal distention) is the effect of diminished pressure on the portion of the spinal marrow which is concerned with the nutrition of the locomotive agents, the lower limbs; greatly increased pressure also produces much the same symptoms. This effect has no relation to the absence of oxygen.

These early Himalyan climbers made no physiological observations, and the first serious studies of man's ability to summit Everest "*without adventitious aids*" were those of mountaineer-chemist Alexander Kellas. Kellas did no laboratory work, but from others' data calculated that a well-acclimatized and trained climber could reach the summit. He was puzzled that the height where AMS becomes a problem differs between individuals and from place to place. He accepted the belief that facing into the wind increases alveolar oxygen by "*packing air into the lungs.*"

Kellas knew that alkalosis resulted from altitude hyperventilation, but, lacking accurate measurements, he hedged a bit:

> At high altitude . . . the quantity of carbon dioxide in the blood is lowered, but the acidity increases (or rather the alkalosis produced by removal of carbon dioxide is diminished correspondingly) and the respiratory center remains adequately stimulated.

Kellas died en route to Everest in 1924, at the start of the expedition on which Mallory and Irvine disappeared near the summit, and Norton reached 8570 m, where the atmospheric oxygen pressure (51 torr) is only two or three torr more than on the summit. Not for almost 50 years would that last thousand feet be climbed breathing only air, as Kellas had predicted would be done.

During the 1924 expedition, surgeon Hingston recorded pulse rates, blood pressure, breath-holding time, and red blood cell counts on eight of the climbers up to 21,500 feet, the first such data collected so high.

However, access to Everest was strictly controlled by the Tibetans, and only a few British parties were allowed, so those who wished to study the effects of altitude turned to smaller, less formidable peaks and to another great Himalayan peak.

In the 1930s, German mountaineers were attempting to climb Nanga Parbat, at 8125 m the seventh highest summit in the world. Although their goal was to reach the top, in 1934 important studies were made there (and in Berlin) by Ulrich Luft. His definitive thesis, *Acclimatization to Altitude,* was published in 1941, but only recently translated into English and made generally available.

The long romance between science and mountaineering has blossomed in the last 50 years, hastened by several forces. First there was the great leap forward in physiology due to the imperatives of air warfare in WWII. Even though mountaineering was stifled, the human responses to high altitude were explored, and this continued after hostilities ended. In 1946, a decompression chamber study called Operation Everest showed that the thin air on the mountain summit need not be fatal and provided clues to the intricacies of acclimatization.

Soon political forces caused the opening of more and more reclusive mountain ranges in central Asia, beginning the Golden Age of Himalayan mountaineering in 1950. Hard-core climbers soon recognized how much the life sciences could contribute to their success, even to their survival on the highest mountains. The powerful synergy between the stresses of hypoxia, hypothermia, hunger, and dehydration was recognized, and when not appreciated, such stresses caused many deaths.

Griffith Pugh's studies on Cho Oyu were helpful to the first oxygen ascent of Everest in 1953. More expeditions combining physiology and climbing soon followed; it became chic to do science **and** climb, and money became available for respectable mountain medical projects. The Silver Hut (1962), the Mt. Logan studies (1967–78), the Denali research laboratory (1977–87), and well-equipped laboratories high on Mont Blanc and Monte Rosa have stimulated state-of-the-art research. In 1981 came AMREE, which collected data on acclimatizing mountaineers, some of it as high as Everest's summit, and similar climbing cum research expeditions have gone to other mountains as well. Another large decompression chamber study (Operation Everest II) in 1985 added more understanding of acclimatization.

A major factor in the explosion of mountain research was the fantastic evolution of instruments that could measure almost anything under almost any conditions. Scientist-mountaineers could do electrocardiograms on the summits, measure cerebral and pulmonary blood flow anywhere any time, and could collect for later analysis fluid from the lungs, blood, urine, and muscle tissue. Just as it seemed there were few frontiers left, the genetic engineers opened a completely new area.

Hand in hand with the onrush of science came increasing expertise in climbing techniques. The limit of the possible stretched so that it seemed the audacious might climb an overhanging wall of glass. Once Everest and K-2 had been climbed from base to summit and back in one day, without oxygen, others tried to beat the time—and some died. Technical mountaineering has mutated to competitive acrobatics on man-made (as well as natural) cliffs of paralyzing difficulty. Equipment and nutrition have kept pace.

Not to be ignored is the increasing flood of tourists, skiers, and hikers who go to mountainous areas where altitude sickness is likely and can even be fatal. This growing recognition has led to more studies on healthy people of all ages, visiting moderate altitude. These activities seem likely to attract an increasing number of ordinary people!

Where will the romance take us? Is old-style exploration/mountaineering dying, now that few areas on earth are unexplored? Will fame and fortune continue to fall to him who does the unbelievable on high mountains? Will competitive climbing discolor the art of mountaineering? Or will fickle humans turn to other games?

What new frontiers will open in genetic and molecular physiology? New instruments of currently unimagined capability will be available. What secrets will be left a few decades from now? We have very far to go before we approach the limits. Exploring normal physiology in humans under abnormal conditions enlightens our comprehension of the patients with hypoxic illness. And it is certain that many lessons will be learned from other forms of hypoxic life.

Even when all the now known mountains have been climbed and we believe we have learned all about life, there will always be more

. . . blue rimmed mountains lined with snow

and other dragons to be found and slain.

ACKNOWLEDGMENTS

I gratefully acknowledge the help and encouragement of Pius Burki (Zurich), Zhou Zheng (Beijing), Nancy Crane (Burlington), and Bob Bates (Exeter).

SUGGESTED READINGS

Acosta, J. *The Natural and Moral Historie of the East and West Indies.* London: Blount and Apley, 1604.

Aldrovandi, Ulysse. *Natural History.* Folio in Library of Congress, circa 1650.

Barcroft, J. *Respiratory Function of the Blood. Part I. Lessons from High Altitude.* New York: Cambridge University Press, 1925.

Barcroft, J., C. A. Binger, A. V. Bock, H. S. Forbes, G. Harrop, et al. Observations upon the effect of high altitude on the physiological process of the human body. *Proc. R. Soc. Lond.* [Series B] 211:352–480, 1923.

Bernier, F. *Travels in the Mogul Empire.* London: Pickering, 1826.

Bert, P. *Barometric Pressure.* Bethesda, MD: Undersea Medical Society, 1978.

Blaschko, H. *Mountain Sickness.* Berlin, 1882.

Bouguer, P. Relation of a voyage to Peru to determine the degree of longitude near the equator. Pinkerton. *A General Collection of the Best and Most Interesting Voyages and Travels.* London; 1813.

Boycott, A. E., and J. S. Haldane. The effects of low atmospheric pressures on respiration. *J. Physiol.* 37:355–377, 1908.

Bruce, C. G. *The Assault on Mount Everest—1922.* London: Arnold, 1923.

Campbell, E. J. The evolution of oxygen. J. R. Sutton, N. L. Jones, and C. S. Houston (eds). *Hypoxia: Man at Altitude.* New York: Thieme-Stratton, 1982, pp. 2–7.

Colburn, C. B. *Journal of a Voyage to Peru.* London; 1828.

Coward, F. A. Mountain sickness as observed in the Andes. *J. S.C. Med. Assoc.* 2:123–125, 1906.

Cunningham, P. Effects of mountain elevations upon the human body. *Lond. Med. Gaz.* 1834:207–208.

De Saussure. In Pinkerton, John. A General Collection of the Best and Most Interesting Voyages and Discoveries in All Parts of the World. London: Longman; 1813.

DeBeer, G. R. *Alps and Men.* London: Arnold, 1932. (*Note:* A rich source for ancient mountain history.)

Dent, C. T. Can Mount Everest be ascended. The Nineteenth Century 32(188):604–613, 1892.

Desideri, I. *An Account of Tibet: the Travels of Ippolito Desideri of Pistoia.* London: Routledge, 1932.

Douglas, C. G.; J. S. Haldane, Y. Henderson, and E. C. Schneider, The physiological effects of low atmospheric pressure as observed on Pikes Peak, Colorado. *Proc. R. Soc. Lond.* [Series B] 85:65–67, 1912.

Fa-Hsien. *The Travels of Fa-Hsien.* Cambridge: Cambridge University Press, 1923.

Fitzgerald, M. P. The changes in the breathing and the blood at various high altitudes. *Proc. R. Soc. Lond.* [Series B] 203:351–371, 1913.

Fitzgerald, M. P. Further observations on the changes in the breathing and the blood at various high altitudes. *Proc. R. Soc. Lond.* [Series B] 88:248–258, 1914–1915.

Frank, R. *Harvey and the Oxford Physiologists.* Berkeley: University of California.

Frith, H. *Ascents and Adventures: A Record of Hardy Mountaineering in Every Quarter of the Globe.* London: Rutledge, 1884.

Gessner, C. *On the Admirtion of Mountains.* (Trans. by J. M. Thorington) San Francisco: Grabhorn Press, 1937.

Gilbert, D. L. The first documented description of mountain sickness: the Andean or Pariacaca story. *Respir. Physiol.* 52:327–347, 1983.

Gilbert, D. L. The first documented report of mountain sickness: the China or headache story. *Respir. Physiol.* 52:315–326, 1983.

Gilbert, D. *Oxygen and Living Processes.* Zurich: Springer-Verlag, 1981.

Green, J. *Voyages and Travels.* London: Astley, 1745–6.

Green, P. *Alexander of Macedon, 356–323 B.C. A Historical Biography.* Berkeley: University of California, 1991.

Gribble, F. *The Early Mountaineers.* London: Fisher Unwin, 1899.

Haidar, M. A history of the Moguls of Central Asia. N. Elias (trans). *The Tarikh-I-Rashida.* Lahore: Book Traders, 1896.

Haldane, J. S., A. M. Kellas, and E. L. Kennaway. Experiments on acclimatisation to reduced atmospheric pressure. *J. Physiol.* 53:181–206, 1919–1920.

Henderson, Y. *Adventures in Respiration. Modes of Asphyxiation and Methods of Resuscitation.* Baltimore: Williams & Wilkins, 1938.

Henderson, Y. The last thousand feet on Everest. *Nature* 143(3631):921–923, 1939.

Henderson, Y. Life at great altitudes. *Yale Rev.* 3NS:759–773, 1914.

Hepburn, M. L. The influence of high altitudes in mountaineering. *Alpine J.* 20:368–441, 1901.

Hepburn, M. L. Some reasons why the science of altitude illness is still in its infancy. *Alpine J.* 21:161–179, 1902.

Hingston, R. W. G. Physiological difficulties in the ascent of Mt Everest. *Geog. J.* 65:4–23, 1925.

Houston, C. S., and R. L. Riley. Respiratory and circulatory changes during acclimatization to high altitude. *Am. J. Physiol.* 149:565–588, 1947.

Houston, C. S. *Going Higher: the Story of Man and Altitude.* Boston: Little, Brown, 1987.

Howard-Bury, C. K. *Mount Everest—The Reconnaissance, 1921.* New York: Longmans Green; 1922.

Hudson, B. Some common mountain ailments and how to combat them. *Lancet* 2:1871, 1921.

Humboldt, A. Personal Narrative of Travels to the Equinoctial Regions of America During the Years 1799–1804: Bohn; 1852–3.

Keay, J. *When Men and Mountains Meet.* London: Murray, 1974.

Kellas, A. M. Possibility of climbing Everest. *Alpine J.* 31:134–138, 1917.

Kellogg, R. H. Altitude acclimatization, a historical introduction emphasizing the regulation of breathing. *Physiologist* 11:37–57, 1968.

Kellogg, R. H. Some high points in altitude physiology. L. J. Folinsbee, J. A. Wagner, J. F. Borgia, R. I., Drinkwater, J. A. Gliner, and J. F. Bedi. (eds). *Environmental Stress: Individual Human Adaptations.* New York: Academic Press, pp. 317–324, 1978.

Kronecker, H. Mountain sickness. *Med. Mag.* 4(7):651–666, 1895.

Longstaff, T. G. *Mountain Sickness and Its Probable Cause.* London: Spottiswoode, 1906.

Longstaff, T. *This My Voyage.* London: Murray, 1950.

Luft, U. *Acclimatization to Altitude—1941.* Albuquerque: Lovelace Medical Foundation; 1993. (Trans. of original (Berlin 1941).)

54. Marcet W. On the use of alcoholic stimulants in mountaineering. *Alpine J.* 13:324–327, 1888.

Mason, K. *Abode of Snow.* London: Hart-Davis, 1955. (*Note:* Extensive review of old history of Himalayan climbing and traveling.)

Maundeville, J. *Travels.* London: 1725.

Morse, W. An unrecognized factor in altitude effects. *Sci. Monthly* 27(8):108–113, 1923.

Mosso, A. *Life of Man on the High Alps.* London: T. Fisher Unwin, 1998.

Murray, H. *Historical Account of Discoveries and Travels in Asia from the Earliest Times to the Present.* Edinburgh: Constable, 1820.

Norton, E. F. *The Fight for Everest 1924.* London: Arnold, 1925.

Quintus, Curtius Rufus. *History of Alexander.* Modern translation London, 1946.

Ravenhill, T. H. Some experiences of mountain sickness in the Andes. *J. Trop. Med. Hyg.* 1620:313–320, 1913.

Irving, R. L. G. *The Mountain Way.* New York: Dutton, 1938. (*Note:* Rich collection of poems, stories, records of mountaineering, old and recent.)

Russell, H. On mountains and mountaineering in general. *Alpine J.* 5:241–248, 1871.

Scheuchzer, J. J. In: Gribble The Early Mountaineers. London: T Fisher Unwin, 1899. (*Note:* Summary of Scheuzcher's dragon studies.)

Schneider, E. C. Physiological effects of altitude. *Physiol. Rev.* 1:631–659, 1921.

Simmler, J. *Die Alpen*. Munich: Alpiner Buchverein [Facsimile], 1931.

Speer, S. T. *On The Physiological Phenomena of Mountain Sickness*. London: T. Richards, 1853.

Strauch, A. Mountain sickness. *Am. J. Med. Sci.* 2:105–117, 1911.

Thorington, J. M. Alpine dangers of the sixteenth century. *Sierra Club Bull.* 18:34–43.

Tissot, J. Study of the causes of mountain sickness. *J. Physiol. Pathol. Gen.* [Paris] 12:520–525, 1910.

Torricelli, E. Torricelli's letters on the pressure of the atmosphere. J. B. West, (ed). *High Altitude Physiology*. Stroudsberg, PA: Hutchinson Ross, pp. 60–63, 1981.

Tyndall, J. *The Glaciers of the Alps, Being a Narrative of Excursions and Ascents, an Account of the Origin and Phenomena of Glaciers, and an Exposition of the Physical Principles to Which They Are Related*. London: Murray, 1860.

Unsworth, W. *Everest: A Mountaineering History*. Boston: Houghton Mifflin, 1981. (*Note:* Excellent history of Everest from the beginning.)

Von Tschudi, J. J. *Travels in Peru during the Years 1838–1842*. New York: Putnam, 1849.

Wessels, C. *Early Jesuit Travellers in Central Asia, 1603–1721*. The Hague: Nijhoff, 1924.

West, J. B. Alexander M. Kellas and the physiological challenge of Mt. Everest. *J. Appl. Physiol.* 63(1):3–11, 1987.

Whymper, E. The first ascent of Chimborazo. J. B. West (ed). *High Altitude Physiology*. Stroudsberg, PA: Hutchinson Ross, 1981, pp. 20–26.

Whymper, E. *A Guide to Chamonix and the Range of Mont Blanc* (Facsimile Edition 1974). London: Gaston, original edition published in 1896.

Woodworth, J. A. Brief notes and bibilography of history of mountain medicine. *Appalachia* 1976:81–93.

Workman, W. H. Some altitude effects at camps above 20,000 feet. Appalachia 13:350–359, 1908.

Wright, M. R. (trans.). *Empedoles: The Extant Fragments*. New Haven: Yale University; 1981.

Yusuf A. *Three Travellers to India: Being a Simple Account of India as Seen by Yuan Chwang (Hiuen Tsang), Ibn Batuta, and Francois Bernier*. London: Al-Biruni.

Zuntz, N., and A. Loewy. *Hohenklima und Bergwanderungen*. Berlin; 1906.

2
Analysis and Simulation of Mechanical Loads on the Human Musculoskeletal System: A Methodological Overview

ANTON J. VAN DEN BOGERT, Ph.D.

The analysis of mechanical loads in the various tissues (bones, joints, ligaments, muscles) of the human body has always been an important topic in biomechanical research. This research is stimulated by questions from sports medicine, ergonomics, and rehabilitation. In each of these disciplines, the underlying assumption is that excessive forces are harmful, potentially leading to injuries, and that a reduction of forces can be beneficial. A good understanding of the factors and mechanisms contributing to excessive loading should therefore lead to improved preventive and therapeutic methods. Forces in the human body can change dramatically as a function of the character and the speed of the movement being performed. Additionally, forces may depend on anthropometrical variables, such as body size and mass, and on the mechanical properties of the tissues and the various (bio)materials; for example, the stiffness of muscles, ligaments, and footwear. Research in this field is aimed at unraveling the complex relationships between mechanical loads and all these variables.

Hypotheses regarding the influence of a certain variable on the internal forces can be tested by experiments in which the variable is systematically varied. This "cause-and-effect" research strategy [59] is typically structured as follows:

1. Formulate a hypothesis about the relationship between mechanical load and controllable experimental conditions.
2. Estimate the relevant internal loads in a group of human subjects, as a function of the experimental condition.
3. Analyze the results statistically to determine if there is a significant effect of the experimental condition on the loads.

A suitable method for step 2 should be selected from the methods presented in this chapter. The statistical analysis will reveal effects that are larger than the uncertainty due to random interindividual variations. This "comparative load analysis" can be successful, despite systematic errors in the methods for load analysis and limited knowledge on "safety limits" for load on living tissue. An "absolute load analysis", i.e., determining whether a certain loading condition is an excessive load or not, is usually much more difficult.

The physiological effects of load on living tissue are usually studied in experimental animals, where the loads can be directly measured by instrumentation, and the tissue properties can be accurately determined in postmortem tests. Some of the methods used for load analysis in animal studies are applicable to humans, but many are too invasive. For this reason, most studies on forces in the human body make use of indirect methods, such as EMG analysis, kinematic analysis, inverse dynamics, or computer simulation. These indirect methods have many limitations and suffer from large inaccuracies. It is the purpose of this paper to provide a comprehensive overview of the methods, with emphasis on recent innovations, and indicate their respective limitations and the main sources of error. The severity of these methodological limitations and errors will depend very much on the particular situation in which a method is applied, and this should be an important consideration when selecting a method for analyzing mechanical loads in the human body.

QUANTITATIVE MEASURES OF LOAD

The term "load" is not well defined and should be replaced by a physical quantity that is suitable as indicator for mechanical "load" in a certain situation. Several quantitative variables can be used. In structural engineering, the mechanical load in materials is quantified by the stress σ, defined as the force F acting on an infinitesimally small area element, divided by the area A of the element:

$$\sigma = \frac{F}{A} \tag{1}$$

The unit of stress is the pascal: $1\ \mathrm{Pa} = 1\ \mathrm{N/m^2}$. In a three-dimensional structure, force is a vector with three components, and the area can be oriented in three different orthogonal planes. This gives six possible combinations of force and area, and the complete loading condition is therefore expressed as a symmetrical stress tensor [52]. The diagonal elements correspond to forces perpendicular to the area element (normal stresses), and the off-diagonal elements represent forces within the plane of the area element (shear stresses). In tendons, muscles, and ligaments, the load is mostly produced by tensile forces in one direction. In this approximation, only a normal stress in the direction of the force will occur, which can be quantified by a single scalar variable according to equation (*1*). In those materials, this equation therefore provides a simple method to predict stress theoretically, if the external force and the geometry of the structure are known. For solid elastic materials such as bone, the complete stress tensor is relevant, and the theoretical relationship between stress, external forces, and geometry becomes more complex. For simple geometries, a "beam model" can be appropriate, but usually a finite element analysis (FEA) is used to predict the stress distribution in bone or orthopaedic implants from external forces and geometry [42].

While stress is the appropriate measure of load in mechanical engineering, other variables may be equally informative and more practical in a biomechanical application. When the geometry is constant, stress is proportional to force. If force is reduced by 50%, stress is also reduced by 50%. Thus, the force on a structure may be sufficient information for a comparative analysis of two conditions. When muscle forces are estimated using inverse dynamics analysis (see *Inverse Dynamics*), they are essentially proportional to the resultant joint moments from which they are calculated. Joint moments can therefore be used to quantify muscle loads, although this will give only one "load" value for an entire group of muscles acting at the joint. The resultant joint moment can also indicate the magnitude of the joint compression force, which depends mostly on muscle forces. Another useful variable is strain, which quantifies deformation. In an elastic material, stress has a well-defined relationship to strain. In a simple one-dimensional loading regime, as discussed before, the strain ε is defined as:

$$\varepsilon = \frac{L - L_0}{L_0} \qquad (2)$$

where L is the length of (part of) the structure and L_0 is the length when not loaded. Strain is dimensionless, but sometimes "microstrain" is used as a unit, being a strain of 10^{-6}. In cases where strain is easier to measure than stress, strain is a more suitable variable for quantification of load.

In a structural engineering design process, the stresses or strains in a particular structure (measured experimentally or calculated theoretically) are compared with the known failure limits for the material. When the internal loads exceed a certain safety margin, the geometry of the structure must be adapted or the external forces reduced. In principle, the same procedure can be applied to biological structures. However, the safety limits of biological materials are not well known. In vitro tests can provide a wide range of results, partly because of the variable quality of the tissue samples. Additionally, maximal stresses obtained from failure tests will not provide information about the level at which irreversible damage occurs. In the living system, minor damage is reversible due to biological repair processes but may also accumulate if the load is frequently repeated as, for example, in an athlete during an intensive training period. Interpretation of mechanical loads in biological materials is therefore not as straightforward as in mechanical engineering. Such an "absolute load analysis," where loads are compared with safety limits, can only be done with a large margin of error. In general, it is impossible to conclude that one condition leads to injuries and the other does not.

A "comparative load analysis," where the same method of analysis is applied to several experimental conditions, is usually more practical. For instance, if a certain analysis shows that the stress in the tibia is 50 Mpa during barefoot running and 40 Mpa while wearing running shoes, the result provides useful information, in spite of the fact that the analysis may be very inaccurate and safety limits are unknown. Another advantage of comparative load analysis is that it is not important which variable is chosen for quantification of load: stress, force, strain, or moment may all be suitable.

DIRECT MEASUREMENT OF LOADS

Direct measurement of forces inside the human body is rare, because it is invasive and requires sophisticated instrumentation and recording techniques. In animals, however, these techniques are widely used. Studies involving invasive measurements in humans are usually quite limited in the number of subjects tested and in the nature of the movements. Nevertheless, such studies provide extremely valuable information which can and should be used to validate some of the noninvasive methods of analysis (see *Inverse Dynamics* and *Computer Simulation*).

Muscle and Ligament Forces

Muscle force can be measured directly using a "buckle transducer" (Fig. 2.1*A*). This transducer consists of a metal element, instrumented with strain gauges, which is deformed by the force in the tendon to which it is attached. This technique has gained widespread use in the cat and other animals, where it is used as a tool to study muscular control of movement [37]. A disadvantage of these transducers is the relatively large size and the fact that they slightly reduce the length of the tendon, thereby possibly altering the functioning of the instrumented structure. For this reason, they cannot be applied where tendons are close together, or on short ligaments. Calibration should ideally be carried out post mortem, by applying known forces and measuring the signals generated by the strain gauges. A less accurate alternative is to remove the transducer from the tendon and calibrate it with an "artificial" tendon. In humans, the buckle transducer has been applied exclusively to measure forces in the Achilles tendon [28]. The results have been compared with a simultaneous inverse dynamics analysis, which showed an excellent agreement in certain phases of a jumping movement and errors up to 50% in other phases. The difference was explained as a contribution by other plantarflexors.

FIGURE 2.1

A. A "buckle transducer" for measuring force in tendons. Adapted from [28]. B. A liquid metal strain gauge for measuring strain in tendons and ligaments. Adapted from [67].

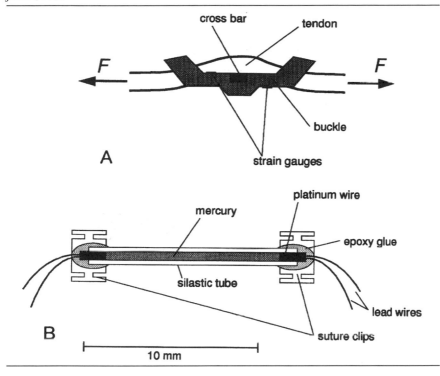

Unfortunately, this type of information is not available for other muscle groups in humans. Extensive animal studies on the distribution of muscle forces suggest that some of the assumptions made in the inverse dynamics analysis, especially those regarding the "distribution problem" (see later in this chapter) may be not valid [37].

An alternative technique for measuring muscle forces is the "liquid metal strain gauge" (LMSG, Fig. 2.1*B*) [67, 56]. This transducer measures the deformation (strain) of the tendon itself, and a postmortem calibration of the force-strain relationship is required if quantification of forces is desired. LMSGs are smaller than buckle transducers and interfere less with the functioning of the tendon. They are therefore also applicable in relatively short ligaments. A major disadvantage of LMSGs is the sensitivity to temperature and to changes in force distribution within the tendon or ligament. This leads to a difficult calibration procedure, especially if quantification of force is the purpose of the measurement. In humans, LMSGs have been applied to measure strain in the patellar tendon [51].

Presumably, other structures are less accessible, and the risk of leakage of mercury from the transducer should also be considered. For injury-related or clinical studies, it could be argued that measuring strain in soft tissue is more appropriate than measuring force, because tissue damage will occur at a certain level of deformation (strain), independent of the dimensions of the actual anatomical structure. Safety limits for force are not so easily established. Strength tests have shown that ligaments and tendons rupture at strains of 10–15%, and minor damage may occur well below those strains [86]. Recently, a miniature transducer that uses the buckle principle but measures locally, similar to the LMSG, has been described [97]. Presently, useful quantitative results can only be obtained from this transducer after a postmortem calibration, and this may prevent it from ever being used in humans.

Bone and Joint Forces
Bone is an elastic material, which makes it possible to estimate local stresses (force per unit area) from local deformations. Typical deformations of bone are between 100 and 1000 microstrains, and these deformations can be accurately measured by strain gauges attached to the bone surface. Strain gauges are widely used in animal studies and for in vitro experiments on human specimens. The only known in vivo measurements on human subjects have been done by Lanyon et al., who measured strain in the human tibia during walking and jogging [54]. Using typical values for the elastic properties of bone, stresses have been estimated from these data [14]. The peak stresses were 3 MPa for walking and 12 Mpa for jogging, which is very low, compared with typical failure stresses for bone of about 100 Mpa [98]. However, it should be kept in mind that stress can depend very much on location, and the location of the strain gauge may not have been the area where maximal stresses occur.

When bone strain is measured simultaneously at several locations and in several directions, the total force and moment vector on the bone can be calculated. When no muscles are attached between the strain gauges and the joint, these variables represent the load transmitted through the joint by articular contact forces and possibly ligaments. This analysis requires a mathematical model that establishes the relationship between the load variables and the measured strains. Such relationships can be based on a beam model for stresses perpendicular to the cross-section [71], but analysis of torsional and shear forces in noncircular cross-sections requires a finite element analysis [31]. Alternatively, a multivariate regression model based on a postmortem calibration can be used [70]. Multiple strain gauge techniques are extremely invasive and therefore hardly applicable to humans. It is, however, feasible to attach strain gauges to a joint prosthesis and perform a similar analysis to obtain the joint loads in a human patient. This technique has been first used in hip prostheses for a short-term measurement and has evolved into long-term implantation of an instrumented prosthesis with telemetric data transmission [3, 19]. The latter method should not cause any discomfort or risk to the patient and is a very promising development. Unfortunately, joints other than the hip are not so easily instrumented.

EMG PROCESSING

Electromyography (EMG) is a noninvasive (when surface electrodes are used) technique to measure muscle activity, and there has been considerable interest in using EMG signals for estimation of muscle forces. While the EMG signal strength obviously depends on the magnitude of the muscle force, the relationship is not simple. Two types of models have been used to estimate muscle forces from EMG: muscle models and regression models. Since EMG amplitude depends not only on the mechanics of the muscle but also on the conduction of the electrical impulses from the muscle fibers to the electrode, there is always the requirement for a calibration procedure, where known loads are applied and the corresponding EMG signals are measured. When the known loads are quantified as joint moments, the resulting (muscle or regression) model will predict muscle moments, rather than muscle forces. EMG analysis may be preferred over the other main noninvasive method, inverse dynamics analysis, for two different reasons. First, EMG can provide information about specific muscles rather than a sum of all muscles acting together at a joint. Secondly, EMG analysis does not require the use of force platforms and kinematic measurements, which are typically only possible in a laboratory environment. The latter aspect may be important for field studies in ergonomics or sports biomechanics.

The use of muscle models for EMG-to-force processing was pioneered by Hof and van den Berg [38], who used an analog electronic computer to simulate a Hill muscle model in real time. The method was applied for quantification of the contributions by the gastrocnemius and soleus muscles to the total plantarflexion moment of the ankle joint. By comparing the predicted total moment with the moment obtained from inverse dynamics [39], for different movements and different subjects, an average error of 29% in the muscle forces, estimated from EMG, was found. A similar approach, using more sophisticated muscle models, was used in studies on vertical jumping [5] and sprinting [44].

Phenomenological relationships, based on regression models, have been used to predict resultant joint moments from EMG and kinematics [61]. Such analyses do not provide more insight and are probably less accurate than the inverse dynamics analysis on which the regression models are based. But it is an attractive technique for research in ergonomics and sport because EMG could provide immediate feedback on the magnitude of muscle forces and thereby, indirectly, of joint forces. This is especially useful for training of coordination in lifting movements, to minimize the risk of injuries [22, 58].

EMG analysis is only applicable for certain muscles that are accessible by surface electrodes. Intramuscular electrodes are invasive and may provide signals from only a (nonrepresentative) part of the muscle. On the other hand, surface electrodes may suffer from cross-talk. In addition, the calibration procedure is an essential part of the analysis, requiring an activity where inverse dynamics provides good estimates for individual muscle forces. For the calf muscles, this was effectively solved by calibrating the soleus during extreme knee flexion, thereby shortening the gastrocnemius and preventing it from generating force [39]. Such a procedure is not always possible, and it is more common to calibrate with respect to the total joint moment, rather than individual muscles [44, 61]. In that case, the individual muscle forces, estimated from EMG, may not be reliable.

KINEMATIC ANALYSIS

The mechanical behavior of ligaments can be approximated by single or multiple elastic line elements with endpoints attached to bones. This implies that the strain in a ligament depends on the spatial positions and orientations of the bones, which can be measured. If necessary, the force can then be calculated from the elastic properties, assuming they are known or estimated. The relationship between bone kinematics and ligament strain can be established by a kinematic model (calculating the distance between insertion points) or, which is less common, by a regression model fitted to in vitro measurements of strain and kinematics [45].

Although the procedure is straightforward, there are many difficulties associated with this approach. First of all, this type of kinematic analysis will provide results in the form of ligament length as a function of time. According to the definition of strain (2), the unloaded length L_0 must be known to calculate strain. When postmortem loading tests cannot be done, the ligament length at one particular time or one particular spatial position and orientation of the bones is used as the "zero-strain" condition. For instance, when analyzing gait, it is often assumed that the ligaments are unloaded at heel strike. Any errors in L_0 will produce a shift in the calculated strains. Such errors are generally not a problem when a comparative analysis is done in the same test subject, as long as the same L_0 is used for the kinematic analysis of all experimental conditions.

A second practical difficulty with kinematic strain analysis is the sensitivity to measuring errors. Physiological ligament strains are quite small (<10%), which means that small measuring errors in the length L can produce a large error in the strain ε, according to equation (2). For instance, at a strain of 5%, an error of only 1% in L will give an error of 20% in ε. Errors in kinematic analysis can be random noise, originating from the digitization process, or can be systematic because of nonlinearity of the measuring system or, more importantly, having markers placed on the skin rather than on the bone. Random errors can be removed by appropriate low-pass filtering techniques [94], but this is not possible for systematic errors. This has important practical implications. In an in vivo kinematic measurement, skin movement is the major problem, and successful in vivo applications have therefore only been developed for long ligaments, where the influence of errors in L is relatively small. The horse has several such long ligaments, as part of the passive stabilization mechanism of the limbs. Kinematic analysis gave satisfactory results for the suspensory ligament [68], located in the distal part of the limb, where skin movement is very small, and for the entirely tendinous peroneus tertius muscle, where the kinematic data were corrected for skin movement errors [89]. In both cases, the noninvasive kinematic analysis was validated by a simultaneous direct measurement by strain gauges.

In humans, an attractive application is the analysis of strains in the knee ligaments during various activities. This has, for instance, been applied to determine the effect of knee braces on ligament load using in vitro kinematics [88]. A sensitivity analysis using in vitro data has shown that the reliability of quantitative results depends on accurate information about the insertion locations of the ligaments [36]. Furthermore, skin movement errors of only several millimeters can make the results entirely unreliable. This means that the analysis can only be done when the actual movements of the bone are measured. Presently, the only available in vivo technique is based on transcutaneous bone pins, which have been used for accurate quantification of knee motion during walking [50]. These results have not been used to estimate ligament loading, but such an interpretation is certainly possible. For instance, the anterior-posterior translation pattern suggests that the posterior cruciate ligament (PCL) is loaded during the first half of the support phase, and the anterior cruciate ligament (ACL) during the second half [50]. Medical imaging techniques (x-ray stereophotogrammetry, computed tomography, or magnetic resonance imaging) could provide less invasive alternatives for these methods, although these can presently only be used in static conditions.

INVERSE DYNAMICS ANALYSIS

Principle of Inverse Dynamics Analysis

Inverse dynamics is the most widely used method for estimating internal loads. The method is essentially the same for all joints in the human body and has become a part of standardized protocols in clinical gait analysis. The analysis is based on a representation of the human body as a set of rigid segments. All forces acting between two adjacent body segments are represented by one resultant joint force $\vec{F}$ and one resultant joint moment $\vec{M}$ (Fig. 2.2). The relationship between loads and movements is given by the Newton-Euler equations of motion. For three-dimensional translation and rotation, respectively, the equations of motion for each segment are [35]:

$$\sum_i \vec{F}_i = m \cdot \mathbf{R}^{-1} \cdot (\ddot{\vec{r}} - \vec{g})$$

(3)

$$\sum_i \vec{M}_i + \sum_i (\vec{p}_i \times \vec{F}_i) = \mathbf{I} \cdot \dot{\vec{\omega}} + \vec{\omega} \times (\mathbf{I} \cdot \vec{\omega})$$

(4)

The vector $\vec{r}$ is the position of the center of mass of the segment with respect to an inertial reference frame, also known as the "laboratory coordinate system." The vector $\vec{g}$ indicates the magnitude and direction of

FIGURE 2.2
Forces (A) and moments (B) acting on a body segment, with the corresponding variables from the equations of motion (3) and (4).

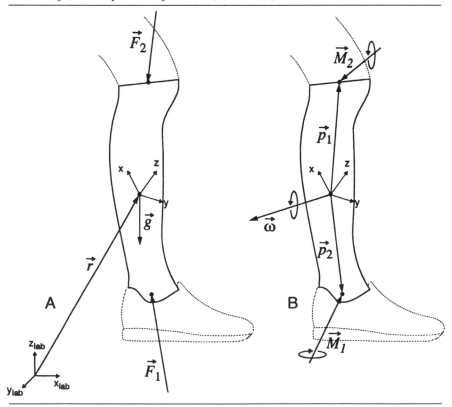

acceleration of gravity. All other vector variables in these equations are defined with help of a "segment coordinate system," which has its origin in the center of mass. $\mathbf{R}$ is the rotation matrix, which, premultiplied to a segment coordinate vector, produces a laboratory coordinate vector. The vector $\vec{p}_i$ is the point of application of the force $\vec{F}_i$, in the segment coordinate system. If $\vec{p}_i$ coincides with the center of rotation of the joint, implying a ball-and-socket joint model, the resultant moment $\vec{M}$ can be interpreted as the sum of the muscle moments with respect to the joint center. The angular velocity vector in the segment coordinate system is $\vec{\omega}$, and the first derivative is the angular acceleration $\dot{\vec{\omega}}$. The inertial properties of the segment are the mass m and the inertia tensor $\mathbf{I}$. The terms in the summations on the left side correspond to the connections (joints) with neighboring body segments or with the ground. In inverse dynamics, the variables on the right side are assumed to be known from measurements, and the unknown forces and moments on the left side are solved. The term *inverse dynamics* refers to the fact that the forces are inferred from the movements caused by them. This is opposite to the actual causality in the system.

When N body segments are included in the analysis, inverse dynamics gives $2N$ vector equations. This means that, at most, $2N$ unknown vector variables can be solved. Since there are two unknown vector variables at each joint, a force and a moment, the number of joints with unknown loads should not be larger than N. It should be noted that each joint force or moment vector occurs twice in the left side of the equations of motion: once in the equations for the first segment, and once (with opposite direction) in the equations for the second segment. If there are more joints in the system than segments, there are more unknowns than equations, and inverse dynamics cannot produce a unique solution. Usually, the number of unknowns can then be reduced by measuring the loads between one of the body segments and the ground with a force transducer or force platform. If this is not possible, there is a "closed loop problem" [82]. Optimization criteria can be used to obtain a unique solution [83], but it is doubtful whether this corresponds to reality. This problem is similar to the distribution problem for a single joint, discussed below.

Inverse dynamics analysis requires data for only a part of the human body. For instance, to estimate the resultant force and moment at the hip, it is sufficient to include the equations of motion of the body segments distal to the hip. Usually, the lower extremity is represented by three segments: thigh, shank, and foot. This gives six vector equations (*3*) and (*4*). If the force between foot and ground is measured, there are six remaining unknown vector variables: the force and moment at the hip, knee, and ankle.

Kinematic and Kinetic Input Variables
The kinematic variables are typically obtained by measuring the coordinates of markers on the body segments, as a function of time. If a marker i

is placed at position $\vec{p}_i$ in a segment-fixed coordinate system, its position r_i in the laboratory coordinate system will depend on the position and orientation of the segment according to:

$$\vec{r}_i = \vec{r} + \mathbf{R} \cdot \vec{p}_i \tag{5}$$

By measuring these $\vec{r}_i$ for $n \geq 3$ noncolinear landmarks on the segment, the position $\vec{r}$ of the center of mass and the orientation matrix $\mathbf{R}$ can be solved using a constrained least-squares method [84]. (A public-domain implementation of this algorithm in Fortran can be obtained by members of Biomch-L [11] by sending the command "SEND DISP3DB FORTRAN" by electronic mail to LISTSERV@NIC.SURFNET.NL or to LISTSERV@HEARN.BITNET.) A least-squares method is appropriate, because the system is overdetermined. There are $3n$ (at least 9) equations for only 6 unknowns; the 3 cartesian components of $\vec{r}$ and the three independent Euler/Cardanic angles that describe the rotation matrix $\mathbf{R}$. The first and second derivatives of (5) are:

$$\dot{\vec{r}}_i = \dot{\vec{r}} + \vec{\omega} \times \vec{p}_i \tag{6}$$

$$\ddot{\vec{r}}_i = \ddot{\vec{r}} + \dot{\vec{\omega}} \times \vec{p}_i + \vec{\omega} \times (\vec{\omega} \times \vec{p}_i) \tag{7}$$

Equation (6) is linear in the components of the velocity and angular velocity vectors. This set of $3n$ equations can be used to obtain $\vec{\omega}$ (and $\dot{\vec{r}}$, which is not needed for inverse dynamics) using a conventional linear least-squares method, after calculating the velocities $\dot{\vec{r}}_i$ of the markers. Similarly, once $\vec{\omega}$ is known, the equations (7) are linear in the components of the acceleration and angular acceleration vectors $\ddot{\vec{r}}$ and $\dot{\vec{\omega}}$. These can then be solved by the same least-squares method [85]. The angular velocity and acceleration vectors should be premultiplied by $\mathbf{R}^{-1}$ to transform them to the segment coordinate system, as required in (4). It is important that least-squares methods are used at this stage, because these make optimal use of all available measurements to minimize error propagation.

The processing of kinematic data, as described above, requires numerical differentiation, which tends to amplify noise in the measurements. This can be avoided by low-pass filtering techniques [94]. An elegant technique is the use of spline functions for this purpose, because the differentiation of the piecewise polynomial functions can be done analytically, once the smoothing is done. A public-domain software package for spline smoothing and differentiation has been developed by Woltring [93]. (The Fortran source code of this package can be obtained by members of Biomch-L [11] by sending the command "SEND GCVSPL FORTRAN" by electronic mail to

`LISTSERV@NIC.SURFNET.NL` or to `LISTSERV@HEARN.BITNET`.)
Spline smoothing is mathematically equivalent to the commonly used But-
terworth digital filter, except for boundary conditions [95]. Boundary
conditions can become important when low cutoff frequencies are used
and the data record is short. Higher-order splines appear to have superior
performance in such cases, compared with digital filters or Fourier analysis
[94].

When external forces are used in the analysis, the errors of measurement
are relatively small. Piezoelectric force platforms are very accurate, as far as
the force is concerned, but significant errors have been found in the
moment, or point of application [6]. It has been suggested that this error
is caused by small deformations of the plate, which shifts the center of
pressure within the individual transducers. Fortunately, this error can be
predicted by a simple equation and is easily corrected, if necessary [6].

Methodological Problems Associated with High-Frequency Loading
Inverse dynamics becomes increasingly inaccurate for analysis of high-
frequency loading, such as impact or vibration. A major source of error is
the filtering and differentiation of kinematic data. Even after optimal
filtering, the derivatives will contain considerable error. A relationship
between the characteristics of the measuring system (noise σ and sampling
interval T) and the accuracy σ_k of the kth derivative of a measured variable
has been derived by Lanshammar [53]:

$$\sigma_k^2 \geq \frac{2^{2k+1}\pi^{2k}}{2k+1}\,\sigma^2 T f^{2k+1}, \tag{8}$$

where f is the highest relevant frequency in the signal that is being analyzed.

When impact in running, containing frequencies of up to 40 Hz, is
analyzed with a typical kinematic analysis system (200 samples per second,
1 mm accuracy after filtering), Lanshammar's formula predicts an error of
18 m/s^2, or almost 2 g, in the accelerations. In equation (*3*), this error is
multiplied by the mass of the body segments. When analyzing forces in the
ankle, the mass of the foot is used, and therefore the error is small and
probably acceptable. But for the hip, the mass of all body segments between
the hip and the ground is involved, and the error may be too large for
successful application of inverse dynamics for load analysis. An elegant
approach to circumvent these problems is the use of accelerometers [49]
and angular rate sensors [96], in combination with conventional marker
kinematics and external force measurements. This allows a direct measurement of the linear acceleration and the angular velocity, and only one
differentiation is required for the angular acceleration. It was shown, using
measurements of normal walking, that severe overestimation as well as

underestimation of the resultant force at the knee can occur when using differentiation of marker data for estimating accelerations [49].

A second source of error is the limited validity of the rigid-body equations of motion. Body segments consist of bone and soft tissue, and some relative movement does occur between the two. As a result, kinematic data obtained from markers on the skin may not represent the movement of the entire segment. Movements between skin and bone can easily reach values of several centimeters [69]. Even when these displacement errors are small, they become an important source of error for high-frequency accelerations; a displacement error of 1 cm at 10 Hz gives an acceleration error of $(2\pi f)^2 \times 1$ cm, or almost 4 g. It is possible to measure the measurements of the bones directly by using transcutaneous pins [50], but this does not prevent errors in inverse dynamics because the soft tissue mass is a significant part of the segment, and its accelerations remain unknown if only bone movement is measured. Correction algorithms to obtain bone movement from skin marker data [10, 90] are equally useless for inverse dynamics and should only be used for pure kinematic analysis. The errors caused by nonrigidity can presumably be minimized by careful selection of marker locations, to measure movements and accelerations that represent a suitable compromise between bone and soft tissue. In a comprehensive test of the validity of rigid-body models for analysis of running [7], this was accomplished by markers attached to a light-weight exoskeleton. The same study showed that the choice of low-pass filter cutoff frequencies is very critical for this application.

An interesting approach to solve the nonrigidity problem is the "wobbling mass model" [32], in which the segments are divided into soft tissue mass and bone mass. The soft tissue mass is attached to the rigid bone segment by a passive viscoelastic connection. The movements of the soft tissue masses are simulated numerically, and the resulting forces in the connection are added to the left side of the inverse dynamics equations. This model has been successfully used for analysis of impact. One difficulty in using this method is the choice of suitable stiffness and damping parameters for the viscoelastic connections; presumably they should be fitted to match observed relative movements between bone and soft tissue.

Distribution Problem
The forces and moment obtained from an inverse dynamic analysis are resultant loads. They represent the sum of all load-carrying structures between two adjacent body segments. It is not always necessary to know the load in the individual structures; the resultant moment can be used as an indicator of muscle function. The resultant *force*, however, is less meaningful because it is the sum of (compressive) joint contact and (tensile) muscle forces, which act mostly in opposite directions and partially cancel out. It is therefore often desirable to separate the resultant force and moment into forces in actual anatomical structures. This may be done at several levels of

complexity (Fig. 2.3). If muscle forces are the variables of interest, the joint is usually considered as a simple kinematic connection such as a spherical (ball-and-socket) joint with three degrees of freedom (DOF). This allows ligaments to be omitted from the model. The relationship between muscle forces $\vec{F}_i$ and resultant moment $\vec{M}$, obtained from inverse dynamics, can be written as:

$$\vec{M} = \sum_i (\vec{r}_i \times \vec{F}_i) \qquad (9)$$

where $\vec{r}_i$ is a vector from the joint center (as defined in the inverse dynamics procedure) to a point on the line of action of the muscle. This "moment arm" vector, and the direction of the muscle force, may depend on the joint angles and should be calculated using a suitable model (see *Muscle Models*). The vector equation (9) therefore has only the magnitude of the muscle forces as (scalar) unknowns. If the analysis involves more than three muscles, the equation does not provide sufficient information. This is known as the *distribution problem*. Once the muscle forces are known, the reaction force $\vec{F}_R$ in the spherical joint can be obtained from the resultant joint force using the equation:

FIGURE 2.3
Simplified diagram of data flow in an inverse dynamics analysis. The upper part *illustrates the calculation of resultant joint loads, according to equations (3) and (4). The* bottom part *represents the "distribution problem", equations (9) and (10).*

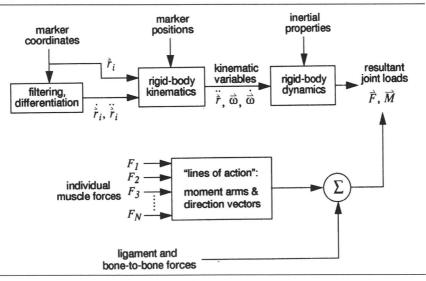

$$\vec{F} = \vec{F}_R + \sum_i \vec{F}_i \qquad (10)$$

The 3-DOF spherical joint model is common in inverse dynamics, but other models are possible. It is sometimes necessary (in 2-D) or desirable (in 3-D) to represent joints as a hinge joint with only one DOF. This means that only one component of the resultant joint moment vector (the component along the joint axis) represents muscle action and that only one muscle force can be solved. In a 3-D hinge joint, the other moment components provide information about the transmission of torsion or bending moments through the joint [13]. It is also possible to consider more than three DOF in the analysis, to obtain information about ligament forces and distribution of the contact pressure on the joint surfaces [57, 66]. In general, the number of unknown forces is larger than the number of equations available, which is equal to the number of degrees of freedom in the joint model. Three methods are available to solve this distribution problem: reduction, optimization, and addition.

In the "reduction" method, the number of unknown forces is reduced until it is equal to the number of equations. This is done by a combination of: (*a*) simplification, or leaving unimportant anatomical structures out of the analysis, (*b*) grouping muscles with similar function into one effective force and line of action, and (*c*) separating the movement into phases where different muscles are active, with the help of EMG. This approach has been used successfully for the hip [64], the knee [57], and the ankle [66]. Some of the assumptions in these studies are questionable, especially where EMG was used to support the assumption that certain muscles were inactive. Although this may result in errors in the muscle forces, the joint contact forces obtained from these studies are considered to be very good and have been used, for example, as criteria for the design of joint prostheses.

Optimization has become popular as a method to select a unique, "optimal" solution from the infinite number of solutions of the underdetermined system of equations (*9*). The optimization criterion is expressed by a "cost function," and a numerical or analytical method is used to find the solution that minimizes the cost function. Linear cost functions, such as the sum of muscle forces [72] or the sum of muscle stresses [16], have been used because they allow the problem to be easily solved by linear programming. Linear criteria have the disadvantage of not predicting load sharing between synergistic muscles; one muscle will deliver the total moment, unless an upper limit is placed on the muscle forces. More recently, nonlinear criteria have been used, such as the sum of squared [65] or cubed [17] muscle stresses. The implications of the various cost functions have been evaluated by Dul et al. [23], who also introduced a new "minimum fatigue" criterion [24]: the maximization of the smallest endurance time of all muscles. The endurance time was assumed to be an empirically determined power function of the muscle stress. The minimum fatigue criterion was tested by predicting speed-related changes peak forces in the gastrocnemius and soleus of the cat. The predictions were found to be in agreement with literature data of measurements using buckle transducers. However, it was shown later that none of these existing static optimization criteria predicts the load sharing during the entire gait cycle [37]. In particular, the "loops" in the force-force diagrams of two synergistic muscles will never be predicted correctly, unless some knowledge about the dynamics of force generation of muscles is included in the analysis. Dynamic optimization (see below) could provide a possibility for achieving this goal.

The *addition* method resembles a mechanical engineering approach to solve a statically indeterminate system. In principle, all load-carrying structures have load-deformation properties, and the distribution of load is determined by those properties. For example, a perfectly symmetric table supported on four legs is statically indeterminate. When placed on a deformable surface, the forces on the legs will depend on the length of the legs; the shortest leg will cause the least deformation and therefore carry the least load. The loads can be calculated if the force-deformation relationships are known. This principle can be applied to the (passive) load distribution in a joint, by using the total reaction load obtained from inverse dynamics (after subtracting the muscle forces) as input for a model of the joint that incorporates discrete elements representing the joint surfaces and the ligaments. This approach is especially useful for a complex joint such as the knee, which has been modeled statically in 3-D [4] and dynamically in 2-D [25].

Mechanical properties of muscles can be used to help solve the distribution problem for muscles, but this is complicated by the fact that muscles are active elements and the activation level is unknown. Replacing each unknown force by an unknown activation level (Fig. 2.3) does not reduce the number of unknowns, but it does reduce the solution space considered by only allowing solutions that are consistent with physiological (activation dynamics) and mechanical (force-length, and force-velocity) properties of the muscles. The system is still indeterminate, so there is still the need for an optimization to obtain a unique solution. These techniques are known as "dynamic optimization" because muscles are mathematically represented by a dynamic model (a set of differential equations), in contrast to the "static optimization" described earlier. Typically, the cost function for dynamic optimization will include a term that depends on muscle activation levels, which is related to minimization of metabolic cost. Dynamic optimization presently offers the best possibilities of obtaining good estimates for muscle forces from noninvasive measurements but has not been widely used [18, 80].

DIRECT DYNAMICS ANALYSIS OR COMPUTER SIMULATION

All methods described in this overview are based on measurements on living test subjects. Not all research questions (what is the influence of X on the force in Y) however, can be answered using the experimental approach. This could be caused by one or more of the following problems:

REPRODUCIBILITY. Measurements on the human body are not perfectly repeatable and are subject to uncontrollable variations. This is essentially the same for measurements of ground reaction forces [21], kinematics [91], and muscle activity [46]. The only possibility for minimizing the influence of these random variations is performing many measurements in the same experimental condition, to increase the power of the statistical analysis.

UNDERSTANDING. Even when statistically significant relationships are found, the underlying mechanical relationships may be too complex to be uncovered. In such a case, experimental research may answer a specific question, but it does not lead to increased knowledge.

CONTROLLABILITY. It is not always possible to introduce controlled variations in an experimental procedure. For example, it is hardly possible to determine the influence of certain changes in muscle coordination on performance, for example in a jumping movement, because muscle activation is not consciously controlled.

COST. The cost of biomechanical experiments may be prohibitive; an extreme example is studies on vehicle crash injuries. In general, experimental research on human movement requires considerable manpower and expensive equipment.

ACCURACY. Estimates of internal forces may be very inaccurate. Often, such inaccuracies are caused by systematic errors that do not depend on the experimental conditions. This type of error is relatively harmless and does not affect the statistical interpretation. Sometimes, however, the errors are very large and partly dependent on the experimental condition. An example is the inaccuracy of inverse dynamics for high-frequency or impact loading. If we are using inverse dynamics to investigate the effect of cushioning properties of footwear, the soft-tissue movement (and the errors it causes in inverse dynamics) will certainly depend on the experimental condition. Extreme caution is therefore required when interpreting experimental results in such cases.

These problems have led to the use of direct dynamics methods, as opposed to inverse dynamics methods, to analyze internal forces for certain types of human movement. In direct dynamics, the experiment is performed on a computer model instead of on a human subject. This is analogous to the common practice in mechanical engineering, specifically in robotics and vehicle dynamics, where new designs are tested by a computer simulation before building a first prototype. In relation to the previously mentioned limitations of experimental research, computer

simulations are perfectly reproducible, provide understanding by including the underlying causal mechanisms, allow control of all variables, cost
little after an initial development effort, and finally can be made as accurate
and complex as desired. The latter aspect is a critical one: unnecessary
complexity in a model should be avoided because it diminishes the validity
of the results [40].

A direct dynamics analysis is a simulation of movement, using the forces
as input (Fig. 2.4). The entire model, muscles and body segments, is
represented by a large set of coupled differential equations. Simulation of
movement is accomplished by simultaneous numerical solution of these
equations. Forces in all anatomical structures included in the model, as a

FIGURE 2.4

Graphical representation of the vector constraint equation (11), *imposed by a spherical joint.*

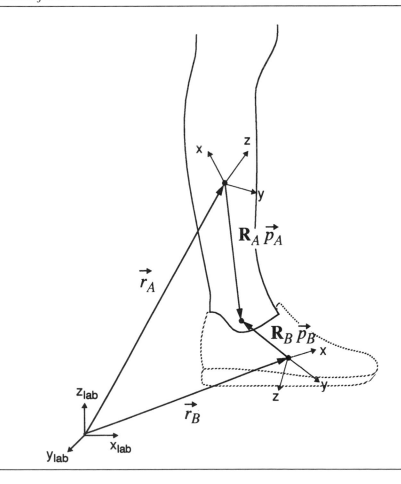

function of time, are obtained as a by-product of the simulation. Musculoskeletal simulation models have become an important tool in theoretical studies of coordination of movement [40, 75, 99], where the internal forces were of lesser importance. Similar models, however, are also suitable to study the forces, rather than movement. Compared with inverse dynamics, direct dynamics requires considerably more knowledge about the muscles, in particular the activation and control of the muscles. For this reason, direct dynamics load analysis has mostly been used for impact-type situations such as vehicle collisions. These events occur on a very short time scale, without significant influence of neural control of muscles. If muscle activation does not change, the muscles can be modeled as passive elements. Interestingly, this is exactly the type of problem where the methodological problems of inverse dynamics are most severe. Besides mathematical (direct dynamics) models, physical models of the human body have occasionally been used to simulate impact events, for instance to determine ligament forces in the knee during lateral impact [26].

Equations of Motion and Solution Methods
Similar to inverse dynamics, the equation of motion for direct dynamics is derived from a multibody model. However, the segments are not treated as independent. The Newton-Euler equations of motion (*3*) and (*4*) are supplemented by kinematic constraint equations that represent the joints. For example, when a spherical joint between two segments is located at $\vec{p}_A$ on segment A and at $\vec{p}_B$ on segment B, the kinematics of the multibody model should always satisfy the equation (Fig. 2.4):

$$\vec{r}_A + \mathbf{R}_A \cdot \vec{p}_A = \vec{r}_B + \mathbf{R}_B \cdot \vec{p}_B \qquad (11)$$

This vector equation represents three (scalar) constraint equations and removes three DOF from the system. Similarly, other types of kinematic connections can be used to restrict the relative movements between segments. The total system of equations describing the multibody model is thus a mixed system of differential and algebraic equations (DAE): the differential equations (*3*) and (*4*) and the algebraic constraint equations such as (*11*). Numerical solution of such systems of equations can be accomplished by some form of "coordinate reduction," i.e., identifying independent kinematic variables corresponding to the DOF and eliminating the other (dependent) kinematic variables from the differential equations. Several methods for coordinate reduction are possible.

First, symbolic manipulation can be used to solve the derivatives of the dependent kinematic variables from the constraint equations and substitute these into (*3*) and (*4*) to obtain a smaller number of differential equations with no constraints. This could also be done by starting out with Lagrange's or Kane's equations, which should give the same result [47]. *N* second-order ordinary differential equations (ODE) will be obtained for N independent kinematic variables, where N is the number of kinematic degrees of freedom in the system. The equations will emerge in the following form:

$$\mathbf{M} \cdot \ddot{q} = Q, \qquad (12)$$

where $\mathbf{M}$ is the "mass matrix," $q = (q_1, q_2, \ldots q_N)$ are the kinematic variables, and $Q = (Q_1, Q_2, \ldots Q_N)$ are the generalized forces and moments corresponding to these kinematic variables, including Coriolis and gravitational terms where applicable. For instance, if q_i is a joint angle, Q_i is the corresponding joint moment. The system of equations (12) can be solved by standard numerical methods [73], if the Q_i are known as a function of q, q̇, and time. These forces and moments may originate from muscles, ligaments, and the environment (Fig. 2.5). Appropriate constitutive equations for these elements are required (see below). Manual derivation of equation (12) is possible for relatively simple models [63]. For more complex models, the amount of work becomes prohibitive. Special-purpose symbolic manipulation software is available to automate the derivation of the equations and help prevent errors [41]. The best known software packages are AUTOLEV (On-line Dynamics, Sunnyvale, California) and SD/FAST (MGA Inc., Concord, Massachusetts), both based on Kane's method for constrained mechanical systems [47]. Recently, SD/FAST has been incorporated in the musculoskeletal modeling package SIMM (Musculographics Inc., Evanston, Illinois), thus providing a user-friendly environment for musculoskeletal simulations including muscle dynamics and visualization using animated 3-D graphics [20].

FIGURE 2.5
Schematic diagram of the causal relationships in a direct dynamics simulation of the musculoskeletal system.

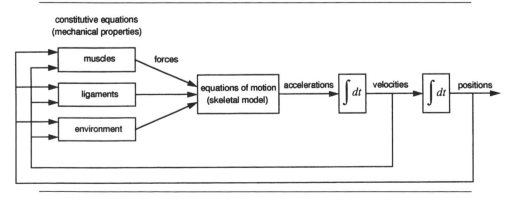

A second class of methods uses purely numerical techniques to solve the dependent kinematic variables, retaining the original differential and algebraic equations [60]. This type of software is widely used in robotics, vehicle dynamics, and machine design. The most common commercially available software packages in this class are ADAMS (Mechanical Dynamics, Ann Arbor, MI) and DADS (CADSI, Coralville, IA). Further details about numerical methods for direct dynamics simulation can be found in [35]. These packages are very user-friendly, because the user constructs a model from a large library of standard model elements (spherical joints, hinge joints, springs, dampers, etc.), without ever seeing any equations or doing any programming. Constitutive behaviour of nonstandard elements, such as muscles, ligaments, or shoes, can be incorporated by linking user-written Fortran code to the main program. This is a nontrivial task, but the code can be developed in such a way that it results in a general-purpose musculoskeletal simulation program [9]. A noncommercial numerical package (SPACAR, Delft University of Technology, The Netherlands) has been used in a simulation study on vertical jumping [74, 75].

External Forces
When external forces (such as air resistance or ground reaction forces) are included in a simulation, mathematical models are required that describe how the forces depend on positions and velocities of the body segments (Fig. 2.5). Aerodynamic forces probably do not contribute significantly to internal forces but may be important in simulating the flight phase of certain activities. Those forces, as a function of position and velocity, can be modeled using empirical equations, obtained from wind tunnel tests, or by using equations derived from theoretical considerations [78]. Ground reaction forces can be modeled by equations describing viscoelastic force-deformation properties and Coulomb-like frictional properties [8]. This idea has been used for ground reaction forces in running [29], where the vertical and horizontal components, respectively, were described by:

$$F_z = -az^3 (1 - b\dot{z}) \tag{13}$$

and

$$F_y = \begin{cases} -c\dot{y} & \text{if } -\dfrac{d}{c}F_z < \dot{y} < \dfrac{d}{c}F_z \\[2ex] -dF_z \cdot \dfrac{\dot{y}}{|\dot{y}|} & \text{elsewhere} \end{cases} \tag{14}$$

where y and z are the horizontal and vertical coordinates of the contact point with respect to the ground surface, a is a stiffness parameter, b is a damping parameter, d is the friction coefficient, and c is a large constant to approximate the discontinuity of the (Coulomb) frictional force at $\dot{y} = 0$. The parameters can be adjusted to give properties similar to a real foot-ground interface.

It may be appropriate for the purpose of the simulation to consider the ground as infinitely rigid. In that case, the ground contact becomes a kinematic connection (a "joint") between foot and ground. This is easiest when the contact is continuous, as in the push-off phase of a jump [75]. When simulating gait, the number of DOF changes at heel strike and at toe off, requiring a restart of the simulation with a different model, taking into account the impulsive forces that are responsible for discontinuities in velocity [33]. A similar approach is possible to simulate the "stiction effect" due to a true Coulomb friction model [48].

Muscle Models
Muscle forces can modify movements and also increase the joint contact forces by compressing the joints. It is therefore important to include muscles in a direct dynamics simulation. The coupling between muscle forces and the skeletal model (Fig. 2.5) requires a model for the "line of action" of the muscles. Relevant variables are the length between origin and insertion, and the moment arms with respect to the joint centers, as a function of the positions and orientations of the bones. Early models used piecewise straight-line models for the line of action [20], but this does not always represent the actual anatomy. These geometrical models can be refined by adding circular arc segments to the line of action [27, 68]. A disadvantage of geometrical models is that moment arms can only be calculated when the center of rotation of the joint is known. This presents a problem for some joints, such as the knee, which have no fixed center of rotation. This problem can be avoided by using the principle of virtual work to define the moment arm d_i with respect to joint i [1]:

$$d_i = \frac{\partial}{\partial \alpha_i} L \, (\alpha_1 \ldots \alpha_N) \tag{15}$$

where α_i is the joint angle and $L()$ is the function describing how origin-insertion length depends on one or more joint angles. This function can be determined by fitting a mathematical equation to results from a geometrical model [34], but it is much more elegant and accurate to measure it directly from tendon displacement in cadavers [30, 76, 77, 87]. This approach only provides information about length and moment arms and not about the "direction of pull" of muscles. The latter is necessary if joint contact forces are to be estimated in the model. A direction vector can be assumed (usually parallel to the long axis of the corresponding bone), or a geometrical origin-insertion model can be used.

During most activities, muscle activation changes continuously and is controlled by the central nervous system. It is undesirable to include the complexity of neural control in a mechanical analysis, and therefore direct dynamics has been mostly used for situations where muscle forces can be neglected or represented by simple passive models. Under impulsive loads, muscles can be represented as linear or nonlinear spring-damper combinations [15, 43, 81]. The stiffness and damping coefficients in these models are rather arbitrary and are usually selected by matching the results of a simulation to real movements. It is better to obtain those parameters from well-known mechanical properties of muscles, such as force-length and force-velocity relationships. In simulations of motor coordination, some type of Hill muscle model is usually included in the simulation model [62, 75]. This can be done at various levels of complexity, and it is important to select the simplest muscle model that is appropriate for the question, to avoid a multitude of model parameters whose values are not known. Complexity of Hill-type muscle models has been discussed by [2, 92]. These muscle models are also used for EMG to force processing and dynamic optimization in inverse dynamics (see the respective sections above). Hill muscle models, with the assumption of constant activation level, have been used to include muscle forces in simulations of impact loads in running [29, 79].

The Hill model is not the only possible representation of mechanical properties. Simpler models are possible when, for instance, the mechanical properties are dominated by the series elastic element. In the distal limb of the horse, the ratio of tendon length to muscle fiber length is extremely high. The influence of (horse) shoe design on internal forces was successfully simulated using a muscle model consisting of a kinematic actuator element (the fibers) and an elastic element (the tendon) [12]. Toward the other extreme, more complex models, based on A. F. Huxley's cross-bridge theory, have been proposed for use in musculoskeletal simulations but have not been applied for this purpose [55]. Researchers in musculoskeletal dynamics probably feel that the Hill model is adequate for their needs.

SUMMARY AND CONCLUSION

Load in the human body can be quantified as force, stress, or strain, depending on the anatomical structure and the measuring technique. Direct measurements of these variables are invasive and only possible in animals or in small-scale in vivo studies in humans. Miniaturization of transducers and electronics may open new possibilities for direct measurements of load in the human body.

Studies with a large number of human subjects, and routine analysis of patients, are done using noninvasive techniques: EMG analysis for muscle forces, kinematic analysis for ligament forces, and inverse dynamics for resultant joint loads. Inverse dynamics is the most general method and is applicable to all joints in the human body. Important limitations of inverse dynamics are due to the "distribution problem": the separation of resultant loads into the individual forces in muscles and other structures. Dynamic optimization is the most promising solution method for this problem. Inverse dynamics also relies heavily on the assumption that body segments are rigid. The errors caused by this simplification are most severe in impact and vibration studies.

Computer simulation is a well-established method for load analysis in mechanical engineering but is relatively rare in biomechanics. Replacing the human test subject by a mathematical model has many advantages, mainly for reproducibility and understanding of the results. Models for mechanical properties and control of muscles are an important and difficult part of computer simulation. For this reason, computer simulation has only been applied for load analysis in impact simulations, where the muscles can be regarded as passive, or for certain special problems where similarly simple muscle models can be used. In the future, we may see more applications of computer simulation for analysis of more complex activities, such as gait and sports.

REFERENCES

1. An, K. N., K. Takahashi, T. P. Harrigan, and E. Y. Chao. Determination of muscle orientations and moment arms. *J. Biomech. Eng.* 106:280–282, 1984.
2. Audu, M. J. Biomech. L. and D. T. Davy. The influence of muscle model complexity in musculoskeletal motion modeling. *J. Biomech. Eng.* 107:147–157, 1985.
3. Bergmann, G., A. Rohlmann, and F. Graichen. In vivo Messung der Hü ftgelenkbelastung. 1. Teil: Krankengymnastik [In vivo measurement of hip joint loading. Part I: Physiotherapy]. *Z. Orthop.* 127:672–679, 1989.
4. Blankevoort, L., and R. Huiskes. Mathematical simulations of passive knee joint motions. G. Bergmann, R. Kölbel, A. Rohlmann (eds). *Biomechanics: Basic and Applied Research.* Dordrecht: Martinus Nijhoff, 1987.
5. Bobbert, M. F., P. A. Huijing, and G. J. van Ingen Schenau. A model of the human triceps surae muscle-tendon complex applied to jumping. *J. Biomech.* 19:887–898, 1986.
6. Bobbert, M. F., and H. C. Schamhardt. Accuracy of determining the point of force application with piezoelectric force plates. *J. Biomech.* 23:705–710, 1990.
7. Bobbert, M. F., H. C. Schamhardt, and B. M. Nigg. Calculation of vertical ground reaction force estimates during running from positional data. *J. Biomech.* 24:1095–1105, 1991.
8. Bogert, A. J. van den, H. C. Schamhardt, and A. Crowe. Simulation of quadrupedal locomotion using a dynamic rigid body model. *J. Biomech.* 22:33–41, 1989.
9. Bogert, A. J. van den. Musculoskeletal modelling: the DADS experience. Newsletter of the International Society of Biomechanics, no. 39, pp. 4–6, 1990.
10. Bogert, A. J. van den, P. R. van Weeren, and H. C. Schamhardt. Correction for skin displacement errors in movement analysis of the horse. *J. Biomech.* 23:97–101, 1990.
11. Bogert, T. van den, K. Gielo-Perczak, and H. J. Woltring. Biomch-L: an electronic mail discussion forum for biomechanics and movement science. *J. Biomech.* 25:1367, 1992.
12. Bogert, A. J. van den, and H. C. Schamhardt. Multi-body modelling and simulation of animal locomotion. *Acta Anat.* 146:95–102, 1993.
13. Bogert, A. J. van den, and B. M. Nigg. Three dimensional stress analysis of the tibia during running. Proceedings XIV Congress of the ISB, Paris, France, 1993.

14. Carter, D. R. Anisotropic analysis of strain rosette information from cortical bone. *J. Biomech.* 11:199–202, 1978.

15. Chuang, T. Y., and D. K. Lieu. A parametric study of the thoracic injury potential of basic taekwondo kicks. *J. Biomech. Eng.* 114:346–351, 1992.

16. Crowninshield, R. D., R. C. Johnston, J. G. Andrews, and R. A. Brand. A biomechanical investigation of the human hip. *J. Biomech.* 11:75–85, 1978.

17. Crowninshield, R. D., and R. A. Brand. A physiologically based criterion of muscle force prediction in locomotion. *J. Biomech.* 14:793–801, 1981.

18. Davy, D. T., and M. L. Audu. A dynamic optimization technique for predicting muscle forces in the swing phase of gait. *J. Biomech.* 20:187–201, 1987.

19. Davy, D. T., G. M. Kotzar, R. H. Brown, K. G. Heiple, V. M. Goldberg, et al. Telemetric force measurements across the hip after total arthroplasty. *J. Bone Joint Surg.* 70-A:45–50, 1988.

20. Delp, S. L., J. P. Loan, M. G. Hoy, F. E. Zajac, E. L. Topp, and J. M. Rosen. An interactive graphics-based model of the lower extremity to study orthopaedic surgical procedures. *IEEE Trans. Biomed. Eng.* 37:757–767, 1990.

21. De Vita, P., and B. T. Bates. Intraday reliability of ground reaction force data. *Hum. Movement Sci.* 7:73–85, 1988.

22. Dolan, P., and M. A. Adams. The relationship between EMG activity and extensor moment generation in the erector spinae muscles during bending and lifting activities. *J. Biomech.* 26:513–522, 1993.

23. Dul, J., M. A. Townsend, R. Shiavi, and G. E. Johnson. Muscular synergism—I. On criteria for load sharing between synergistic muscles. *J. Biomech.* 17:663–673, 1984.

24. Dul, J., G. E. Johnson, R. Shiavi, and M. A. Townsend. Muscular synergism—II. A minimum-fatigue criterion for load sharing between synergistic muscles. *J. Biomech.* 17:675–684, 1984.

25. Engin, A. E., and M. H. Moeinzadeh, "Dynamic modelling of human articulating joints. *Math. Modelling* 4:117–141, 1983.

26. France, E. P., L. E. Poulos, G. Jayaraman, and T. D. Rosenberg. The biomechanics of lateral knee bracing. Part II: Impact response of the braced knee. *Am. J. Sports Med.* 15:430–438, 1987.

27. Frigo, C., and A. Pedotti. Determination of muscle length during locomotion. E. Asmussen and K. Jorgensen (eds). *Biomechanics VI-A,* pp. 355–360, Baltimore: University Park Press, 1978.

28. Fukashiro, S., P. V. Komi, M. Jaervinen, and M. Miyashita. Comparison between the directly measured achilles tendon force and the tendon force calculated from the ankle joint moment during vertical jumps. *Clin. Biomech.* 8:25–30, 1993.

29. Gerritsen, K. G. M., A. J. van den Bogert, and B. M. Nigg. Direct dynamics simulation of the impact phase in heel-toe running. Proceedings 4th International Symposium on Computer Simulation in Biomechanics, Paris, 1993.

30. Grieve, D. W., S. Pheasant, and P. R. Cavanagh. Prediction of gastrocnemius length from knee and ankle joint posture. In E. Asmussen and K. Jorgensen (eds). *Biomechanics VI-A,* pp. 405–412, Baltimore: University Park Press, 1978.

31. Gross, T. S., K. J. McLeod, and C. T. Rubin. Characterizing bone strain distributions in vivo using three triple rosette strain gauges. *J. Biomech.* 9:1081–1087, 1992.

32. Gruber, K., J. Denoth, H. Ruder, and E. Stuessi. Zur Mechanik der Gelenkbelastung [The mechanics of joint loading]. *Z. Orthop.* 129:260–267, 1991.

33. Hatze, H., and A. Venter. Practical activation and retention of locomotion constraints in nueromusculoskeletal control system models. *J. Biomech.* 14:873–877, 1981.

34. Hawkins, D., and M. L. Hull. A method for determining lower extremity muscle-tendon lengths during flexion/extension movements. *J. Biomech.* 23:487–494, 1990.

35. Haug, E. J. *Computer-Aided Kinematics and Dynamics of Mechanical Systems. Volume I: Basic Methods.* Boston: Allyn and Bacon, 1989.

36. Hefzy, M. S., and E. S. Grood. Sensitivity of insertion locations on length patterns of anterior cruciate ligament fibres. *J. Biomech. Eng.* 108:73–81, 1986.
37. Herzog, W., and T. R. Leonard. Validation of optimization models that estimate the forces exerted by synergistic muscles. *J. Biomech.* 24(Suppl. 1):31–39, 1991.
38. Hof, A. L., and Jw. van den Berg. EMG to force processing—I. An electrical analogue of the Hill muscle model. *J. Biomech.* 14:747–758, 1981.
39. Hof, A. L., C. N. A. Pronk, and J. A. van Best. Comparison between EMG to force processing and kinetic analysis for the calf muscle moment in walking and stepping. *J. Biomech.* 20:167–178, 1987.
40. Hubbard, M. Computer simulation in sport and industry. *J. Biomech.* 26, (Suppl.1):53–61, 1993.
41. Hubbard, M. Review of symbolic manipulation software. Newsletter of the International Society of Biomechanics, no. 39, pp. 4–6, 1990.
42. Huiskes, R., and E. Y. S. Chao. A survey of finite element analysis in orthopedic biomechanics: the first decade. *J. Biomech.* 16:385–409, 1983
43. Huston, R. L., and J. W. Kamman. On parachutist dynamics. *J. Biomech.* 14:645–652, 1981.
44. Jacobs, R. Coordinated Muscle Functioning. Thesis, Vrije Universiteit Amsterdam, The Netherlands, 1992.
45. Jansen, M. O., A. J. van den Bogert, D. J. Riemersma, and H. C. Schamhardt. In vivo tendon forces in the forclimb of ponies at the walk, validated by ground reaction force measurements. *Acta Anat.* 146:162–167, 1993.
46. Kadaba, M. P., H. K. Ramakrishnan, M. E. Wootton, J. Gainey, G. Gorton, and G. V. B. Cochran. Repeatability of kinematic, kinetic, and electromyographic data in normal adult gait. *J. Orthop. Res.* 7:849–860, 1989.
47. Kane T. R., and D. A. Levinson. *Dynamics: Theory and Applications.* New York: McGraw-Hill, 1985.
48. Karnopp, D. Computer simulation of stick-slip friction in mechanical dynamic systems. *J. Dyn. Syst. Meas. Contr.* 107:100–103, 1985.
49. Ladin, Z., and G. Wu. Combining position and acceleration measurements for joint force estimation. *J. Biomech.* 24:1173–1187, 1991.
50. Lafortune, M. A., P. R. Cavanagh, H. J. Sommer, and A. Kalenak. Three-dimensional kinematics of the human knee during walking. *J. Biomech.* 25:347–357, 1992.
51. Lamontagne, M., J. J. Dowling, and E. D. Lemaire. Validation of a musculoskeletal model to predict force in human quadriceps muscles. Proceedings XII Congress of the ISB, Los Angeles, California, abstract #235, 1989.
52. Landau, L. D., and E. M. Lifshitz. *Theory of Elasticity.* London: Pergamon, 1959.
53. Lanshammar, H. On precision limits for derivatives numerically calculated from noisy data. *J. Biomech.* 15:459–470, 1982.
54. Lanyon, L. E., W. G. J. Hampson, A. E. Goodship, and J. S. Shah. Bone deformation recorded in vivo from strain gauges attached to the human tibial shaft. *Acta Orthop. Scand.* 46:256–268, 1975.
55. Ma, S., and G. I. Zahalak. A distribution-moment model of energetics in skeletal muscle. *J. Biomech.* 24:21–35, 1991.
56. Meglan, D., N. Berme, and W. Zuelzer. On the construction, circuitry and properties of liquid metal strain gages. *J. Biomech.* 21:681–685, 1988.
57. Morrison, J. B. Bioengineering analysis of force actions transmitted by the knee joint. *Biomed. Eng.* 3:164–170, 1968.
58. Mouton, L. J., A. L. Hof, H. J. de Jongh, and W. H. Eisma. Influence of posture on the relation between surface electromyogram amplitude and back muscle moment: consequences for the use of surface electromyogram to measure back load. *Clin. Biomech.* 6:245–251, 1991.
59. Nigg, B. M., and M. F. Bobbert. On the potential of various approaches in load analysis to reduce the frequency of sports injuries. *J. Biomech.* 23, (Suppl. 1):3–12, 1990.

60. Nikravesh, P. E. Some methods for dynamic analysis of constrained mechanical systems: a survey. E. J. Haug (ed). *Computer Aided Analysis and Optimization of Mechanical System Dynamics (NATO ASI-F9)*, Berlin: Springer, 1984.
61. Olney, S. J., and D. A. Winter. Predictions of knee and ankle moments of force in walking from EMG and kinematic data. *J. Biomech.* 18:9–20, 1985.
62. Pandy, M. G., and F. E. Zajac. Optimal muscular coordination strategies for jumping. *J. Biomech.* 24:1–10, 1991.
63. Pandy, M. G., and N. Berme. A numerical method for simulating the dynamics of human walking. *J. Biomech.* 21:1043–1051, 1988.
64. Paul, J. P. Forces transmitted by joints in the human body. *Proc. Instn. Mech. Engrs.* 181:8–15, 1967.
65. Pedotti, A., V. V. Krishnan, and L. Stark. Optimization of muscle force sequencing in human locomotion. *Math. Biosci.* 38:57–76, 1978.
66. Procter, P., and J. P. Paul. Ankle joint biomechanics. *J. Biomech.* 15:627–634, 1982.
67. Riemersma, D. J., and J. L. M. A. Lammertink. Calibration of the mercury-in-Silastic strain gauge in tendon load experiments. *J. Biomech.* 21:469–476, 1988.
68. Riemersma, D. J., A. J. van den Bogert, H. C. Schamhardt, and W. Hartman. Kinetics and kinematics of the equine hind limb: in vivo tendon strain and joint kinematics. *Am. J. Vet. Res.* 49:1353–1359, 1988.
69. Ronsky, J. R., and B. M. Nigg. Error in kinematic data due to marker attachment methods. Proceedings of the XIIIth congress of the ISB, Perth, Australia, pp. 390–392, 1991.
70. Roszek, B., H. Weinans, P. van Loon, and R. Huiskes. In vivo measurements of the loading conditions on the tibia of the goat. *Acta Anat.* 146:188–192, 1993.
71. Schamhardt, H. C., W. Hartman, and J. L. M. A. Lammertink. Forces loading the tarsal joint in the hind limb of the horse, determined from in vivo strain measurements of the third metatarsal bone. *Am. J. Vet. Res.* 50:728–733, 1989.
72. Seireg, A., and R. J. Arvikar. A mathematical model for evaluation of forces in lower extremities of the musculo-skeletal system. *J. Biomech.* 6:313–326, 1973.
73. Shampine, L. F., and M. K. Gordon. *Computer Solution of Ordinary Differential Equations: The Initial Value Problem.* San Francisco: Freeman, 1975.
74. Soest, A. J. van, A. L. Schwab, M. F. Bobbert, and G. J. van Ingen Schenau. SPACAR: a software subroutine package for simulation of the behavior of biomechanical systems. *J. Biomech.* 25:1219–1226, 1992.
75. Soest, A. J. van, A. L. Schwab, M. F. Bobbert, and G. J. van Ingen Schenau. The influence of the biarticularity of the gastrocnemius muscle on vertical-jumping achievement. *J. Biomech.* 26:1–8, 1993.
76. Spoor, C. W., J. L. van Leeuwen, C. G. M. Meskers, A. F. Titulaer, and A. Huson. Estimation of instantaneous moment arms of lower-leg muscles. *J. Biomech.* 23;1247–1259, 1990.
77. Spoor, C. W., and J. L. van Leeuwen. Knee muscle moment arms from MRI and from tendon travel. *J. Biomech.* 25:201–206, 1992.
78. Sprigings, E. J., and J. A. Koehler. The choice between Bernouilli's or Newton's model in predicting dynamic lift. *Int. J. Sport Biomech.* 6:235–245, 1990.
79. Stacoff, A., J. Denoth, X. Kaelin, and E. Stuessi. Running injuries and shoe construction: some possible relationships. *Int. J. Sport Biomech.* 4:342–357, 1988.
80. Thunissen, J. G. M. Muscle force prediction during human gait. Thesis, University of Twente, The Netherlands, 1993.
81. Tien, C. S., and R. L. Huston. Numerical advances in gross-motion simulations of head-neck dynamics. *J. Biomech. Eng.* 109:163–168, 1987.
82. Vaughan, C. L., J. G. Hay, and J. G. Andrews. Closed loop problems in biomechanics. Part I—A classification system. *J. Biomech.* 15:197–200, 1982.
83. Vaughan, C. L., J. G. Hay, and J. G. Andrews. Closed loop problems in biomechanics. Part II—An optimization approach. *J. Biomech.* 15:201–210, 1982.
84. Veldpaus, F. E., H. J. Woltring, and L. J. M. G. Dortmans. A least-squares algorithm for the equiform transformation from spatial marker co-ordinates. *J. Biomech.* 21:45–54, 1988.

85. Verstraete, M. C., and R. W. Soutas-Little. A method for computing the three-dimensional angular velocity and acceleration of a body segment from three-dimensional position data. *J. Biomech. Eng.* 112:114–118, 1990.
86. Viidik, A. Functional properties of collagenous tissues. D. Hall and D. Jackson (eds). *International Reviews of Connective Tissue Research.* New York: Academic Press, pp 127–215, 1973.
87. Visser, J. J., J. E. Hoogkamer, M. F. Bobbert, and P. A. Huijing. Length and moment arm of human leg muscles as a function of knee and hip-joint angles. *Eur. J. Appl. Physiol.* 61:453–460, 1990.
88. Walker, P. S., J. S. Rovick, and D. D. Robertson. The effects of knee brace hinge design and placement on joint mechanics. *J. Biomech.* 21:965–974, 1988.
89. Weeren, P. R. van, M. O. Jansen, A. J. van den Bogert, and A. Barneveld. A kinematic and strain gauge study of the reciprocal apparatus in the equine hind limb. *J. Biomech.* 25:1291–1301, 1992.
90. Weeren, P. R. van, A. J. van den Bogert, and A. Barneveld. Correction models for skin displacement in equine kinematic gait analysis. *J. Equine Vet. Sci.* 12:178–192, 1992.
91. Winter, D. A. Kinematic and kinetic patterns in human gait: variability and compensating effects. *Hum. Movement Sci.* 3:51–76, 1984.
92. Winters, J. M., and L. Stark. Muscle models: what is gained and what is lost by varying model complexity. *Biol. Cybern.* 55:403–420, 1987.
93. Woltring, H. J. A FORTRAN package for generalized, cross-validatory spline smoothing and differentiation. *Adv. Eng. Software* 8:104–113, 1986.
94. Woltring, H. J. On optimal smoothing and derivative estimation from noisy displacement data in biomechanics. *Hum. Movement Sci.* 4:229–245, 1985.
95. Woltring, H. J. Release notes for GCVSPL software, 1986. (Retrievable by electronic mail with the request "SEND GCVSPL MEMO" from LISTSERV@NIC.SURFNET.NL)
96. Wu, G., and Z. Ladin. The kinematometer—An integrated kinematic sensor for kinesiological measurements. *J. Biomech. Eng.* 115:53–62, 1993.
97. Xu, W. S., D. L. Butler, D. C. Stouffer, E. S. Grood, and D. L. Glos. Theoretical analysis of an implantable force transducer for tendon and ligament structures. *J. Biomech. Eng.* 114:170–177, 1992.
98. Yamada, H. *Strength of Biological Materials.* F. G. Evans (ed). Baltimore: Williams and Wilkins, 1970.
99. Zajac, F. Muscle coordination of movement: a perspective. *J. Biomech.* 26(Suppl.1):109–124, 1993.

3
Preemployment Physical Evaluation

ANDREW S. JACKSON, P.E.D., F.A.C.S.M.

Employers have always used some method to select an employee among potential job applicants. The rapid rise in the use of standardized tests for job placement can be traced to this country's need for rapid mobilization and utilization of human resources during the first and second World Wars. The goal was to match military personnel to jobs on the basis of test performance. The development of preemployment tests grew out of the discipline of psychology and the early success in measuring differences among people. The common theme of this work was that persons differ from each other in reasonable, stable ways, on some number of attributes and that patterns of individual attributes are more or less suited to particular patterns of job requirements [44].

Much of the early preemployment testing focused on cognitive abilities, but with the rise in women seeking jobs that were once male dominated, the need for preemployment physical abilities tests increased. In 1982, Campion [25] suggested that there was a need for better methods of selecting personnel for physically demanding jobs for at least three reasons. First, equal employment opportunity legislation resulted in greater numbers of females and handicapped individuals seeking employment in occupations requiring high levels of physical ability. Second, there was evidence suggesting that physically unfit workers had higher incidences of lower back injuries. Lastly, preemployment medical evaluations used alone are inadequate for personnel selection for a physically demanding job. The disciplines most prominent in this research are industrial-organizational (I/O) psychology, industrial engineering, ergonomics, biomechanics, and exercise physiology.

Preemployment test research must not only meet the demands of traditional peer review but also potential legal review, because physical ability tests are likely to have adverse impact against females [64]. (Some governmental literature uses the term *physical agility*. The term *physical ability* will be used in this document.) In this context, adverse impact is a selection rate for females less than 80% of the male rate [48]. This potential for adverse impact can be traced to the well-documented male and female differences in strength [60, 94, 109], maximal oxygen uptake (VO_2max) [5, 75, 131], and percentage body fat [84, 85, 103, 131]. If hiring practices produce adverse impact, federal law requires a completed validation study to support the selection method. These forces have led to the development of a body of knowledge that integrates classic psychometric measurement theory, biomechanics, ergonomics, and work physiology. This chapter reviews these issues and research.

LEGAL AND LEGISLATIVE FORCES

The current interest and research on preemployment test methodology for physically demanding jobs has its roots not only in work physiology [45, 103, 115] and psychometric test theory [42], but also federal civil rights legislation and court decisions on employment practices. In 1964, Congress passed the Civil Rights Act. Title VII of this act prohibits employment discrimination based on race, color, religion, sex, or national origin. In 1966, the Equal Employment Opportunity Commission (EEOC) published the first set of guidelines on employment testing, which were revised in 1970. This led, in 1978, to the publication of the Uniform Guidelines on Employee Selection Procedures [47]. These federal standards and rules were jointly agreed upon by the EEOC, Civil Service Commission, and Departments of Labor and Justice. The American with Disabilities Act extended legal protection from employment discrimination to handicapped Americans [47] will have on preemployment testing.

Although some form of selection method has been always used to select employees for a job, the legal controversy surrounding employment testing is only about 30 years old. The initial and majority of legal cases concerning preemployment testing involved racial and ethnic discrimination by paper and pencil cognitive tests [3], but with the increasing interest of women in seeking jobs traditionally held by men, the litigation of cases concerning physical requirements has increased. A major source of this gender discrimination litigation has been with public safety jobs, police officer, fire fighter, and correctional officer jobs.

Uniform Guidelines on Employee Selection
The uniform guidelines incorporate a set of principles to judge the use of tests and other selection procedures for employment decisions. They provide a framework for determining the proper use of tests and other selection procedures [48]. Federal law prohibits employment practices that discriminate because of race, color, religion, sex, and national origin, and with the passage of ADA, disabilities.

Discrimination, as defined by the guidelines, is the use of any selection procedure that has an adverse impact on the hiring (or promotion) of a defined minority group. The four-fifths rule determines adverse impact. A selection rate for any race, sex, or ethnic group that is less than four-fifths (80%) of the rate for the group with the highest rate is considered by federal enforcement agencies as evidence of adverse impact. To illustrate, assume that 60% of the male applicants pass a physical abilities test, but only 15% of the female applicants pass. This is adverse impact because the pass rate for females is only 9% of the rate for men, (i.e., 0.15 × 0.60 = 0.09). To satisfy the four-fifths rule in this example, a minimum of 48% of women would need to pass the physical abilities test.

According to the uniform guidelines, a preemployment test with adverse impact is discriminatory and inconsistent with the guidelines unless the test has been validated in a manner consistent with the guidelines. In practice this means that the employer must conduct a validation study to show that the test measures important job behaviors. The guidelines may be met by conducting a criterion-related, content, or construct validation study that is consistent with established test validation methods [1, 42]. The test validation section of this chapter describes these three general validation strategies.

The American with Disabilities Act
The American with Disabilities Act (ADA) passed into law on July 26, 1992, and promises to have wide-reaching implications for preemployment tests. ADA goes beyond traditional equal employment law and affirmative action principles by requiring individualized treatment on a better-than-equal basis [47]. A disabled person is someone with a substantial impairment that significantly limits or restricts a major life activity such as hearing, seeing, speaking, walking, breathing, performing manual tasks, caring for oneself, learning, or working. The exact number of Americans covered under this law is not known, but many believe it exceeds 43 million.

Under ADA, employment tests or other selection methods cannot be used to screen out individuals with a disability unless the test or selection method is shown to be job-related. The testing procedures cannot be used to disqualify disabled individuals if the test requires knowledge, skills, or abilities not required to perform essential job functions. Employers must now show that the preemployment screening test measures only those abilities required to perform essential job functions. Under ADA, medical examinations cannot be given until an offer of employment is made. This suggests that one possible consequence of ADA is that validated physical ability tests will play a greater role in employee selection.

Court Rulings
Much of the controversy in employment practice can be traced to court rulings on employment practices. Arvey [3] maintains that the landmark case of Myart v. Motorola in 1963 was the first signal that the court system became involved in the employment process. Leon Myart, a black with previous job-related experience, was refused a job in a Motorola plant because his score on a five-minute intelligence test was too low. Myart filed a complaint with the Illinois Fair Employment Practices Commission and charged racial discrimination. The Illinois Commission ruled that Mayart be offered a job and ruled that the test could no longer be used for

selection decisions. This landmark case motivated employers to develop preemployment tests that did not discriminate against a protected group [3].

Hogan and Quigley [63] provide an excellent review of court cases related to physical testing and physical standards. The cases reviewed include the use of height and weight standards and physical ability testing. Of the 44 cases reviewed, 34 involved height and weight standards and 10 cases involved physical ability tests for employee selection. Of these cases, most (37) involved law enforcement and firefighter employee selection procedures.

The law is clear: if there is adverse impact, the employment practice is open for legal examination, and the employer needs competent evidence showing that the preemployment test is valid [3, 48]. In the 1960s, height and weight standards were a condition of employment for many public safety jobs, and these standards clearly have adverse impact on women. Arvey [3] reported that in 1973, nearly all the nation's large police departments had a minimum height requirement. The average requirement was 68 inches. More than 90% of women and 45% of men would be expected to fail the 68-inch height requirement. The rationale for the standard was that size was related to physical strength, and the effectiveness of a police officer's job performance depended upon strength.

Arvey [3] maintains that the most important case on the use of a height and weight requirement was decided in June, 1977, by the United States Supreme Court. In Dothard v. Rawlinson, a female was refused employment as a correctional-counselor trainee because she did not meet the minimum height and weight requirements of 62 inches and 120 pounds. The standard was found to have adverse impact because it excluded 33.3% of females and only 1.3% of males. The defendants argued that the height and weight requirements were job-related because they have a relationship to strength, which is job related. The Supreme Court ruled that if strength is a real job requirement, then a direct measure of strength should have been adopted.

Only under rare circumstances has a height or weight requirement been supported in the courts. A key issue in these cases is establishing that the height or weight requirement is job related. One case (Boyd v. Ozark Airlines) was ruled in favor of a height requirement. The court ruled that a minimum height is necessary for a pilot to see properly and reach all the controls in an airplane cockpit [3, 63].

Of the 10 cases involving physical tests, all involved police and firefighter preemployment tests, and 8 were won by the defendants, who were job applicants [63]. The common test development approach that emerged from these cases was the use of general physical ability and fitness tests such as sit-ups, push-ups, pull-ups, squat thrusts, and various strength tests. Arvey [3] maintains that these tests are less likely to be legally supported because they do not represent "samples" of actual work behavior. This was especially evident in the classic 1982 New York City firefighter case, Berkman v. City of New York. The physical agility test items were selected using the constructs defined by Fleishman [49]. None of the women tested passed the New York City firefighter test, while 46% of the men did. The court stated: "Nothing in the concepts of dynamic strength, gross body equilibrium, stamina, and the like, has such a grounding in observable behavior of the way firefighters operate that one could say with confidence that a person who possesses a high degree of these abilities as opposed to others will perform well on the job" [3, p. 279].

Another requirement that courts ruled discriminatory are lifting requirements. In response to the deleterious working conditions encountered by women during the industrial revolution, many states passed laws that "protected" women from physical labor. The lifting requirement was ruled discriminatory in the 1969 case, Weeks v. Southern Bell Telephone & Telegraph Company. The company did not consider a female employee's bid for a job vacancy as switchman because the job had a 30-pound lifting requirement. While Southern Bell contended that the switchman's job was "strenuous," the court ruled that Southern Bell did not show that the job was so strenuous that most women could not perform it and that the lifting requirement was based on a "stereotyped characterization." Southern Bell lost the case because they did not establish the validity of the lifting requirement [3, 63].

Physiological test principles helped decide a 1992 case involving a preemployment test for entry-level mill workers in a company's logging and sawmill operations (*Findings of Fact and Conclusions of Law as to Liability, EEOC v. Simpson Timber Company,* US District Court, Western District of Washington, 1992). The preemployment test used by the timber company was ruled illegal because it disproportionately excluded women qualified for the jobs. The test had three items: board pull ergometer to measure strength (pulling 30-, 50-, and 70-pound weights for specified durations), a six-minute step test using an 11-inch bench, and a visual assessment of the applicant's gross body coordination. During the test, the applicant wore a heart rate monitor, and the test was stopped and the applicant failed if the heart rate exceeded 85% of estimated maximum aerobic capacity. Since the female passing rate on the test was 42.4% of the male passing rate, the test showed adverse impact under the uniform guidelines 80% rule. The judge stated: "Simpson has met its burden of showing that the test is job-related and serves, in a significant way, the company's legitimate employment goal of hiring a physically fit work force, in that those who pass the test, as a group, are likelier to be able to do the jobs adequately and safely than are those, as a group, who do not pass the test. The test nonetheless unnecessarily excludes qualified applicants, a disproportionate number of whom are women."

The judge ruled that methods used to administer a step test introduced gender bias and that the step test cut score of 10 METs be reduced to 8.5

METs, the cut score used in testing existing employees who sought a transfer from one division of the company to another. The judge further ruled that part of the adverse impact was caused by the failure to use an adjustable height bench or different height benches for male and females and that this would not change the selection device except to increase accuracy. Lastly, part of the adverse impact was attributed to poor test administration. The judge stated that in some instances, women applicants were not given timely instructions about what they should eat or drink before the test; males and females were required to wait together while the test was administered; and female applicants were treated in ways that caused tension and anxiety.

INJURY RATES

Another major force motivating companies to initiate preemployment physical tests is reducing work-related injuries and containing workers' compensation costs. Many occupations have a high incidence of musculoskeletal injuries, of which a very high proportion affect the low back [123]. Most back injuries are not usually serious, with employees returning to work within 3 weeks; the problem is with their prevalence [87]. About 80% of Americans will experience a low back disorder at some time in their lives, and the total compensable cost for low back disorders in the United States during 1988 was $15.3 billion. In 1988, 16.4% of workers' compensation claims of a major insurance company were for low back disorders [122]. Back problems are the most common reason for a worker's decreased work capacity and reduced leisure time activity in Americans below the age of 45. In a comprehensive survey of insurance claims for back injuries, Snook and associates [123] reported that the major occupational acts associated with low back injury were lifting, 49%; twisting and turning, 18%; bending, 12%; and pulling 9%. There are three ergonomic approaches used to reduce the number of industrial back injuries: (a) redesign physically demanding jobs; (b) use preemployment tests for workers of physically demanding jobs; and (c) education and training [122].

Job Redesign
Job redesign represents an engineering approach to reduce the worker's exposure to the risk factors of low back disorders. Some examples of job redesign are lowering stacking heights to shoulder or below and using equipment (e.g., hydraulic lifts, air hoists,) to move heavy containers and equipment [6]. A second ergonomic job redesign approach used is to establish "safe" lifting loads. Definitions of "safe" lifting loads come from psychophysical, biomechanical, and physiological research.

PSYCHOPHYSICAL LIFTING STANDARDS. Snook and associates [123] completed a major, retrospective epidemiologic study seeking the causal factors related to industrial insurance claims for low back pain. They reported that a worker was three times more susceptible to low back injury if the job demands exceeded the level that 25% of the working population felt they could do. It was estimated that the injury rate associated with materials-handling tasks could be reduced by 67% by using work loads that fit the physical capabilities of the working population, supporting the value of redesigning materials-handling jobs to fit the perceived lifting levels of the industrial population.

The psychophysical approach involves having workers rate the maximum weight that can be lifted for various job conditions. This research produced maximum acceptable lifting loads and work rates [10, 34, 110, 124, 126] for men and women and various work conditions. The work conditions considered were the width of object; vertical distance moved (*a*) floor-to-knuckle height, (*b*) knuckle-to-shoulder height, (*c*) shoulder-to-arm height); and rate of movement (number of lifts per hour). These studies give load lift standards for selected percentages of the industrial male and female populations [121, 124, 126].

BIOMECHANICAL LIFTING MODELS. Another method of redesigning the job is to use biomechanical models to define "safe" lifting loads. Industrial engineers developed models to estimate the strain capabilities of the musculoskeletal structure, particularly the spinal cord. The objective of these models is to define "safe" job conditions, based on the compressive forces that work tasks place on the spine. Two-dimensional biomechanical models are available for estimating the low back compression forces on L5/S1 disc for various lifting positions [27, 109, 114]. The factors used are (*a*) horizontal location at the start of lift; (*b*) vertical location of origin of lift (e.g., on the floor); (*c*) vertical travel distance between origin and destination of lift; and (*d*) lift frequency.

The most obvious factor that increases spine compression forces is the weight of the lifted object. Less obvious, but very important, is the position of the object at the start of the lift. The longer the horizontal distance between the load's center of gravity and the location of the L5/S1 disc, the higher the compression forces. The validity of the model was empirically supported by data from 400 industrial workers [32]. They showed that the incidence of low back pain was related to L5/S1 disc compression forces estimated by the biomechanical model. Jobs that placed more than 650 kilograms of compression forces on the low back were considered hazardous to all but the most fit workers. In terms of job design, a level of 350 kilogram forces is viewed as the upper limit for industrial workers [110]. These current biomechanical lifting standards are presently being debated and under review [86, 132].

Ayoub [8] developed a simplified method of estimating low back compression force for three different lifting tasks. He published multiple regression equations that estimate the maximum L5/S1 compression force from weight of load (kilograms), and body weight (kilograms). The equations for the three lifts are:

Floor-to-knuckle height:
L5/S1 compression forces = 4.6153 (body weight) + 12.2923 (load weight)

Floor-to-shoulder height:
L5/S1 compression forces = 4.8600 (body weight) + 10.6654 (load weight)

Knuckle-to-shoulder height:
L5/S1 compression forces = 2.8119 (body weight) + 14.6556 (load weight)

Marras and associates [100] reported that the two-dimensional bi-omechanical models do not consider all the potential causal factors that increase the risk of back problems. They developed a multiple logistic regression model that defined the industrial low back risk associated with a variety of work tasks. They studied 403 industrial jobs from 48 manufacturing companies. The jobs were divided into low-risk jobs (no injuries and no turnover for 3 years) and high-risk jobs defined by at least 12 back injuries per 200,000 hours worked. The variables related to low back risk were lifting frequency (lifts/hour), average twisting velocity (deg/sec), maximum moment (Nm), maximum sagittal flexion (degrees), and maximum lateral velocity (deg/sec). Maximum moment is the product of the weight of the object lifted and distance from the object's center of gravity and the worker's L5/S1 region of the back. Adding the trunk motion variables increased the predictive power of this model three times over the current recommended model [110]. The logistic risk model provides not only a means of identifying the jobs with high risk but also insight into the redesign of jobs.

PHYSIOLOGICAL WORK STANDARDS. Most research focused on the effects of muscular strength on back injuries, but several investigators reported that the lack of muscular endurance causes low back injuries. Low back pain patients and normals not only differ in muscle strength, but also in muscle endurance. Suzuki and Endo [129] studied 90 male patients using isokinetic trunk-strength testing methods. Significant flexion and extension differences were found between patients and healthy controls on both strength and endurance measures. Nicolaisen and Jorgensen [108] found that isometric endurance was lower in patients with low back problems than in healthy controls. Hultman and associates [67] reported that trunk endurance was related to low back problems. Their data showed a gradual loss of isometric trunk endurance from a back-healthy group of men to those with intermittent low back pain to men with chronic low back pain. Lee [95] reported that in fatigue overloading, series of repetitive loads to the spine may be at a submaximal level, but once beyond the fatigue capacity of one's muscles, the spinal column becomes overloaded to the level of injury. For example, "one can sustain a back injury from shoveling snow" [95, p. 275].

Another method of redesigning the job is defining the maximum permissible lifting limits with metabolic energy expenditure models. The National Institute of Occupational Safety and Health (NIOSH) recommends a maximum permissible lifting limit of 5 kilocalories per minute [110]. This standard is presently being debated [8, 86, 132]. Ayoub [8] provides regression equations for estimating the energy cost of lifting (VO_2 (ml · min^{-1}) from F, frequency of lift (lifts · min^{-1}); L, weight of load (kilograms); and B, body weight (kilograms); and the interaction of these factors. The equations for three common lift heights are:

$$\text{Floor-to-knuckle height:}$$
$$VO_2 \text{ (ml · min}^{-1}) = 3.8941(B) + 0.5211(F \times B) + 3.0072(L) + 3.0577(F \times L)$$

$$\text{Floor-to-shoulder height:}$$
$$VO_2 \text{ (ml · min}^{-1}) = 5.7152(B) + 0.3087(F \times B) + 0.1976(L) + 5.2392(F \times L)$$

$$\text{Knuckle-to-shoulder height:}$$
$$VO_2 \text{ (ml · min}^{-1}) = 3.7471(B) + 0.1896(F \times B) + 3.7880(L) + 3.1313(F \times L)$$

Preemployment Testing
Preemployment testing is the preferred ergonomic approach for those physically demanding jobs that cannot be redesigned [122]. The goal is to match the worker's physiological capabilities with the physical demands of the job. The strategy to control injury is one of selecting only those individuals with the capacity to perform a given job without excessive risk [7, 29, 31, 89, 122].

Strength testing is the most effective job placement technique for materials-handling tasks [122]. The hypothesis behind this approach is that there is a relationship between the probability of injury and percentage of strength capacity used by the worker in job performance. If a job required lifting a 100-pound object using the back, the individual with a capacity of 100 pounds would be more prone to injury than one with a 200-pound lifting capacity [7].

Chaffin and associates [29, 31, 89] showed that strength is related to injury rate and that a worker's likelihood of sustaining a musculoskeletal injury increased when job lifting requirements approached or exceeded the worker's strength capacity. Their approach compared the worker's strength with the strength required by the work task. Using 410 current employees in 103 jobs, they found a significant relationship between the ratio of strength required on the job and the worker's strength and the incidence of low back injury during the year of the study [29].

In a second study [31], with 551 employees from six plants, the likelihood of sustaining back injuries was a function of isometric arm, leg, and torso strength. As the strength demands of the job approached the subject's maximum strength capacity, the chances of injury increased. In a third study [88], a biomechanical analysis quantified the strength demands on production jobs in an aluminum reduction plant. The biomechanical data served as the model for designing strength tests that simulated the job activities with the greatest strength demands. A cross-section of employees assigned to the physically demanding jobs was strength tested and monitored for medical incidents for more than 2 years. The data analysis showed that workers with strength abilities below the job strength requirements suffered a significantly higher rate of medical incidents than workers whose strength matched or exceeded job demands.

Cady and associates [23] found a relationship between the incidence of firefighter back injuries and level of physical fitness. The reported injury rates for fitness groups were least fit, 7.1%; middle fit, 3.2%; and most fit, 0.8%. The back injuries of physically fit firefighters were less costly than injuries of those who were less fit. Doolittle and associates [43] found similar results with electrical lineworkers. They reported a significant correlation between worker scores on strength and endurance tests and the incidence of lost work days due to on-the-job injuries. In contrast, Battie and associates [12] did not find a relationship between aerobic fitness and the incidence of back injuries of industrial workers.

Battie and associates [13] studied the relationship between isometric back lift strength and the incidence of back injuries in a cohort of industrial workers who perform a variety of manual tasks. They administered isometric strength tests to 2178 workers. A total of 172 workers reported back problems during the 4-year study. They reported that those with the greatest strength were at significantly greater risk of low back problems than were weaker workers, but this depended on age; younger workers had more injuries than older employees. Once age was statistically controlled, the strength-injury rate was no longer statistically significant. Although older men had fewer injuries than younger men, the cost of the claim for the older men was significantly higher. Women had fewer injuries than men, but the claim was more likely to become a high-cost injury claim (i.e., >$10,000) [17].

The conflicting results reported by Battie et al. [13] and the work of Chaffin and associates [29, 31, 89] are likely due to matching the worker with the demands of the work task. It has been our experience that workers may have the same job classification but not do the same work. In the task analysis phase of extremely demanding materials-handling tasks, we observed employees who could not lift some of the heavier boxes. These heavy boxes were lifted by stronger employees [81].

Training and Education
Education and training is the third ergonomic method used to reduce back injuries. Many companies train their workers to lift "properly," but this

approach has not proven to be successful. Workers taught safe lifting methods do not follow the methods; likely because it is harder and more difficult to lift by these methods [122]. Kishino and associates[91] maintained that they can teach patients the safe mechanics of lifting, but it is difficult to get them to comply and incorporate the technique into daily living. They observed that patients initially lift gingerly, using the "proper lifting technique" of bent knee and straight back taught to them by so many industrial training and "back school" programs. Yet, when given permission to lift in the way that "feels right" and allows most efficient lifting, patients select any of several modes of lifting technique. They have observed that some general rules about lifting appear appropriate, but when given the freedom to choose, the lifting patterns of individuals differ dramatically. Factors that affect lifting patterns besides the weight of the object, are the speed of the lift, size and shape of the object lifted, and the lifter's physical characteristics.

Brown [20] examined programs designed to train workers to lift "properly." Their summary of published data showed that training on safe lifting procedure did not effectively control low back injuries. The injury rate of those employers who provided training was as high as that for those who did not. One may argue that perhaps the proper lifting procedures are not being used effectively. But, in a Swedish study [40], nursing aides received instruction on the "correct" lifting technique, and these instructions were repeated every third month to ensure compliance. Yet, this did not reduce the occurrence of low back injury.

Fitness level and exercise training appear to be related to injury. High levels of aerobic fitness, strength, and flexibility were inversely related to workers' compensation costs of firefighters [23, 24] and lineworkers [43]. These data suggest that fitness programs would likely reduce musculoskel-etal injuries. The major problem with this approach is that most do not comply with exercise training. In the typical supervised exercise setting, about 50% of the clients will drop out of the program within 6 months to 1 year [41], and those most likely to continue an exercise program are those who are most physically fit and have an active lifestyle [133]. Of those employees given the opportunity to be involved in an exercise program, most will not participate at a beneficial level. Only about 20–40% of the employees eligible to use worksite exercise facilities will do so, and only about 33% of these users will exercise on a regular basis at desirable intensity levels [41].

VALIDATION STUDY METHODOLOGY

A likely outcome of implementing a physical abilities test is that it will have adverse impact on women. When adverse impact is documented, test validation is essential because the employment testing procedures are more likely to be examined for compliance with the Uniform Guidelines on Employee Selection Procedures [48]. Much of the preemployment test validation methodology comes from psychometric theory, and the legal standards of judging a test's validity use psychological criteria [1, 42].

The first important component of a preemployment test validation study is the job analysis. The goal of the job analysis is to identify the important work behaviors demanded by the job. The job analysis gives foundation for the preemployment test items to be validated according to established guidelines [47, 48] and professional procedures [1, 42]. After completing the validation study, the final step is to define the cut score for selecting qualified employees.

Job Analysis

A job analysis is an essential component in the development of a preemployment test. Job analysis, broadly defined, is the collection and analysis of any type of job-related information by any method for any purpose [53, p. 3]. It is the process of reducing to words what people do. The uniform guidelines clearly require that a validity study must include a job analysis. The objective of a job analysis is to find measures of work behavior(s) or performance that are used for the job and determine the extent to which they represent critical or important job duties, work behaviors, or work outcomes [48].

The outcomes of court cases on physical testing [3, 63] clearly document the importance of the job analysis. When the job analysis did not tap relevant physical duties and performance requirements adequately, it tended to be legally challenged. Other challenges raised in court cases are that the sample used for the job analysis was not sufficiently large and did not represent the appropriate population of workers. Lastly, the job analysis data and test item(s) selected lacked congruence.

Many different methods are available for conducting a job analysis. These methods include observing work, recording work activities, interviewing workers or supervisors, using questionnaires to collect data, or using various combinations of these methods [53]. The general methods commonly used to validate tests for physically demanding tasks usually come from combinations of psychophysical, biomechanical, and physiological data sources. Examples of validation studies that used all three data sources appear in the literature [7, 43].

PSYCHOPHYSICAL METHODS. An easy and efficient method of quantifying the work demands is to have workers rate tasks in some systematic manner. The research on the rating of perceived exertion (RPE) [18, 19, 111] gives theoretical foundation for this method. Although Borg's RPE scales can be used to rate tasks, a more common approach is to rate work tasks using some form of Likert scale. Examples of these scales can be found in another source [64].

Fleishman and associates [50, 65, 66] found that perceived physical effort ratings provided reliable and valid estimates of the metabolic cost of work tasks. Hogan and Fleishman [65] showed that personnel specialists discriminated among tasks of known energy cost differences. Using trained specialists and untrained male and female students, they reported a 0.80 correlation between their average rating and textbook listing of the estimated energy costs of 30 occupational tasks. The most difficult task was "lift and carry objects weighing 85–100 pounds." The work task in the middle of metabolic demand was "cut wood with a power saw," and the least demanding tasks were "ride a lawn mower" and "sit at a desk, using a hand calculator." They showed that the ratings of perceived effort were not a function of either training or gender.

Hogan and associates [66] extended this work and showed that metabolic ratings can be used by subjects performing tasks to predict actual physical work. They reported correlations of 0.75 and 0.72 between indices of average metabolic costs of work tasks and ratings of physical effort. In a second study, they had 20 subjects perform 24 separate materials-handling tasks whose ergonomic costs (work = force X distance) were calculated. They reported a correlation of 0.88 between psychophysical rating and work of the 24 tasks.

The taxonomy of physical abilities developed by Fleishman [49] is often used by I/O psychologists to develop psychophysical scales to rate job demands. The nine physical dimensions include four strength components (static, explosive, dynamic, and trunk strength), two flexibility components (extent and dynamic), and factors of coordination, balance, and stamina. These published psychophysical scales [51, 64] provide a method for evaluating and categorizing work tasks by the nine dimensions. Hogan [61] suggests that only three constructs are needed: (*a*) muscular strength; (*b*) cardiovascular endurance; and (*c*) movement quality. The movement quality factor combined Fleishman's balance and flexibility into a single dimension. The physiological validity of these factors lacks verification.

BIOMECHANICAL METHODS. The task analysis for physically demanding jobs often includes biomechanical data. The types of data collected include heights that objects are lifted, weights of the objects lifted or transported, and forces needed to complete work tasks such as opening and closing valves or pushing and pulling objects. Biomechanical models provide a means of evaluating the stresses that materials-handling and lifting tasks place on the spine [27, 110, 114].

PHYSIOLOGICAL METHODS. Work tasks such as climbing stairs and fighting fires have a significant aerobic endurance component. Physiological methods document the cardiovascular response of these work tasks. A tradition of work physiology has been to define the energy cost of work tasks by oxygen uptake [45, 115, 127]. Because of the expense for equipment and work environment restrictions, oxygen uptake data are typically not collected during a job analysis. The more common method is measuring exercise heart rate during actual or simulated work tasks and using heart rate data to estimate the intensity of the task [11, 38, 81, 96, 99, 112, 127].

Validation Strategies

Validity of a preemployment test involves determining the accuracy with which a test or other selection device measures the important work behaviors identified with the job analysis. Validity depends on reliability and relevance [14]. Reliability reflects the test's ability to differentiate among the true levels of performance within the tested population. Relevance involves defining the qualities being tested. The job analysis defines the relevance of a preemployment tests. Since validity depends on reliability, statistical estimates of reliability should be made whenever feasible. The Uniform Guidelines on Employee Selection Procedures [48] lists three acceptable types of studies by which preemployment tests may be validated: criterion-related validity, content validity, or construct validity studies.

CRITERION-RELATED VALIDITY. According to the uniform guidelines, a criterion-related validly study should consist of empirical data showing that the preemployment test is predictive of, or significantly correlated with, important elements of job performance. The sample subjects should represent the candidates normally available in the relevant labor market for the job and should, insofar as feasible, include the races, sexes, and ethnic groups normally available in the relevant job market. Statistical significance at the 0.05 level is accepted as a relationship between criterion and predictor. The performance on a test or other selection device is compared with job effectiveness and may be divided into concurrent and predictive methods. Concurrent methods use current employees and relate test results to current job performance. In the predictive approach, test data are obtained on people prior to hire and compared with performance data obtained at a later date [48].

Although not related to preemployment testing, exercise physiologists used the criterion-related method to establish the validity of field measures of body composition [21, 46, 84, 85, 116] and aerobic capacity [52, 75, 117]. The goal of the validation study is to find field tests that accurately predict an established criterion, hydrostatically determined body density and VO_2max in the exercise physiology context. In the preemployment setting, the criterion is an important element of job performance. The types of job performance criteria listed in the Uniform Guidelines that may be suitable are supervisory ratings, production rate, error rate, tardiness, absenteeism, and success in training. Supervisory ratings are often used, but due to the possible bias of these subjective evaluations, they need to be carefully devised to show that they do not unfairly deny opportunities to members of protected groups. According to the guidelines, this is not an inclusive list of criteria. Other examples of criteria used include injury rates [43], accidents [118], field performance [118], and job-related work tasks [2, 77, 78, 80].

An important issue of a criterion-related study is the "fairness" of the preemployment test. Unfairness exists when members of a minority group obtain lower scores on a preemployment test than members of another group, but the difference in scores is not reflected in differences in the criterion of job performance [48]. This is the Cleary test of fairness [3] and affirmed by showing that the regression line that defines the relationship between the preemployment test and criterion is common to both groups. The statistical procedure is to test for homogeneity of regression slopes and intercepts. Other sources [3, 70, 90] provide the statistical foundation and illustrate this statistical test. The literature provides examples of the use of tests of fairness in the employment setting [2, 118].

CONTENT VALIDITY. Content validity is a rational process that involves gathering evidence that shows a logical relationship between the preemployment tests and important duties or job behaviors. There is no index of content validity that is agreed upon, and professional judgment is usually the basis for estimating content validity. According to the uniform guidelines, a content validity study needs to present data showing that the content of the selection procedure represents important aspects of performance on the job for which the candidates are to be evaluated [48]. A preemployment test can be judged to be content valid to the extent that it represents the content of the job. The job analysis gives essential job content data.

A content validation strategy usually results in a work-sample test or some type of test that simulates the important aspects of job performance. Work-sample tests potentially have high content validity because they sample the actual work performed in the job. A common example is using a typing test for a secretarial position. The tests are directly and logically related to the job behaviors [3].

CONSTRUCT VALIDITY. The construct validity approach is more theoretical than content validity because it is necessary to establish that a construct is required for job success and that the selection device measures the same construct. The data from a construct validation study should show that the preemployment test measures the degree to which candidates have identifiable characteristics that are important for successful job performance [48].

Content validation involves linking the job and test domains, while construct validation is more complete and tests theoretical and empirical relationships. The goal is to establish linkage between the important constructs and multiple indicators of job performance [4]. It is the process of developing evidence and confirming inferences regarding these constructs and indicants of job performance. It is the process of confirming and disconfirming hypotheses regarding the relationship between physical ability and job constructs.

Construct validation is used extensively to develop psychological tests. Factor analysis [119] is the statistical procedure commonly used to identify constructs and the tests that measure it. This statistical method reduces several correlated variables to a smaller number of factors or dimensions. A factor is a linear combination of the original variables used in the analysis. The factor loadings or coefficients form a linear combination of the original variables that define the factor. In theory, each variable's factor loading represents the relationship (in a correlational sense) between the variable and the theoretical construct. The variables with the highest coefficients identify and define the construct.

The user should show empirically that the selection procedure validly relates the constructs to the performance of critical or important work behavior(s). This often also requires a criterion-related study to show that the construct is related to job performance. The physical ability test developed for the New York Fire Department used constructs defined by Fleishman [49]. The test was ruled discrimatory against women (Berkman v. City of New York, 1982) because the test developers did not establish that the constructs of dynamic strength, gross body equilibrium, and stamina were related to the work of firefighters [3, 63].

Physical Ability Test Selection
The types of tests used in physical ability preemployment tests can be put into two general categories. The type of tests used for content validation studies are job-sample tests or tests that simulate important work tasks identified with the job analysis. The second general type of tests are those that comprise motor ability and physical fitness batteries. As previously discussed in the section on litigation, the use of motor ability and physical fitness tests is likely to increase the chance that a preemployment test will be challenged in the courts. A work-sample test represents observable job behaviors; it is more difficult to show that the capacity to do pull-ups or sit-ups, for example, is job related.

WORK-SAMPLE TESTS. The advantage of work-sample tests is that they simulate the actual working conditions and are more likely to have content validity. Lifting and carrying boxes a specified distance is an example of a materials-handling work-sample test. Arnold and associates [2] used work-sample tests to simulate the physical work demands required of steelworkers. Work-sample tests are commonly used to screen applicants for police officer and firefighter jobs. Arvey [4] reported that most police and firefighter physical ability tests consist of some combination of job-sample tests. Some common work-sample tests for police officer jobs are scaling a wall, usually 6 feet in height; long (broad) jumping a set distance; crawling though openings at ground level; running a set distance, usually a quarter mile; dragging a heavy object a set distance; and running a course consisting of various obstacles. Tests often found in firefighter preemployment batteries are climbing a ladder; pushing and pulling a ceiling hook; dragging a dummy a set time period; and running up stairs carrying hose bundles.

While work-sample tests have the advantage of appearing to be valid, Ayoub [7] maintains that they have at least two limitations. The first is safety. Applicants seeking employment are likely to be highly motivated to pass the work-sample test. A highly motivated applicant who lacks the physical capacity to perform the task is likely to increase the risk of injury [29, 31, 88, 123]. Outdoor telephone craft jobs require employees to climb telephone poles, and accident data showed that this was a dangerous task [118]. Using a pole-climbing test to screen applicants would have content validity, but likely be too dangerous for untrained employees. This injury risk was the reason why a physical ability test was validated to screen employees seeking to enroll in pole-climbing school [16, 118].

A second limitation of job-simulation tests is they do not give any information about the applicant's maximum work capacity [7]. A work-sample test is often scored by pass or fail (e.g., lifted a 95-pound jackhammer and carried it a specified distance). Some can easily complete the test, while others may just pass and be working near their maximum. If it can be assumed that there is a liner relationship between job performance and the preemployment test performance, applicants with the highest test scores can be expected to be the more productive workers. Testing for maximum capacity not only identifies the most potentially productive workers, but also provides the opportunity to define a level of reserve that may reduce the risk of musculoskeletal injury.

MOTOR ABILITY AND FITNESS TEST ITEMS. Numerous investigators [15, 16, 35–37, 49, 57, 69, 83, 93, 98, 104, 105, 135] have conducted factor analysis studies that identified the constructs of human physical performance. The work of Fleishman [49], an I/O psychologist, has become the most common construct validation model used in preemployment validation studies. Listed next is a description of the more common physical ability constructs defined by Fleishman and tests used in preemployment validation studies. (See [14] Chapter 8, Measuring Physical Abilities for a more complete description of the factors.) Hogan [64] provides an excellent review of motor ability and fitness test items used in preemployment test batteries.

Static strength is the ability to exert maximum force. Isometric strength, isotonic strength (1–repetition maximum), and isokinetic strength tests measure this construct. This factor is positively correlated with fat-free weight and absolute endurance tests. An example of an absolute endurance test is the bench press test of the YMCA adult fitness battery [55].

Dynamic strength involves the capacity to move or maintain the body weight to exhaustion. Common tests of this construct are pull-ups and flexed arm hang. Test performance is negatively correlated with body weight and percentage body fat.

Explosive strength, often termed power, involves rapidly moving total body weight. The most common tests of this factor are standing long jump, vertical jump, and short sprints. This factor is negatively correlated with body weight and percentage body fat.

Trunk strength involves the capacity to use the abdominal muscle groups to move or maintain the body's upper extremity to exhaustion, using either isometric or isotonic contractions. Sit-ups and leg lifts are common tests of this factor. This factor is negatively correlated with body weight and percentage body fat.

There are two balance factors. The first, gross body equilibrium, is the ability to balance with the eyes closed. The second is the capacity to balance with visual cues. The tests used to measure these constructs involve balancing on an object (e.g., small board) with the eyes either opened or closed.

Flexibility has two factors, dynamic and extent flexibility. Dynamic flexibility is the ability to change direction with the body parts rapidly and efficiently. The squat thrust test measures this construct. The second flexibility factor, extent flexibility, is the ability measured by common fitness tests such as the sit and reach.

Fleishman [49] uses the term stamina to define the factor of physical working capacity, or VO_2max[5]. The tests used to sample this factor are field tests of aerobic fitness, usually a distance run or step test that estimates VO_2max from heart rate response to bench-stepping power output.

Cut Scores

After completing the validation study, the next, difficult step is to set a cut score. The cut score is the test score that an applicant must obtain to be considered for the job. The uniform guidelines merely specifies that cut scores should be reasonable and consistent with normal expectations of acceptable proficiency within the work force [48]. The consensus in the professional literature is that there is no single method of determining a cut score that is optimal in all situations [26]. The decision of where to set a cut score for a physical ability preemployment test should be a business decision that depends not only upon the available labor pool but also other factors such as desired level of work productivity, worker safety, and level of adverse impact.

The primary concern when setting a cut score is to find the extent to which the test correctly classifies candidates [26, 92]. Those applicants that exceed the cut score and are successful employees are termed "true positives." "True negatives" are those who cannot perform the job and fall below the established cut score. Since all tests lack perfect validity, some applicants will be misclassified. Those applicants that exceed the established cut scores but cannot adequately perform the job are termed "false positives." "False negatives" are applicants who were eliminated by the test but can perform the job. This is the theoretical decision model used in medical research to quantify the accuracy of a medical test in terms of test sensitivity and specificity. In the employment decision model, "test sensitivity" is the proportion of those who cannot do the job and fail the cut score. "Test specificity" is the percentage of those who exceed the cut score and can do the job. Altering the cut score changes test sensitivity and specificity. The cut score decision-making process considers not only test sensitivity and specificity but also the degree of adverse impact.

The cut score should be based on a rational process and valid selection system that is flexible and meets the needs of the organization. Based on legal, historical, and professional guidelines, Cascio and associates [26] offer several recommendations. The cut score should be based upon the results of the job analysis. The validity and job-relatedness of the testing procedure are crucial. The cut score should be sufficiently high to ensure minimally accepted job performance. The performance level associated with a cut score should be consistent with the normal expectations of acceptable proficiency within the work force. Lastly, a warranted concern is the utility of the decision process [68]. Utility in this context, concerns the cost savings for eliminating unqualified applicants [2].

The strategies used to set cut scores evolved largely from preemployment studies using psychological paper-and-pencil tests. In physical testing, a tradition of work physiology and ergonomics is to match the worker to the physiological demands of the task. Maximum oxygen uptake and strength are the physiological variables often used to evaluate a worker's capacity. Biomechanical and psychophysical data used to define "safe" material handling tasks provide another source of data to define cut scores for industrial jobs.

CUT SCORES BASED ON ENERGY COST. Many work tasks are defined by their energy cost expressed in kilocalories per minute, oxygen consumption, or metabolic equivalents (METs). Energy cost tables for common work tasks and recreational activities are published in several sources [5, 45, 103, 115]. This approach involves measuring the energy cost of the work tasks and selecting people whose maximum aerobic power is high enough so they can perform the job without excessive fatigue [25].

A current, important research focus is to define the energy cost needed to fight fires. This research effort can be attributed to the amount of litigation leveled at the validity of firefighter preemployment tests and the use of age to terminate employment. Several investigators [11, 38, 96, 99, 112, 127] published data showing that fire-suppression work tasks have a substantial aerobic component. In an important study, Sothmann and a team of researchers [128] provide strong evidence that the minimum VO_2max required to meet the demands of firefighting is 33.5 ml/kg/min. The authors used a work-sample test involving seven job-related firefighter tasks. The sensitivity (percentage of correctly classified unsuccessful performers) and specificity (percentage of correctly classified successful performers) for a VO_2max cut score of 33.5 ml/kg/min were 67% and 83%, respectively. Lowering the cut score to 30.5 ml/kg/min, dropped the sensitivity to 25% and increased the specificity to 95%.

While the 33.5 ml/kg/min value reflects an important benchmark in defining a firefighter cut score for aerobic capacity, it likely will not be the only source of data considered. Research [22] clearly shows that VO_2max declines with age, and that this decline depends somewhat on lifestyle [74]. Selecting young applicants who just meet this minimum standard would likely result in hiring employees who would find that firefighting exceeded their physiological limits as they age. Given these conditions, recommended entry-level VO_2max cut scores in the low 40s are more likely [38, 97, 112, 128].

A problem with using published energy cost data for defining cut scores is that the values typically represent average values for the general population, and many aerobic work tasks allow employees to pace themselves. This was shown in a study examining endurance work tasks required of coal miners [77]. The two work tasks involved shoveling a material with the density of coal over a 3.5-foot wall and transporting 50-pound bags. The subjects were instructed to work at a rate that was comfortable for their level of fitness. The average exercise heart rate of the males and females did not differ, but the work rate of the males was significantly higher than that of the females. The female subjects simply worked at a lower power output. Unless a minimum work productivity power output can be defined and supported by the job analysis, making a cut score based on energy cost estimates may be difficult to defend.

CUT SCORE BASED ON STRENGTH. Many materials-handling and industrial work tasks depend on the worker's strength. The work of Chaffin and his associates [28–31, 33, 58, 89] showed the importance of matching the strength of workers with the job demands. They used isometric strength tests to determine whether a worker physically met the work demands. Although the primary focus of their research was to examine the role of strength on the incidence of musculoskeletal injury, the approach provides a sound method for establishing a cut score. If a 75-pound load must be lifted and transported, a worker must have sufficient strength to complete the task.

Several studies [71–73, 76–82] focused on defining the level of strength required by different industrial tasks. The approach relates work-sample performance to isometric strength level defined by the sum of several strength tests. The results of these studies show that strength is highly correlated with many industrial work-sample tasks, and regression equations provide empirical models to define the level of strength needed to meet the work-task demands. This can be illustrated with data from a recently completed validation study involving materials handling and push-pull tasks [81].

The job analysis [81] showed that one physically demanding job was pushing or pulling containers loaded with freight. As part of the job analysis, an electronic load cell defined the peak force required to move freight containers that varied in weight. The subject's peak push force was measured with an isometric push test that stimulated the position used to push containers. Figure 3.1 presents the linear relationship between the simulated push test and the sum of arm, shoulder, torso, and leg lift

FIGURE 3.1

A scatterplot with male and female regression lines defining the relationship between isometric strength and push force. The slopes and intercepts of the male and female regression slopes and intercepts do not differ significantly. The general equation that defined push force (PF) from the sum of arm, shoulder, torso, and leg lift strength (ΣIS) was: PF = 0.198(ΣIS) + 2.031, R = 0.78.

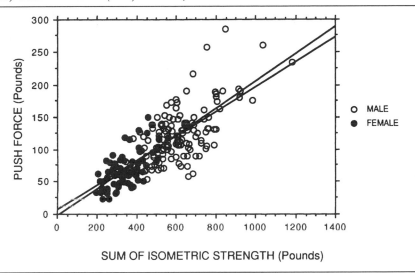

isometric tests. Since the weight distributions of the containers and the relation between push force and container weight were known, regression equations provided models for defining the level of strength needed to generate the push forces needed to move containers that varied in weight. The decision model used these data to define an isometric-strength cut score.

Other physically demanding tasks identified by the task analysis were lifting boxes from the floor and placing them on shelves 30 and 69 inches high [81]. The work-sample tests required the subjects to lift boxes from the floor and place them at these two heights. The task analysis defined the lift heights and the distribution of box weights handled by workers. To ensure safety, the simulated test started with a light (25-pound) box and progressively worked up to the 75-pound box. The test was scored by pass or fail. Data analysis showed that the sum of arm, shoulder, torso, and leg lift tests were significantly related to the capacity to complete the lifts. As expected, stronger individuals were more likely to complete the lift. Logistic regression analysis provides a method of quantifying the relationship between dichotomous and continuously scaled variables [120]. Figure 3.2 presents the logistic models that defined the probability of completing the lift for levels of strength. These data helped establish the strength cut score.

FIGURE 3.2

Logistic probability curves for defining the ability to lift a 75-pound box to heights of 30 and 69 inches. The logistic equations are 30-inch lift, LS = 0.0244(ΣIS) − 6.7996; and 69-inch lift, LS = 0.0284(ΣIS) − 13.3171. The equation to estimate the probability of completing the lift is: p = [e^{LS}/(1 + e^{LS})] × 100, where e is the base of the natural logarithm function (≈ 2.718), and LS is the logistic value estimated from ΣIS. The logistic probability curves documented the expected, the lift to the 69-inch height required more strength than the 30-inch lift.

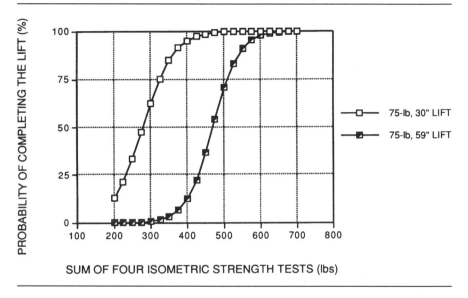

CUT SCORES BASED ON "SAFE" WORK LEVELS. The previously discussed biomechanical models [8, 27, 54, 86, 100, 101, 110, 114, 132] and psychophysical methods [8, 106, 107, 121, 124–126] for redesigning materials-handling tasks offer data for setting cut scores. This research focused on defining "safe" work loads for the industrial population and provide another source of data for defining cut scores for physically demanding materials-handling tasks.

PUBLISHED VALIDATION STUDIES

Although many preemployment tests have been completed, most are not in the published literature. The completed validation study often is a technical report to the governmental agency or private company that funded the project, and many organizations consider these privileged. Hogan [64] provides an extensive list of these unpublished reports. Summarized next are validation studies that are in the literature.

Outside Craft Jobs

One of the first published concurrent validation studies was for outdoor telephone craft jobs that involved pole-climbing tasks [16, 118]. The issues leading to the development of this study were the large differences between male and female workers in turnover and accident rates. After 6 months, 43% of the women left the outdoor craft jobs, compared with only 8% of the males. More important, women sustained substantially more injuries than men from falls while climbing or working on poles.

An extensive job analysis showed that pole climbing was an essential, physically demanding work task. Bernauer and Bonanno [16] evaluated the factor composition of 40 tests and anthropometric measures on a sample of 241 job applicants. They developed a six-item battery consisting of reaction time, grip strength, percentage body fat, step test performance, balance, and sit-ups. They found that the balance and step tests significantly differentiated the successful and unsuccessful students enrolled in pole-climbing school.

Reilly and associates [118] extended this work by completing two concurrent validation studies. In the first experiment, several anthropometric and physical performance tests were administered to 83 male and 45 female candidates for outdoor telephone craft jobs. There were two validation criteria used in this experiment. The first, general task performance, was the average of two supervisor performance ratings of the candidate's performance during the 5-day pole-climbing school. Job analysis data were used to construct the rating scale. The second criterion was a dichotomy of those who were on the job 6 months after placement and those who were not. Using the criterion of general task performance, stepwise multiple regression isolated a three-predictor battery consisting of dynamic arm-strength (i.e., the number of revolutions completed in one minute of arm ergometer cranking with a 3-kilogram resistance), reaction time, and Harvard bench step time. The analysis yielded a multiple correlation of 0.45. The statistically significant zero-order correlations between the job tenure criterion and these tests were dynamic arm strength, 0.36; reaction time, 0.19; and bench step time, 0.18. Further analysis showed that a common regression line defined male and female performance, meeting the important criteria of job fairness.

The second experiment used a larger sample of employees, who represented the whole company. The criterion of pole-climbing training success was changed to be consistent with changes introduced in the pole-climbing course. The second study included four different criteria of job performance: (*a*) time to complete the pole-climbing school; (*b*) completion of pole-climbing school (a number withdrew from the course); (*c*) field observations of pole-climbing proficiency; and (*d*) accidents for 6 months after entering outdoor craft work. The second sample consisted of 78 female and 132 male pole-climbing school applicants.

Using the criterion time to complete the course, multiple regression selected a three-item battery: body density estimated from skinfold fat; balance; and an isometric arm-strength test. The significant correlations between the three tests and the four criteria were, time to complete the course, 0.46; training dropout, 0.38; field observations for the female sample, 0.53; and accidents, 0.15. Further analysis showed that the same regression equation was equally valid for both males and females.

Firefighters
Nearly all major fire departments have a physical ability preemployment test [92]. Considine and associates [35] published a physical test battery for screening firefighter applicants. The test battery evolved from an occupational task analysis that surveyed, rated, and analyzed 81 tasks performed by firefighters. The authors selected a construct validation strategy. The constructs identified through the task analysis were dynamic strength, static strength, agility, total body coordination, cardiorespiratory endurance, muscular endurance, eye-hand coordination, and total body speed.

The sample of the first study consisted of 191 males who were tested on body composition measures, general physical performance tests, and eight job-sample tests. A factor analysis of these data produced three general factors. The factor names and tests representing each factor were, factor 1, the ability to handle the body weight, measured by percentage body fat, obstacle run, and flexed-arm hang; factor 2, muscle power, measured by the hose lift, man-lift-and-carry, and stair-climb work-sample tests; and factor 3, body structure, measured by fat-free weight and height.

A major purpose of the second study was to analyze the test battery for racial bias. Based on the results of the first study, nine tests were administered to 165 firefighters and 19 candidates. Data analysis showed that black and white subjects did not differ on any of the tests. These data were factor analyzed, producing three common factors. The final recommended battery consisted of four work-sample tests, and one fitness test, the flexed-arm hang. The work-sample tests were modified man-lift-and-carry, which simulated rescuing a trapped victim; stair climb, which simulated climbing the stairs in a building; obstacle run, which simulated moving the body through confined spaces; and hose couple, which involved coupling three hoses to a hose couple.

Davis and associates [39] examined the relationship between simulated firefighting tasks and physical performance measures. The sample consisted of 100 randomly selected men from the population of Washington, D.C., firefighters. The physical performance measures included body composition, general fitness, aerobic fitness, and cardiovascular variables. The five work-sample tests came from the job analysis of firefighter work tasks and involved handling a ladder; lifting and transporting a 33.1-kg load up five flights of stairs; pulling a 23.5-kg hose roll from the ground up to and through the fifth-floor window; carrying and dragging a 53-kg dummy down five flights of stairs; and using a sledge hammer to simulate forceful entry.

Canonical correlation showed that two independent dimensions defined the relationship between the physical performance variables and firefighter work-sample tests. The first canonical dimension (Rc = 0.79) represented a physical work capacity factor that reflected the muscular strength and endurance, and maximal aerobic capacity elements of the simulated work-sample tests. The second dimension (Rc = 0.63) represented a resistance to fatigue factor and the ability to complete the work tasks quickly. Multiple regression selected two physical performance batteries (laboratory and field batteries) to estimate each work-sample dimension. The field-test battery for the physical work capacity factor consisted of push-ups, sit-ups, and grip strength. The validity of the field battery (R = 0.73) was lower than that of the five-item laboratory battery (R = 0.95), which added submaximal oxygen pulse and maximum heart rate to the battery. The three-item field test of the second factor included estimated percentage body fat, lean body weight, and VO_2max estimated with a step test (R – 0.77). The laboratory test added maximum heart rate and treadmill performance and increased the validity (R = 0.89) of the resistance-to-fatigue work-sample factor.

The physiological response of firefighting has been the focus of many investigators. Exercise heart rate responses elicited by simulated and actual firefighting tasks confirmed that these tasks have a significant cardiovascular effect [11, 38, 96, 99, 112, 127]. In a study during actual fire-suppression emergencies, Sothmann and associates [127] measured exercise heart rate and oxygen uptake of 10 male firefighters. Their data showed that firefighters worked at an average of 88% (± 6%) of their measured maximum heart rate for an average duration of 15 (±7) minutes. The average energy cost of the firefighter emergency work task was a VO_2 of 25.6 ± 8.7 ml $\cdot$ kg^{-1} $\cdot$ min^{-1}, representing an intensity of 63 % (± 14%) of VO_2max.

Sothmann and associates [128] examined the relationship between VO_2max and firefighting work tasks. A seven-item content-valid fire-suppression test was administered to 20 experienced firefighters. The average energy cost of the firefighter simulation tests was 30.5 (± 5.6) ml $\cdot$ kg^{-1} $\cdot$ min^{-1}. The work simulation required the firefighters to work at an intensity of 76% (± 8) of VO_2max. The correlation between the elapsed time required to complete the firefighter work-simulation test and measured VO_2max was −0.55. In a cross-validation study with 32 different male firefighters, successful work-simulation performance was a function of VO_2max. Of the 32 tested, seven firefighters could not complete the work-sample tests. The VO_2max of five of the seven was below 32.5 ml $\cdot$ kg^{-1} $\cdot$ min^{-1}.

Highway Patrol Officers

With an increasing number of women seeking employment as highway patrol officers, the objective of the study published by Wilmore and Davis [134] was to find the minimum physical qualifications and develop a job-related preemployment test. They administered three different batteries of tests to 140 male and 16 female patrol officers. The laboratory and field-test batteries included strength, flexibility, body composition, and cardiorespiratory endurance items. The job-sample tests included a barrier surmount and arrest simulation, and a dummy drag that simulated dragging an injured victim 50 feet to safety.

The major difference between the field and laboratory batteries was that the 1.5-mile run replaced the maximum treadmill test and body fat was estimated from skinfolds rather than measured by hydrostatic weighing. The laboratory test battery was significantly correlated with the dummy drag (R= 0.66) and barrier surmount and arrest simulation tests (R= 0.68). Replacing the laboratory tests with the field tests resulted in slightly lower correlations, 0.57 and 0.62 for the dummy drag, and barrier surmount and arrest simulation tests, respectively. Although the fitness tests estimated work-simulation test performance, test performance was not related to job performance, consisting of supervisor ratings on 16 critical job tasks.

The data analysis showed that the officers were like the normal population in strength, body fat, flexibility, and cardiorespiratory endurance. Importantly the study showed that the predominantly sedentary officer's job leads to a rapid deterioration in physical fitness following their academic training, suggesting the need for an in-service physical conditioning program.

Steel Workers

Arnold et al. [2] developed a preemployment test for selecting entry-level steel workers. The task analysis documented that entry-level steel workers must do several different physically demanding tasks. The investigators used a combination of content and construct validation strategies. The job analysis identified the physically demanding work tasks required of the entry-level workers and categorized them by Fleishman's constructs of static strength, dynamic strength, and endurance [49]. The selected physical performance test candidates were those that theoretically measured these constructs.

The objective of the study was to determine whether the physical performance tests were related to the work-sample tests developed from the job analysis. The sample included 168 men and 81 women who were in their first 6 months of employment at three different plant locations. The job analysis showed that work tasks differed somewhat across the three sites, resulting in 11 work-sample tests at one site and 12 at the other two. The average work-sample test performance was the criterion of work performance. Besides the work-sample tests, each subject completed 10 physical performance tests sampling strength, flexibility, agility, balance, and cardiorespiratory endurance.

Multiple regression selected the physical performance tests most highly correlated with the work sample criterion. For all three work sites, arm dynamometer strength was the most important predictor of work-sample test performance. The zero-order correlations between arm strength and work-sample test performance was consistently high—0.82, 0.85, and 0.85 for the three sites. Adding two more tests to the multiple regression models added little to the validity, the multiple correlations for the three predictor models increased to 0.87, 0.88, and 0.89.

The authors completed a utility analysis for the single arm-strength test [68], estimating the amount of money the company would save by hiring workers who could do the work. Utility estimates are based on test validity and the monetary value related to the variability of work performance. Using 1982 wage standards, Arnold et al. estimated that using the single arm-strength test to select employees would save about $5000 per year for each employee selected. Based on the number of employees hired, the estimated company savings exceeded $9 million/year.

Underground Coal Mining
A job analysis showed that the work of underground coal miners was physically demanding and could be represented with four work-sample tests [76–78]. The first work-sample simulation test, roof bolting, measured maximum isokinetic torque and simulated straightening a steel roof bolt. The block-carry test involved lifting, transporting, and placing 82-pound concrete blocks in positions commonly used to built retaining walls in the mine. The shoveling simulation test involved shoveling polyvinyl chloride from the floor over a 3.5-foot wall. Polyvinyl chloride has the density of coal, and the task was to shovel 800 pounds at a rate consistent with fitness. The bag-carry simulation test measured the number of 50-pound bags that were lifted and transported 9 feet during a five-minute period.

The four work-sample tests and three isometric strength tests, grip, arm lift, and torso lift [109], were administered to 25 male and 25 female subjects. The validation strategy was similar to that followed by Arnold et al. with steelworkers [2]. The correlations between the sum of the isometric strength tests and four work-sample tests ranged from 0.68 for the bag-carry test to 0.91 for the roof-bolting test. Multiple regression analysis showed that neither gender nor the gender by isometric strength interaction accounted for additional significant variance. This showed that a common male and female regression line defined the relationship between strength and work-sample test performance.

Both exercise heart rate and rating of perceived exertion data showed that the shoveling and bag-carry tests had a significant aerobic component [77]. Besides the isometric strength tests, the subject's maximal arm-cranking oxygen uptake was metabolically determined. The zero-order

FIGURE 3.3

Nonlinear regression lines estimating endurance coal mining work task performance from the sum of isometric grip, arm lift, and torso lift strength [77]. The polynominal regression equations estimating that defined the relationship between shoveling and bag carry power output are

$$\text{Shoveling rate } (lb \cdot min^{-1}) = 0.8078(\Sigma IS) - 0.0007(\Sigma IS)^2 - 43.4463$$
$$\text{Bag transport } (lb \cdot min^{-1}) = 3.0055(\Sigma IS) - 0.0026(\Sigma IS)^2 - 126.1211$$

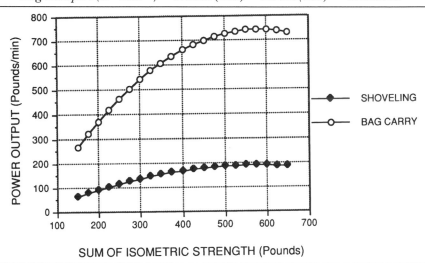

correlations between the sum of isometric strength and the work-sample shoveling and bag-carry tests were higher than the correlations found with arm VO_2max (ml/min). The strength correlations were 0.71 for shoveling and 0.63 for the bag-carry test, compared with 0.68 and 0.46 for arm VO_2max (ml/min). Multiple regression analysis showed that arm VO_2max accounted for an additional 9% of shoveling variance beyond that of isometric strength, but it did not account for additional bag-carry variance. Polynomial regression analysis showed that the relationship between these two endurance work-sample tests and isometric strength was quadratic, not linear. Figure 3.3 shows the quadratic regression lines. Strength was more important for differentiating work-sample performance at the lowest levels.

Chemical Plant Workers

Job analyses documented that the physically demanding tasks required of chemical and refining plants workers included cracking, opening, and closing valves [79, 113]. Osburn [113] developed a valve-turning work-simulation test administered on a specially developed ergometer consisting of a disc brake mechanism turned by a 12-inch value handwheel. The unit was calibrated to a power output of 1413.5 foot-pounds/minute. The objective of the work-sample test was to complete 250 revolutions in 15 minutes. The job analysis showed this level of work would open or close 75% of the emergency valves in 15 minutes.

The distribution of the valve-turning test was bimodal. Physically fit workers easily completed the 15-minute test, but it was too demanding for many, who stopped before reaching 50 revolutions [80]. The test elicited maximal cardiovascular responses in many applicants [113]. This led to a second study, designed to determine whether isometric strength tests validly predicted valve-turning performance [73, 80]. The valve-turning work-sample test and three isometric strength tests—grip, arm lift, and torso lift—were administered to 26 men and 25 women. The zero-order correlation between the tests was 0.82. Because of the bimodal valve-turning distribution, a logistic regression model [120] defined the probability of completing the test by levels of isometric strength. The logistic equations and probability curves are published [80].

In a second study, a task analysis questionnaire completed by operators at a major chemical plant identified valve cracking as the most physically demanding work task [79]. An electronic load cell measured the peak cracking torque on 217 randomly selected valves in the plant. The sampled valves included those with horizontal and vertical orientations, positioned close to the ground and overhead, those in awkward or hard-to-reach positions, and valves of various sizes. The results of this biomechanical job analysis showed that 100 pounds of force applied to the end of a 36-inch valve wrench generated sufficient torque to crack 93% of the plant valves.

A valve-cracking, work sample test simulated cracking valves in eight different ways. The eight cracking torques were obtained by varying the action (push and pull), direction (horizontal and vertical), and height (high and low). A computerized torque wrench measured the torque applied to four nuts placed in vertical and horizontal positions at two heights.

The valve-cracking test and isometric strength tests (grip, arm lift, and torso lift) were administered to 118 men and 66 women. The intercorrelations among the eight measures of valve-cracking torque were high, ranging from 0.66 to 0.89. Because of the high intercorrelations, the eight valve-cracking scores were averaged and used as the work-sample measure. The correlation between the sum of the three isometric strength tests and average valve-cracking torque was 0.65. A logistic regression equation [120] defined a probability model for estimating the chances of generating the 100-pound criterion for levels of isometric strength. These data are published elsewhere [80].

Electrical Transmission Lineworkers
Doolittle et al. [43] developed a preemployment test for selecting electrical transmission lineworkers. The study included an extensive job analysis of electrical transmission lineworker jobs. The initial stage of the task analysis surveyed workers using scales designed to answer three questions: (*a*) How often was the task performed? (*b*) How much time was spent completing

each task? (*c*) How physically demanding was the task for the individual? The identified critical, physically demanding tasks were studied in detail to define the forces needed to perform them safely and efficiently. This involved defining standard anatomical movements for lifting, pushing, and hoisting; measuring the masses lifted and forces exerted; and estimating the metabolic costs of various work tasks.

Using the task-analysis data, five strength tests that duplicated the muscular action were selected and administered to 48 incumbents. The tests required the subject to move a weight that represented loads linemen moved. The weights ranged from 7 to 61 kilograms. The final two tests selected were chins and VO$_2$max estimated from bench stepping and exercise heart rate. The seven tests were combined into a single performance measure. Criterion-related validity was examined by comparing physical test performance with two criteria, supervisor ratings and accident rates. The crew chiefs confidentially evaluated each incumbent on the following six dimensions of job performance: (*a*) productivity; (*b*) working with others; (*c*) supervision; (*d*) safety; (*e*) physical ability; and (*f*) technical skills. The correlation between the composite physical test criteria of supervisor ratings and lost work days due to on-the-job injuries averaged over five years were 0.59 and 0.46, respectively.

Diver Training
There have been two validation studies [56, 62] designed to estimate successful completion of military underwater diver training programs. Gunderson and associates [56] used successful completion of underwater demolition training as the criterion of performance. They found a multiple correlation of 0.54 between success defined by the completion of training and five variables: squat-jumps, pull-ups, sit-ups, body weight, and the Cornell Medical Index. Using these tests, they predicted about 70% of those who passed training.

Hogan [62] used 46 male, Naval personnel who volunteered for diver training. The criteria of success included nine performance rating scales that reflected physical condition, swimming training, leadership potential, teamwork, and overall performance. A second criterion was successful completion of training. The predictor measures included three anthropometric measurements and 23 fitness tests. She reported a multiple correlation of 0.63 between the average performance rating and three physical tests, 1-mile run, sit and reach, and muscular endurance measured with an arm ergometer. The multiple correlation between these three tests and successful completion of the course was 0.64. Hogan suggested that the validity coefficients were likely an overestimate because of an unfavorable ratio of the number variables and subjects [90].

Demanding Military Jobs
The United States military services examined methods of matching enlisted personnel with physically demanding jobs. The Air Force adopted a

preinduction dynamic one-repetition maximum (1-RM) strength test [9]. The Army and Navy examined the relationship between body composition variables and physically demanding work tasks [102].

The United States Air Force developed a Strength Aptitude Test (SAT) to match the general strength abilities of individuals with the specific strength requirements of Air Force jobs filled by enlisted personnel [9]. The Air Force SAT measures the subject's voluntary 1-RM lift to a height of 6 feet. The SAT starts with a 40-pound lift. The lift load is increased by 10 pound increments until the subject reaches maximum voluntary lift or a maximum weight of 200 pounds. The SAT is administered to Air Force recruits as part of their preinduction physical examination. Each enlisted Air Force career field has a prerequisite SAT cut score.

An area of concern expressed by the Committee on Military Nutrition Research of the Institute of Medicine, National Academy of Sciences is the role that body composition plays on physical performance. This relationship is important not only for making decisions of acceptance or rejection of recruits for the military service, but also for retention and advancement of those in the service [102]. Hodgdon et al. [59] examined the relationship between body composition, fitness, and materials-handling tasks required of naval enlisted men. The two materials-handling tasks were (a) the maximum box weight that could be lifted to elbow height and (b) the total distance a 34-kg box could be carried during two 5 min work bouts. The variables most highly correlated with maximum box lift were push-ups (r = 0.63) and fat-free mass (r = 0.80). The variables most highly correlated with the box-carry test were push-ups (r = 0.56), 1.5-mile run time (r = −0.67), and fat-free mass (r = 0.44). Fat-free mass was highly correlated with muscular strength measures, suggesting the possibility of using fat-free mass as an approximation of general strength in job assignment.

Vogel and Friedl [130] examined the relationship between body composition and absolute lifting capacity. They reported significant correlations between maximum lifting capacity and fat-free mass for male and female soldiers. Although they did not test for homogeneity of male and female regression lines, they published separate equations for men and women. The male and female equations for estimating maximum lifting capacity in pounds (MLC) from kilograms of fat-free mass (FFM) are

Males: MLC = 2.107(FFM) + 0.502 (r = 0.62, SEE = 20.55 pounds)

Females: MLC = 0.945(FFM) + 23.158 (r = 0.38, SEE = 11.75 pounds)

A limitation of military testing programs is that they lack job-related materials-handling performance tests. While recognizing the need to develop content valid tests, the Committee on Military Nutrition Research concluded that there is a direct relationship between military materials-handling tasks and fat-free mass. In view of this relationship and the lack of job-related tests, the military should seriously consider establishing a minimum standard for fat-free mass [102]. Such a recommendation might be implemented for the military, but using body composition variables in preemployment tests in the private sector would likely meet an immediate legal challenge.

SUMMARY

There is a growing trend toward using preemployment tests to select employees for physically demanding jobs. Women are, in increasing numbers, entering physically demanding occupations that were traditionally dominated by men. Under current Federal employment law, it is illegal to disqualify an employee for a job because of race, color, religion, sex, national origin, and with the recent passage of the American Disabilities Act (ADA), handicap. Because of gender differences in strength, body composition, and VO_2max, preemployment tests for physically demanding jobs tend to screen out more females than males. Employers are using preemployment tests not only to enhance worker productivity, but also to minimize the threat of litigation for discriminatory hiring practices and to reduce the risk of musculoskeletal injuries. The primary ergonomic methods used in industry to reduce the risk of back injuries are preemployment testing and job redesign. When a test results in adverse impact, the validity of the test must be established. Validity in this context means that the test represents or predicts the applicant's capacity to perform the job. Criterion-related, content, and construct validation studies are the means used to establish validity. The validity of preemployment hiring practices for physically demanding jobs has been decided in the courts. The most common reason for ruling an employment practice invalid is the failure to show that the test measured important job behaviors. Much of this litigation has involved height and weight requirements for public safety jobs. The courts have generally ruled that using height and weight standards as a criteria for employment is illegal because they were not job related. If fitness tests comprise part or all of the preemployment test, it is essential to demonstrate that the fitness component is related to job performance. Although there are many factors to consider when establishing a cut score, there is a growing trend toward establishing the cut score on the basis of the job's physical demands, defined by VO_2max and strength. This literature is limited because most validation studies are not published. They more typically take the form of a technical report to the governmental agency or company that funded the project. There are published preemployment validation studies for outdoor telephone craft jobs involving pole-climbing tasks; firefighters;

highway patrol officers; steel workers; underground coal miners; chemical plant workers; electrical transmission lineworkers; and various military jobs.

REFERENCES

1. A.P.A, *Standards for Educational and Psychological Testing.* Washington, D.C.: American Psychological Association, 1985.
2. Arnold, J. D., J. M. Rauschenberger, W. G. Soubel, and R. M. Guion. Validation and utility of a strength test for selecting steelworkers. *J. Appl. Psychol.* 67:588–604, 1982.
3. Arvey, R. D., and R. H. Faley, *Fairness in Selecting Employees,* 2nd ed. Reading, MA: Addison-Wesley, 1988.
4. Arvey, R. D., S. M. Nutting, and T. E. Landon. Validation strategies for physical ability testing in police and fire settings. *Pub. Pers. Mgt.* 21:301–312, 1992.
5. Åstrand, P.-O., and K. Rodahl. *Textbook of Work Physiology.* 3rd ed. New York: McGraw-Hill, 1986.
6. Ayoub, M. A. Control of manual lifting hazards: II. job redesign. *J.O.M.* 24:688–676, 1982.
7. Ayoub, M. A. Control of manual lifting hazards: III. pre-employment screening. *J.O.M.* 24:751–761, 1982.
8. Ayoub, M. M. Determining permissible lifting loads: an approach. *Proceedings of the Human Factors Society 35th Annual Meeting* 35:825–829, 1991.
9. Ayoub, M. M., J. D. Denardo, J. L. Smith, N. J. Bethea, B. K. Lambert, et al. *Establishing Physical Criteria for Assigning Personnel to Air Force Jobs (Contract No. F19620-79-C0006.,* Lubbock, TX: Texas Tech University, 1982.
10. Ayoub, M. M., A. Mital, G. M. Bakken, S. S. Asfour, and N. Bethea. Development of strength and capacity norms for manual materials handling activities: the state of the art. *Hum. Factors* 22:271–283, 1980.
11. Barnard, R. and H. W. Duncan. Heart rate and ECG responses of firefighters. *J.O.M.* 17:247–250, 1975.
12. Battie, M., S. Bigos, L. Fisher, T. Hansson, A. Nachemson, et al. A prospective study of the role of cardiovascular risk factors and fitness in industrial back pain complaints. *Spine* 14:141–147, 1989.
13. Battie, M., S. Bigos, L. Fissher, T. Hansson, M. Jones, and M. Wortley. Isometric lifting strength as a predictor of industrial back pain reports. *Spine* 14:851–856, 1989.
14. Baumgartner, T. A., and A. S. Jackson, *Measurement for evaluation in Physical Education and Exercise Science.* 4th ed Dubuque, IA: Wm. C. Brown, 1991.
15. Baumgartner, T. A., and M. A. Zuidema. Factor analysis of physical fitness tests. *Res. O.* 43:443–450, 1972.
16. Bernauer, E. M., and J. Bonanno. Development of physical profiles for specific jobs. *J.O.M.* 17:22–33, 1975.
17. Bigos, S., D. Spengler, N. Martin, J. Zeh, L. Fisher, and A. Nachemson. Back injuries in industry: a retrospective study. III *Spine* 3:252–256, 1986.
18. Borg, G. *Physical Work and Effort. Proceedings of the First International Symposium, Wenner-Gren Center, Stockholm, Sweden.* Oxford, England: Pergamon, 1977.
19. Borg, G., and D. Ottoson, *The Perception of Exertion and Physical Work.* Stockholm: The Wenner-Gren Center, 1986.
20. Brown, J. R., *Manual Lifting and Related Fields: An Annotated Bibliography.* Toronto: Ontario Ministry of Labour, 1972.
21. Brozek, J. and A. Keys. The evaluation of leanness-fatness in man: norms and intercorrelations. *Br. J. Nutr.* 5:194–206, 1951.
22. Buskirk, E. R. and J. L. Hodgson. Age and aerobic power: the rate of change in men and women. *Fed. Proc.* 46:1824–1829, 1987.
23. Cady, L. D., D. P. Bishoff, E. R. O'Connell, P. C. Thomas, and J. H. Allan. Back injuries in firefighters. *J.O.M.* 21:269–272, 1979.

24. Cady, L. J., P. Thomas, and R. Karwasky. Program for increasing health and physical fitness of firefighters. *J.O.M.* 27:110–114, 1985.
25. Campion, M. A. Personnel selection for physically demanding jobs: Review and recommendations. *Pers. Psych.* 36:527–550, 1983.
26. Cascio, W. F., R. A. Alexander, and G. V. Barrett. Setting cutoff scores: Legal, psychometric, and professional issues and guidelines. *Pers. Psych.* 41:1–24, 1988.
27. Chaffin, D. B. Biomechanical Strength Models in Industry. D. B. Chaffin (Ed). Chap. 3. *Ergonomic Interventions to Prevent Musculoskeletal Injuries in Industry.* Chelsea, MI. Lewis Publishers, 1987, pp. 27–45.
28. Chaffin, D. B. Ergonomics guide for the assessment of human static strength. *Am. Ind. Hyg. Assoc. J.* 36:505–511, 1975.
29. Chaffin, D. B. Human strength capability and low-back pain. *J.O.M.* 16:248–254, 1974.
30. Chaffin, D. B., R. O. Andres, and A. Garg. Volitional postures during maximal push/pull exertions in the sagittal plane. *Hum. Factors* 25:541–550, 1983.
31. Chaffin, D. B., G. D. Herrin, and W. M. Keyserling. Pre-employment strength testing. *J.O.M.* 67:403–408, 1978.
32. Chaffin, D. B., and K. S. Park. A longitudinal study of low-back pain as associated with occupational weight lifting factors. *Am. Ind. Hyg. Assoc. J.* 34:513–525, 1973.
33. Chaffin, D. B., and K. S. Park. A longitudinal study of low-back pain as associated with occupational weight lifting factors. *Am. Ind. Hyg. Assoc. J.* 34:513–525, 1973.
34. Ciriello, V. M., and S. H. Snook. A study of size, distance, height, and frequency effects on manual handling tasks. *Hum. Factors* 25:1983.
35. Considine, W., J. E. Misner, R. A. Boileau, C. Pounian, J. Cole, and A. Abbatieilo. Developing a physical performance test battery for screening Chicago firefighting applicants. *Pub. Pers. Mgt.* 5:7–14, 1976.
36. Cousins, G. F. A factor analysis of selected wartime fitness tests. *Res. Q.* 26:277–288, 1955.
37. Cumbee, F. A factorial analysis of motor coordination. *Res. Q.* 25:412–420, 1954.
38. Davis, P. and C. Dotson. Heart rate responses to firefighting activities. *Ambulatory Electrocariol.* 1:15–18, 1978.
39. Davis, P. O., C. O. Dotson, and D. L. SantaMaria. Relationship between simulated firefighting and physical performance measures. *Med. Sci. Sports Exerc.* 14:65–71, 1982.
40. Dehlin, O., B. Hendenrud, and J. Horal. Back symptoms in nursing aids in a geriatric hospital. *Scand. J. Rehabil. Med.* 8:47–53, 1976.
41. Dishman, R. K. (ed) *Exercise Adherence: Its Impact on Public Health.* Champaign, IL: Human Kinetics, 1988.
42. Division of Industrial-Organizational Psychology and A. P. Association. *Principles for the Validation and Use of Personnel Selection Procedures.* Washington, D.C.: Division of Industrial-Organizational Psychology, American Psychological Association, 1987.
43. Doolittle, T. L., O. Spurlin, K. Kaiyala, and D. Sovern. Physical demands of lineworkers. *Proceedings of the Human Factors Society, 32nd Annual Meeting* 32:632–636, 1988.
44. Dunnette, M. D., and L. M. Hough (eds). *Handbook of Industrial and Organizational Psychology,* 2nd ed. Vol. 2. Palo Alto: Consulting Psychologists Press, 1991.
45. Durnin, J. V., and R. Passmore. *Energy, Work and Leisure.* London: Heineman, 1967.
46. Durnin, J. V. G. A. and J. Wormsley. Body fat assessed from total body density and its estimation from skinfold thickness: measurements on 481 men and women aged from 16 to 72 years. *Br. J. Nutr.* 32:77–92, 1974.
47. Equal Employment Opportunity Commission. Equal employment opportunity for individuals with disabilities: Final Rule. *Federal Register* 56(144):29 CRF Parts 1602 and 1627, 1991.
48. Equal Employment Opportunity Commission, Civil Service Commission, Department of Labor, and Department of Justice. Uniform Guidelines on employment selection procedures. *Federal Register* 43:1978.
49. Fleishman, E. A., *The Structure and Measurement of Physical Fitness.* Englewood Cliffs, NJ: Prentice-Hall. 1964.

50. Fleishman, E. A., D. L. Gebhardt, and J. C. Hogan. The measurement of effort. *Ergonomics* 27:947–954, 1984.
51. Fleishman, E. A. and M. D. Mumford. Ability requirement scales. S. Gael (ed.) *The Job Analysis Handbook for Business, Industry, and Government.* New York: John Wiley & Sons, 1988, pp. 917–935.
52. Foster, C., A. S. Jackson, M. L. Pollock, et al. Generalized equations for predicting functional capacity from treadmill performance. *Am. Heart J.* 107:1229–1234, 1984.
53. Gael, S. *The Job Analysis Handbook for Business, Industry, and Government,* Vol. I. New York: John Wiley & Sons, 1988.
54. Garg, A., D. B. Chaffin, and G. B. Herrin. Prediction of metabolic rates for manual materials handling jobs. *Am. Ind. Hyg. Assoc. J.* 39:661–674, 1978.
55. Golding, L. A., C. R. Meyers, and W. E. Sinning. *The Y's Way to Physical Fitness,* 3rd ed. Chicago: National Board of YMCA, 1989.
56. Gunderson, E. K. E., R. H. Rahe, and R. J. Arthur. Prediction of performance in stressful underwater demolition training. *J. Appl. Psychol* 56:1972.
57. Harris, M. A factor analytic study of flexibility. *Res. Q.* 40:62–70, 1969.
58. Herrin, G. D., D. B. Chaffin, and R. S. Mach, *Criteria for Research on the Hazards of Manual Materials Handling.* Washington, D.C.: U.S. Government Printing Office: NIOSH, 1974.
59. Hodgdon, J. A. Body composition in the military services: standards and methods. B. M. Marriott and J. Grumstrup-Scott (eds). *Body Composition and Physical Performance: Applications for the Military Services,* Washington, D.C.: National Academy Press, 1992, pp. 57–70.
60. Hoffman, T., R. Stouffer, and A. S. Jackson. Sex differences in strength. *Am. J. Sports Med.* 7:265–267, 1979.
61. Hogan, J. Structure of physical performance in occupational tasks. *J. Appl. Psychol.* 76:495–507, 1991.
62. Hogan, J. Tests for success in diver training. *J. Appl. Psychol.* 70:219–224, 1985.
63. Hogan, J. and A. M. Quigley. Physical standard for employment and courts. *Am. Psychol.* 41:1193–1217, 1986.
64. Hogan, J. C. Physical Abilities. In: Dunnette, M.D., and L. M. Hough (eds). *Handbook of Industrial and Organizational Psychology,* 2nd ed. Vol. 2. Chap. 11. Palo Alto: Consulting Psychologists Press, 1991, pp. 743–831.
65. Hogan, J. C. and E. A. Fleishman. An index of the physical effort required in human task performance. *J. Appl. Psychol.* 64:197–204, 1979.
66. Hogan, J. C., G. D. Ogden, D. L. Gebhardt, and E. A. Fleishman. Reliability and validity of methods for evaluating perceived physical effort. *J. Appl. Psychol.* 65:672–679, 1980.
67. Hultman, G., M. Nordin, H. Saraste, and H. Ohlsen. Body composition, endurances, strength, cross-sectional area, and density of MM erector spinae in men with and without low back pain. *J. Spinal Disorders* 6:114–123, 1993.
68. Hunter, J. E., F. L. Schmidt, and R. Hunter. Differential validity of employment tests by race: a comprehensive review and analysis. *Psychol. Bull.* 86:721–735, 1979.
69. Ismail, A., H. Falls, and D. MacLeod. Development of a criterion for physical fitness tests from factor analysis results. *J. Appl. Psychol.* 20:991–999, 1965.
70. Jackson, A. S. Chap. 9. Application of regression analysis to exercise science. M. J. Safrit and T. M. Wood (eds.), *Measurement Concepts in Physical Education and Exercise Science,* Human Kinetics: Champaign, IL: 1989, pp. 181–205.
71. Jackson, A. S., *Pre-Employment Isometric Strength Testing Methods—Medical and Ergometric Values and Issues.* Lafayette, IN: Lafayette Instrument Company, 1990.
72. Jackson, A. S., *Validity of Isometric Strength Tests for Predicting Work Performance in Offshore Drilling and Producing Environments. Houston: Shell Oil Company, 1986.* Houston: Shell Oil Company, 1986.
73. Jackson, A. S., *Validity of Isometric Strength Tests for Predicting Work Performance of Refinery Workers.* Houston: Shell Oil Company, 1987.
74. Jackson, A. S., E. F. Beard, L. T. Wier, and J. E. Stuteville. Multivariate model for defining

changes in maximal physical working capacity of men, ages 25 to 70 years. *Proceedings of the Human Factors Society 36th Annual Meeting* 1:171–174, 1992.

75. Jackson, A. S., S. N. Blair, M. T. Mahar, L. T. Wier, R. M. Ross, and J. E. Stuteville. Prediction of functional aerobic capacity without exercise testing. *Med. Sci. Sports Exerc.* 22:863–870, 1990.

76. Jackson, A. S., and H. G. Osburn. *Pre-Employment Physical Test Development for Coal Mining Technicians. Technical Report to Shell Oil Co.* Houston: Shell Oil Company, 1983.

77. Jackson, A. S., H. G. Osburn, and K. R. Laughery. Validity of isometric strength tests for predicting endurance work tasks of coal miners. *Proceedings of the Human Factors Society 35th Annual Meeting* 1:763–767, 1991.

78. Jackson, A. S., H. G. Osburn, and K. R. Laughery. Validity of isometric strength tests for predicting performance in physically demanding jobs. *Proceedings of the Human Factors Society 28th Annual Meeting* 28:452–454, 1984.

79. Jackson, A. S., H. G. Osburn, K. R. Laughery, and K. P. Vaubel. *Validation of Physical Strength Tests for the Texas City Plant—Union Carbide Corporation.* Houston: Center for Psychological Services, Rice University. 1990.

80. Jackson, A. S., H. G. Osburn, K. R. Laughery, and K. P. Vaubel. Validity of isometric strength tests for predicting the capacity to crack, open and close industrial valves. *Proceedings of the Human Factors Society 36th Annual Meeting* 1:688–691, 1992.

81. Jackson, A. S., H. G. Osburn, K. R. Laughery, and S. L. Young. *Validation of Physical Strength Tests for the Federal Express Corporation.* Houston: Center of Applied Psychological Services, Rice University, 1993.

82. Jackson, A. S., H. G. Osburn, K. R. Laughery, Sr., and K. P. Vaubel. Strength demands of chemical plant work tasks. *Proceedings of the Human Factors Society 35th Annual Meeting* 1:758–762, 1991.

83. Jackson, A. S., and M. L. Pollock. Factor analysis and multivariate scaling of anthropometric variables for the assessment of body composition. *Med. Sci. Sports Exerc.* 8:196–203, 1976.

84. Jackson, A. S., and M. L. Pollock. Generalized equations for predicting body density of men. *Br. J. Nutr.* 40:497–504, 1978.

85. Jackson, A. S., M. L. Pollock, and A. Ward. Generalized equations for predicting body density of women. *Med. Sci. Sports Exerc.* 12:175–182, 1980.

86. Karwowski, W. and N. Brokaw. Implications of the proposed revisions in a draft of the revised NIOSH lifting guide (1991) for job redesign: a field study. *Proceedings of the Human Factors Society 36th Annual Meeting* 36:659–663, 1992.

87. Kelsey, J. An epidemiological study of the relationship between occupations and acute herniated lumbar intervertebral discs. *Int. J. Epidemiol* 4:179–205, 1975.

88. Keyserling, W., G. Herrin, D. Chaffin, T. Armstrong, and M. Foss. Establishing an industrial strength testing program. *Am. Ind. Hyg. Assoc. J.* 41:730–736, 1980.

89. Keyserling, W. M., G. D. Herrin, and D. B. Chaffin. Isometric strength testing as a means of controlling medical incidents on strenuous jobs. *J.O.M.* 22:332–336, 1980.

90. Kirlinger, F. N., and E. J. Pedhazur. *Multiple Regression in Behavioral Research.* New York: Holt, Rinehart and Winston, 1973.

91. Kishino, N. D., T. G. Mayer, R. J. Gatchel, and More. Quantification of lumbar function: Part 4: Isometric and isokinetic lifting simulation in normal subjects and low-back dysfunction patients. *Spine* 10:921–927, 1985.

92. Landy, F. J., and P. Investigator. *Alternatives to Chronological Age in Determining Standards of Suitability for Public Safety Jobs: Volume I: Technical Report.* The Pennsylvania State University: Center for Applied Behavioral Sciences, 1992.

93. Larson, L. A. A factor analysis of motor ability variables and tests with for college men. *Res. Q.* 12:499–517, 1941.

94. Laubach, L. L. Comparative muscular strength on men and women: a review of the literature. *Aviat. Space Environ. Med.* 47:534–542, 1976.

95. Lee, C. K. The use of exercise and muscle testing in the rehabilitation of spinal disorders. *Clin. Sports Med.* 5:271–276, 1986.

96. Lemon, P. and R. Hermiston. Physiological profile of professional firefighters. *J.O.M.* 19:337–340, 1977.
97. Lemon, P., and R. T. Hermiston. The human energy cost of firefighting. *J.O.M.* 19:558–562, 1977.
98. Liba, M. R. Factor analysis of strength variables. *Res. Q.* 38:649–662, 1967.
99. Manning, J., and T. Griggs. Heart rates in firefighters using light and heavy breathing equipment: similar near-maximal exertion in response to multiple work load conditions. *J.O.M.* 25:215–218, 1983.
100. Marras, W. S., S. A. Lavender, S. E. Leurgans, S. L. Rajulu, G. Allreae, et al. Industrial quantification of occupationally-related low back disorder risk factors. *Proceedings of the Human Factors Society 36th Annual Meeting* 36:757–760, 1992.
101. Marras, W. S., C. M. Sommerich, and K. P. Granata. A three-dimensional motion model and validation of loads on the lumbar spine. *Proceedings of the Human Factors Society 35th Annual Meeting* 35:795–799, 1991.
102. Marriott, B. M., and J. Grumstrup-Scott. *Editors: Body Composition and Physical Performance: Application for the Military Services.* Washington, D.C.: National Academy Press, 1992, p. 356.
103. McArdle, W. D., F. I. Katch, and V. L. Katch. *Exercise Physiology: Energy, Nutrition, and Human Performance.* 3rd ed. Philadelphia: Lea & Febiger, 1991.
104. McCloy, C. H. A factor analysis of tests of endurance. *Res. Q.* 27:213–216, 1956.
105. Meyers, D. C., D. L. Gebhardt, C. E. Crump, and E. A. Fleishman. *Factor Analysis of Strength, Cardiovascular Endurance, Flexibility, and Body Composition Measures (Tech. Rep. R83–9).* Bethesda, MD: Advanced Research Resources Organization, 1984.
106. Mital, A. The psychophysical approach in manual lifting—a verification study. *Hum. Factors* 25:485–491, 1983.
107. Mital, A., and I. Manivasagan. Maximum acceptable weight of lifts a function of material density, center of gravity location, hand preference, and frequency. *Hum. Factors* 25:33–42, 1983.
108. Nicolaisen, T. and K. Jorgensen. Trunk strength, back muscle endurance and low-back trouble. *Scand J. Rehabil. Med.* 17:121–127, 1985.
109. NIOSH. *Pre-employment Strength Testing.*, Washington, D.C.: U.S. Department of Health and Human Services, 1977.
110. NIOSH. *Work Practices Guide for Manual Lifting, Washington.* Washington, D.C.: U.S. Department of Health and Human Services, 1981.
111. Noble, B. J., G. A. V. Borg, E. Cafarelli, R. J. Robertson, and K. B. Pandolf. Symposium on recent advances in the study and clinical use of perceived exertion. *Med. Sci. Sports Exerc.* 14:376–411, 1982.
112. O'Connell, E., P. Thomas, L. Caddy, and R. Karwasky. Energy costs of simulated stair climbing as a job-related task in firefighting. *J.O.M.* 28:282–284, 1986.
113. Osburn, H. G., *An Investigation of Applicant Physical Qualifications in Relation to Operator Tasks at the Deer Park Manufacturing Complex.* Houston: Employee Relations, Shell Oil Company, 1977.
114. Park, K., and D. B. Chaffin. Biomechanical evaluation of two methods of manual load lifting. *AIIE Trans.* 6(2):1974.
115. Passmore, R., and J. V. G. A. Durnin. Human energy expenditure. *Physiol. Rev.* 35:801–840, 1955.
116. Pollock, M. L., E. E. Laughridge, B. Coleman, A. C. Linnerud, and A. S. Jackson. Prediction of body density in young and middle-aged women. *J. Appl. Psychol.* 38:745–749, 1975.
117. Pollock, M. L., R. L. Bohannon, K. H. Cooper, J. J. Ayres, A. Ward, et al. A comparative analysis of four protocols for maximal treadmill stress testing. *Am. Heart. J.* 92:39–42, 1976.
118. Reilly, R. R., S. Zedeck, and M. L. Tenopyr. Validity and fairness of physical ability tests for predicting craft jobs. *J. Appl. Psychol.* 64:267–274, 1979.

119. Rummel, R. J., *Applied Factor Analysis*. Evanston: Northwestern University Press, 1970.
120. SAS. *JMP User's Guide: Version 2 of JMP*. Cary, NC: SAS Institute, 1989.
121. Snook, S. H. The design of manual handling tasks. *Ergonomics* 21:963–985, 1978.
122. Snook, S. H. Low back disorders in industry. *Proceedings of the Human Factors Society 35th Annual Meeting* 35:830–833, 1991.
123. Snook, S. H., R. A. Campanelli, and J. W. Hart. A study of three preventive approaches to low back injury. *J.O.M.* 20:478–481, 1978.
124. Snook, S. H., and B. M. Ciriello. Maximum weights and work loads acceptable to female workers. *J.O.M.* 16:527–534, 1974.
125. Snook, S. H. and C. H. Irvine. Psychophysical studies of physiological fatigue criteria. *Hum. Factors* 11:291–299, 1969.
126. Snook, S. H., C. H. Irvine, and S. F. Bass. Maximum weights and work loads acceptable to male industrial workers. *Am. Ind. Hyg. Assoc. J.* 31:579–586, 1970.
127. Sothmann, M. S., K. Saupe, D. Jasenor, and J. Blaney. Heart rate response of firefighters to actual emergencies. *J.O.M.* 34:797–800, 1992.
128. Sothmann, M. S., K. W. Saupe, D. Jasenof, J. Blaney, S. Donahue-Fuhrman, and T. Woulfe. Advancing age and the cardiorespiratory stress of fire suppression: determining a minimum standard for aerobic fitness. *Hum. Perf.* 3:217–236, 1990.
129. Suzuki, N., and S. Endo. A quantitative study of trunk muscle strength and fatigability in the low-back pain syndrome. *Spine* 8:69–74, 1983.
130. Vogel, J. A., and K. E. Friedl. Army data: body composition and physical capacity. B. M. Marriott and J. Grumstrup-Scott (eds). *Body Composition and Physical Performance: Applications for the Military Services*. Washington, D.C.: National Academy Press, 1992, pp. 89–104.
131. Vogel, J. A., J. F. Patton, R. P. Mello, and W. L. Daniels. An analysis of aerobic capacity in a large United States population. *J. Appl. Psychol.* 60:494–500, 1986.
132. Waters, T. R. Strategies for assessing multi-task manual lifting jobs. *Proceedings of the Human Factors Society 35th Annual Meeting* 35:809–813, 1991.
133. Wier, L. T. and A. S. Jackson. Factors affecting compliance in the NASA/JSC fitness program. *Sports Med.* 8:9–14, 1989.
134. Wilmore, J. H. and J. A. Davis. Validation of a physical abilities field test for the selection of state traffic officers. *J.O.M.* 21:33–40, 1979.
135. Zuidema, M. A. and T. A. Baumgartner. Second factor analysis of physical fitness tests. *Res. Q.* 45:247–256, 1974.

4
Aging Skeletal Muscle: Response to Exercise

GREGORY D. CARTEE, Ph.D.

Skeletal muscle is a highly malleable tissue which, in youth, can respond to altered patterns of contractile activity with remarkable adaptations. Since a reduction in adaptive capacity is commonly attributed to aging, an obvious question is, How does skeletal muscle respond and adapt to exercise during old age? The answer to this question has important implications that extend beyond scientific curiosity, impacting the health and quality of life of older individuals, the most rapidly growing segment of the population of the U.S.

The primary purpose of this review is to evaluate the literature that characterizes the response of aging skeletal muscle to exercise. The reader is referred to earlier reviews [32, 36, 69] for detailed assessment of the age-related changes in muscle. The most recent edition (Vol. 22) of this series included an excellent review that emphasized the influence of age and exercise on human skeletal muscle [83]. Longitudinal studies of human aging are problematic for a number of reasons, including the length of time required, the inability to perform some invasive procedures, and the limited control of the subjects. Therefore, the appropriate use of animal models is especially valuable for gerontological research. This review will highlight knowledge about several species (predominantly rats, but also mice, hamsters, and dogs) and compare these data with information from human experimentation.

Age-related changes that occur during the early portion of the life span (before ~6–10 mo of age for rats) are not generally considered by gerontologists to represent senescence [36]. Although the attainment of sexual maturity is sometimes used as an indicator of adulthood, use of this criteria can be misleading in the study of skeletal muscle. Rats reach sexual maturity at <2 mo of age [86], but skeletal muscle mass is still rapidly growing, having attained only ~25–50% of peak values [4, 39]. By 6–10 mo of age, skeletal muscle mass reaches ~80–100% of the peak values [39, 102]. Therefore, this review focuses on age-related changes that occur in rats ≥6 mo of age. It is also important to be aware that the term "old" is sometimes inappropriately used to describe rats as young as 6–12 mo of age. While there is no universally accepted standard for correct use of the term "old," Walford [96] suggested that the 50% survival point is an indicator of the onset of the senescent portion of the life span, provided that the housing conditions are good and epidemic disease is avoided. Under optimal conditions, the median and maximal life spans of most commonly used strains of laboratory rats exceed 21–30 and 30–40 mo, respectively [74]. Of course, the precise values depend on the strain employed and nutritional and environmental conditions.

Researchers would do well to consider the advise from Gutmann: "Research on muscle in old age should take into account the marked diversity among muscles with different functions, as well as the heterogeneity of muscle fibers constituting an individual muscle" [44]. Careful examination of this heterogeneity can offer valuable insight into the etiology of age-related changes.

SKELETAL MUSCLE FIBER COMPOSITION

Using histochemical staining procedures (based on myofibrillar ATPase activity), many laboratories studying rats have reported little effect of aging on fiber type composition in various muscles, including the extensor digitorum longus (EDL), flexor digitorum longus (FDL), and lateral omohyoideus (LOMO) [2, 13, 29, 30, 36, 37, 70, 97]. Florini and Ewton [37] made similar observations for the EDL and soleus from C57B1/NNia mice. There was no effect of age (2–3 vs. 10–13 yr) on the proportion of type I and II fibers in the gastrocnemius, triceps, or semitendinosus muscles of female beagles [45]. Holloszy et al. [47] found that the proportion of type I fibers increased from 15% to 26% in the plantaris of old (28–30 mo) Long Evans rats, while there was a nonsignificant trend for a decrease in the percentages of type IIa fibers. In contrast, some investigators have reported a large reduction in the proportion of type IIb along with an increase in the proportion of type I fibers with advancing age. Florini [36] speculated that marked shifts in fiber type composition were related to the failure to use specific pathogen-free animals and/or to animal housing conditions, but the explanation for this discrepancy has not been conclusively determined.

Larsson et al. [62, 63] evaluated the myosin heavy chains (MHC) in fibers from the tibialis anterior muscle of rats (3–6 vs. 20–24 mo) using antibodies specific for types I, IIA, IIB, and the newly identified type IIX. Fibers that were immunologically recognized as type IIX were histochemically identified as type IIB. Although the fiber type composition was unaltered, based on ATPase staining, the abundance of fibers expressing type IIX MHC was greatly increased in old rats. Old, but not young, rats had some motor units containing type IIX along with type IIB or type IIA fibers; these motor units were designated as IIXB and IIXA, respectively. The authors proposed that type IIX represents a transitional fiber type, with type IIB motor units undergoing the following sequential shift in old age: IIB → IIXB → IIX → IIXA → IIA. If this scenario is true, the absence of large shifts in fiber composition across a large portion of the life span as determined histochemically suggests that this progression is completed only in very old age.

Klitgaard et al. [59] found little effect of strength or swim training on the fiber composition of the soleus or plantaris of old rats. Stebbins et al. [90] observed no effect of 5 mo of treadmill running, initiated at 21 mo of age, on the proportion of fiber types in the gastrocnemius. However, they found that training led to a small increase in the percentage of type I fibers. Kovanen [61] also reported that treadmill running led to a small increase in the percentage of type I fibers in the soleus of young (10 mo) and old (24 mo) rats. The trained animals at each age also had a greater percentage of type I and IIa fibers and lesser percentage of IIb fibers in the rectus femoris.

Reviewing the human literature, Rogers and Evans [83] reported that although some studies using biopsy samples provided evidence for a decline in the percentage of type II fibers and a reciprocal increase in the proportion of type I fibers, recent studies using larger sample sizes have not supported these results. Lexell et al. [65] evaluated whole vastus lateralis muscles taken from men at autopsy and found no effect of age on fiber type composition. With endurance training, the percentage of type I fibers is unaltered in humans, regardless of age, while the percentages of type IIa and IIb fibers increase and decrease, respectively. Apparently, the effects of age and endurance training on histochemically determined fiber composition are similar in humans and rats.

SKELETAL MUSCLE ATROPHY

Skeletal muscle atrophy is often considered a hallmark of aging, and this deficit has profound implications for function and health. Changes in muscle mass must be secondary to altered fiber number, altered fiber size, and/or altered amount of extramyofibrillar components. Several investigators have observed a significant decline in muscle mass despite little or no detectable decline in fiber number of various muscles (soleus, EDL) in rats between 9 and 27–30 mo of age [11, 13, 25, 29]. Alnaqeeb and Goldspink [2] found no reduction in type I or type II fiber number, or cross-sectional area (CSA) of type I fibers in the soleus of male rats (10 vs. 24 mo), but they did find a significant decline in the cross-sectional area of type II fibers. Between 9–10 and 28–30 mo of age, Holloszy et al. [47] found that plantaris mass declined by 24% compared with a 30% reduction in the average CSA of fibers, also consistent with the interpretation that little or no decrease in fiber number had occurred. The decline in CSA was greater in the type IIb fibers (37%) than in the type I fibers (21%). Taken together, these studies indicate that the decreased muscle mass in rats between ~23 and 30 mo of age is largely secondary to fiber atrophy, particularly of type II fibers.

There is also evidence that the type II fibers of dogs are more susceptible to age-related atrophy. The CSA of type II fibers was significantly lower (22–31%) in the triceps and gastrocnemius of old (10–13 yr) than young (2–3 yr) female beagles [45]. No difference was seen in the type II fibers from the semitendinosus. The CSA of type I fibers was unchanged in the triceps and gastrocnemius, but significantly increased (14%) in the semitendinosus. The reduced size of type II fibers would be expected to cause a significant decline in the mass of the gastrocnemius and triceps, since type II fibers account for 65–88% of fibers in these muscles, but muscle mass and fiber number were not assessed.

Lexell et al. [65] counted the fiber number in cross-sections from the whole vastus lateralis obtained from men at autopsy. The decline in muscle mass could be primarily attributed to a 39% reduction in fiber number between 20 and 80 yr of age. Fiber number appeared to decline progressively, with the decrease beginning at ~30 yr of age. The CSA of fibers also declined, particularly in type IIb fibers. Coggan et al. [21] observed an age-related reduction (13–30%) in the CSA of types IIa and IIb, but not type I, in biopsies obtained from the gastrocnemius of older men and women. Apparently, a reduction in fiber CSA, particularly of type II fibers, occurs commonly in various muscles from humans, dogs, and rats. A diminished fiber number appears to be more important in old humans than in old rats.

Quadriceps, soleus, plantaris, and gastrocnemius mass decreases significantly in old age [47]. However, some small muscles (LOMO, FDL, adductor longus, and epitrochlearis) do not atrophy in rats up to 27–30 mo of age [47, 70, 97]. The heterogeneity of effects of age suggests that systemic changes (e.g., growth hormone) are insufficient to explain the age-related changes in some skeletal muscle. Apparently, some factor(s) in the affected muscle or its α-motoneuron works alone or in concert with the systemic factor(s).

There is less information about selective atrophy humans, since human studies seldom evaluate more than one muscle. One study indicated that the atrophy was more pronounced in certain muscles of old humans (65–92 yr) at autopsy, but the comparisons were not quantitative [53]. The relative decrease in muscle CSA determined by computed tomography in old (68 yr) compared with young (28 yr) men was similar for the quadriceps (24%) and elbow flexors (20%) [60]. The CSAs for several muscles (the gastrocnemius and soleus or the quadriceps) were reported to decrease by 23–35% between ~20–30 and ~ 65–80 yr [106, 112]. The magnitude of these changes is comparable to the decline in mass of the quadriceps (26%), gastrocnemius (32%), and soleus (11%) in male Long-Evans rats between 9–10 and 27–28 mo [47].

Some of the age-related changes in muscle might be caused by reduced locomotor activity rather than being a primary effect of aging. Supporting this contention, spontaneous activity declines with advancing age [101], and the voluntary running of rats provided with running wheels declines markedly throughout adulthood [13, 33, 43]. Holloszy et al. [47] noted that atrophy is especially marked in weight-bearing muscles. These observations are consistent with the hypothesis that disuse contributes to some of the age-related changes in muscle.

The precise mechanism for age-related atrophy has not been identified, but there is considerable evidence for a loss in the number of functional α-motoneurons [5, 32, 54, 69]. Apparently, an adaptive process that involves axonal sprouting of the remaining α-motoneurons can lead to the reinnervation of at least some fibers. Consistent with this idea, motor unit size is increased in both humans and rats with aging [54, 94]. Ansved and Larsson [5] reported a decline in the number of large myelinated nerve fibers in the L5 ventral roots of old animals, along with morphological evidence of degeneration of α-motoneurons. The effect of exercise on the motor unit size and α-motoneuron number and morphology of old animals has apparently not been evaluated. Several studies have indicated that treadmill training protocols can alter neuromuscular remodeling in old rats. Rosenheimer [84] observed a decline in number of nerve terminal branches per endplate in the soleus and EDL of old (25 mo) compared with young (10 mo) rats. Treadmill running, initiated at 3 mo of age, resulted in an increase in the number of sprouting nerve terminals in both muscles from old animals. Stebbins et al. [90] found that treadmill running initiated at 21 mo of age increased growth configurations (defined as "all end plates innervated by 2 or more myelinated or unmyelinated branches from the same terminal axon") in the soleus but not the gastrocnemius of 26-mo-old rats. Andonian and Fahim [3] found that 8 wk of training (treadmill running) by male C57GL/6NNia mice (12, 18, or 24–25 mo) led to significantly larger nerve terminals in the soleus and EDL from 12-mo-old mice. In the 18- and 24–25-mo-old groups, the same exercise training resulted in smaller nerve terminals than in age-matched controls.

SKELETAL MUSCLE HYPERTROPHY

Relatively few experiments have been designed primarily to evaluate the effect of age on the hypertrophic response in animals. Tomanek and Woo [93] studied compensatory hypertrophy of the plantaris by bilateral denervation of the synergistic gastrocnemius in rats aged 45 d or 19 mo. Beginning 1 wk after surgery, animals were exercised by walking on a treadmill (40° incline) for 85–90 days. Mean fiber diameter was increased ~13% in the experimental animals at each age. This experiment demonstrates that moderately old rats retain the capacity for muscle hypertrophy, but this model has little in common with the typical resistance training protocol used by humans.

Klitgaard et al. [57–59] used a more physiological model of resistance training. Male Wistar rats were trained to rise to their hindlimbs inside a Plexiglas tube and perform a maximum plantar flexion while lifting a weight attached to a shoulder collar. Training was initiated at 19 mo of age and consisted of performing ~10 lifts/d for 4 d/wk. Fiber number declined in the soleus from sedentary rats between 9 and 24 mo of age. Training prevented the decline in fiber number at 24 mo of age but not in the 29-mo-old rats. However, strength training eliminated most of the decrease in fiber CSA between 24 and 29 mo. Strength training attenuated the decline in plantaris mass to a lesser degree than in the soleus. CSA of type IIb fibers of the plantaris was significantly increased above age-matched controls in strength-trained rats at 24 and 29 mo. Fiber number was not determined in the plantaris.

Brown [12] studied the effect of exercise initiated at several ages late in the life of female Sprague-Dawley rats. Training consisted of 3 mo of training (3 sets of 10 repetitions, twice/d, 5 d/wk) that required elbow flexion executed against resistance. In the trained 30-mo-old rats, the CSA of type II fibers of the palmaris muscle was elevated by 27%, while the CSA of type I fibers was not altered. The results were similar at 21 and 24 mo.

Voluntary wheel running can elicit skeletal muscle hypertrophy in old rats. Rats are housed in cages with free access to running wheels. Unlike treadmill training that typically consists of 30–120 minutes of steady-state exercise, voluntary wheel cage running by rats (~3 mo of age) consists of many (~100–200) brief bouts (40–90 sec) of high-speed running (averaging 40–45 m/min) each day [82]. The main disadvantages of this exercise model are the considerable variation in the amount of voluntary activity [82] and the marked decline in volitional exercise with advancing age [13, 33, 43]. When female Long-Evans rats lived in a running-wheel cage, their average running distance declined by 75% between 9 and 27 mo of age [13]. Soleus mass was elevated in the young and old exercise-trained groups compared with age-matched controls, and the mass and cross-sectional fiber areas of the old trained group were comparable to those of the young controls. Voluntary running initiated at 3 mo of age also prevented soleus atrophy in 28-mo-old male rats, but the soleus did not hypertrophy in 9-mo-old males [33].

Unlike wheel running, motorized treadmill running does not typically elicit muscle hypertrophy in the soleus of young rats [25, 92]. However, Daw et al. [25] found that treadmill running initiated at 3 mo of age led to a 13% increase in soleus mass of 27-mo-old male F344 rats without any change in fiber number, implicating an increase in fiber size. Soleus mass was unaffected in identically trained 12-mo-old rats. Treadmill run training for 6 mo caused a 15% enlargement in the soleus mass of 24-mo-old male F344 rats without significantly affecting the soleus from 10-mo-old animals (unpublished observation).

Resistance training can lead to increased muscle CSA in young and old humans, as determined by computed tomography [80]. The relative increases in fiber CSA reported for older humans tend to be greater in type II (20–52%) than type I (8–17%) fibers [83]. In two studies that have used resistance training in older rats [12, 59], there were no striking differences in the relative amount of hypertrophy found in type I (5–49%) and type II (10–54%) fibers. This apparent difference might be more related to variations in the training protocols and/or muscles studied than to the species.

CONNECTIVE TISSUE IN SKELETAL MUSCLE

The active shortening of muscle depends on the contractile proteins, and the provision of ATP is accomplished by various proteins in the cytosol and the mitochondria. Generally less appreciated are the roles of connective tissue proteins. The collagenous matrix performs many functions in muscle, including the alignment of muscle fibers, providing structural support and strength, conferring elasticity, storing elastic energy during stretching, and participating in muscle remodeling during growth and regeneration [61]. During atrophy with aging, or hypertrophy after resistance training, the proteins that constitute the extracellular matrix must accommodate these alterations.

In rats, muscle collagen concentration increases with advancing age, and endurance training (treadmill running) causes a greater accretion in collagen in the soleus muscle. The activity of prolyl hydroxylase (an enzyme of collagen biosynthesis) was higher in endurance-trained old men [91] and rats [61] than in age-matched controls. Kovanen [61] evaluated mechanical properties of the soleus, including ultimate tensile strength, the tangent modulus, and elastic efficiency. Each increased with training in young and old rats. Extensive posttranslation modification of collagen fundamentally alters its mechanical properties. Little is known about the interaction between age and exercise on postranslational modification of collagen.

SKELETAL MUSCLE CAPILLARITY

Several studies have indicated no age-related change in the capillarity of rat skeletal muscles. Capillarity is unchanged in the FDL muscle of male F344 rats between 6 and 28 mo of age, whether results are expressed as capillaries around each fiber, capillaries/fiber, or capillaries/mm^2 [97]. Capillary/fiber ratios are unchanged in the soleus and EDL of female Long-Evans (9–27 mo) and Wistar (6–24 mo) rats [11, 13]. In contrast to the results with rats, Haidet and Parsons [46] noted in female beagles a significant age-related decline (2–3 vs. 10–13 yr) in capillarity expressed as capillary/fiber ratio or capillaries/mm^2 in the gastrocnemius, semitendinosus, and triceps muscles.

In humans, there have been conflicting reports about the influence of age on skeletal muscle capillarity. Parízkova et al. [78] reported a decline in the capillary/fiber ratio (20 vs. 70 yr), but because of the reduced CSA of fibers in old age, there was no change in capillaries/mm^2. Coggan et al. [21] reported an age-related (25 vs 65 yr) decrement in capillarity of the gastrocnemius (expressed as capillary/fiber ratio or number of capillaries in contact with each fiber). Grimby et al. [41] found no change in the capillarity (capillaries/mm^2 or capillary/fiber ratios) of the vastus lateralis of people of up to 81 yr of age.

Exercise training can lead to increased capillarity of skeletal muscle of rats and humans regardless of age. Voluntary wheel running initiated at 4 mo of age increased the capillary/fiber ratios of the soleus of 9- and 28-mo-old rats to a similar extent, despite the substantial reduction in training volume by the old rats [13]. Endurance-trained young and old humans had similar levels of muscle capillarity, even when the young subjects ran longer distances at a faster pace [25].

SKELETAL MUSCLE BLOOD FLOW

Irion et al. [51] used microspheres to measure muscle blood flow in anesthetized F344 rats (12 or 24 mo of age) during electrical stimulation of the plantar flexor muscles. Muscle blood flow during contractile activity was significantly reduced in each fiber type of old, male rats, compared with young animals. No reduction in blood flow was found in old female rats during an identical stimulation procedure [52]. Because the old male rats also had a reduction in the response to a nonspecific vasodilator (diazoxide), the authors proposed that the reduced blood flow in the old group was caused by a change in muscle vasculature.

Haidet and Parsons [46] used microspheres to measure blood flow in female beagles (2–3 v. 10–14 yr) during treadmill running. There was no age-related effect on blood flow to locomotory (triceps, deltoid, flexor carpi ulnaris, flexor digitorum superficialis, gastrocnemius, gracilis, semimembranosus, and semitendinosus) or nonlocomotory (temporalis) muscles during maximal exercise. Maximal cardiac output was reduced in the old dogs because of the decline in blood flow to splanchnic organs.

Wahren et al. [95] measured leg blood flow (constant-rate intra-arterial indicator infusion technique) of trained young (25–30 yr) and older (52–59 yr) men during bicycle ergometery at progressively increasing work rates. Leg blood flow was lower in older (52–59 yr) men at every submaximal workload. Leg blood flow was 4.46 liters/min in maximal exercise for the older men, compared with 5.57 liters/min in the younger men at a lower, submaximal workload. The young men were not studied during maximal exercise, but since leg blood flow increases linearly during submaximal exercise with increasing oxygen consumption and workload, the highest leg blood flow of the young men would be expected to be considerably greater than that in the older group. It is difficult to compare the results found with rats, dogs, and humans because of the diversity of techniques and exercise protocols. However, at least in old rats and humans, there is evidence for attenuated blood flow during contractile activity. The effect of training on muscle blood flow during exercise has not been reported for old animals or humans.

SKELETAL MUSCLE OXIDATIVE CAPACITY

Oxidative capacity declines in some skeletal muscles with advancing age. Farrar et al. [31] measured O_2 consumption by mitochondria isolated from gastrocnemius and plantaris muscles and found an age-related decline in the amount of mitochondrial protein. This decline was not due to a change in the mitochondrial yield in the old animals. The ADP/O and respiratory control ratios were unaffected by age. These results indicate that the mitochondria from old animals were not damaged by isolation and suggest that the effect of age is primarily on the number rather than the quality of the mitochondria.

Several researchers have reported that the activities of numerous mitochondrial enzymes decrease in muscle from rats during old age. Citrate synthase (CS), NAD-isocitrate dehydrogenase, 2-oxoglutarate dehydrogenase, succinate dehydrogenase (SDH), fumarase, cytochrome oxidase (Cytox), carnitine acetyltransferase, carnitine palmitoyltransferase, acyl-CoA dehydrogenase, 3-hydroxyacyl-CoA dehydrogenase (β-HAD), and 3-ketoacid-CoA transferase decline in the soleus [45, 47]. CS, Cytox, and β-HAD decreased in the gastrocnemius [18]. CS, SDH, and fumarase were reduced in the plantaris [47]. These decreases were noted between 6–10 and 24–28 mo of age, and the relative declines ranged from 14- to 56%. In contrast, several investigators [43, 47, 97, 100] reported no significant effect of age on mitochondrial enzyme levels in the epitrochlearis, deep red portion of the vastus lateralis, superficial white portion of the vastus lateralis muscle, flexor digitorum brevis, or the FDL. The epitrochlearis [100] and the FDL [97] also exhibit unaltered mass up to 26–31 mo of age. SDH activity tended (12–28%) to be lower in the gastrocnemius and semitendinosus of old dogs. Unexpectedly, SDH activity was greater in the triceps of old dogs than in young dogs, perhaps because of the decrease in CSA of type II, but not type I, fibers [45].

The capacity to oxidize fatty acids is preferentially depressed relative to other substrates in the aged rat heart [1, 45], but it is uncertain if such an effect exists in skeletal muscle. The respiratory capacity of homogenates prepared from the quadriceps from old hamsters was reduced (29%) with palmitoyl-carnitine as a substrate, but unchanged with pyruvate-malate as substrate [75]. Beyer et al. [7] observed a greater age-linked decline in O_2 utilization by gastrocnemius homogenates supplied with palmityl-CoA as a substrate than with pyruvate-malate (39% vs. 16%, respectively). In contrast, Holloszy et al. [47] found a 15% decline with each of these substrates in the plantaris. Cartee and Farrar [17] found a 45% reduction in gastrocnemius palmitate oxidation between 10 and 24 mo of age, compared with a 14–24% decline in markers of the Krebs cycle (CS), electron transport chain (Cytox) and β-oxidation (β-HAD). Beyer et al. [7] found that the oxidation of palmitoyl-CoA, but not palmitoyl carnitine, is depressed in the hindlimb muscle of old rats, indicating that age-related defects distal to palmitoyl carnitine transferase I did not cause the decreased palmitate oxidation. Of the two enzymes implicated: (*a*) carnitine palmitoyl transferase activity was decreased by 44% in the soleus [45] but not in the plantaris [47] of old rats, and (*b*) palmitoyl-CoA synthase activity has apparently not been evaluated in muscles from old rats.

Endurance-type training during youth is characterized by an increase in the mitochondrial content of the active skeletal muscle [92]. This adaptation is functionally important because the ability of skeletal muscle to regenerate ATP by oxidative metabolism is closely related to endurance capacity [33]. The magnitude of the training-induced increase in muscle oxidative capacity depends on the intensity and amount of exercise performed [33, 82, 92]. It is not, therefore, surprising that when a comparison is made between young rats that are exercising at higher absolute workloads and old animals performing significantly less work, the young animals attain a higher level of oxidative capacity [40, 43, 88]. More revealing are the experiments that have compared young and old animals subjected to identical exercise training protocols (which are, of course, limited by the exercise capacity of the old animals). Table 1 summarizes the results of the studies that have used this experimental design [17, 31, 79, 100]. The most striking observation is that in each study the old animals attained levels of oxidative capacity quite similar to those of the identically trained young rats. However, this level of adaptation falls well short of the adaptations young rats can achieve when they train more vigorously. This situation presents a dilemma for researchers hoping to compare the maximal adaptability of skeletal muscle from young and old animals: work capacity decreases with advancing age, so old animals cannot exercise train at the maximal work rates achieved by young animals.

Walters et al. [98] attempted to circumvent this problem with an approach that is unique in gerontological research. An electrode cuff was placed around the tibial nerve of young (6–8 mo) and old (26–28 mo) rats, and muscles were electrically stimulated to contract (10 Hz, 8 hr/d) for 10 to 90 d. The CS activity was measured in the FDL. The young animals had a greater increase in CS activity during the first 35 d of stimulation, but thereafter the values for the two groups converged, so that by 90 d, CS activity was virtually identical in the stimulated groups (40% above controls).

It is not necessary to exercise throughout life to induce adaptations in mitochondrial enzymes above the levels in young, sedentary animals. After 2.5 mo of training initiated at 21–24 mo of age, old rats attained values exceeding those of both the young and old sedentary groups [40, 79].

Furthermore, the magnitude of the increase in mitochondrial markers in these animals was similar to that achieved by old rats that had trained for 6–21 mo [17, 31, 87, 100].

Rogers and Evans [83] summarized the results from several Scandinavian studies that have found little evidence for an age-related decline in muscle oxidative capacity in humans. They also described other studies that have reported significant (14–30%) reductions in oxidative enzyme activities in older men and women. They noted that those studies that found a decrement had carefully selected truly sedentary subjects. This interpretation is consistent with the notion that the age-associated decline in oxidative capacity is secondary to reduced physical activity. The magnitude of the age-related decrements in oxidative enzyme activities in humans is comparable to the changes reported in old rats.

Coggan et al. [23] compared the enzymatic profile of muscle biopsy samples from endurance-trained master athlete distance runners (63 yr) and a group of younger men (26 yr) who were matched to the older men for training and performance. The activities for mitochondrial enzymes (CS, SDH, and β-HAD) in the gastrocnemius were ~25% higher in the old runners than in training-matched young men. These higher values might have been because the master athletes had been training longer than the younger men. A second group of young runners (28 yr), who were training at faster speeds (24%) and for longer distances (55%) than the master athletes, was also studied. Mitochondrial enzyme activities were 14–23% higher in these young runners than in master athletes. These findings are congruous with the observations made for rats: i.e., vigorous exercise training in older age can lead to levels of muscle oxidative capacity as high as those in young individuals undergoing similar training, but when young individuals train at higher workloads, their muscles attain higher activities for mitochondrial enzymes.

SKELETAL MUSCLE CARBOHYDRATE METABOLISM

Skeletal muscle carbohydrate metabolism has profound implications not only for the function of the muscle but also for the well-being of the whole organism. Carbohydrate is a key fuel for muscle during contractile activity, and skeletal muscle plays a pivotal role in maintaining glucose homeostasis, since it accounts for as much as 85% of insulin-stimulated removal of blood glucose [26]. Muscle insulin resistance is an early event in the development of glucose intolerance by old humans and rats [76, 85].

Glucose enters muscle cells via facilitated diffusion, mediated by glucose transporter proteins [56], and glucose transport is the rate-limiting step for muscle glucose metabolism [104]. The GLUT-4, or insulin-regulatable, glucose transporter is the predominant glucose transporter protein expressed by skeletal muscle [56]. Both insulin and exercise increase glucose transport rate by stimulating the translocation of GLUT-4 transporters from an intracellular site to the plasma membrane, where they are accessible to extracellular glucose. This translocation process is reversible, and the transporters are resequestered inside the cell when the stimulus is removed [56].

GLUT-4 levels in rats decrease early in life (between 1–4 and 10–13 mo) in several muscles (epitrochlearis, red quadriceps, and plantaris), with no further decline between 10–13 and 25 mo (16, 42, 43). The maximal capacity of insulin to stimulate glucose transport activity in isolated epitrochlearis muscle appears to track the age-related decline in GLUT-4, with a significant reduction occurring early in life (between 1–4 and 10–13 mo), and no further change is evident between 10–13 and 25 mo [16, 42]. Advancing age does not have a universal effect on all muscles, as there is no age-related change in GLUT-4 in the flexor digitorum brevis or soleus between 1 and 25–29 mo of age [42, 43, 55].

A single bout of exercise can markedly increase the rate of glucose transport in the exercised muscle. This change is intrinsic to the muscle itself, as evidenced by the increased glucose transport found in muscles dissected out of the body after exercise and studied in vitro [19]. Following exercise, glucose transport is enhanced in the absence of insulin, but most of this effect is lost 1–3 hr after the cessation of exercise. More long-lasting is the enhancement of insulin-stimulated glucose transport, which can persist the day after the exercise bout. The increased insulin sensitivity for glucose transport probably contributes to the improved whole body insulin-sensitivity after a bout of exercise and to the glycogen supercompensation process (i.e., the acquisition of supranormal glycogen stores when carbohydrate feeding follows strenuous exercise).

Because previous investigations into the exercise effect on muscle glucose transport had used very young rats (~ 1–4 mo of age), we recently examined the effect of a single bout of exercise on insulin-stimulated glucose transport in young (3.5 mo), adult (13 mo), and old (25 mo) rats [16]. Isolated epitrochlearis muscles were studied 4 hr after completion of exercise. At this time, insulin sensitivity determined with a physiological, submaximally effective insulin concentration was increased by 50–75% at each age. With a maximally effective insulin concentration (20,000 μU/ml), muscle glucose transport was enhanced in the young group, in agreement with previous research [19]. In contrast, there was no increase in glucose transport with this amount of insulin in the adult or old groups. Muscle is not normally exposed to such a high insulin concentration, so the demonstration that exercise leads to an improvement insulin sensitivity regardless of age has more physiological relevance.

Exercise training can lead to elevated GLUT-4 concentration in the muscles from young rats [81]. Kern et al. [55] studied rats after 10–15 wk of endurance training (60 min/d, 5 d/wk, at 75% of VO_2max) and found substantial increases in soleus and gastrocnemius GLUT-4 levels in rats at

6–8 and 15–17 mo of age. No significant increase was found in old (27–29 mo) rats after training. However, the training speed for the old rats was only 57% of that for the young group. Gulve et al. [43] measured GLUT-4 concentration in the epitrochlearis and muscles of adult (10 mo) and old (25 mo) rats that had been living in cages fitted with running wheels beginning at 4 mo of age. GLUT-4 levels was increased ~50% above sedentary control values in the adult, but not the old, runners. Running distance of the old rats had fallen to levels <50% of the value found in the adult animals. The lack of any increase in GLUT-4 in exercising old animals in both of these studies might indicate a reduced adaptability in old age or simply reflect the substantial decrease in the amount of exercise the old animals were performing. Consistent with this second possibility, Gulve et al. [43] found that CS activity increased in the young, but not the old, runners.

The effect of training on muscle GLUT-4 in middle-aged and older humans has also been reported recently. Houmard et al. [48] reported that the GLUT-4 levels in gastrocnemius biopsy samples of endurance-trained (running 3–7 d/wk for an average of 10 yr) middle-aged (49 yr) men were ~2-fold higher than values found for age-matched sedentary men. Subsequently, the same group [49] measured gastrocnemius GLUT-4 levels before and after 14 wk of training (walking, running, stair climbing up to 45 min/day, 4 d/wk at ≈80% of maximum heart rate) by middle-aged men (47 yr). After only 14 wk of training, these previously unfit men achieved a relative increase in GLUT-4 (1.8-fold) quite similar to that found in the long-term runners. Short-term training increased VO₂max (2.8 vs 3.4 liters/min) and reduced the percentage of body fat (26.3% vs. 28.7%), but these values did not approach those in long-term runners (4.03 liters/min and 14.1%). Hughes et al. [50] extended these results further, demonstrating that even older men and women (64 yr) could increase GLUT-4 in the vastus lateralis by 1.6-fold after 12 wk of training (cycle ergometry at 50% or 75% of heart rate reserve) despite no change in percentage body fat. Based on data from rats [82], this increase in GLUT-4 content was probably accompanied by an increased capacity for insulin-stimulated muscle glucose transport. In all of these experiments, whole body insulin sensitivity was improved with exercise training [48–50].

After glucose enters the muscle cell, it is rapidly phosphorylated by hexokinase (HK). Goodman et al. [39] found a significant decline in HK in the EDL during the growth phase (1–11 mo) but no further decline from 11–22 mo. HK activity was unaffected by age in a variety of muscles (plantaris, soleus, red portion of the vastus lateralis, white vastus lateralis, epitrochlearis, and flexor digitorum brevis) between 9–10 and 24–28 mo [43, 47, 100]. Klitgaard et al. [59] found no change in HK activity in the soleus and plantaris between 9 and 24 mo, but a 22–31% decline was seen at 29 mo, while Sanchez et al. [88] reported that HK decreased by 10% and 26%, respectively, in the soleus and EDL between 6 and 24 mo.

Swimming or voluntary wheel running caused significant increases in HK activity in the epitrochlearis of 9–10 and 24–25-mo-old rats [43, 100]. As discussed above, voluntary running induced an increase in epitrochlearis GLUT-4 levels only in the young rats, suggesting that the amount and/or intensity of exercise needed to induce an increase in HK activity is below the threshold for upregulation of GLUT-4. Endurance and strength training increased HK activity in old rats [59, 88].

The product of HK, glucose 6-phosphate, has two primary metabolic fates in skeletal muscle: incorporation into glycogen or degradation by the glycolytic pathway. Dall'Aglio et al. [24] reported that total glycogen synthase activity, the rate-limiting enzyme for glycogen synthesis, decreases by 15–42% between 12 and 24 mo of age in the tensor fascia latae, biceps femoris, and soleus. Such a decrease could potentially slow the rate of muscle glycogen resynthesis following a bout of exercise.

During vigorous exercise, glycogenolysis is critical for muscle function. the maximal activity of phosphorylase, the rate-limiting enzyme of glycogenolysis, was unchanged between 9–10 and 24–28 mo in the epitrochlearis, soleus, or red portion of the vastus lateralis, but it decreased (14–21%) in the plantaris and white portion of the quadriceps [47, 100]. The production of ATP from carbohydrate depends on the glycolytic pathway. The maximal activity of phosphofructokinase (PFK), the rate-limiting step in glycolysis, declines (14–28%) in the plantaris, red and white portions of the vastus lateralis, EDL, and gastrocnemius between 9–11 and 22–28 mo of age [39, 47, 87], but no decline was observed in the soleus [47]. The activity of lactate dehydrogenase (LDH) has been consistently shown to decrease by 19–39% between 9–11 and 22–28 mo in several muscles, including the soleus, EDL, plantaris, and red and white portions of the vastus lateralis [39, 47, 59, 87]. The age-related reduction in glycolytic potential would be likely to be detrimental during high-intensity exercise requiring very rapid ATP production.

Consistent with earlier findings with young animals, endurance training did not alter muscle phosphorylase or PFK activity in old rats [87, 100]. Klitgaard et al. [59] reported that both swim and strength training elevated LDH activity in the soleus of old rats, but only strength training increased the LDH activity in the plantaris. Sanchez et al. [88] found no evidence that treadmill running attenuated the age-related decline in soleus LDH activity.

Coggan et al. [22] reported that 10 mo of endurance exercise training by 60–70-yr-old men and women reduced gastrocnemius LDH activity but did not alter gastrocnemius activities for PFK or phosphorylase. Örlander and Aniansson [77], however, reported that exercise training led to an increase in the LDH activity determined in biopsy samples from the vastus lateralis of 70–75-yr-old men. This apparent discrepancy might be related to their training protocol, which included a combination of endurance and strength training. Taken together, these results indicate that the muscle enzymes of glycolysis and glycogenolysis from old rats and humans respond to exercise training in a similar fashion.

The availability of muscle glycogen is important for endurance capacity. Many studies have found that aging does not alter muscle glycogen in rodents [14, 16, 18, 34, 39, 75], but other investigators [6, 24] have reported an age-related decline. One of these studies also found a reduction in glycogen synthase activity [24].

An experiment by Fitts et al. [34] offers important insight into the effect of age on glycogen metabolism during contractile activity. They studied the metabolic and contractile response of young (9 mo) and old (28 mo) male Long-Evans rats that were submitted to identical stimulation protocols (30 min of in situ isometric contractile activity). Resting soleus glycogen concentration was not significantly affected by age, but the poststimulation glycogen values were reduced by 72% in the old muscle. This result represents a 2.3-fold greater glycogen depletion in the old animals (Figure 4.1). Resting ATP and CP levels were unaffected by age. Following contractile activity, ATP was similarly reduced in both ages, but CP concentration declined more in old animals. Poststimulation muscle lactate concentration was >2-fold higher in the old rats.

What factors are most likely to account for these energetic disparities? Muscle metabolic profile is an important determinant for substrate selection and utilization. The same laboratory group reported that

FIGURE 4.1

Estimated soleus glycogen depletion during 30 min of electrically stimulated in vitro contractile activity. Total bar height *equals resting glycogen concentration.* Hatched portion of the bar *equals the glycogen remaining in the muscle poststimulation.* Open portion of the bar *equals the estimated glycogen depletion (resting glycogen concentration minus poststimulation glycogen concentration) during the contractile activity. Drawn from data in Fitts et al. [34].*

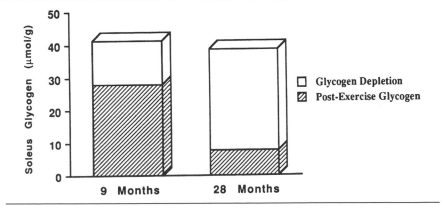

maximal activities for phosphorylase, HK, and PFK are not different in the soleus of 9- and 28-mo-old rats, and LDH activity is 23% lower in the old soleus [47]. This scenario suggests that the greater depletion of glycogen and accumulation of lactate were secondary to altered allosteric or covalent activation of these regulatory enzymes. The degradation of CP liberates inorganic phosphate, which is necessary for glycogenolysis [20]. Dudley and Fleck [27] measured ATP, CP, and lactate concentrations in several muscles of young (7 mo) and old (23 mo) male F344 rats at rest and after moderate or intense in situ contractile activity. Depletion of ATP and CP after contractile activity was greater for old rats in all of the muscles studied (soleus, superficial and deep gastrocnemius). During moderate-intensity contractile activity, lactate accumulation was greater in the superficial gastrocnemius (predominantly type IIb) and deep gastrocnemius (predominantly type IIa) of old rats, compared with young rats. During high-intensity contractile activity, lactate accumulation was significantly higher in the deep gastrocnemius and soleus of the old animals. The authors suggested that these differences were because of the reduced mitochondrial content in the old muscle. It seems likely that the reduction in mitochondrial enzymes in the soleus [47] contributed to the greater glycogen use observed by Fitts et al. [34], since glycogen utilization during exercise correlates with muscle oxidative capacity [33].

The dependence on muscle glycogen for fuel would be expected to increase if the availability of alternative energy sources is diminished. An important energy source is muscle triglycerides, but muscle triglyceride concentration is unchanged or increased in old age [15, 39]. The most important blood-borne energy sources are glucose and FFA, but their blood concentrations do not decrease with aging [18, 39, 76]. However, the delivery of blood-borne substrates depends on blood flow as well as the substrate concentration. Irion et al. [51] found a 44% reduction in soleus blood flow of old male rats during contractile activity under experimental conditions very similar to those employed by Fitts et al. [34]. It would be interesting to compare the rate of glycogen depletion during contractile activity in young and old female F344 rats, since blood flow is not impaired in old female rats.

Cartee and Farrar [18] studied the effect of 30 min of treadmill running (at 75% of VO_2max) in young (10 mo) and old (24 mo) male F344 rats. In addition to untrained animals, rats were studied at each age after undergoing an identical endurance-training protocol. Resting gastrocnemius glycogen levels were very similar among the groups. A reduced depletion of muscle glycogen during exercise is a well-documented adaptation to endurance exercise in youth [33], and this experiment demonstrated that this adaptation also occurs in trained, old rats (Figure 4.2).

Interestingly, the amount of gastrocnemius glycogen depletion was similar in the two trained groups. It is important to recognize that during

FIGURE 4.2

Estimated gastrocnemius glycogen depletion during 30 min of treadmill running at 75% of maximal oxygen consumption. YUT, *young untrained;* YT, *young trained;* OUT, *old untrained;* OT, *old trained. Treadmill speeds were 20, 27, 13.8, and 20 m/min in the YUT, YT, OUT, and OT groups, respectively.* Total bar height *equals resting glycogen concentration.* Hatched portion of the bar *equals the glycogen remaining in the muscle postrun.* Open portion of the bar *equals the estimated glycogen depletion (resting glycogen concentration minus postrun glycogen concentration) during the exercise. Drawn from data in Cartee and Farrar [18].*

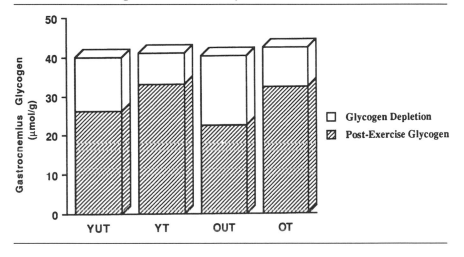

the final bout of exercise, animals were exercising at the same percentage of VO_2max. Despite identical training, VO_2max was lower in the old rats. As a result the old trained (OT) rats ran at a slower treadmill speed (20 m/min) than the young trained (YT) rats (27 m/min) during the final exercise test. Had the OT group also run at 27 m/min, they would have been expected to deplete more gastrocnemius glycogen.

What might account for this greater glycogen depletion in the OT group? It would not be caused by reduced muscle oxidative capacity, since this was very similar in the YT and OT groups (Table 4.1). Serum glucose and FFA levels were also very similar in the YT and OT groups (18, unpublished observation), so delivery of blood-borne substrates would be decreased only if muscle blood flow was reduced. Another possible factor would be changes in the levels of hormones that regulate metabolism. Fleg et al. [35] noted an exaggerated plasma catecholamine response to submaximal exercise by untrained older humans, which would be expected to elicit a greater rate of glycogenolysis, provided there is no change in muscle adrenergic receptors or postreceptor events. The effect of training on blood catecholamine levels during exercise has not been reported for old rats or humans.

TABLE 4.1
Comparison of Markers of Skeletal Muscle Oxidative Capacity in Identically Trained Young and Old Rats

Ages (mo)	Exercise	Muscle	Group	CS (%)	SDH (%)	β-HAD (%)	β-KAT (%)	CytOx (%)	SS Mito (%)	IMF Mito (%)	Palmitate Oxidation (%)	Reference
Y = 10 O = 24	Treadmill running 5d/wk 60 min/d 25m/min 0% grade	Gastrocnemius and Plantaris	YT OUT OT	— — —	— — —	— — —	— — —	— — —	172 106 158	171 70 159	— — —	31
Y = 9 O = 24	Swimming 5d/wk 3h/d	Epitrochlearis	YT OUT OT	121 92 120	139 88 126	121 112 137	152 95 152	— — —	— — —	— — —	— — —	100
Y = 10 O = 24	Treadmill running 5d/wk 60min/d 20m/min 0% grade	Gastrocnemius	YT OUT OT	115 86 121	— — —	101 76 99	— — —	114 81 117	— — —	— — —	123 55 107	17
Y = 6 O = 26	Treadmill running 5d/wk 60min/d 20m/min 6% grade	Plantaris	YT OUT OT	133 85 181	— — —	137 76 157	— — —	— — —	— — —	— — —	— — —	79

Values are expressed as percentages, relative to the young untrained group = 100%. YT, young trained; OUT, old untrained; OT, old trained. CS, citrate synthase; SDH, succinate dehydrogenase; β-HAD, β-hydroxyacyl-CoA dehydrogenase; β-KAT, β-ketoacid-CoA transferase; CytOX, cytochrome oxidase; SS Mito, subsarcolemmal mitochondria; IMF Mito, intermyofibrillar mitochondria.

Nichols and Borer [75] compared quadriceps muscle glycogen utilization of young (3 mo) and old (16–17 mo) female golden hamsters during 60 min of treadmill running at 60% of VO_2max. Although the young animals ran 19% faster than the old hamsters, muscle glycogen depletion was similar in the age groups. Serum catecholamine and muscle triglyceride concentrations were unaffected by age or exercise.

Campbell et al. [14] studied the effect of age (11 vs. 25 mo) on glycogenolysis under conditions where anaerobic metabolism predominates (electrically stimulated contractile activity with occluded blood flow). In the white portion of the gastrocnemius, glycogenolysis and lactate accumulation during contractile activity were greater in the young rats. These results demonstrate that when the age-related decrement in blood flow and oxidative capacity are made irrelevant, aging does not accelerate the rate of glycogenolysis during contractile activity.

Little information is available regarding muscle glycogen in elderly humans. Meredith et al. [72] found that glycogen concentration measured in the vastus lateralis was 61% higher in young (24 yr) than in old (65 yr) sedentary men and women. After 12 wk of endurance training, muscle glycogen levels had increased by 27% but were still less than those in trained young subjects. Hughes et al. [50] also observed an elevation (24%) in muscle glycogen after 12 wk of training by older individuals (62 yr), but the values were still below those typically reported for young people. The age difference in muscle glycogen might be related to a deficit in glucose transport or glycogen synthase activity, but these possibilities have not been tested in humans. Regardless of the mechanism, the lower muscle glycogen concentration would be a disadvantage in endurance-type activity, particularly in older individuals with significant muscle atrophy, where the decrement in the total amount of stored glycogen would exceed the reduction in glycogen concentration.

SKELETAL MUSCLE FATIGUE AND EXERCISE CAPACITY

Is old muscle more easily fatigued than young muscle? Several laboratories have evaluated the effect of age on muscle function, using preparations in which contractile activity was elicited by electrical stimulation. The stimulation protocols commonly used are very demanding, resulting in a 40–80% decrement in tension developed after only 1–4 min [14, 34, 51, 52, 97]. Fitts et al. [34] studied male rats, using a similar in situ stimulation protocol, and reported no age-related difference in the degree of muscle fatigue over the course of 30 min. However, after 1 min of contractile activity, the decrement in developed tension was almost twice as great in the old than in the young rats. Thereafter, the rate of decline was nearly identical for the two groups. Irion et al. [51], using a similar stimulation protocol, found a significantly greater reduction in tension development during electrically stimulated in situ contractile activity in old (24 mo) male, compared with young (12 mo), F344 rats, and all of this decline had occurred during the first min. The same researchers studied female rats of the same ages, using an identical stimulation protocol, and saw no evidence for greater fatigue in the old females [52]. As described above, muscle blood flow during contractile activity was reduced in old male, but not old female, rats.

Several investigators [70, 97] found no effect of age on fatigability of certain muscles (FDL, LOMO, and soleus) in male F344 rats between 6 and 30 mo old. Campbell et al. [14] reported a lower initial tetanic tension in old (25 mo), compared with young (11 mo), male F344 rats, but both ages showed similar relative decreases in tension developed during 60 sec of contractile activity performed with occluded blood flow. Muscle levels for various metabolic parameters commonly cited as potentially relevant to the development of fatigue (glycogen, lactate, ATP, CP) were more profoundly affected in the young animals, suggesting either that old muscle is more susceptible to the fatiguing effects of these parameters or that other parameters contributed to the fatigue.

Brooks and Faulkner [10] determined sustained power (defined as the product of shortening velocity, the average force developed, the train rate, and the duration of the contraction) in situ using the EDL from C57BL/6 mice. This protocol measured sustained power lasting at least 30 min. Sustained power declined between 2 and 12 mo of age and further still between 12 and 26 mo of age. The authors speculated that the reduced power output was secondary to compromised ability to maintain energy balance, which in turn might have been the result of reduced oxidative capacity and/or reduced muscle blood flow.

These in vitro and in situ preparations are useful, but more important are the functional consequences of age and training during physiological exercise. Mazzeo et al. [68] observed a marked and progressive age-related decline in the ability of female F344 rats (3, 12, or 24 mo) to perform a treadmill endurance test (treadmill running at 27 m/min and 15% grade). Physical training (treadmill running at 75% of VO_2max) led to considerable increases in endurance time (300–800%), compared with age-matched controls. Even more impressive, the endurance time for the trained 24-mo-old rats was >3-fold higher than in the untrained 12-mo-old animals. Nonetheless, the 24-mo-old group showed the smallest relative improvement in endurance following training. Rumsey et al. [87] and Farrar et al. [31] began training (treadmill running) rats at 10 and 18 mo of age, respectively. At 22–25 mo of age, however, the old rats in each study had difficulty maintaining the training pace, so the speed had to be reduced. Skeletal muscle function is, of course, only one of many determinants of work capacity, so the failure to maintain exercise capacity, despite continued training, might be caused by changes in other tissues (e.g., the cardiovascular system).

In humans, age reportedly has little effect on muscle endurance during brief (<60 sec) contractile activity at a given relative workload [83]. Because the maximal work capacity is reduced, the older individual cannot sustain exercise at the same absolute workload as long as a younger person. These observations are in agreement with some, but not all, of the studies using rodents. Perhaps the most compelling evidence that physical performance deteriorates in humans with advancing age is the unmistakable fact that world record performances in track and field decline progressively with advancing age [73].

SKELETAL MUSCLE CONTRACTILE PROPERTIES

Since maximal tension development is closely related to muscle CSA, the age-related muscle atrophy leads to a reduction in strength. It seems possible that the decline in strength exceeds the decrease in mass, suggesting that muscle is qualitatively diminished in old age. A great deal of research with rats has indicated that specific isometric tension, expressed as the ratio of tension developed to CSA, is stable across the adult life span. Specific tension was well-maintained in the soleus [34, 70], EDL [34], superficial vastus lateralis [34], FDL [97], plantaris [58], and LOMO [70] of old rats. McCarter and McGee [70] used in vitro preparations; the remaining studies were conducted in situ. Klitgaard et al. [58] found a significant (29%) decrease in the specific tension in the soleus between 9 and 24 months, with no further change at 29 mo. Larsson and Edstrom [64] studied the tibialis anterior (TA) and soleus of young (6 mo) and old (20–24 mo) male rats and found in both muscles from old rats a lower tetanic force-generating capacity expressed per unit muscle weight. The authors attributed this decline to the age-related increase in adipose and connective tissue. Supporting this assertion, when the results were expressed per CSA of the muscle fibers, specific tension was unaffected by age in the TA or soleus. Eddinger et al. [28] found no influence of age (9 vs. 30 mo) on the specific tension determined in vitro for isolated fiber bundles or skinned fibers from the EDL, but an increase in the specific tension of the soleus from old rats with each preparation.

Irion and co-workers found that the capacity of the gastrocnemius-soleus-plantaris muscles to develop isometric tension is well-maintained in old male and female F344 rats [51–52]. Campbell et al. [14], studying the same muscles, found a 28% decline in tetanic tension developed per g of muscle in old (25 mo), compared with young (11 mo), male F344 rats.

Faulkner and colleagues have reported that specific tension measured in situ is not significantly affected by age (2–3, 12–13, and 26–27 mo) in the EDL of male C57BL/6 mice [8, 103]. The same group reported a significant (22%) decrease in the specific tension of EDL measured in vitro in old (26–27 mo), compared with young (2–3 mo), or adult (9–10 mo), mice [8]. They suggested that the in situ measures are less precise, and this lack of precision might account for the failure to detect an age-related decline in specific tension.

Rogers and Evans [83] concluded "the decrease in muscle size with aging can account for much of the reduction in muscle strength," indicating that the muscle does not become "intrinsically weaker with age." The reduction in muscle mass is clearly the dominant reason for reduced strength in humans, but several investigators [60, 94, 99] have noted a significant (15–38%) reduction in specific tension in men. It is possible that some of this difference is accounted for by a reduction in the proportion of muscle that is contractile protein, secondary to increased lipid and connective tissue content. In women, there is little or no decline in specific tension in old age [60, 99].

In studies where age-associated changes in the temporal aspects of contraction have been noted, these changes would contribute to slower movement in the old animals. Several studies have indicated no effect of age on contraction time (CT) for various muscles [28, 70, 97], but there are reports of an increase in CT in muscles from old animals [34, 64]. Brooks and Faulkner [8] found that half-relaxation time (HRT) was lengthened in the soleus but not the EDL of old mice. Fitts et al. [34] reported a longer HRT in the soleus, EDL, and superficial vastus lateralis (SVL) of old rats. Others have observed no effect of age on HRT [64, 70, 97]. There is little or no effect of age on shortening velocity, i.e., Vmax [28, 34, 70, 97]. Walters et al. [97], studying the FDL of rats (6–28 mo), found no evidence for an age-related change in any of the contractile properties measured, demonstrating that reduced function cannot be assumed to occur in every muscle.

The specific tension for the soleus and plantaris from old (24 or 29 mo) strength-trained rats exceeded that of age-matched controls and equaled that of untrained 9-mo-old rats [58]. Soleus HRT of 29-mo-old rats was increased and decreased in strength- and swim-trained rats, respectively [58]. Voluntary wheel running did not affect specific tension of the soleus, EDL, or SVL at any age [34]. The CT was increased in the soleus of old, but not young, runners [34]. The HRT was prolonged in the soleus and SVL of old rats and in the soleus and EDL of young rats. Regardless of age, voluntary running did not alter the V_{max} of any muscle.

Vandervoort and McComas [94] evaluated contractile properties of ankle dorsiflexor and plantarflexor muscles of 111 men and women from 20 to 100 yr of age and found an age-related prolongation of CT and HRT in both muscle groups and both genders. As described above, when an age-related effect on these parameters occurred in rats, it has consistently been in this direction. A 6-mo strength-training program resulted in an increased time to peak tension without altering HRT in the triceps brachii of men aged 65–78 yr [80]. Resistive training by older humans can lead to significant increases in the CSA of the whole muscle (determined with computed tomography) as well as the CSA of individual fibers (determined histologically in biopsy samples). The human studies that have measured the effect of resistance training in older humans have demonstrated that increases in strength (41–174%) greatly exceeded the increases in muscle CSA (8–15%). Human strength is generally assessed by maximal voluntary contractions, where the coordination of muscle and neural processes must be intact. The proportionally larger increases in strength than in muscle size presumably reflect, at least in large part, neural adaptations (recruitment, synchronization, coordination, learning, and neural drive). In contrast, strength is typically measured in anesthetized animals by electrically stimulating the nerve or muscle, so changes in strength indicate adaptations distal to the central nervous system. Klitgaard et al. [60] compared sedentary young (28 yr) and old (69 yr) men with 3 groups of older men (68–70 yr) that had been physically active (swimming, running, or weight lifting) for 12–17 yr before being studied. Specific tension for the quadriceps and elbow flexors decreased in the older sedentary men but not in the older trained groups.

EXERCISE-INDUCED SKELETAL MUSCLE DAMAGE

Most of the previous discussion has centered around apparently beneficial effects of exercise in old age on skeletal muscle. However, one group of researchers has published a series of reports [66, 89] indicating that muscles from old mice are damaged by exercise, based on morphological changes in the t-tubules, sarcoplasmic reticulum, and mitochondria, as well as reductions in the activities of several enzymes (aldolase, superoxide dismutase, and creatine kinase). Some of these studies used an exceptionally mild protocol of motorized treadmill running (30 min/d, 6 d/wk at 3.5 m/min), compared with other training regimens [3] that have been used with mice (60 min/d, 5 d/wk at 28 m/min). A great deal of evidence in rats and humans indicates positive adaptations in skeletal muscle with common forms of exercise training. Nonetheless, there are data suggesting that muscles from old rats and humans are also more susceptible to exercise-induced damage with certain types of contractile activity.

When rats (6–28 mo) underwent tonic electrical stimulation (10 Hz, 8 hr/d) of the tibial nerve for up to 90 d, CSA fibers in the FDL muscle declined regardless of age, but the magnitude of this change was greater in the old animals [98]. Furthermore, specific tension of the FDL was reduced by chronic electrical stimulation only in the old rats.

Faulkner and co-workers have evaluated the effect of age (2–3, 11–12, or 26–27 mo) on skeletal muscle damage in mice [9]. When the EDL was studied after a relatively brief period (5 min) of injurious in situ lengthening contractions, the decline in maximum tetanic force (P_o) measured 10 min or 3 d postinjury was more pronounced in the old than in the 2 younger groups. When the duration of the lengthening contractions was increased to 15 min, mice of all ages developed similar decrements in P_o and fiber number at 3 d postinjury [103]. By 28 d postinjury, muscle mass was significantly reduced only in the old animals. These results suggest a greater susceptibility for contraction-induced muscle injury and an altered time-course for recovery from the injury in old mice.

The replacement and repair of myofibers after injury depends on satellite cells. Gibson and Schultz [38] found that the number of satellite cells declines in the EDL and soleus of rats between 12 and 24 mo. McCormick and Thomas [71] observed that the mitotic activity of satellite cells is doubled in the soleus of endurance-trained (10 wk of treadmill running), old (26–27 mo) rats, compared with age-matched controls. Histological examination revealed that the proportion of damaged fibers increased from 2% in controls to 4% in trained rats. The authors concluded that the level of mitotic activity was appropriate for the small amount of damage. This damage might be a normal part of the response and adaptation to exercise. Since young animals were not included in this study, the effect of age on the susceptibility to exercise-induced damage cannot be evaluated.

Manfredi et al. [67] evaluated muscle damage after eccentric exercise in sedentary young (20–30 yr) and older (59–63 yr) men. Histochemical evaluation of muscle biopsy samples indicated that immediately after exercise, >90% of fibers from older men showed evidence of focal damage, compared with only 5–50% in young men. The authors speculated that the difference might be related to a reduced muscle mass or to the habitually lower level of physical activity in the older men. As described above, old mice are more susceptible to muscle damage after a protocol (in situ lengthening contractions) where reduced mass would not be expected to lead to greater injury [9].

SUMMARY AND CONCLUSIONS

The mass of many weight-bearing muscles declines in old rats, secondary to the atrophy of fibers, particularly of type IIb, with relatively little loss of muscle fibers during most of the adult life span. In humans, muscle atrophy is the result of a combination of progressive fiber loss and fiber atrophy. In both species, the proportion of histochemically determined fiber types is relatively stable across the adult portion of the life span. The loss of strength in old age is predominantly accounted for by reduced muscle mass in humans and rats. Resistance training leads to increased muscle mass and strength in old humans and rats, primarily by increasing fiber CSA. Muscle capillarity is unchanged in old rats but decreases in old dogs. Apparently, capillarity declines in truly sedentary older people. Endurance training enhances capillarity, and old rats and humans can attain levels of capillarity comparable to their active young counterparts, even when performing considerably less exercise. Blood flow during contractile activity is reduced in male rats and humans but not in old female rats or dogs. Oxidative capacity declines in many muscles of sedentary old rats and humans. With endurance training, old individuals from both species attain levels of muscle oxidative capacity quite similar to those in identically training young individuals. Muscle insulin-stimulated glucose transport is enhanced in rats after a bout of exercise, regardless of age. Endurance training elevates muscle GLUT-4 levels in young and middle-aged, but not old, rats, perhaps because the old rats trained at slower treadmill speeds. Middle-aged (47–62 yr) men and women can substantially increase muscle GLUT-4 with relatively brief (12–14 wk) endurance training; older humans (>70–80 yr) have not been studied. Endurance training leads to reduced LDH activity without altering PFK or phosphorylase in old rats and humans. Muscle glycogen depletion, CP depletion, and lactate accumulation during contractile activity are exaggerated in old rats, apparently secondary to reduced muscle oxidative capacity and blood flow. Resting muscle glycogen concentration is diminished in older humans, probably in part because of a more sedentary lifestyle. Although several months of endurance training raises muscle glycogen concentration in older people, it does not restore it to youthful levels. Endurance training can greatly improve endurance in old age, at least in part by the same mechanism originally described in youth, i.e., an increase in muscle oxidative capacity, which contributes to reduced glycogen depletion. Muscles from old individuals appear to be more susceptible to muscle damage by eccentric exercise.

It is apparent that the adaptability of muscle to exercise remains robust even in very old age. The response to exercise and training are generally similar in young and old individuals. At least some of the deterioration of muscles appears to be secondary to disuse. Of particular interest is the identification of several muscles that appear to be highly resistant to age-related decline. Further examination of these muscles, along with muscles known to respond to aging, should offer insight into the age-related changes. The research reviewed has been largely descriptive because that is the nature of most of the currently available information on the topic. Future researchers should benefit from this foundation. Some very important descriptive work remains to be completed, but knowledge and technology have progressed sufficiently to allow more mechanistic experimentation.

ACKNOWLEDGMENTS

Work from the author's laboratory was supported by NIH grant AG10026 and a grant from the American College of Sports Medicine Foundation.

REFERENCES

1. Abu-Erreish, F. H., J. R. Neely, J. T. Whitmer, V. Whitman, and D. R. Sanadi. Fatty acid oxidation by isolated perfused working hearts of aged rats. *Am J. Physiol.* 232:E258–E262, 1977.
2. Alnaqeeb, M. A., and G. Goldspink. Changes in fibre type, number and diameter in developing and ageing skeletal muscle. *J. Anat.* 153:31–45, 1986.
3. Andonian, M. H., and M. A. Fahim. Effects of endurance exercise on the morphology of mouse neuromuscular junctions during ageing. *J. Neurocytol.* 16:589–599, 1987.
4. Ansved, T., and L. Larsson. Effects of ageing on enzyme-histochemical, morphometrical and contractile properties of the soleus muscle in the rat. *J. Neurol. Sci.* 93:105–124, 1989.
5. Ansved, T., and L. Larsson. Quantitative and qualitative morphological properties of the soleus motor nerve and the L5 ventral root in young and old rats. *J. Neurol. Sci.* 96:269–282, 1990.
6. Bastien, C., and J. Sanchez. Phosphagens and glycogen content in skeletal muscle after treadmill training in young and old rats. *Eur. J. Appl. Physiol.* 52:291–295, 1984.
7. Beyer, R. E., J. W. Starnes, D. W. Edington, R. J. Lipton, R. T. Compton III, and M. A. Kwasman. Exercise-induced reversal of age-related declines of oxidative reactions, mitochondrial yield, and flavins in skeletal muscle of the rat. *Mech. Ageing Dev.* 24:309–323, 1984.
8. Brooks, S. V., and J. A. Faulkner. Contractile properties of skeletal muscles from young, adult and aged mice. *J. Physiol.* 404:71–82, 1987.
9. Brooks, S. V., and J. A. Faulkner. Contraction-induced injury: recovery of skeletal muscles in young and old mice. *Am. J. Physiol.* 258:C436–C442, 1990.
10. Brooks, S. V., and J. A. Faulkner. Maximum and sustained power of extensor digitorum longus muscles from young, adult, and old mice. *J. Gerontol. Biol. Sci.* 46:B28–33, 1991.
11. Brown, M. Change in fibre size, not number, in ageing skeletal muscle. *Age and Ageing* 16:244–248, 1987.
12. Brown, M. Resistance exercise effects on aging skeletal muscle in rats. *Phys. Ther.* 69:46–53, 1989.
13. Brown, M., T. P. Ross, and J. O. Holloszy. Effects of ageing and exercise on soleus and extensor digitorum longus muscles of female rats. *Mech. Ageing Dev.* 63:69–77, 1992.
14. Campbell, C. B., D. R. Marsh, and L. L. Spriet. Anaerobic energy provision in aged skeletal muscle during tetanic stimulation. *J. Appl. Physiol.* 70(4):1787–1795, 1991.
15. Carlson, L., S. Froberg, and E. Nye. Effect of age on blood and tissue lipid levels in the male rat. *Gerontologia,* 14:65–79, 1968.
16. Cartee, G. D., C. Briggs-Tung, and E. W. Kietzke. Persistent effects of exercise on skeletal muscle glucose transport across the life-span of rats. *J. Appl. Physiol.* 75:972–978, 1993.
17. Cartee, G. D., and R. P. Farrar. Muscle respiratory capacity and $\dot{V}O_2$max in identically trained young and old rats. *J. Appl. Physiol.* 63:257–261, 1987.
18. Cartee, G. D., and R. P. Farrar. Exercise training induces glycogen sparing during exercise by old rats. *J. Appl. Physiol.* 64:259–265, 1988.
19. Cartee, G. D., D. A. Young, M. D. Sleeper, J. Zierath, H. Wallberg-Henriksson, and J. O. Holloszy. Prolonged increase in insulin-stimulated glucose transport in muscle after exercise. *Am. J. Physiol.* 256:E494–E499, 1989.
20. Chasiotis, D. The reguation of glycogen phosphorylase and glycogen breakdown in human skeletal muscle. *Acta Physiol. Scand. Suppl.* 518:1–68, 1983.
21. Coggan, A. R., R. J. Spina, D. S. King, et al. Histochemical and enzymatic comparison of the gastrocnemius muscle of young and elderly men and women. *J. Gerontol. Biol. Sci.* 46:B71–76, 1992.
22. Coggan, A. R., R. J. Spina, D. S. King, et al. Skeletal muscle adaptations to endurance training in 60- to 70-yr-old men and women. *J. Appl. Physiol.* 72:1780–1786, 1992.
23. Coggan, A. R., R. J. Spina, M. A. Rogers, et al. Histochemical and biochemical characteristics of skeletal muscle in master athletes. *J. Appl. Physiol.* 68:1896–1901, 1990.

24. Dall'Aglio, E., H. Chang, G. M. Reaven, and S. Azhar. Age-related changes in rat muscle glycogen synthase activity. *J. Gerontol.* 42:168–172, 1987.
25. Daw, C. K., J. W. Starnes, and T. P. White. Muscle atrophy and hypoplasia with aging: impact of training and food restriction. *J. Appl. Physiol.* 64:2428–2432, 1988.
26. DeFronzo, R. A., E. Jacot, E. Jequier, E. Maeder, J. Wahren, and J. P. Felber. The effect of insulin on the disposal of intravenous glucose. *Diabetes.* 30:1000–1007, 1981.
27. Dudley, G. A., and S. J. Fleck. Metabolite changes in aged muscle during stimulation. *J. Gerontol.* 39:183–186, 1984.
28. Eddinger, T. J., R. G. Cassens, and R. L. Moss. Mechanical and histochemical characterization of skeletal muscles from senescent rats. *Am. J. Physiol.* 251:C421–C430, 1986.
29. Eddinger, T. J., R. L. Moss, and R. G. Cassens. Fiber number and type composition in extensor digitorum longus, soleus, and diaphragm muscles with aging in Fisher 344 rats. *J. Histochem. Cytochem.* 33:1033–1041, 1985.
30. Edstrom, L., and L. Larsson. Effects of age on contractile and enzyme-histochemical properties of fast- and slow-twitch single motor units in the rat. *J. Physiol.* 392:129–145, 1987.
31. Farrar, R. P., T. P. Martin, and C. M. Ardies. The interaction of aging and endurance exercise upon the mitochondrial function of skeletal muscle. *J. Gerontol.* 36:642–647, 1981.
32. Faulkner, J. A., S. V. Brooks, and E. Zerba. Skeletal muscle weakness and fatigue in old age: Underlying mechanisms. X. V. J. Cristofalo and M. P. Lawton (eds). *Annual Review of Gerontology and Geriatrics.* New York:Springer, 1990, pp. 147–166.
33. Fitts, R. H., F. W. Booth, W. W. Winder, and J. O. Holloszy. Skeletal muscle respiratory capacity, endurance, and glycogen utilization. *Am. J. Physiol.* 228:1029–1033, 1975.
34. Fitts, R. H., J. P. Troup, F. A. Witzmann, and J. O. Holloszy. The effect of ageing and exercise on skeletal muscle function. *Mech. Ageing Dev.* 27:161–172, 1984.
35. Fleg, J. L., S. P. Tzankoff, and E. G. Lakatta. Age-related augmentation of plasma catecholamines during dynamic exercise in healthy males. *J. Appl. Physiol.* 59:1033–1039, 1985.
36. Florini, J. R. Effect of aging on skeletal muscle composition and function. *Rev. Biol. Res. Aging* 3:337–358, 1987.
37. Florini, J. R., and D. Z. Ewton. Skeletal muscle fiber types and myosin ATPase activity do not change with growth hormone administration. *J. Gerontol. Biol. Sci.* 44:B110–117, 1989.
38. Gibson, M. C., and E. Schultz. Age-related differences in absolute numbers of skeletal muscle satellite cells. *Muscle Nerve* 6:574–580, 1983.
39. Goodman, M. N., S. M. Dluz, M. A. McElaney, E. Belur, and N. B. Ruderman. Glucose uptake and insulin sensitivity in rat muscle: changes during 3–96 weeks of age. *Am. J. Physiol.* 244:E93–E100, 1983.
40. Gosselin, L. E., M. Betlach, A. C. Vailas, and D. P. Thomas. Training-induced alterations in young and senescent rat diaphragm muscle. *J. Appl. Physiol.* 72:1506–1511, 1992.
41. Grimby, G., B. Danneskiold-Samsoe, K. Hvid, and B. Saltin. Morphology and enzymatic capacity in arm and leg muscles in 78–81 year old men and women. *Acta Physiol. Scand.* 115:125–134, 1982.
42. Gulve, E. A., E. J. Henriksen, K. J. Rodnick, J. H. Youn, and J. O. Holloszy. Glucose transporters and glucose transport in skeletal muscles of 1- to 25-mo-old rats. *Am. J. Physiol.* 264:E319–E327, 1993.
43. Gulve, E. A., K. J. Rodnick, E. J. Henriksen, and J. O. Holloszy. Effects of wheel running on glucose transporter (glut4) concentration in skeletal muscle of young adult and old rats. *Mech. Ageing Dev.* 67:187–200, 1993.
44. Gutmann, E. Muscle. C. E. Finch and L. Hayflick (eds.). *Handbook of the Biology of Aging.* New York: Van Nostrand Reinhold, 1977, pp. 445–469.
45. Hansford, R. G., and F. Castro. Age-linked changes in activity of enzymes for the tricarboxylate cycle and lipid oxidation, and of carnitine content, in muscles of the rat. *Mech. Ageing Dev.* 19:191–201, 1982.

46. Haidet, G. C., and D. Parsons. Reduced exercise capacity in senescent beagles: an evaluation of the periphery. *Am. J. Physiol.* 260:H173–H182, 1991.

47. Holloszy, J. O., M. Chen, G. D. Cartee, and J. C. Young. Skeletal muscle atrophy in old rats: differential changes in the three fiber types. *Mech. Ageing Dev.* 60:199–213, 1991.

48. Houmard, J. A., P. C. Egan, P. D. Neufer, J. E. Friedman, W. S. Wheeler, et al. Elevated skeletal muscle glucose transporter levels in exercise-trained middle-aged men. *Am. J. Physiol.* 261:E437–E443, 1991.

49. Houmard, J. A., M. H. Shinebarger, P. L. Nolan, et al. Exercise training increases GLUT-4 protein concentration in previously sedentary middle-aged men. *Am. J. Physiol.* 27:E896–E901, 1993.

50. Hughes, V. A., M. A. Fiatarone, R. A, Fielding, et al. Exercise increases muscle GLUT-4 levels and insulin action in subjects with impaired glucose tolerance. *Am. J. Physiol.* 27:E855–E862, 1993.

51. Irion, G. L., U. S. Vasthare, and R. F. Tuma. Age-related change in skeletal muscle blood flow in the rat. *J. Gerontol.* 42:660–665, 1987.

52. Irion, G. L., U. S. Vasthare, and R. F. Tuma. Preservation of skeletal muscle hyperemic response to contraction with aging in female rats. *Exp. Gerontol.* 23:183–188, 1988.

53. Jennekens, F. G. I., B. E. Tomlinson, and J. N. Walton. Histochemical aspects of five limb muscles in old age. *J. Neurol. Sci.* 14:259–276, 1971.

54. Kanda, K., and K. Hashizume. Changes in properties of the medial gastrocnemius motor units in aging rats. *J. Neurophysiol.* 61:737–746, 1989.

55. Kern, M., P. L. Dolan, R. S. Mazzeo, J. A. Wells, and G. L. Dohm. Effect of aging and exercise on GLUT-4 glucose transporters in muscle. *Am. J. Physiol.* 263:E362–E367, 1992.

56. Klip, A., and M. Paquet. Glucose transport and glucose transporters in muscle and their metabolic regulation. *Diabetes Care* 13:228–2243, 1990.

57. Klitgaard, H. A model for quantitative strength training of hindlimb muscles of the rat. *J. Appl. Physiol.* 64:1740–1745, 1988.

58. Klitgaard, H., R. Marc, A. Brunet, H. Vandewalle, and H. Monod. Contractile properties of old rat muscles: effect of increased use. *J. Appl. Physiol.* 67:1401–1408, 1989.

59. Klitgaard, H., A. Brunet, B. Maton, C. Lamaziere, C. Lesty, and H. Monod. Morphological and biochemical changes in old rat muscles: effect of increased use. *J. Appl. Physiol.* 67:1409–1417, 1989.

60. Klitgaard, H., M. Mantoni, S. Schiaffino, et al. Function, morphology and protein expression of ageing skeletal muscle: a cross-sectional study of elderly men with different training backgrounds. *Acta Physiol. Scand.* 140:41–45, 1990.

61. Kovanen, B. Effects of ageing and physical training on rat skeletal muscle. *Acta. Physiol. Scand.* 135 (Suppl. 577):1–56, 1989.

62. Larsson, L., T. Ansved, L. Edstrom, L. Gorza, and S. Schiaffino. Effects of age on physiological immunohistochemical and biochemical properties of fast-twitch single motor units in the rat. *J. Physiol.* 443:257–275, 1991.

63. Larsson, L., D. Biral, M. Campione, and S. Schiaffino. An age-related type IIB to IIX myosin heavy chain switching in rat skeletal muscle. *Acta Physiol. Scand.* 147:227–234, 1993.

64. Larsson, L., and L. Edstrom. Effects of age on enzyme-histochemical fibre spectra and contractile properties of fast- and slow-twitch skeletal muscles in the rat. *J. Neurol. Sci.* 76:69–89, 1986.

65. Lexell, J., C. C. Taylor, and M. Sjostrom. What is the cause of the ageing atrophy? Total number, size and proportion of different fiber types studied in whole vastus lateralis muscle from 15- to 83-year-old men. *J. Neurol. Sci.* 84:275–294, 1988.

66. Ludatscher, R., M. Silbermann, D. Gershon, and A. Reznick. The effects of enforced running on the gastrocnemius muscle in aging mice: an ultrastructural study. *Exp. Gerontol.* 18:113–123, 1983.

67. Mandfredi, T. G., R. A. Fielding, K. P. O'Reilly, C. N. Meredith, H. Y. Lee, and W. J. Evans. Plasma creatine kinase activity and exercise-induced muscle damage in older men. *Med. Sci. Sports Exerc.,* 23:1028–1034, 1991.

68. Mazzeo, R. S., G. A. Brooks, and S. M. Horvath. Effects of age on metabolic responses to endurance training in rats. *J. Appl. Physiol.* 57:1369–1374, 1984.
69. McCarter, R. J. M. Age-related changes in skeletal muscle function. *Aging* 2:27–38, 1990.
70. McCarter, R., and J. McGee. Influence of nutrition and aging on the composition and function of rat skeletal muscle. *J. Gerontol.* 42:432–441, 1987.
71. McCormick, K. M., and D. P. Thomas. Exercise-induced satellite cell activation in senescent soleus muscle. *J. Appl. Physiol.* 72:888–893, 1992.
72. Meredith, C. N., W. R. Frontera, E. C. Fisher, et al. Peripheral effects of endurance training in young and old subjects. *J. Appl. Physiol.* 66:2844–2949, 1989.
73. Moore, D. H. A study of age group track and field records to related age and running speed. *Nature* 253:264–265, 1975.
74. National Research Council. *Mammalian Models for Research on Aging.* Washington, D. C.: National Academy, 1981, pp. 75–81.
75. Nichols, J. F., and K. T. Borer. The effects of age on substrate depletion and hormonal responses during submaximal exercise in hamsters. *Physiol. Behav.* 41:1–6, 1987.
76. Nishimura, H., H. Kuzuya, M. Okamoto, et al. Change of insulin action with aging in conscious rats determined by euglycemic clamp. *Am. J. Physiol.* 254:E92–98, 1988.
77. Örlander, J., and A. Aniansson. Effects of physical training on skeletal muscle metabolism and ultrastructure in 70 to 75-year-old men. *Acta Physiol. Scand.* 109:149–154, 1980.
78. Parízkova, J., E. Eiselt, S. Sprynarova, and M. Wachtlova. Body composition, aerobic capacity, and density of muscle capillaries in young and old men. *J. Appl. Physiol.* 31:323–325, 1971.
79. Powers, S. K., J. Lawler, D. Criswell, F. Lieu, and D. Martin. Aging and respiratory muscle metabolic plasticity: effects of endurance training. *J. Appl. Physiol.* 72:1068–1073, 1992.
80. Rice, C. L., D. A. Cunningham, D. H. Paterson, and J. R. Dickinson. Strength training alters contractile properties of the triceps brachii in men aged 65–78 years. *Eur. J. Appl. Physiol.* 66:275–280, 1993.
81. Rodnick, K. J., E. J. Henriksen, D. F. James, and J. O. Holloszy. Exercise training, glucose transporters, and glucose transport in rat skeletal muscles. *Am. J. Physiol.* 262:C9–C14, 1992.
82. Rodnick, K. J., G. M. Reaven, W. L. Haskell, C. R. Sims, and C. E. Mondon. Variations in running activity and enzymatic adaptations in voluntary running rats. *J. Appl. Physiol.* 66:1250–1257, 1989.
83. Rogers, M.A., and W. J. Evans. Changes in skeletal muscle with aging: effects of exercise training. XXI. J. O. Holloszy (ed). *Exercise and Sports Science Reviews.* Baltimore: Williams & Wilkins, 1993, pp. 65–102.
84. Rosenheimer, J. Effects of chronic stress and exercise on age-related changes in end-plate architecture. *J. Neurophysiol.* 53:1582–1589, 1985.
85. Rowe, J. W., K. L. Minaker, J. A. Pallotta, and J. S. Flier. Characterization of the insulin resistance of aging. *J. Clin. Invest.* 71:1581–1587, 1983.
86. Rowett, H. G. Q. *The Rat as a Small Mammal.* London: John Murray, 1965, p. 85.
87. Rumsey, W. L., Z. V. Kendrick, and J. W. Starnes. Bioenergetics in the aging Fischer 344 rat: effects of exercise and food restriction. *Exp. Gerontol.* 22:271–287, 1987.
88. Sanchez, J., C. Bastien, and H. Monod. Enzymatic adaptations to treadmill training in skeletal muscle of young and old rats. *Eur. J. Appl. Physiol.* 52:69–74, 1983.
89. Steinhagen-Thiessen, A., Z. Reznick, and H. Hilz. Negative adaptation to physical training in senile mice. *Mech. Ageing and Dev.* 12:231–236, 1980.
90. Stebbins, C. L., E. Schultz, R. Smith, and E. L. Smith. Effects of chronic exercise during aging on muscle and end-plate morphology in rats. *J. Appl. Physiol.* 58:45–51, 1985.
91. Suominen, H., and E. Heikkinen. Enzyme activities in muscle and connective tissue of m. vastus lateralis in habitually training and sedentary 33 to 70-year-old men. *Eur. J. Appl. Physiol.* 34:249–254, 1975.
92. Terjung, R. L. Muscle fiber involvement during training of different intensities and durations. *Am. J. Physiol.* 230:946–950, 1976.

93. Tomanek, R. J., and Y. K. Woo. Compensatory hypertrophy of the plantaris muscle in relation to age. *J. Gerontol.* 25:23–29, 1970.

94. Vandervoort, A. A., and A. J. McComas. Contractile changes in opposing muscles of the human ankle joint with aging. *J. Appl. Physiol.* 61:361–367, 1986.

95. Wahren, J., B. Satlin, L. Jorfeldt, and B. Pernow. Influence of age on the local circulatory adaptation to leg exercise. *Scand. J. Clin. Lab. Invest.* 33:79–86, 1974.

96. Walford R. L. When is a mouse old? *J. Immunol.* 117:352–353, 1976.

97. Walters, T. J., H. L. Sweeney, and R. P. Farrar. Aging does not affect contractile properties of type IIb FDL muscle in Fischer 344 rats. *Am. J. Physiol.* 258:C1031–C1035, 1990.

98. Walters, T. J., H. L. Sweeney, and R. P. Farrar. Influence of electrical stimulation on fast-twitch muscle in aging rats. *J. Appl. Physiol.* 71:1921–1928, 1991.

99. Young, A., M. Stokes, and M. Crowe. The size and strength of the quadriceps muscles of old and young men. *Clin. Physiol.* 5:145–154, 1985.

100. Young, J. C., M. Chen, and J. O. Holloszy. Maintenance of the adaptation of skeletal muscle mitochondria to exercise in old rats. *Med. Sci. Sports Exerc.* 15:243–246, 1983.

101. Yu, B. P., E. J. Masoro, and C. A. McMahan. Nutritional influences on aging of Fischer 344 rats I. Physical, metabolic, and longevity characteristics. *J. Gerontol.* 40:657–670, 1985.

102. Yu, B. P., E. J. Masoro, I. Murata, J. A. Bertrand, and F. T. Lynd. Life span study of SPF Fischer 344 male rats fed ad libitum or restricted diets: longevity, growth, lean body mass and disease. *J. Gerontol.* 37:130–141, 1982.

103. Zerba, E., T. E. Komorowski, and J.A. Faulkner. Free radical injury in skeletal muscles of young, adult, and old mice. *Am. J. Physiol.* 258:C429–C435, 1990.

104. Ziel, F. H., N. Venkatesan, and M. B. Davidson. Glucose transport is rate limiting for skeletal muscle metabolism in normal and STZ-induced diabetic rats. *Diabetes.* 37:885–890, 1988.

5
The Potential Role of Physical Activity in the Prevention of Non-Insulin-Dependent Diabetes Mellitus: The Epidemiological Evidence

ANDREA M. KRISKA, Ph.D.
STEVEN N. BLAIR, P.E.D.
MARK A. PEREIRA, M.S.

The purpose of this chapter is to evaluate epidemiological evidence related to the hypothesis that physical activity influences the development of non-insulin-dependent diabetes mellitus (NIDDM). Specifically, after it is briefly acknowledged that such a causal relationship between physical activity and NIDDM is biologically plausible and coherent with physiological knowledge provided by metabolic research, the existing epidemiological studies that examine this issue are presented. Included are specific discussions regarding whether or not the relationship between inactivity and NIDDM differs between males and females and whether this relationship depends upon the intensity of the activity. This chapter also includes a section covering specific issues concerning the development of a physical activity intervention program for the purpose of preventing or delaying the onset of NIDDM.

The reader is referred to a review paper "An Epidemiological Perspective of the Relationship Between Physical Activity and NIDDM: From Activity Assessment to Intervention" [49] to supplement the information provided here.

DEFINITION AND DIAGNOSIS OF NIDDM

NIDDM is the most common type of diabetes, accounting for 90–95% of all diabetic cases in the United States. Based upon national self-reported survey data, the annual incidence rate is 32 cases/10,000 per year in individuals aged 20 or older [21]. This translates to about 500,000 new cases annually. With a total of 2.5–3.4% of United States adults having NIDDM diagnosed by a physician, the population estimate for the disease amounts to 5.8 million people. Unfortunately, this number does not include the estimated 4–5 million undiagnosed cases of NIDDM in the general population, because the individual with NIDDM often does not display symptoms at the onset of the disease [26, 27]. The undiagnosed cases become a major issue when examining diabetes in relation to potential risk factors.

Depending upon the population studied and the definition of obesity, an estimated 60–90% of NIDDM patients are obese at disease onset [66]. NIDDM is also more prevalent in older age groups, with an incidence that increases with advancing age [21, 69]. Survival rates in individuals with NIDDM are generally lower than those of similarly aged nondiabetic individuals, with the magnitude of difference in the survival rates varying, depending upon the number of years since diagnosis of the disease, age at diagnosis, gender, and the population in question [26].

Diagnosis of NIDDM is typically based upon an oral glucose tolerance test (OGTT) in which the venous plasma glucose concentrations are determined after an overnight fast and two hours after ingestion of a 75-gram carbohydrate load [92]. Diabetes is diagnosed if the two-hour postload plasma glucose concentration is at least 11.1 mmol/liter [92]. Individuals with postload glucose responses of 7.8–11.1 mmol/liter are considered to have impaired glucose tolerance. Impaired glucose tolerance is predictive of diabetes development, although its presence does not guarantee disease development [35, 38, 77].

BIOLOGICAL PLAUSIBILITY OF A CAUSAL RELATIONSHIP BETWEEN PHYSICAL ACTIVITY AND NIDDM

NIDDM is actually considered to be a heterogeneous group of disorders with two major subgroups, obese and nonobese [3]. The former is much more prevalent and forms the basis for most of the research in the field.

The major factors thought to be involved in the pathogenesis of NIDDM as a whole are obesity (and more recently, fat distribution), insulin resistance/sensitivity, insulin secretion, and hepatic glucose production. Little is known about the natural history of "nonobese" NIDDM, although it is thought that environmental components play a much weaker role than genetic factors in predicting disease onset for this type of NIDDM. (For a comprehensive epidemiological review of the pathogenesis of NIDDM, see Bennett et al., [3]).

Insulin resistance (or hyperinsulinemia) is thought to be the most likely candidate for the hypothetical primary defect of "obese" NIDDM, since hyperinsulinemia [78, 82] and insulin resistance [9] predict the development of impaired glucose tolerance among those with normal glucose tolerance. Although obesity and fat distribution (specifically, the distribution of body fat in the central rather than the peripheral regions, commonly determined by comparing waist to hip or waist to thigh circumferences or subscapular to tricep skinfolds) have also been shown to be related to glucose intolerance [6, 7, 18, 23, 28, 43, 44, 63, 68, 83], these conditions alone are not enough to cause NIDDM [3].

Early observations were made that athletes had lower plasma glucose and insulin levels in response to a glucose load than nonathletes [60]. Later metabolic studies demonstrated an effect of physical activity on carbohydrate metabolism and glucose tolerance, mainly through its influence on insulin sensitivity/resistance [5, 33, 46, 88]. In fact, physical activity may be most influential in regards to the progression of NIDDM at earlier stages of glucose intolerance, under conditions in which insulin resistance appears to be the major cause of the abnormal glucose tolerance [32]. In support of this, training studies with small sample sizes, examining the effect of activity in individuals with mild glucose intolerance, have suggested a positive role for physical activity in preventing NIDDM, through its beneficial influence on glucose tolerance and insulin sensitivity [51, 58, 76, 79, 80, 86].

Physical activity is also inversely associated with obesity and central fat distribution, and recent studies demonstrate that physical training can reduce both parameters [4, 10, 15, 52]. Thus, physical activity may also prevent or delay NIDDM by decreasing the deposition of total fat or specifically intra-abdominal fat.

Therefore, the metabolic literature supports the hypothesis that physical activity can influence glucose intolerance directly through altered sensitivity to insulin or indirectly through prevention of obesity or centrally distributed body fat. Whether or not the epidemiological literature agrees with this hypothesis is addressed below.

ASSESSMENT OF PHYSICAL ACTIVITY IN EPIDEMIOLOGICAL STUDIES

Physical activity is a very complex behavior that has been measured in a variety of ways [55]. This complexity can be partially explained by the fact that there are several health-related components of physical activity, such as overall caloric expenditure, aerobic intensity, weight bearing, flexibility, and strength [12]. Examining the relationship between physical activity and a disease or condition requires focusing on the component(s) of physical activity that is most likely to be associated with the outcome of interest.

The physical activity survey is typically the method of choice for population studies. Reasons for its popularity include its nonreactiveness (lack of alteration of the individual's behavior as a direct result of the assessment technique), practicality (generally determined by cost and participant convenience), applicability (ability to modify the instrument to suit the population in question), and its acceptable accuracy (both reliability and validity) relative to other methods [55, 65]. More objective measurements of energy expenditure, such as the activity monitor, the graded exercise test, or the doubly labeled water technique, are not practical in most epidemiological studies but have been used to validate the physical activity questionnaire [55, 65].

The survey approaches used to measure physical activity vary from activity diaries to self-administered or interviewer-administered activity questionnaires. The time frame and complexity of the activity question-naire can range from a single question about usual activity to a recall survey with a time frame of one week, one year, or even a lifetime [29, 55, 65]. The advantages of assessing activity by using a survey with a short time frame are that the estimate is easier to validate and less likely to suffer from recall bias. In contrast, assessment over a short time period is less likely to reflect "usual" behavior, as activity levels may vary with season, as a result of an acute health condition, or because of sudden time pressures.

One activity questionnaire that is currently being used in epidemiology research around the world, such as the Pima Indian Study [1], the Strong Heart Study [56], and studies of diabetes in the South Pacific [95] and Mauritius [17], is the Pima Physical Activity Questionnaire [49]. This questionnaire is comprehensive in that it assesses current (past year and past week) occupational and leisure activities, as well as extreme levels of inactivity due to disability. It's original version [48] also assessed historical (over a lifetime) physical activity, which has been used for retrospective studies. (A copy of this questionnaire along with instructions for its administration and summary calculations is provided in Kriska and Bennett [49]).

Physical activities assessed by questionnaire are usually limited to those that require an energy expenditure above that of daily living. The assumption is that the activities of daily living, such as bathing or feeding, are similar among most individuals within the population and that accurate measurement of such typical activities shared by all participants is not feasible or necessary. Likewise, two important components of total energy expenditure, basal metabolic rate and the thermic effect of food [74], are obviously not taken into consideration when assessing activity levels by this method. Therefore, the physical activity estimates obtained by activity questionnaire do not reflect total energy expenditure for a particular individual. Determination of total energy expenditure can only be obtained by more exact measures such as the respiratory chamber or the doubly labeled water technique [73]. However, the estimates obtained by the activity questionnaire are valuable in relative terms and can be used to rank individuals or groups of subjects within a population from the least to the most active. The result is a relative distribution of individuals, based upon their reported levels of physical activity, which can then be examined in relation to physiological parameters (such as postload glucose or insulin values) and disease outcome (such as the development or occurrence of NIDDM).

EPIDEMIOLOGICAL STUDIES OF PHYSICAL ACTIVITY AND NIDDM

Early Observations

Some of the earliest suggestions that physical activity may be associated with NIDDM originated from observations that societies that had abandoned their traditional way of life had experienced major increases in NIDDM [90]. Further evidence of this association came from studies that examined the effect of environmental change such as migration or modernization on the health status of a population.

Migration studies found that individuals who left their homeland and migrated to a more westernized environment developed more NIDDM than those who remained in their native land [25, 37, 75]. For example, a migration study by Kawate et al. [37] compared Japanese living in Hiroshima with those who migrated to Hawaii. Despite the similar genetic background, the prevalence of diabetes was almost two times higher, after adjusting for age, sex, and obesity, in Japanese Hawaiians than in those in Hiroshima. Crudely classifying individuals according to their preretirement levels of occupational physical activity (Fig. 5.1) showed that more Japanese females and males than Hawaiian individuals had engaged in moderate/ heavy work. This suggested that the difference in occupational physical activity levels between these two populations might have partially accounted for the difference in diabetes prevalence.

Studies of the consequences of habitation in a rural, compared with an urban, environment also support the hypothesis of a protective effect of a more active lifestyle [14, 40, 93, 94]. In Kiribati, a Central Pacific nation, the age-standardized prevalence of diabetes in urban residents was more than twice that of rural residents [39]. The urban sample was also less physically active (based upon a crude four-point activity scale) than their rural counterparts for each age and sex group, suggesting that the difference in prevalence of diabetes between the two might be at least partially due to differences in physical activity levels.

Extreme Inactivity Studies

An increase in NIDDM was observed in persons with extreme levels of inactivity. Lipman et al. [59] demonstrated that induced inactivity, consisting of 35 days of absolute bed rest in eight healthy young males, caused a decrease in glucose tolerance. This decrease, however, was less severe in those permitted one hour of vigorous supine exercise per day.

This same phenomenon was observed cross-sectionally, in the finding that glucose and insulin values during an oral glucose tolerance test (OGTT) were higher in both spinal cord–injured diabetic and nondiabetic

FIGURE 5.1

Levels of occupational physical activity during preretirement years in males and females from Hiroshima and Hawaii. (Adapted from Kawate et al. 1979 [37].)

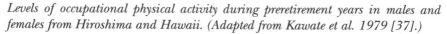
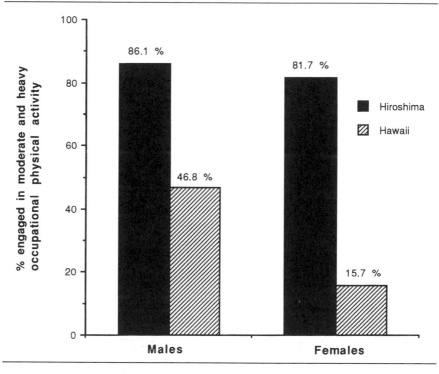

patients than in age-matched controls [19]. Among the spinal cord–injured patients, those with diabetes had the cord lesion for a longer time than those with a normal OGTT. The author suggested that a potential explanation for the effect of duration of cord lesion on glucose tolerance is that muscle wasting increases as duration of the lesion increases.

Similarly, diabetes mortality in army veterans suffering from limb amputation was higher than diabetes mortality in veterans who lost part of the hand or foot or who had a disfigurement without loss of a body part [34]. The physical activity of the veterans with an amputation would be involuntarily lowered below that of the other groups, supporting an association between inactivity and diabetes.

Cross-Sectional and Retrospective Studies of Diabetes and Physical Activity
In general, most cross-sectional and retrospective findings demonstrate a significant relationship between physical activity and NIDDM development. A brief summary of the findings from the epidemiological literature as well as an example of each type of study design is presented below.

Cross-sectional studies collect information about the health outcome (glucose intolerance or NIDDM) and the potential risk factor (physical inactivity) at the same time within the same group. This type of epidemiological design is limited, because it is not possible to establish causality (i.e., did inactivity cause the glucose intolerance or did the condition cause the inactivity?).

For example, in a cross-sectional study, Dowse et al. [18] examined the prevalence of glucose intolerance by level of physical activity in 5080 individuals from the island nation of Mauritius. Physical activity was determined by a trained interviewer and was based upon reported levels of both occupational and leisure activity. The prevalence of both impaired glucose tolerance and NIDDM was higher in the inactive than in the active, for both males and females of all major ethnic groups (Table 5.1). This relationship remained significant in many of the gender-ethnic groups after stratifying (low, medium, high) by either body mass index or fat distribution estimated by waist-to-hip ratio [18]. The observation that this relationship exists both in those individuals with impaired glucose tolerance and in those with diagnosed NIDDM strengthens the possibility that activity affected the disease rather than the disease influencing the activity levels.

Most other studies that have examined the association between diabetes presence and inactivity report similar results. Groups of individuals with NIDDM are usually found to be less currently active than those without the disease [39, 50, 84, 85]. Likewise, cross-sectional studies that examine the continuous relationship between physical activity and postload glucose values (determined by an OGTT) in nondiabetic individuals generally show that postload glucose [13, 18, 50, 57, 81, 89] and insulin values [18, 57, 89] are significantly higher in those less active. However, these results are not consistent across all subgroups within a population [18, 40, 50] or across all studies [36, 64].

TABLE 5.1
Crude Prevalence of NIDDM and IGT by Total Physical Activity Level*

		Hindu		Muslim		Creole		Chinese	
		Male	Female	Male	Female	Male	Female	Male	Female
NIDDM	Active	10.2	4.5	7.1	7.7	4.1	10.5	13.0	8.1
	Inactive	19.3	12.2	16.7	14.1	13.2	15.8	21.4	14.6
IGT	Active	11.1	12.9	7.1	11.5	8.9	12.3	10.1	18.9
	Inactive	15.5	21.0	15.3	19.9	24.0	21.3	22.1	20.7

*The physical activity index is a combination of reported leisure and occupational physical activity.
Adapted from Dowse, G. K., P. Z. Zimmet, H. Gareeboo, K. G. M. M. Alberti, J. Tuomilehto, et al. Abdominal obesity and physical inactivity are risk factors for NIDDM and impaired glucose tolerance in Indian, Creole, and Chinese Mauritians. *Diabetes Care* 14:271–282, 1991.

In case-control (or retrospective) studies, individuals with and without diabetes are asked questions about their past, particularly their exposure to the specific risk factor in question (physical activity level). Although this type of study design is valuable in cases where the disease outcome is rare, it does suffer from potential recall bias, in which the diseased or high-risk individual may remember or recall past events differently.

FIGURE 5.2
Physical activity recall over a lifetime.

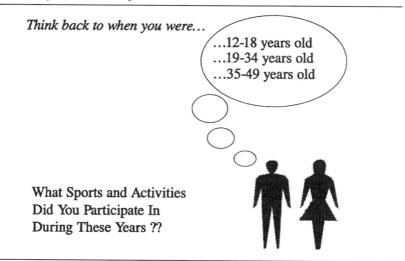

For example, in one retrospective study individuals over the age of 37 were asked to recall being a teenager (12–18 years of age), a young adult (19–34 years of age), or a middle-aged adult (35–49 years of age) and then estimate their participation in various popular sports and leisure activities during each time period [50]. Although the short-term reproducibility of this method was shown to be good [48], because of the extreme potential for recall bias, physical activity was handled as a dichotomous variable (low/high activity levels) in these analyses. As shown in Figure 5.3, both males and females with diabetes reported less physical activity over their lifetime than those individuals without diabetes. This relationship between reported physical activity as a teenager or as an adult and NIDDM remained significant after controlling for age, body mass index, fat distribution, parental history, and current levels of physical activity.

Most of the cross-sectional and retrospective studies that have examined this question found a significant negative relationship between physical activity and diabetes. One of the limitations of these types of study designs is that they prohibit any assumption of a causal relationship. In other words, with a cross-sectional or retrospective design, it can be concluded that physical activity and diabetes are significantly associated. However, whether

FIGURE 5.3

Reported historical (over a lifetime) leisure physical activity in diabetic and nondiabetic Pima Indian males (left) and females (right) aged 37–59 years. (Adapted from Kriska et al., 1993[50].)

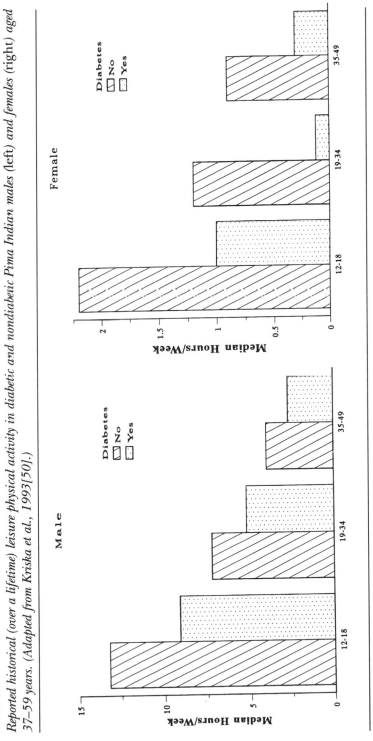

physical inactivity is causing the diabetes or whether diabetes is influencing the inactivity or the reporting of the inactivity cannot be differentiated by this type of study design. In contrast, prospective studies provide stronger evidence of a casual relationship between activity and glucose intolerance or NIDDM.

Prospective Studies of NIDDM and Physical Activity

The most powerful observational study design is the prospective or longitudinal study. This design identifies and follows individuals initially free of the health outcome of interest (diabetes) and seeks to establish whether initial physical activity levels differentiate those who do and do not subsequently develop the disease. Because of the sample size that is often required to carry out this study and the length of time that the participants need to be followed, this study design is usually the most costly of the observational study designs. Four of the most recent prospective studies examining the relationship between physical inactivity and development of non-insulin-dependent diabetes mellitus are described below.

Frisch et al. [22]. In support of the potential importance of historical physical activity to occurrence of diabetes, Frisch [22] reported that for most age groups, women college alumni who were former college athletes had lower rates of diabetes after age 20 than nonathletes. The criterion for athletic status in this study was belonging to at least one varsity, house, or other intramural team for at least one year or achieving some athletic distinction such as receiving a college letter. Also included in the athletic category were those individuals who were not on a team but trained regularly (e.g., running at least 2 miles per day for 5 days per week [22]). Nevertheless, since more former athletes than nonathletes claimed to be currently exercising regularly and were estimated to be leaner, the potential effect of current activity and body fat on diabetes outcome cannot be discounted.

Helmrich et al. [31]. The physical activity levels of 5990 male University of Pennsylvania alumni were measured in 1962 and examined again, along with the development of NIDDM, 14 years later [31]. All men who attended the university between 1928 and 1947 and completed both "mailed" questionnaires (sent in 1962 and in 1976) were eligible. Following a true prospective study design, anyone at baseline of the study who reported physician-diagnosed diabetes was eliminated from the study. Physical activity (total kilocalories expended per week by walking, stair climbing, and sports participation) was assessed by a questionnaire included in the 1962 mailing. Height and weight were asked on both questionnaires and were also obtained from each individual's college entrance examination, to determine change in body mass index between college and 1962.

After the 14 years of follow-up, 202 men reported that they had developed diabetes. As hypothesized, the age-adjusted incidence rates of diabetes in these college alumni decreased as the reported total kilocalories of physical activity expended per week increased from the lowest to the highest levels. This relationship remained significant after adjusting for age, current body mass index, history of hypertension, and parental history of diabetes. If the variable "change of body mass index since college" was also controlled for, the relationship between physical activity and diabetes incidence was weaker but remained significant [31]. This suggests that at least part of the protective effect of physical activity on NIDDM development was due to less weight gain in the more active male alumni.

Interestingly, the protective effect of physical activity was mainly noted in those men who were initially at high risk for diabetes development (defined as "those with a body-mass index of 25 or more, a history of hypertension, a positive parental history of diabetes, or any combination of these factors"). This suggests that it would be most effective to target a high-risk group when planning physical activity intervention to prevent diabetes.

Finally, when the summary estimate of total kilocalories of physical activity expended per week was separated into its various components (i.e., walking, stair climbing, and moderate and vigorous sports participation), sports participation was most strongly and consistently related to a reduced risk of NIDDM. The finding that walking was one of the least reliable activities was in agreement with other research findings, with reasons that were discussed in detail elsewhere [48].

Manson et al. [61, 62]. In a prospective study of 87,253 female registered nurses, aged 34–59 years, nondiabetic women were initially asked about their regular physical activity patterns and then followed for eight years to determine subsequent incidence of NIDDM [61]. Physical activity was determined by the question, "At least once a week, do you engage in any regular activity similar to brisk walking, jogging, bicycling, etc., long enough to work up a sweat? If yes, how many times per week?" Disease outcome was determined by a positive response to the question, "Have you had diabetes mellitus diagnosed?"

Women who reported engaging in vigorous exercise at least once a week were found to have a lower incidence of self-reported NIDDM during the 8 years of follow-up and were leaner than women who did not exercise at least once a week. Statistically controlling for body mass index as well as age, family history, and duration of follow-up did not eliminate this relationship.

Similar results were reported in a prospective study of 21, 271 U.S. male physicians, aged 40–84 years [62]. With a design similar to that of the previous study, nondiabetic males were initially asked about their regular physical activity patterns and then followed for five years to determine subsequent risk for NIDDM development. Physical activity was determined by the question, "How often do you exercise vigorously enough to work up a sweat?" Disease outcome was self-reported and obtained by a medical questionnaire.

Physicians who reported engaging in vigorous exercise at least once a week were found to have a lower incidence of self-reported NIDDM during the 5 years of follow-up and also were leaner than the men who did not. Adjusting for body mass index and age as well as other variables did not eliminate this relationship.

In both of these studies by Manson [61, 62], when examining the association between frequency of reported vigorous physical activity per week (<1, 1, 2, 3, or 4+ times per week in the females; <1, 1, 2–4, and 5+ in the males) and subsequent incidence of NIDDM, there was no clear dose-response gradient by frequency of exercise in the females and a significant but nonimpressive trend in the males (Table 5.2). Examining the age- and body mass index–adjusted relative risk of NIDDM development by frequency of exercise, the largest and most consistent difference in risk occurs between those females or males who reported relatively no activity per week (less than once per week) and those who reported doing something on a weekly basis (at least once per week). This suggests that the population that would benefit the most from any public health effort to prevent NIDDM is the most sedentary individuals.

Although the results of all of the prospective epidemiological studies are quite suggestive of a causal relationship between physical inactivity and NIDDM, the strength of their findings is weakened because diabetes is determined by self-report. Since national data show that almost half of the cases of NIDDM are undetected [26], the extent and strength of the relationship between physical inactivity and NIDDM need to be examined in a population-based study that determines diabetes by oral glucose tolerance tests.

Finally, support of the hypothesis that physical fitness may provide some

TABLE 5.2

Incidence of NIDDM in Nurses and Physicians by Reported Physical Activity Level

Nurses*		Physicians**	
Vigorous Activity (times per week)	*Relative Risk [#]*	*Vigorous Activity (times per week)*	*Relative Risk [#]*
<1	1.0	<1	1.0
1	0.89	1	0.78
2	0.71	2–4	0.68
3	0.93	≥5	0.71
≥4	0.86		

*Adapted from Manson, J. E., E. B. Rimm, M. J. Stampfer, G. A. Colditz, W. C. Willett, et al. Physical activity and incidence of non-insulin-dependent diabetes mellitus in women. *Lancet*338:774–778, 1991.
**Adapted from Manson, J. E., D. M. Nathan, A. S. Krolewski, M. J. Stampfer, W. C. Willett, and C. H. Hennekens. A prospective study of exercise and incidence of diabetes among US male physicians. *JAMA* 268:63–67, 1992.
[#]Adjusted for age and body mass index.

protection against mortality in men at all levels of glucose intolerance was provided by Kohl et al. [45]. In this study, 8715 middle-aged men (mean age = 42 years) were followed for an average of 8.2 years (range, 1–15 years) after a baseline clinical examination. Physical fitness was assessed at baseline by a maximal-exercise test on a treadmill, and low physical fitness was defined as the lowest quintile of treadmill test tolerance. Blood glucose was measured after an overnight fast, and men were assigned to three strata of glucose tolerance (<6.4 mM, 6.4–7.8 mM and > 7.8 mM or clinical evidence of NIDDM).

There were 190 deaths during follow-up. Age-adjusted all-cause death rates were 82.5/10,000 man-years of follow-up in the low-fit men and 45.9/10,000 in fit men (top four quintiles of treadmill test tolerance). The relative risks for all-cause mortality for unfit men, compared with fit men, were 1.93, 3.42, and 1.80 across the three strata of glucose tolerance. This relationship between low fitness and mortality generally held after adjustment for other potential confounding variables (age, resting systolic blood pressure, serum cholesterol level, body mass index, family history of heart disease, smoking habit, and length of follow up).

Physical Activity Intervention Trials to Prevent or Delay the Development of NIDDM
The most powerful and by far the most labor-intensive epidemiological study design is that in which efforts are made to prevent or delay the onset of the disease outcome (diabetes) by manipulating the risk factor of interest (in this case, physical activity levels). In this design, the initially healthy sample (initially free of NIDDM) is randomly assigned to receive either the intervention (the physical activity intervention group) or no intervention (the control group). Subsequent follow-up of the two groups over time determines whether the groups differ, by the percentage who eventually develop the disease outcome.

Evidence of a potentially favorable effect of physical activity intervention is available from two community-based studies involving diabetic volunteers from two high-risk populations, Australian Aborigines [67] and the Zuni Indians [30]. In an attempt to recreate the ancestral environment, O'Dea [67] took 10 middle-aged, overweight, diabetic Aborigines into an isolated location in their traditional country to live as hunter-gathers for 7 weeks. The metabolic abnormalities of NIDDM greatly improved in these individuals, and the change was ascribed to the changes in lifestyle, namely, the increase in physical activity, changes in diet composition, and substantial decreases in body weight.

Likewise, an exercise program was made available to members of the Zuni Indian community because of the extremely high rates of diabetes found in that population [30]. Comparing 30 diabetic individuals in the program with 56 who chose not to participate, the former had a greater drop in their fasting blood glucose concentrations, were more likely to have decreased or stopped medications, and lost more weight than the latter.

However, an obvious limitation of these two studies is that the participants were not randomly chosen, thus raising the possibility of self-selection bias.

The most promising of all the diabetes studies that have included physical activity as part of their intervention regimen was a 6-year feasibility study of diabetes prevention in Malmö, Sweden [20]. From a community screening program, 181 individuals with impaired glucose tolerance and 41 with mild nonsymptomatic NIDDM were identified and enrolled in the intervention program. In contrast, 79 nonrandomized subjects with impaired glucose tolerance at baseline were not enrolled in the intervention program and served as the reference group.

The first 1–1.5 years of the intervention program included dietary advice and physical activity training, with the choice of group participation or following the protocol on their own after initial instructions. After that time, participants were asked to continue to follow the protocol either on their own, with previous group partners, or at local sports clubs. The physical activity training consisted or two 60-min sessions per week, with activities that included walking, jogging, calisthenics, soccer, and badminton, performed under the guidance of a physiotherapist [79]. More intense physical activities were not a major part of the activity intervention until late in the training period [79]. Testing was performed 0.5, 1, 1.5, 2, 3, 4, and 5 years after enrollment and included an oral glucose tolerance test, a submaximal bicycle ergometer test (to estimate maximal oxygen uptake), and height and weight measures.

Focusing on the subjects who had impaired glucose tolerance (IGT) at baseline, IGT individuals who took part in the intervention program had an increased maximal oxygen uptake, decreased body weight, and lower 2-hour glucose and insulin values than the nonparticipating IGT individuals, after 5 years of follow-up (Fig. 5.4). Most exciting was that the percentage of IGT individuals from the intervention group who developed diabetes by the 5-year follow-up was less than half that in the nonparticipating reference group (10.6% vs. 28.6%).

Since the participants were not randomized at baseline in the Malmö study, the hypothesis that physical activity intervention may prevent or delay the onset of NIDDM has not been adequately tested. The Malmö intervention study, along with metabolic, epidemiological, and clinical studies in the field, all suggest that such a prevention trial would be worthwhile.

Role of Physical Activity in the Prevention of NIDDM
The last section of this review examines some of the issues to be considered relative to developing a NIDDM prevention study with physical activity as part of the intervention. Such important issues as what populations should be targeted, which health-related components of physical activity should be considered, and what exercise should be prescribed are discussed below.

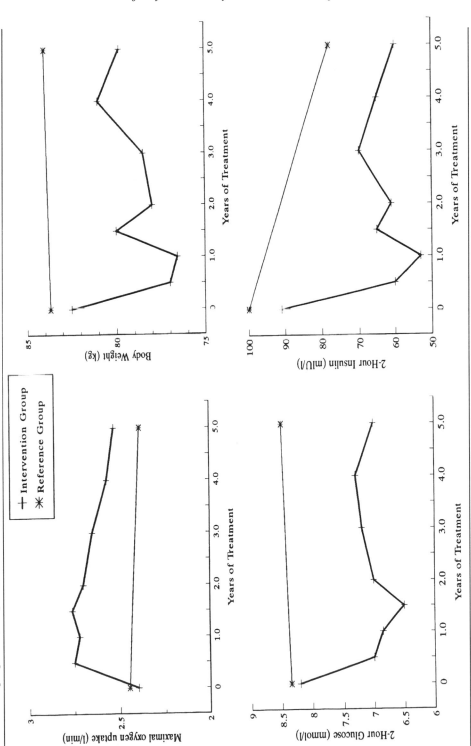

Baseline and follow-up values of maximal oxygen uptake, body weight and 2-hour glucose and insulin values for individuals with baseline impaired glucose tolerance that did (intervention group) and did not (reference group) participate in the diet and physical activity intervention program. (Adapted from Eriksson et al., 1991[20].)

WHO SHOULD BE TARGETED FOR THE PREVENTION PROGRAM? As discussed above, individuals at highest risk of developing NIDDM are those with impaired glucose tolerance [2, 35, 38] and are more likely to be obese [66], hyperinsulinemic [78, 82], insulin-resistant [9], older [21, 69], and sedentary [18]. In addition, since these individuals are older, they may also have competing health problems that may negatively affect physical function and so limit the ability to perform certain physical activities.

Not only are these individuals at high risk for diabetes development, but they seem to be the population that would benefit the most from physical activity intervention [31, 61, 62]. Physical activity conceivably could decrease NIDDM incidence directly, through altered sensitivity to insulin, or indirectly, through prevention of obesity or centrally distributed body fat.

In addition, there is no reason to assume that physical activity intervention would have different effects in men and women. Unfortunately, NIDDM [27], obesity [53], and inactivity [11] are all prevalent in both sexes. Neither the metabolic nor the epidemiologic literature provides any reason to suspect that the basic mechanisms through which physical activity would influence the progression of NIDDM (i.e., insulin sensitivity and resistance, obesity, centrally distributed body fat, etc.) would differ between the two sexes. However, the relative importance of each pathway may not be exactly equal in men and women. For example, in some populations the influence of central fat distribution on the development of NIDDM is greater in women than in men [18, 24]. Therefore, it is possible that the influence of physical activity on NIDDM may be explained to a larger degree by the role of physical activity on fat distribution in women than in men.

WHAT HEALTH-RELATED COMPONENTS OF PHYSICAL ACTIVITY SHOULD BE TARGETED IN THE NIDDM PREVENTION PROGRAM? When considering physical activity intervention by itself, the issue of what physical activity to recommend to the participants of the diabetes prevention program is a complicated one with no clear answer.

On one hand, the potential improvements in glucose tolerance and insulin resistance with exercise are believed to be partly due to the *cumulative* effect of a frequent lowering of the blood glucose level with each specific bout of exercise [46, 80]. In addition, physical training studies suggest that higher-intensity exercises are more likely to bring about the desired metabolic changes than are lower-intensity activities [32]. Therefore, to maximize the success of the training program, an intense program of long duration would most likely be prescribed.

On the other hand, the profile of the individuals who will probably be targeted for this prevention program must be kept in mind. As described above, they will most likely be obese and inactive, both which are negatively related to compliance with exercise participation [16, 41, 47]. An intense exercise training program of relatively long duration may not be successful in this population.

The logical answer to this dilemma can be gained from considering the population that will be targeted. As mentioned previously, they are more likely to be overweight/obese [66] and somewhat older. In addition, the adaptation caused by exercise training that appears to consistently affect insulin resistance over the long term (especially in the older adult) is the change in body composition [42]. Therefore, logically, the diabetes prevention program should combine diet and exercise for the main purpose of changing body composition.

In fact, studies have demonstrated that the combination of a dietary component and mild physical training is more effective in improving glucose tolerance and insulin sensitivity than either component alone [8, 54, 72, 91]. Furthermore, physical activity plays an important role in long-term weight maintenance [70, 87, 91]. Since the combination of physical activity and diet intervention appears more likely to succeed in preventing NIDDM than either component alone, and since such a combination is feasible and potentially applicable to the public health arena, it seems reasonable to investigate both simultaneously.

Therefore, if the basic design of the diabetes prevention program is a combination of diet and exercise for the main purpose of changing body composition, the specific health related component of physical activity of interest, is *overall caloric expenditure.* In other words, the main goal of the activity portion of the intervention should be to "burn more calories." Based upon this premise, the exercise recommended prescription for the intervention program is described below.

WHAT WILL BE PRESCRIBED FOR EXERCISE? An important consideration for the activity portion of a proposed intervention trial is the kind of physical activity that should be used. This trial will need to extend over a period of years to demonstrate convincingly that the behavioral intervention can significantly reduce or delay the onset of NIDDM. This means that the physical activity intervention will also be required for a long time and raises the greatest concern for physical activity intervention trials, the issue of long-term compliance with the activity intervention.

Since intervention studies that include lower-intensity exercise have demonstrated good compliance [47, 91] and are relatively less likely to result in injury [71], a low-intensity activity such as walking, moderate-intensity cycling, or gardening should be considered. Since the activity intervention is intended to create and maintain weight loss, the physical activity or activities selected should be performed for a substantial amount of time throughout the week. When setting up the exercise intervention, the adequacy of the physical activity prescription in achieving its goal must be carefully weighed against compliance with the exercise and risk of injury (Fig. 5.5).

FIGURE 5.5

Balancing the adequacy of the physical activity prescription against compliance issues and risk for injury.

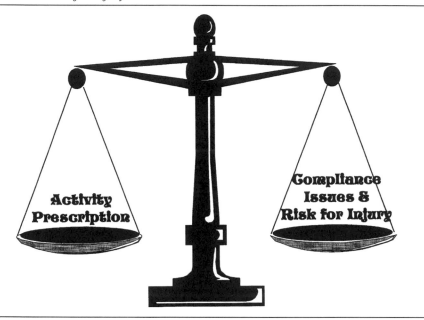

SUMMARY

Examining the epidemiological literature, a relationship between physical activity and the development of NIDDM seems not only plausible but likely. What is needed is a randomized clinical trial to confirm the metabolic and epidemiological research findings to date. To maximize success of a diabetes prevention trial, both diet and physical activity should be part of the intervention. The relative importance of diet or physical activity as components of the intervention will vary, depending upon the participant. However, it is critical that compliance with the physical activity and diet intervention be maintained, for this question to be answered. If the intervention is successful, the participants will have made lifestyle changes that have the potential of lasting beyond the closure of the clinical trial.

REFERENCES

1. Bennett, P. H., N. B. Rushforth, M. Miller, and P. M. LeCompte. Epidemiologic studies of diabetes in the Pima Indians. *Recent Prog. Horm. Res.* 32:333–375, 1976.
2. Bennett, P. H., W. C. Knowler, D. J. Pettitt, M. J. Carraher, and B. Vasquez. Longitudinal studies of the development of diabetes in the Pima Indians. *Advances in diabetes epidemiology.* New York: Elsevier Biomedical Press B.V., 1982.
3. Bennett, P. H., C. Bogardus, J. Tuomilehto, and P. Zimmet. Epidemiology and natural

history of NIDDM: non-obese and obese. K. G. M. M. Alberti, R. A. DeFronzo, H. Keen, and P. Zimmet (eds). *International Textbook of Diabetes Mellitus.* New York: John Wiley & Sons, 1992, pp. 147–176.

4. Björntorp, P., L. Sjöström, and L. Sullivan. The role of physical exercise in the management of obesity. JF Munro (ed). *The Treatment of Obesity.* Lancaster, England: MTP Press, 1979.

5. Björntorp, P., and M. Krotkiewski. Exercise treatment in diabetes mellitus. *Acata Med. Scand.* 217:3–7, 1985.

6. Björntorp, P. Abdominal obesity and the development of non-insulin-dependent diabetes mellitus. *Diabetes Metab. Rev.* 4:615–622, 1988.

7. Björntorp, P. Metabolic implications of body fat distribution. *Diabetes Care* 14:1132–1143, 1991.

8. Bogardus, C., E. Ravussin, D. C. Robbins, R. R. Wolfe, E. S. Horton, and E. A. Sims. Effects of physical training and diet therapy on carbohydrate metabolism in patients with glucose intolerance and non-insulin dependent diabetes mellitus. *Diabetes* 33:311–318, 1984.

9. Bogardus, C., S. Lillioja, and P. Bennett. Pathogenesis of NIDDM in Pima Indians. *Diabetes Care* 14:685–690, 1991.

10. Brownell, K. D., and A. J. Stunkard. Physical activity in the development and control of obesity. A. J. Stunkard (ed). *Obesity.* Philadelphia: WB Saunders, 1980, pp. 300–324.

11. Caspersen, C. J., G. M. Christenson, and R. A. Pollard. Status of the 1990 physical fitness and exercise objectives—evidence from NHIS 1985. *Public Health Rep.* 101:587–593, 1986.

12. Caspersen, C. J. Physical activity epidemiology: concepts, methods, and applications to exercise science. *Exerc. Sports Sci. Rev.* 17:423–473, 1989.

13. Cederholm, J., and L. Wibell. Glucose tolerance and physical activity in a health survey of middle-aged subjects. *Acta Med. Scand.* 217:373–378, 1985.

14. Cruz-vidal, M., R. Costas, M. Garcia-Palmieri, P. Sorlie, and E. Hertzmark. Factors related to diabetes mellitus in Puerto Rican men. *Diabetes* 28:300–307, 1979.

15. Despres, J. P., A. Tremblay, A. Nadeau, and C. Bouchard. Physical training and changes in regional adipose tissue distrubution. *Acta Med. Scand.* (Suppl.) 723:205–212, 1988.

16. Dishman, R. K., J. F. Sallis, and D. R. Orenstein. The determinants of physical activity and exercise. *Public Health Rep.* 100:158–171, 1985.

17. Dowse, G. K., H. Gareeboo, P. Z. Zimmet, K. G. M. M. Alberti, J. Tuomilehto, et al. High prevalence of NIDDM and impaired glucose tolerance in Indian, Creole and Chinese Mauritians. *Diabetes* 39:390–396, 1990.

18. Dowse, G. K., P. Z. Zimmet, H. Gareeboo, K. G. M. M. Alberti, J. Tuomilehto, et al. Abdominal obesity and physical inactivity are risk factors for NIDDM and impaired glucose tolerance in Indian, Creole, and Chinese Mauritians. *Diabetes Care* 14:271–282, 1991.

19. Duckworth, W. C., S. S. Solomon, P. Jallepalli, C. Heckemeyer, J. Finnern, and A. Powers. Glucose intolerance due to insulin resistance in patients with spinal cord injuries. *Diabetes* 29:906–910, 1980.

20. Eriksson, K. F., and F. Lindgärde. Prevention of type 2 (non-insulin-dependent) diabetes mellitus by diet and physical exercise. *Diabetologia* 34:891–898, 1991.

21. Everhart, J., W. C. Knowler, and P. H. Bennett. Incidence and risk factors for non-insulin-dependent diabetes. MI Harris and RF Hamman (eds). *Diabetes in America.* Washington, D.C.: National Diabetes Data Group. USDHHS, NIH Publication no. 85–1468. U.S. Gov. Printing Office. pp. IV, 1–35, 1985.

22. Frisch, R. E., G. Wyshak, T. E. Albright, N. L. Albright, and I. Schiff. Lower prevalence of diabetes in female former college athletes compared with nonathletes. *Diabetes* 35:1101–1105, 1986.

23. Haffner, S. M., M. P. Stern, H. P. Hazuda, M. Rosenthal, J. A. Knapp, and R. M. Malina. Role of obesity and fat distribution in non-insulin-dependent diabetes mellitus in Mexican Amercans and non-Hispanic whites. *Diabetes Care* 9:153–161, 1986.

24. Haffner, S. M., B. D. Mitchell, H. P. Hazuda, and M. S. Stern. Greater influence of central

distribution of adipose tissue on incidence of non-insulin-dependent diabetes in women than men. *Am. J. Clin. Nutr.* 53:1312–1317, 1991.

25. Hara, H., T. Kawase, M. Yamakido, and Y. Nishimoto. Comparative observation of micro- and macroangiopathies in Japanese diabetics in Japan and U.S.A. H Abe and M Hoshi (eds). *Diabetic Microangiopathy.* Tokyo: University of Tokyo Press, 1983.

26. Harris, M. I. Prevalence of non-insulin-dependent diabetes and impaired glucose tolerance. MI Harris and RF Hamman (eds). *Diabetes in America.* Washington, D.C.: U.S. Gov. Printing Office. National Diabetes Data Group, USDHHS, NIH Publication no. 85–1468. pp. VI, 1–31, 1985.

27. Harris, M. I., W. C. Hadden, W. C. Knowler, and P. H. Bennett. Prevalence of diabetes and imparied glucose tolerance and plasma glucose levels in U.S. population aged 20–74. *Diabetes* 36:523–534, 1987.

28. Hartz, A. J., D. C. Rupley, R. D. Kalkhoff, and A. A. Rimm. Relationship of obesity to diabetes. Influence of obesity and body fat distribution. *Prev. Med.* 12:351–357, 1983.

29. Haskell, W. L., A. S. Leon, C. J. Caspersen, V. F. Froelicher, J. M. Hagberg, et al. Cardiovascular benefits and assessment of physical activity and physical fitness in adults. *Med. Sci. Sports Exerc.* 24:S201–S220, 1992.

30. Heath, G. W., B. E. Leonard, R. H. Wilson, J. S. Kendrick, and K. E. Powell. Community-based exercise intervention: Zuni Diabetes Project. *Diabetes Care* 10:579–583, 1987.

31. Helmrich, S. P., D. R. Ragland, R. W. Leung, and R. S. Paffenbarger. Physical activity and reduced occurrence of non-insulin-dependent diabetes mellitus. *N. Engl. J. Med.* 325:147–152, 1991.

32. Holloszy, J. O., J. Schultz, J. Kusnierkiewicz, J. M. Hagberg, and A. A. Ehsani. Effects of exercise on glucose tolerance and insulin resistance. *Acta Med. Scand.* (Suppl.) 711:55–65, 1986.

33. Horton, E. S. Exercise and decreased risk of NIDDM. *N. Engl. J. Med.* 325:196–198, 1991.

34. Hrubec, Z., and R. Ryder. Traumatic limb amputations and subsequent mortality from cardiovascular disease and other causes. *J. Chron. Dis.* 33:239–250, 1980.

35. Jarrett, R. J., H. Keen, J. H. Fuller, and M. McCartney. Worsening to diabetes in men with impaired glucose tolerance. *Diabetologia* 16:25–30, 1979.

36. Jarrett, R. J., M. J. Shipley, and R. Hunt. Physical activity, glucose tolerance, and diabetes mellitus: the Whitehall Study. *Diabetic Med.* 3:549–551, 1987.

37. Kawate, R., M. Yamakido, Y. Nishimoto, P. H. Bennett, R. F. Hamman, and W. C. Knowler, Diabetes mellitus and its vascular complications in Japanese migrants on the island of Hawaii. *Diabetes Care* 2:161–170, 1979.

38. Keen, H., R. J. Jarrett, and P. McCartney. The ten-year follow-up of the Bedford Survey (1962–1972): glucose tolerance and diabetes. *Diabetologia* 22:73–78, 1982.

39. King, H., R. Taylor, P. Zimmet, K. Pargeter, L. Raper, et al. Non-insulin-dependent diabetes in a newly independent pacific nation: the republic of Kiribati. *Diabetes Care* 7:409–415, 1984.

40. King, H., P. Zimmet, L. Raper, and B. Balkau. Risk factors for diabetes in three Pacific populations. *Am. J. Epidemiol.* 119:396–409, 1984.

41. King, A. C., S. N. Blair, D. E. Bild, R. K. Dishman, P. M. Dubbert, et al. Determinants of physical activity and interventions in adults. *Med. Sci. Sports Exerc.* 24:S221–S236, 1992.

42. Kirwan, J. P., W. M. Kohrt, D. M. Wojta, R. E. Bourey, and J. O. Holloszy. Endurance exercise training reduces glucose-stimulated insulin levels in 60 to 70 year old men and women. *J. Gerontol* 48:M84–M90, 1993.

43. Kissebah, A. H., and A. N. Peiris. Biology of regional body fat distribution: relationship to non-insulin-dependent diabetes mellitus. *Diabetes Metab. Rev.* 5:83–109, 1989.

44. Knowler, W. C., D. J. Pettitt, M. F. Saad, M. A. Charles, R. G. Nelson, et al. Obesity in the Pima Indians: its magnitude and relationship with diabetes. *Am. J. Clin. Nutr.* 53:1543S–1551S, 1991.

45. Kohl, H. W., N. F. Gordon, J.A. Villegas, and S. N. Blair. Cardiorespiratory fitness, glycemic status, and mortality risk in men. *Diabetes Care* 15:184–192, 1992.
46. Koivisto, V. A., H. Yki-Jarvinen, and R. A. DeFronzo. Physical training and insulin sensitivity. *Diabetes Metab. Rev.* 1:445–481, 1986.
47. Kriska, A. M., C. Bayles, J. A. Cauley, R. E. LaPorte, R. B. Sandler, and G. Pambianco. A randomized exercise trial in older women: increased activity over two years and the factors associated with compliance. *Med. Sci. Sports Exerc.* 18:557–562, 1986.
48. Kriska, A. M., W. C. Knowler, R. E. LaPorte, A. L. Drash, R. R. Wing, et al. Development of questionnaire to examine the relationship of physical activity and diabetes in the Pima Indians. *Diabetes Care* 13:401–411, 1990.
49. Kriska, A. M., and P. H. Bennett. An epidemiological perspective of the relationship between physical activity and NIDDM: from activity assessment to intervention. *Diabetes Metab. Rev.* 8:355–372, 1992.
50. Kriska, A. M., R. E. LaPorte, D. J. Pettitt, M. A. Charles, R. G. Nelson, et al. The association of physical activity with obesity, fat distribution and glucose intolerance in Pima Indians. *Diabetologia* 36:863–869, 1993.
51. Krotkiewski, M. Physical training in the prophylaxis and treatment of obesity, hypertension and diabetes. *Scand. J. Rehabil. Med.* Suppl:55–70, 1983.
52. Krotkiewski, M. Can body fat patterning be changed? *Acta Med. Scand.* 723(Suppl.):213–223, 1988.
53. Kuczmarski, R. J. Prevalence of overweight and weight gain in the United States. *Am. J. Clin. Nutr.* 55:495S 502S, 1992.
54. Lampman, R. M., and D. E. Schteingart. Effects of exercise training on glucose control, lipid metabolism, and insulin sensitivity in hypertriglyceridemia and non-insulin dependent diabetes mellitus. *Med. Sci. Sports. Exerc.* 23:703–712, 1991.
55. LaPorte, R. E., H. J. Montoye, and C. J. Caspersen. Assessment of physical activity in epidemiologic research: problems and prospects. *Public Health Rep.* 100:131–146, 1985.
56. Lee, E. T., T. K. Welty, R. Fabsitz, L. D. Cowan, N. A. Le, et al. The Strong Heart Study; a study of cardiovascular disease in American Indians: design and methods. *Am. J. Epidemiol.* 132:1141–1155, 1990.
57. Lindgärde, F., and B. Saltin. Daily physical activity, work capacity and glucose tolerance in lean and obese normoglycaemic middle-aged men. *Diabetologia* 20:134–138, 1981.
58. Lindgärde, F., J. Malmquist, and B. Balke. Physical fitness, insulin secretion, and glucose tolerance in healthy males and mild type-2 diabetes. *Acta Diabetol Lat* 20:33–40, 1983.
59. Lipman, R. L., P. Raskin, T. Love, J. Triebwasser, F. R. Lecocq, and J. J. Schnure. Glucose intolerance during decreased physical activity in man. *Diabetes* 21:101–107, 1972.
60. Lohmann, D., F. Liebold, W. Heilmann, H. Senger, and A. Pohl. Diminished insulin response in highly trained athletes. *Metabolism* 27:521–524, 1978.
61. Manson, J.E., E. B. Rimm, M. J. Stampfer, G. A. Colditz, W. C. Willett, et al. Physical activity and incidence of non-insulin-dependent diabetes mellitus in women. *Lancet* 338:774–778, 1991.
62. Manson, J. E., D. M. Nathan, A. S. Krolewski, M. J. Stampfer, W. C. Willett, and C. H. Hennekens. A prospective study of exercise and incidence of diabetes among US male physicians. *JAMA* 268:63–67, 1992.
63. Modan, M., A. Karasik, H. Halkin, Z. Fuchs, A. Lusky, et al. Effect of past and concurrent body mass index on prevalence of glucose intolerance and type 2 diabetes and on insulin response. *Diabetologia* 29:82–89, 1986.
64. Montoye, H. J., W. D. Block, H. Metzner, and J. B. Keller. Habitual physical activity and glucose tolerance: males age 16–64 in a total community. *Diabetes* 26:172–176, 1977.
65. Montoye, H. J., and H. L. Taylor. Measurement of physical activity in population studies: a review. *Hum. Biol.* 56:195–216, 1984.
66. National Diabetes Data Group. Classification and diagnosis of diabetes and other categories of glucose intolerance. *Diabetes* 28:1039–1057, 1979.

67. O'Dea, K. Marked improvement in carbohydrate and lipid metabolism in diabetic Australian Aborgines after temporary reversion to traditional lifestyle. *Diabetes* 33:596–603, 1984.

68. Ohlson, L. O., B. Larsson, K. Svärdsudd, L. Welin, H. Eriksson, et al. The influence of body fat distribution on the incidence of diabetes mellitus: thirteen and one-half years of follow-up of the participants in the study of men born in 1913. *Diabetes* 34:1055–1058, 1985.

69. Palumbo, P. J., L. R. Elveback, C. P. Chu, D. C. Connolly, and L. T. Kurland. Diabetes mellitus: incidence, prevalence, survivorship and causes of death in Rochester, Minnesota, 1945–1970. *Diabetes* 25:566–573, 1976.

70. Pavlou, K. N., S. Krey, and W. P. Steffe. Exercise as an adjunct to weight loss and maintenance in moderately obese subjects. *Am. J. Clin Nutr.* 49:1115–1123, 1989.

71. Pollock, M. L., J. F. Carroll, J. E. Graves, S. H. Leggett, R. W. Braith, et al. Injuries and adherence to walk/jog and resistance training programs in the elderly. *Med. Sci. Sports Exerc.* 23:1194–1200, 1991.

72. Rauramaa, R. Relationship of physical activity, glucose tolerance, and weight management. *Prev. Med.* 13:37–46, 1984.

73. Ravussin, E., and R. Rising. Daily energy expenditure in humans: measurements in a respiratory chamber and by doubly labeled water. JM Kinney and HN Tucker (eds). *Energy Metabolism: Tissue Determinants and Cellular Corollaries.* New York: Raven Press, 1992.

74. Ravussin, E., and B. A. Swinburn. Pathophysiology of obesity. *Lancet* 340:404–408, 1992.

75. Ravussin, E., M. E. Valencia, L. O. Schulz, J. Esparza, and P. H. Bennett. Effect of a traditional life style on the physical and metabolic characteristics of Pima Indians living in northern Mexico. *Diabetes* 41:(Abstract #2), 1992.

76. Rönnemaa, T., K. Mattila, A. Lehtonen, and V. Kallio. A controlled randomized study on the effect of long-term physical exercise on the metabolic control in type 2 diabetic patients. *Acta Med. Scand.* 220:219–224, 1986.

77. Saad, M. F., W. C. Knowler, D. J. Pettitt, R. G. Nelson, D. M. Mott, and P. H. Bennett. The natural history of impaired glucose tolerance in the Pima Indians. *N. Engl. J. Med.* 319:1500–1506, 1988.

78. Saad, M.F., D. J. Pettitt, D. M. Mott, W. C. Knowler, R. G. Nelson, and P. H. Bennett. Sequential changes in serum insulin concentration during development of non-insulin-dependent diabetes. *Lancet* i:1356–1359, 1989.

79. Saltin, B., F. Lindgärde, M. Houston, R. Horlin, E. Nygaard, and P. Gad. Physical training and glucose tolerance in middle-aged men with chemical diabetes. *Diabetes* 28:30–32, 1979.

80. Schneider, S. H., L.F. Amorosa, A. K. Khachadurian, and N. B. Ruderman. Studies on the mechanism of improved glucose control during regular exercise in type 2 diabetes. *Diabetologia* 26:355–360, 1984.

81. Schranz, A., J. Toumilehto, B. Marti, R. J. Jarrett, V. Grabauskas, and A. Vassallo. Low physical activity and worsening of glucose tolerance: results from a 2-year follow-up of a population sample in Malta. *Diabetes Res. Clin Pract.* 11:127–136, 1991.

82. Sicree, R. A., P. Z. Zimmet, H. O. M. King, and J. S. Coventry. Plasma insulin response among Nauruans: prediction of deterioration in glucose tolerance in 6 years. *Diabetes* 36:179–186, 1987.

83. Stern, M. P. Kelly West lecture; Primary prevention of type II diabetes mellitus. *Diabetes Care* 14:399–410, 1991.

84. Taylor, R. J., P. H. Bennett, G. LeGonidec, J. Lacoste, D. Combe, et al. The prevalence of diabetes mellitus in a traditional-living Polynesian population: the Wallis Island Survey. *Diabetes Care* 6:334–340, 1983.

85. Taylor, R. J., P. Ram, P. Zimmet, L. Raper, and H. Ringrose. Physical activity and prevalence of diabetes in Melanesian and Indian men in Fiji. *Diabetologia* 27:578–582, 1984.

86. Trovati, M., Q. Carta, F. Cavalot, S. Vitali, C. Banaudi, et al. Influence of physical training

on blood glucose control, glucose tolerance, insulin secretion, and insulin action in non-insulin-dependent-diabetes patients. *Diabetes Care* 7:416–420, 1984.

87. Van Dale, D., W. H. M. Saris, and F. T. Hoor. Weight maintenance and resting metabolic rate 18–40 months after a diet/exercise treatment. *Int. J. Obesity* 14:347–359, 1990.

88. Wallberg-Henriksson, H. Exercise and diabetes mellitus. JO Holloszy (ed). *Exercise and Sport Sciences Reviews*. Baltimore: Williams & Wilkins, 1992, pp. 339–368.

89. Wang, J. T., L. T. Ho, K. T. Tang, L. M. Wang, Y. D. I. Chen, and G. M. Reaven. Effect of habitual physical activity on age-related glucose intolerance. *J. Am Geriatr. Soc.* 37:203–209, 1989.

90. West, K. M. *Epidemiology of Diabetes and Its Vascular Lesions*. New York: Elsevier, 1978.

91. Wing, R. R., L. H. Epstein, M. P. Bayles, A. M. Kriska, M. P. Nowalk, and W. Gooding. Exercise in a behavioural weight control programme for obese patients with type 2 (non-insulin-dependent) diabetes. *Diabetologia* 31:902–909, 1988.

92. World Health Organization Expert Committee. *Second Report on Diabetes Mellitus*. Technical Report Series No. 646, Geneva, Switzerland, 1980.

93. Zimmet, P. Z., S. Faauiso, S. Ainuu, S. Whitehouse, B. Milne, and W. DeBoer. The prevalence of diabetes in the rural and urban Polynesian population of Western Samoa. *Diabetes* 30:45–51, 1981.

94. Zimmet, P. Z., R. Taylor, P. Ram, H. King, G. Sloman, et al. Prevalence of diabetes and impaired glucose tolerance in the biracial population of Fiji: a rural-urban comparison. *Am. J. Epidemiol.* 118:673–688, 1983.

95. Zimmet, P. Z., G. K. Dowse, S. Serjeantson, C. F. Finch, and H. King. The epidemiology and natural history of NIDDM—lessons from the South Pacific. *Diabetes Metab. Rev.* 6:91–124, 1990.

6
Maternal Exercise, Fetal Well-Being and Pregnancy Outcome

LARRY A. WOLFE, Ph.D.
INGRID K. M. BRENNER, M.Sc.
MICHELLE F. MOTTOLA, Ph.D.

There is an urgent need for scientific information on maternal-fetal responses to both acute and chronic physical activity. Traditional medical advice has been for pregnant women to rest throughout gestation. However, during the past decade there has been increasing participation of women in sports and fitness activities [132], as well as employment of women in nontraditional occupations (e.g., police work, military service, fire fighting) that involve strenuous physical activities [155, 167]. When such women become pregnant, it is important to know the modalities, intensities, and durations of physical activity that help to promote maternal and fetal health. It is also important to know the effects of pregnancy on maternal exercise capacities, to maintain a safe and productive working environment.

From a biological viewpoint, pregnancy is a unique process in which the function of virtually all of the body's control systems is modified to maintain both maternal and fetal homeostasis [193, 196, Table 6.1]. The ability to preserve maternal-fetal well-being in the face of metabolic or environmental stresses depends on the existence of an adequate level of maternal-fetal physiological reserve. The extent of this reserve has not yet been adequately defined, but it can be expected to vary in relation to factors such as maternal health status, age, nutrition, and level of physical fitness. Therefore, from a theoretical viewpoint, acute bouts of exercise may represent a significant challenge to maternal-fetal well-being. Conversely, chronic maternal exercise, if properly prescribed, has the potential of enhancing physiological reserve and can be fetoprotective.

In attempting to analyze the risk:benefit ratio for exercise in pregnancy, much attention has been focused on the concept that contracting maternal skeletal muscle may compete with the fetus for blood flow and oxygen delivery, access to the maternal blood glucose pool, and dissipation of heat [106, 110, 193–196]. Some evidence also exists for increased epinephrine-mediated uterine contractile activity following strenuous maternal exercise [61, 202]. Thus, the most important hypothetical risks of chronic maternal exercise are intrauterine growth retardation, altered fetal development, and induction of premature labor [12]. Again, the validity of these

145

TABLE 6.1
*Important Maternal Metabolic and Cardiorespiratory Adaptations to Pregnancy**

- Increased blood volume of 40–50%, reduced hemoglobin concentration
- Cardiac dilation
- Slight increase in oxygen uptake at rest and during standard submaximal exercise (e.g., cycling)
- Substantial increase in oxygen uptake during weight-dependent exercise (e.g., walking, jogging)
- Increased heart rate at rest and during submaximal exercise
- "Hyperkinetic" cardiac output at rest and during submaximal exercise; reduced venous return, decreased cardiac output and arterial hypotension in the third trimester (especially in supine posture)
- Blunted sympathetic nervous system responses to exercise in late gestation; possible reduction in maximal heart rate
- Increased tidal volume, minute ventilation ($\dot{V}_E$) and ventilatory equivalent ($\dot{V}_E{:}\dot{V}O_2$), and oxygen cost of breathing at rest and during submaximal exercise
- Insulin resistance and reduced maternal carbohydrate utilization at rest in late gestation

---

*Changes are relative to the nonpregnant state.

concerns depends on the existence and capacity of both maternal and fetal mechanisms of adaptation to acute and chronic exercise as well as the characteristics (modality, quality, quantity) of the exercise stimulus.

A growing body of evidence also supports the hypothesis that moderate aerobic-type fitness programs can enhance maternal metabolic and cardiorespiratory reserve [119, 193–196]. Appropriate muscular conditioning programs may also help to facilitate labor and prevent conditions such as gestational low back pain, urinary incontinence, and diastasis recti [4]. Thus, a global view of existing information supports the existence of dose-response relationships between exercise quantity and quality and both maternal and fetal well-being. It appears that an optimal exercise stimulus promotes maternal health and fetoprotective capacities, whereas overexertion may jeopardize fetal well-being.

The purpose of this communication is to provide a critical review of existing research on the interactions between maternal exercise, fetal well-being, and pregnancy outcome and to make recommendations for future study. Particular attention is given to the identification of maternal-fetal adaptive mechanisms that may protect fetal well-being during maternal exertion.

FETAL CARDIOVASCULAR DEVELOPMENT

At the beginning of gestation, the metabolic demands of the embryo are met by diffusion of substrate between maternal capillaries and the embryonic disc. As these demands increase, a primitive cardiovascular system develops. During the third week, blood vessels are formed [124].

In the fourth week of gestation, the heart begins to pump, and by the fifth week, blood begins to circulate through a single heart tube. Initially, myocardial contractions occur in peristaltic waves [124] originating in the ventricular cells. The sinoatrial node (SA node) gradually exerts greater influence with maturation of the cardiac conduction system. The sixth week is characterized by rhythmic and coordinated activity of the heart [124, 164]. By midgestation, fetal heart rate (FHR) is controlled primarily by the SA node and is modulated by the autonomic nervous system [72]. Sympathetic control of FHR exists early in fetal life, and parasympathetic input gradually increases as the fetus matures [72, 88, 135, 183].

Fetal myocardial cells do not normally exhibit the Frank-Starling mechanism. As a result, FHR is the main determinant of cardiac output [81, 142, 198] and regulates blood flow and oxygen supply to fetal organs and tissues. Chemoreceptors, baroreceptors, and higher brain centers send afferent impulses to the vasomotor center that integrates this information and modulates FHR through the autonomic output [199]. Chemoreceptors and baroreceptors become functional in the third trimester [59, 165, 184].

The interactions between baroreceptors and chemoreceptors are complex. In the hypoxic fetus, decreased arterial oxygen tension is detected by aortic chemoreceptors. The chemoreceptors stimulate the sympathetic vasomotor center in the midbrain (medulla oblongata). FHR, peripheral vasoconstriction, and blood pressure increase with increased sympathetic activity. The increased blood pressure is detected by baroreceptors that function to decrease FHR by increasing parasympathetic activity (i.e., increased vagal activity) [114, 142, 176, 186]. Chemoreceptors and baroreceptors can have antagonistic effects on autonomic function, and the final response is difficult to predict except in the case of severe hypoxia when FHR decreases [2, Figure 6.1].

Various hormones can also exert an influence on FHR. In response to hypoxia, the fetal adrenal medulla secretes catecholamines [142]. Norepinephrine is released faster and in greater quantities from the adrenal gland than epinephrine [47]. Catecholamines increase heart rate and myocardial contractility and contribute to peripheral vasoconstriction, blood pressure elevation, and blood flow redistribution during fetal hypoxia. Smaller quantities of epinephrine from the adrenal gland maintain cardiac output and counteract the increased vagal activity that acts to decrease the FHR in response to hypoxia [141]. Other hormones such as aldosterone and vasopressin act on the circulation by altering plasma volume and redistribution of blood flow, respectively [140, 142].

The fetal and maternal circulations are related to each other through the placenta, where gas exchange, nutrient transport, metabolite excretion, and endocrine production occur. Since oxygenation occurs at the

FIGURE 6.1
Autonomic nervous system influences on fetal heart rate.

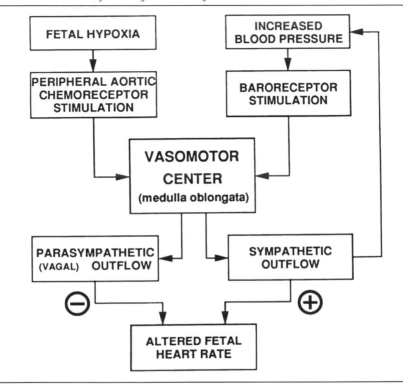

placenta, a parallel circulatory design is present in the fetus, in which both sides of the heart contribute to the systemic circulation [140]. This pattern is facilitated by three temporary shunts (ductus venosus, ductus arteriosus, and the foramen ovale) that close at birth [140, Figure 6.2].

Blood in the umbilical arteries is oxygenated at the placenta and returns to the fetus in the umbilical vein, which enters the liver and divides into the portal vein, which traverses the hepatic parenchyma and the ductus venosus, which by-passes the liver [140]. These streams reunite with blood returning from the lower extremities at the inferior vena cava and ascend to the heart. Preferential flow and streaming compensate for the mixing of oxygenated and deoxygenated blood [81]. An interatrial septum (the crista dividens) divides blood flow into two streams. One stream flows ("via sinistra") through the foramen ovale into the left atrium where it joins with blood returning from the nonfunctional lungs and moves into the left ventricle to be ejected into the ascending aorta and aortic arch, which supplies the coronary arteries, the upper body parts, and the head [140, 187]. The other stream ("via dextra") enters the right atrium, flows into

FIGURE 6.2
Organization of the fetal circulation.

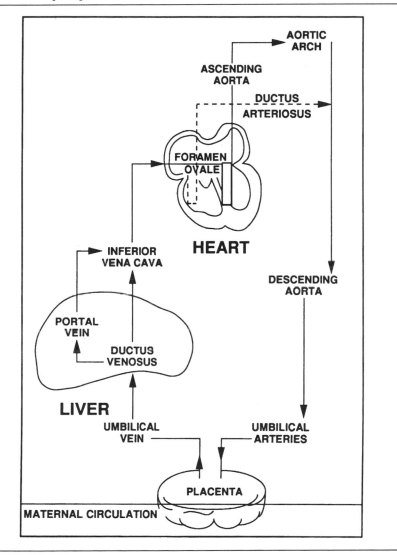

the right ventricle, and is ejected into the pulmonary artery [187]. Due to the high pulmonary vascular resistance, much of this blood is rediverted through the ductus arteriosus to enter the descending aorta, which supplies the gut and kidneys. The descending aorta further branches into the iliac arteries to supply the lower body parts and the umbilical arteries, which travel to the placenta [140].

INDICES OF FETAL WELL-BEING

Fetal Heart Rate (FHR) Patterns

Fetal well-being can be evaluated by monitoring FHR patterns. In this regard, FHR is the most important determinant of fetal cardiac output, and various specific changes in FHR patterns are correlated with fetal distress or decompensation [142]. Doppler ultrasound has been used most frequently to monitor FHR. Other methods include two-dimensional real-time echocardiography, M-mode echocardiography, electronic monitoring, and auscultation. Doppler ultrasound provides clear, easy to analyze FHR tracings and can be used to evaluate fetal well-being during exercise as well as following exercise. The major disadvantage associated with this method is that motion artifact is sometimes recorded [138]. This phenomenon can occur during the exercise phase when poor contact between the transducer and maternal abdomen results in the recording of pedaling frequency, walking cadence, and/or maternal heart rate. Echocardiographic methods provide measurements of FHR during maternal exercise that are free of such artifact [11, 138].

Doppler FHR tracings have baseline and periodic features (Table 6.2). Baseline features include the average heart rate and variability. Periodic features are temporary alterations in the pattern of the tracing and often occur in response to stimulation of the fetus [31, 140, 142]. In a normal, healthy fetus, FHR ranges between 120 and 160 beats·min⁻¹ [31, 72, 140, 142, 176, 199]. The average FHR decreases with increasing gestational age [62, 88, 199]. Heart rates above or below this range, which continue for at

TABLE 6.2
Characteristics of a Normal Fetal Heart Rate Tracing [31,140,142,176,198]

Feature	Description	Comments
Baseline characteristics		
Heart rate	≈120–160 beats · min⁻¹	Deviations from normal rate: Tachycardia—HR > 160 beats ·min⁻¹ for ≥ 120 seconds Bradycardia—HR < 120 beats · min⁻¹ for ≥ 120 seconds May indicate hypoxia
Long-term variability	≈5–25 beats · min⁻¹	Short term variability is difficult to monitor using the conventional Doppler ultrasound technique
Periodic features		
Accelerations	↑ in FHR > 15 beats · min⁻¹ from previous baseline, lasting 15–120 seconds	May be associated with fetal movement Presence indicates fetal well-being
Decelerations	↓ in FHR < 15 beats · min⁻¹ from previous baseline, lasting 15–120 seconds	May be associated with mild hypoxia

↑ = increase; ↓ = decrease; ≈ = approximately; HR = heart rate; FHR = fetal heart rate.

least two minutes, are referred to as tachycardia or bradycardia, respectively [31, 72, 140, 142, 176, 199]. FHR may briefly increase or decrease from its average rate. Accelerations and decelerations are identified when FHR changes at least 15 beats from the previous FHR baseline and lasts for 15–120 seconds [31, 140, 142]. Accelerations occur in association with fetal movement, although they also occur during REM sleep. Periodic accelerations indicate fetal well-being, however, FHR decelerations are often associated with fetal hypoxia or distress [31, 140, 142].

FHR can vary between beats (short-term variability, STV) and over time (long-term variability, LTV). LTV arises from cyclic changes in heart rate from 5 to 25 beats·min^{-1} due to fluctuation in parasympathetic tone [140]. LTV indicates CNS integrity, adequate oxygenation, and fetal well-being [140, 143], whereas absence of LTV suggests fetal compromise [31]. The causes of STV have not been adequately described, but its presence is a valuable index of fetal viability [142].

Specific FHR patterns are associated with fetal hypoxia or asphyxia. The acute response of a fetus to hypoxia is a reflex bradycardia [140, 142]. However, decelerations, reduced LTV (less than 5 beats·min^{-1}), tachycardia, or absence of fetal movements are other signs that may indicate fetal hypoxia [140, 142].

Fetal Activity
Other biophysical variables that have been used to assess fetal well-being include fetal movements (FM) and fetal breathing movement (FBM) patterns. The presence of periodic FM is a sign of fetal well-being [73]. A normal, healthy fetus will move within the uterus, and FHR will accelerate in response to this movement. The nonstress test (NST) often used clinically involves monitoring FHR and FM over time in the absence of an oxytocin challenge. The number of fetal movements, degree of FHR acceleration (beats·min^{-1}), duration of acceleration (seconds), and time to reactivity are the variables that are used to quantify fetal reactivity [101].

EFFECTS OF ACUTE MATERNAL EXERCISE ON FETAL WELL-BEING

Maternal exercise could in theory influence embryonic and fetal growth and development. Three different mechanisms have been proposed to explain how fetal growth and development may be altered by exposure to maternal exercise (Figure 6.3). First, as a result of increased sympathetic neural activity and an increased concentration of circulating catecholamines, maternal cardiac output is redistributed in response to acute exercise [161]. Studies of exercising human subjects have shown that blood flow to the maternal splanchnic and visceral region as well as the uterus and placenta may be reduced [125, 126, 157]. The fetus might then be exposed to transient periods of hypoxia. In theory, repeated exposure of the fetus to brief periods of hypoxia during aerobic conditioning could cause de-

FIGURE 6.3

Hypothetical effects of aerobic exercise on fetal development (Reproduced with permission from Wolfe, L. A., P. J. Ohtake, M. F. Mottola, and M. J. McGrath. Exercise and Sport Sciences Reviews, Vol 17. *Baltimore: Williams & Wilkins, 1989, p. 327.)*

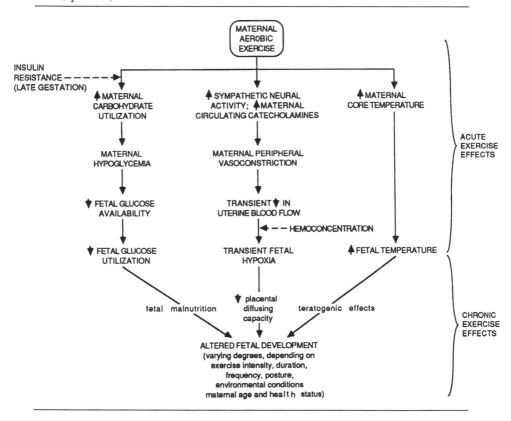

velopmental abnormalities such as neurologic damage or cerebral palsy [74].

Strenuous maternal exercise significantly increases utilization of carbohydrate as a metabolic fuel compared with the resting state. A reduction in maternal blood glucose levels, associated with augmented carbohydrate utilization by contracting skeletal muscle or reduced catecholamine-mediated liver glycogenolysis, could reduce fetal glucose availability. Since the fetus relies primarily on glucose as a metabolic substrate [80, 90], regular exposure to maternal hypoglycemia could lead to fetal malnutrition, intrauterine growth retardation, and reduced birth weight [39].

Finally, an increase in maternal core body temperature occurs with exercise. This increase could reduce and even reverse the temperature gradient so that the fetus now receives heat from the mother [109]. This can increase fetal body temperature and may cause pathological changes in fetal development—especially if the exercise is performed during the first trimester [64–67, 70, 102]. Data from animal research have also indicated that neural tube defects can result from fetal exposure to hyperthermia [64–67, 70, 102].

Uterine Blood Flow/Fetal Oxygen Delivery
In both static and aerobic maternal exercise, blood flow to the exercising muscles increases and blood flow to the visceral region including the uterus and placenta decreases [14, 86, 161]. Local metabolites produced in the muscle appear to be the key factors regulating this blood flow redistribution. Increased levels of inorganic phosphate or potassium produced in response to either aerobic or static exercise, respectively, are detected by free nerve endings (small afferent C-fibers) that elicit a central reflex leading to an increase in sympathetic vasomotor activity. Blood flow to the splanchnic region, uterus, kidneys, and inactive skeletal muscle beds is reduced because of the sympathetic vasoconstriction, whereas blood flow to the active muscle is increased as a result of local vasodilator substances that override the increased sympathetic output. Although the placenta contains a high concentration of catecholamine-metabolizing enzymes (carboxymethyl transferase and monoamine oxidase), approximately 10–15% of maternal catecholamines may reach the fetus [8, 10, 137, 169]. Therefore, the increase in catecholamine concentrations which occurs in response to exercise could, in theory, reduce both uterine and umbilical blood flow. However, some studies have reported that umbilical blood flow remains constant during maternal exercise [162, 180].

ANIMAL STUDIES OF UTERINE BLOOD FLOW. Studies using electromagnetic flow meters or radioactive microspheres injected into exercising animals (sheep and goats) have demonstrated that uterine blood flow either remains constant [36, 56, 136] or decreases in proportion to increasing exercise intensity and/or duration [32, 33, 82, 108]. In response, the fetus experiences only moderate alterations in blood gases and pH [32, 68, 109, 137].

HUMAN STUDIES OF UTERINE BLOOD FLOW. Morris et al., [125] were the first to demonstrate that uterine blood flow decreases in response to maternal exercise in humans. A 25% reduction in uterine blood flow occurred during moderate exercise in women with normal pregnancies. They analyzed the clearance rate of radioactive sodium (^{24}Na) ions from the uterus in response to moderate short-term cycle ergometer exercise in the supine position. Clearance rates decreased during and increased following maternal exercise, compared with preexercise values. It was concluded that uterine blood flow decreased during maternal exercise and that a compensatory increase in uterine blood flow occurred following exercise (flush-back phenomenon). This response was greater in preeclamptic subjects, suggesting greater vascular reactivity.

Rauramo and Forss [157] and Morrow et al. [126] found similar results. Rauramo and Forss [157] observed a reduction in placental blood flow following maternal exercise in patients with preeclampsia, cholestasis, and diabetes. The clearance rate of radioactive labeled xenon from the placenta was used to measure placental blood flow. Subjects were studied in the left lateral position, at rest, and at 1 and 30 minutes following 6 minutes of moderate cycle ergometer exercise (target HR = 140 beats·min^{-1}). Morrow and associates [126] observed a reduction in uterine blood flow in healthy, pregnant subjects (gestational age, 36–41 weeks) following 5 minutes of semirecumbent cycling. An elevation in the systolic to diastolic blood velocity in the uterine artery was recorded by Doppler ultrasound, indicating that uteroplacental vascular resistance increased.

In contrast, several researchers have reported that maternal exercise in normal, healthy pregnancies does not alter uteroplacental blood flow at late gestation [14, 123, 158, 172]. Three of these studies examined uteroplacental blood flow by the continuous wave Doppler technique [14, 123, 172]. In two studies, no change was observed after short-term stationary cycling of moderate intensity, as expressed by either the relation of systolic to end-diastolic maximum velocity [123] or pulsatile index, defined as the difference between peak systolic and end-diastolic flow divided by mean flow [14]. Steegers and associates [172] observed no change in pulsatility index following 10 minutes of treadmill exercise (HR = 130 beats·min^{-1}). Using a different method, Rauramo and Forss [158] examined placental clearance rates of radioactive labeled Xe following 6 minutes of cycling exercise (HR = 140 beats·min^{-1}) and also found no difference in placental blood flow before and after the cessation of exercise.

The varying results obtained by the different studies may be explained by inconsistencies in methodology. Studies that have demonstrated a reduction in uteroplacental blood flow associated with maternal exercise [125, 126, 157] either had the subjects lying in the supine position during the measurements [125, 126] or included subjects with complicated pregnancies [157]. Since venous return may be occluded by the gravid uterus when subjects lie in the supine or semirecumbent position, diminishing cardiac output and uterine blood flow may occur regardless of the effect of maternal exercise [1]. In addition, subjects with preeclampsia, pregnancy-induced hypertension, and diabetes often have a reduced uterine blood flow due to arterial vasospasm [154], and this would bias or confound the data obtained on uterine blood flow in response to maternal exercise.

Many factors are involved in the regulation of uterine blood flow [18]. An increase in maternal PaCO$_2$ leads to increased uterine blood flow, whereas increases in maternal body temperature, blood pH, catecholamine concentration, and sympathetic activity lead to a decrease in uterine blood flow [18]. In addition, compensatory mechanisms exist within the mother and fetus to protect the fetus from hypoxia. Research on animals has shown that during exercise uterine blood flow is redistributed favoring uterine cotyledons over the myometrium [82, 136], hemoconcentration occurs [77], and arteriovenous uterine oxygen extraction is augmented [33, 82, 108]. In the fetus, umbilical blood flow may increase slightly [48], cardiac output is redistributed favouring vital organs (heart, brain, adrenal gland, and placenta) [48], and muscle activity is decreased [144].

FHR Studies in Humans
As discussed above, the most useful noninvasive method currently available for the study of fetal well-being in humans is via FHR monitoring. The study of FHR during and following maternal exercise has several important clinical and theoretical applications:

1. Maternal aerobic exercise can reduce uterine blood flow, may induce changes in FHR indicative of fetal hypoxia, and may be useful to identify women with previously undetected uteroplacental insufficiency.
2. The study of changes in FHR characteristics in response to various modalities, intensities, and durations of exercise in healthy women will help to evaluate the safety of different forms of occupational and recreational physical activity.
3. Serial studies of FHR responses to standard maternal exercise are useful to investigate the development of the neural, humoral, and chemical factors that control fetal heart rate.

Although completed studies of FHR responses to maternal exercise are numerous [11, 193], there has, until recently, been considerable confusion concerning what represents the normal range of fetal responses to maternal exercise. Inconsistent results from early investigations were due at least in part to the use of inadequate measurement devices, lack of standardization of FHR analysis criteria, failure to accurately quantify the exercise stimulus, and failure to provide a complete description of the clinical and physical characteristics of the subject sample under study.

A comprehensive review of completed studies that involved women with healthy pregnancies indicates that the most common fetal response to strenuous maternal aerobic exercise is a moderate ($5–25$ beat·min^{-1}) increase in FHR followed by a gradual return to preexercise baseline during the 20–30 minute postexercise period [10, 38, 45, 60, 145, 179, 192]. Available data suggest that the degree of FHR elevation varies with the modality, intensity, and duration of aerobic exercise in healthy women. In this regard, Clapp et al. [45] studied the FHR responses of 120 recreational athletes during 20-minute physical conditioning sessions between 16 and 39 weeks gestation. FHR was measured using real-time ultrasonography before, during, and following upright cycle ergometry (60% preconceptual $\dot{V}O_2$max) or incline treadmill walking (40, 60% preconceptual $\dot{V}O_2$max).

Other studies measured FHR using Doppler ultrasound before and immediately following routine workouts at the individual's customary exercise intensity. Exercise modalities included swimming, aerobics, and stair climbing. FHR increased during exercise in 97% of the studies, and the effect was significant for all forms of exercise. However, observed changes were lower during cycle ergometry than with other forms of exercise. The magnitude of FHR elevation increased significantly with greater intensity and duration of maternal exercise.

It is noteworthy that FHR responses to static-type exercise performed by healthy pregnant women appear to be different from those to dynamic exercise. Webb et al. [191] compared the FHR responses of 12 pregnant women to static handgrip exercise (30% maximum voluntary contraction to fatigue) with responses to upright cycling (15 minutes, heart rate target = 145 beats·min^{-1}). The subjects were healthy women studied at 37 weeks gestation. Mean FHR increased 9 beats·min^{-1} in response to dynamic exercise but did not change during static exertion. Similar responses to static exercise were also reported in the earlier investigation of Maršál et al. [113].

A number of factors may contribute to exercise-induced FHR elevation in response to dynamic exercise. These include an augmented state of fetal wakefulness or activity [96], increased fetal temperature [181], or a moderate reduction in fetal PO$_2$ related to reduced uterine blood flow during strenuous exercise [50, 59, 108, 137, 182]. All of these factors could trigger increased fetal sympathoadrenal catecholamine output leading in turn to elevation of FHR [46, 47]. Maternal catecholamine output increases as a function of exercise intensity [7], and transfer of maternal catecholamines across the placenta during heavy exertion is also possible in theory [122, 169].

The findings of Clapp et al. [45], cited above, generally support the hypothesis that FHR increases occur as a response to mild transient fetal hypoxia. In this regard, increases in FHR in response to 20-minute exercise bouts were poorly correlated with changes in maternal rectal temperature and circulating norepinephrine levels. Increased fetal activity was not observed during real-time ultrasonography performed on 37 subjects during the first minute following exercise cessation. Also, available evidence suggests that maternal-fetal transfer of catecholamines in active form is probably minimal [169].

Direct proof does not exist which shows conclusively that FHR elevation with maternal exercise is caused by mild transient hypoxia. However, this hypothesis is supported by several lines of indirect evidence. First, as described above, studies of both humans and laboratory animals have demonstrated that uterine blood flow is reduced as a result of redistribution of maternal cardiac output during strenuous exertion. The magnitude of the decrease appears also to be related directly to the intensity and duration of maternal exercise [108]. The effect on reduced uterine blood flow is probably compensated at least in part by redistribution of uterine blood flow favouring the cotyledons versus myometrium [56], exercise-induced hemoconcentration [77], and increased arteriovenous oxygen extraction [110]. Nevertheless, several studies of laboratory animals have confirmed small reductions in fetal PO_2 in association with variable effects on PCO_2 and pH during maternal exercise [32, 109, 137].

The direction and magnitude of fetal autonomic responses to hypoxia at different gestational ages also depends on the integrated input from central and peripheral chemoreceptors and baroreceptors [17, 183–185] as well as the magnitude of PO_2 reduction (Figure 6.2). It is well documented that the usual fetal response to acute hypoxia is bradycardia accompanied by hypertension and blood flow redistribution to vital organs [139, 142]. However, several studies have also suggested that the normal fetal response to mild reductions in PO_2 is to increase FHR [50, 159, 182]. Thus, the hypothesis of Clapp et al. [45] that exercise-induced increases in FHR represent the normal fetal response to mild hypoxia is well-supported from a theoretical viewpoint. However, additional study is needed to verify this hypothesis.

A central area of controversy in the study of fetal responses to acute maternal exercise has been the frequency and clinical significance of fetal bradycardia during or following maternal exercise in healthy women undergoing normal pregnancies. Since bradycardia is a well-accepted indicator of fetal distress during labor and delivery, it is logical to assume that exercise-induced bradycardia is an autonomic reaction associated with increased fetal catecholamine release related in turn to acute fetal hypoxia caused by reduced uterine blood flow.

As summarized in Table 6.3, several laboratories have reported episodes of exercise-induced bradycardia in apparently healthy fetuses [10, 28, 57, 97, 156, 189, 192], whereas others have reported no evidence of this phenomenon [22, 100, 171, 179]. The true incidence of exercise-induced bradycardia has not yet been clarified because of difficulties in obtaining artifact-free data during vigorous maternal activity and inconsistent criteria for the identification of bradycardia.

First, it should be clarified that fetal bradycardia (or tachycardia) represents a change in FHR baseline rather than a periodic change from an established baseline (i.e., accelerations or decelerations). The generally accepted clinical definition of fetal bradycardia is a reduction in FHR below 120 beats·min^{-1} lasting for at least 2 minutes [142, Table 6.2]. However, definitions of fetal bradycardia used in completed studies of exercise during pregnancy have included FHR < 110 beats·min^{-1} for more than 10s [28] and a decrease in FHR of $\geq$ 20 beats·min^{-1} from a previous baseline [189]. Most other reports of exercise-induced fetal bradycardia did not describe their criteria for identification of bradycardia. Thus, the true incidence of exercise-induced bradycardia is difficult to estimate because of varying measurement criteria for its detection. In some published studies,

TABLE 6.3
Fetal Bradycardia Reported with Maternal Aerobic Exercise

Author	Exercise Test	Monitor Type	Sample Size (n)	Fetal Bradycardia (n) During	After
Hon and Wohl-gemuth [85]	Master step-test	Abdominal ECG	26	NA	3
Dale et al. [57]	Submax tread-mill	Doppler ultra-sound	4	3	0
Jovanovic et al. [97]	Submax—cycle ergometer	Doppler ultra-sound	6	4	0
Artal et al. [8, 10]	Submax and symptom-lim-ited max—treadmill	Doppler ultra-sound	30	2 (sub-max) 3 (max)	0
Rauramo [156]	Submax—cycle ergometer	Ultrasound and abdominal ECG	61	2	5
Carpenter et al. [28]	Submax and max—cycle ergometer	Linear array 2-D ultrasound	45	1 (sub-max)	1 (sub-max) 15 (max)
Webb et al. [192]	Submax—cycle ergometer	Doppler ultra-sound	38	1	2
Watson et al. [189]	Cycle ergometer and tethered swim	Continuous-wave Doppler	45	0	6
Total			255	14	32

FHR changes described as fetal bradycardia probably represent FHR decelerations (a periodic feature) rather than time bradycardia (a change in FHR baseline) as defined in major obstetric textbooks [142]. Both the clinical and physiological significance of such decelerations are questionable [13, 120].

Another problem in identifying the true prevalence of exercise-induced fetal bradycardia has been the presence of artifact, which is often detected when FHR is measured during vigorous motion by Doppler ultrasound. Modern Doppler ultrasound FHR monitors use autocorrelation circuits that can record rhythmic maternal cycling or stepping motions during exercise tests. These may be mistaken for FHR recordings representing fetal bradycardia [11, 138]. Again, this probably leads to overestimation of the true prevalence of exercise-induced fetal bradycardia.

One method of overcoming the problem of motion artifact in FHR studies during exercise is to use either M-mode [138] or two-dimensional echocardiography [28, 45] to image fetal cardiac anatomy and function. Carpenter et al. [28] used two-dimensional echocardiography to study FHR responses to cycle ergometer exercise performed by 45 healthy women between 20 and 34 weeks gestation. Data were collected during and following 85 submaximal tests (maternal HR ≤148 beats·min⁻¹) and 79 "maximal" tests terminated at volitional fatigue. The criteria for identification of fetal bradycardia was FHR <110 beats·min⁻¹ for ≥ 10 sec. Bradycardia was observed during exercise on only one occasion. This occurred during a submaximal test in association with a maternal vasovagal hypotensive reaction. The same fetus became bradycardic during postexercise recovery from a maximal test conducted on a different day. No other occurrences of fetal bradycardia were detected, resulting in an incidence of 1.2%. Fetal bradycardia was observed during recovery from 15 "maximal" tests (16.2%). Fetal bradycardia during or following maternal exercise was not associated with clinically significant perinatal complications or fetal mortality.

Another method of obtaining valid FHR data during maternal exercise is to recognize and control for motion artifact when Doppler ultrasound FHR monitors are used. In this regard, Webb et al. [192] examined the fetal responses of two groups of healthy, previously sedentary pregnant women before (20 min), during, and following (20 min) two submaximal cycle ergometer tests conducted at 28±1 and 37±1 weeks gestation, respectively. An experimental group (n=27) participated in an individually prescribed cycle ergometer conditioning regimen during the second and third trimesters, and the other group (n=22) acted as controls and remained sedentary. Exercise tests involved 15 minutes of upright cycling at a maternal heart rate of 140 beats·min⁻¹. Cycling tests were interrupted briefly after both 5 and 10 minutes of exercise to obtain tracings that were free of potential motion artifact. Fetal bradycardia was defined as FHR < 120 beats·min⁻¹ for ≥ 120 sec. FHR recordings during exercise were considered technically acceptable only if they were continuous with those recorded during nonexercising periods. Analysis of 87 technically satisfactory tests revealed only 3 episodes of fetal bradycardia (3.4% of tests). One was observed during exercise in a test conducted in late gestation. The other two were observed following exercise (a second trimester control subject and a third trimester exercising subject). All three women subsequently delivered healthy infants.

Considered together, the results of Carpenter et al. [28] and Webb et al. [192] suggest several important conclusions concerning the incidence of exercise-induced fetal bradycardia. First, it appears that significant fetal deceleratory responses occur infrequently (< 5% incidence) in association with moderate (maternal HR < 150 beats·min⁻¹) exercise performed by healthy pregnant women. It is noteworthy that the incidence of 3.4% reported by Webb et al. [192] was similar to that reported by Carpenter et al. [28] for submaximal exercise (1.2%), despite the longer duration of exercise (15 versus 6 min). However, the criteria for identification of fetal bradycardia used by Webb et al. [192] were also more stringent (FHR ± 120 beats·min⁻¹ for ≥ 120 sec versus FHR < 110 beats·min⁻¹ for ≥ 10 sec).

The findings of Carpenter et al. [28] and Webb et al. [192] further suggest that the most common time of onset of fetal bradycardia is within the first 2–3 minutes of postexercise recovery. The reduction in FHR is usually moderate (FHR, 75–120 beats·min⁻¹) and transient (< 10 min). Both the onset and recovery from exercise-induced bradycardia are often rapid, and compensatory tachycardia may also occur later in the recovery period [100, 192]. Furthermore, fetal bradycardia is much more likely after maximal maternal exertion than during moderate exercise (maternal HR ≤ 150 beats·min⁻¹), presumably because of greater reduction in uterine blood flow at higher exercise intensities [108]. Finally, parallel studies by Watson et al. [189] also suggest that fetal bradycardia (defined as a decrease in FHR of 20 beats·min⁻¹ from preexercise FHR baseline) is less likely to occur following exercise in the water (tethered swimming), compared with maximal exercise on land (upright cycling).

The most reasonable explanation for findings described above is a reduction in uterine blood flow and uteroplacental oxygen delivery, which occurs in the immediate postexercise period. When strenuous exercise is suddenly discontinued, there is a rapid decline in cardiac output. However, at the same time, peripheral vascular resistance remains low because of persistent vasodilation of skeletal muscle vascular beds. The resulting tendency toward venous pooling and postexercise hypotension may be further augmented by the increase in venous capacitance that occurs during pregnancy [75, 76]. Thus, a temporary reduction in maternal cardiac output following strenuous exercise can lead to a significant reduction in maternal cardiac output and uterine blood flow. If this reaction is severe enough, the decrease in fetal PO_2 may be large enough to elicit a fetal vagal response, leading in turn to bradycardia. The lower incidence of fetal bradycardia reported following exercise in the water versus land exercise may be the result of less exercise-induced reduction in maternal blood volume and enhanced preservation of uteroplacental perfusion following maternal exercise [189].

Since fetal bradycardia is a well-accepted indicator of fetal hypoxia or asphyxia during labor and delivery, its occurrence during or following strenuous maternal exercise has been a subject of serious concern and controversy. However, several lines of experimental evidence suggest that sporadic occurrences of moderate exercise-induced bradycardia in the fetuses of women experiencing healthy pregnancies are usually unimportant from a clinical viewpoint. First, it should be recognized that fetal bradycardia is a normal fetoprotective reflex, which is accompanied by hypertension and redistribution of fetal cardiac output to favor vital organs including the brain, heart, adrenal gland, and placenta [48, 49, 142]. The reduction in FHR also appears to be partly compensated by an increased stroke volume [48, 49]. The apparent purpose of these autonomic reactions is to minimize fetal oxygen utilization.

The ability of a healthy fetus to tolerate reduced oxygen availability, hypoxia, and associated bradycardia without decompensation has also been examined in experimental preparations involving pregnant sheep [16, 71,

92, 190]. These studies demonstrate that fetal oxygen delivery under normal homeostatic conditions is approximately twice that required to maintain an adequate fetal O_2 uptake and to prevent metabolic acidosis [190]. When fetal O_2 delivery is reduced, cerebral O_2 utilization remains constant across a broad range of arterial oxygen tensions, as a result of increases in cerebral blood flow [92]. During hypoxia, myocardial blood flow is also increased, and both myocardial O_2 utilization and function are unchanged relative to normoxic conditions [71]. Parer [142] estimated that the circulatory adaptation described above enable the human fetus to survive periods of moderate hypoxia of up to one hour without decompensation. Exercise-induced fetal bradycardia in apparently healthy subjects has not been associated with significant perinatal morbidity or fetal mortality in any published study.

Existing research also indicates that fetal bradycardia is of much greater concern when it is accomplished by a significant reduction or loss of FHR variability. As described above, STV cannot be measured accurately by conventional Doppler ultrasound fetal monitors [142]. To our knowledge, no information is available concerning the effects of acute maternal exercise on STV. Only a few studies have reported the effects of acute maternal exercise on LTV in healthy women [22, 28, 68, 191, 192]. These studies uniformly indicate maintenance of normal LTV following prolonged submaximal exercise [192], following graded near-maximal exercise testing [22], and following static handgrip exercise to fatigue [191]. In the investigation of Carpenter et al. [28] and Webb et al. [192], cited above, all episodes of exercise-induced bradycardia were accompanied by maintenance of normal FHR variability.

Another important indicator of fetal well-being is normal reactivity. Specific criteria to confirm normal reactivity vary across available medical literature. However, it is generally accepted that FHR accelerations (> 15 beats·min^{-1}) should be observed in association with periodic fetal movements. Existing information again supports the general viewpoint that a clinically acceptable level of fetal reactivity is maintained following various forms and intensities of acute maternal exercise performed during a healthy pregnancy [22, 28, 79, 99, 191, 192].

The influence of fetal maturation on the FHR characteristics discussed above is also important to consider in studies of fetal adaptability to acute maternal exercise. The most fundamental change is a progressive reduction in FHR baseline, which occurs with advancing gestational age and development of the fetal autonomic nervous system [62, 88, 168]. This also applies to FHR values measured during and/or following standard exercise [22, 38, 45, 192]. Two recent studies [45, 192] also suggest that the degree of FHR elevation in response to dynamic exercise increases with advancing gestational age. The data of Webb et al. [192] also support the hypothesis that postexercise recovery of FHR to preexercise baseline occurs more rapidly in late- than in mid-gestation. All of these effects can be attributed to development of the fetal autonomic nervous system and enhanced vagal control of FHR [184]. Finally, both fetal reactivity and the frequency of FHR accelerations increase with advancing gestational age at rest [168] and following maternal exercise [192].

Since acute dynamic exercise reduces uterine blood flow and since changes in FHR are correlated with varying degrees of fetal hypoxia or asphyxia, FHR monitoring following a standard maternal exercise test was evaluated in early investigations as a method of detecting uteroplacental insufficiency prior to labor and delivery [85, 151, 153, 170, 173]. Common causes of uteroplacental compromise include toxemia, preeclampsia, postmaturity, multiple pregnancy, diabetes, and umbilical cord compression [50]. Although exercise-induced FHR abnormalities were generally found to be more frequent in women with complicated pregnancies, these studies were often compromised by the use of relatively crude FHR measurement methods, small or heterogeneous study samples, inconsistent criteria for identifying abnormal FHR responses, or failure to standardize the exercise modality, posture, intensity, and duration.

More recently, Brotenak and Sureau [23] performed 1558 exercise tests on 375 women with either healthy or complicated pregnancies (gestational age ≥ 35 weeks). Three to six consecutive exercise tests were performed on each pregnant woman. The exercise test consisted of FHR monitoring in the supine tilted position for 10 minutes immediately following 3 minutes of stair climbing. The FHR response to exercise was considered normal or negative, regardless of maternal health status, when its pattern either remained the same or exhibited one of two variants, depending upon gestational age. In fetuses 35–38 weeks of gestation, some fetuses exhibited a mild saltatory FHR pattern. At 39–41 weeks, some FHR patterns were characterized by a slight temporary acceleration and/or diminished variability. Negative results indicated uteroplacental sufficiency and fetal well-being. In contrast, an abnormal (or positive) exercise test result, characterized by a deceleration in FHR following maternal exercise, indicated compromise in uteroplacental circulation. In some patients with preeclampsia or who had prolonged pregnancies, FHR decelerations following maternal exercise were observed. The FHR abnormalities progressively worsened as the severity of the uteroplacental insufficiency increased. In contrast to earlier investigations, these results support the usefulness of postexercise FHR monitoring for the early detection of uteroplacental insufficiency.

Maternal exercise as an antepartum stress test has several potential advantages. Uteroplacental and umbilical circulation can be evaluated indirectly through FHR monitoring. Moderate exercise can be well tolerated by most pregnant women and, depending upon FHR responses to maternal exercise, limitations for maternal exertion during pregnancy could be identified. However, its safety, sensitivity, and specificity have yet to be verified. Also, technical difficulties encountered in obtaining satisfactory FHR tracings during the exercise test are inherent to such testing [138] and limit the test's specificity or ability to accurately detect noncompromised fetuses. The exercise test can detect fetuses at risk; however, it may also erroneously indicate fetuses in distress (e.g., false positives). Further research is needed to determine the intensity, duration and modality of exercise that would be most useful for diagnostic purposes. In addition, research is needed on the sensitivity and specificity of such a test in evaluating fetal status by correlating test results with labor, delivery, and birth outcome records.

Fetal Activity
Only a few studies have examined the influence of maternal exercise on FM [38, 99, 148]. Platt et al. [148] studied the FM patterns in 17 pregnant women (gestational age = 34.2 ± 0.6 weeks) following 15 minutes of mild treadmill exercise. No statistical difference was observed in the number of fetal movements recorded before and after maternal exercise. Using underwater real-time ultrasound imaging, Katz and associates [99] observed no change in FM (gross body movement, fetal limb movements, and fetal breathing) in fetuses 15–35 weeks of gestation with maternal immersion and exercise on a modified cycle ergometer in water. In contrast, Clapp [38] recorded a decrease in fetal motion within the initial 7 minutes of recovery after having the subjects (gestational ages = 20 and 32 weeks) run on a treadmill at an intensity of 36–79% $\dot{V}O_2$max for 20 minutes.

In theory, fetal hypoxia could increase the frequency of FBM, although, many other factors (e.g., mechanical stimuli, blood glucose levels, pH, hormonal factors, and altered maternal arterial gas concentrations) may be involved in the alterations of FBM patterns associated with maternal exercise. The mechanisms that may be responsible for this alteration are enigmatic [112, 113, 148]; however it is believed that in the fetus, as in adults, increased levels of $PaCO_2$ play a major role in the regulation of breathing [53, 113].

Maršál and associates [112, 113] suggested that compared with FHR patterns, FBM may be a more sensitive indicator of the physiological state of the fetus following maternal exercise. They observed a significant increase in the incidence of irregular breathing and a reduction in periods of apnea and periodic breathing following five minutes of mild maternal bed-type cycle ergometer exercise, whereas FHR baseline and variability were not altered. Regular breathing patterns were reestablished within five minutes of recovery. In contrast, Bousfeild et al. (cited in [148]) observed a reduction in fetal breathing movements following a two-minute step-test, and Platt and associates [148] found no significant change in FBM after their subjects engaged in 15 minutes of mild treadmill exercise (Table 6.4).

Only one study has examined the influence of static maternal exercise on FBM patterns. Maršál et al. [113] studied the FBM responses of 10 normal, healthy pregnant women in their third trimester (gestational ages = 30–40

TABLE 6.4
Studies on fetal Breathing Movement Patterns (FBM) during and following Maternal Aerobic Exercise

Authors	Subjects	Length of Gestation (weeks)	Fetal Monitor	Maternal Aerobic Exercise			FBM Response to Maternal Exercise	
				Modality	Intensity	Duration (min)	During	After
Maršál et al. [112]	n = 30 27 normal 1 mild cholestasis 1 ABO isoimmunization	30–42 (median = 35th week)	A-mode ultrasound	Bed-type cycle ergometer	80 watts	5	NA	↑ irregular breathing ↓ apnea ↓ periodic breathing
Maršál et al. [113]	n = 10 9 normal 1 slight cholestasis	30–40	A-mode ultrasound	Bed-type cycle ergometer	80 watts	5	NA	↑ FBM
Bousfield, 1980 (cited in Platt et al. [148])	n = NA mixed sample	NA	Real-time ultrasound	Bench-step	200 kg-m/min, hypertensives 400 kg-m/min, normotensives	2	NA	→
Platt et al. [148]	n = 17 normal	34.2 ± 0.6	linear array real-time scanner	Treadmill	2 mph (2.33 METS)	15	NA	↔

NA = data not available; ↓ = decrease; ↔ = no change; ↑ = increase.

weeks) to sustained hand-grip exercise at one-third maximum voluntary contraction. No change in FBM was observed following this challenge.

Since normal FBM patterns are episodic and interspersed with irregular periods of apnea, measurement of human fetal breathing patterns has not normally been used clinically as an indicator of fetal well-being [144]. However, it may be used in combination with other biophysical parameters. Further research is needed to determine the usefulness of FBM monitoring to assess fetal well-being during maternal exercise.

Maternal-Fetal Fuel Homeostasis
Accurate information on the effects of exercise on maternal fuel homeostasis is essential in view of fetal dependence on maternal blood glucose as a primary energy source [80, 90]. Indeed, several laboratories have reported significant reductions in maternal blood glucose concentrations following strenuous exertion in late gestation [20, 39, 148]. In theory, such hypoglycemic responses are of serious concern, since fetal glucose availability may be temporarily compromised. If such exercise is repeated on a chronic basis (i.e., physical conditioning), then intrauterine growth retardation or other developmental problems may occur (Figure 6.4).

Currently, significant controversy exists concerning the causes of postexercise hypoglycemic responses in late pregnancy. The data of Clapp and colleagues [35, 39] suggest that carbohydrate versus fat utilization by contracting maternal skeletal muscle is increased during submaximal exercise during pregnancy, compared with the nonpregnant state. This hypothesis is based on values for the respiratory exchange ratio (RER = $\dot{V}CO_2:\dot{V}O_2$) during standard submaximal exercise. Increased maternal carbohydrate utilization may, in theory, result from the additive hyperinsulinemia in pregnancy, in addition to increased glucose uptake resulting from muscle contraction [19, 149, 150]. However, the development of substantial insulin resistance in late pregnancy may tend to negate this effect. Several other laboratories have reported no significant change in RER during standard submaximal work rates in late gestation, compared with the nonpregnant state [103, 146, 163, 197].

An alternative explanation for hypoglycemic responses to maternal exercise is impairment of the liver's usual glucostatic function in late pregnancy. In this regard, Mottola and Christopher [128] reported reduced liver glycogen concentrations in sedentary pregnant rats in the resting state. This could result from insulin resistance or other endocrine factors that tend to reduce glycogen storage and enhance glycogenolysis in the resting state in late pregnancy [83]. Reduced liver glycogen breakdown during strenuous exertion in late pregnancy could also result from blunted sympathoadrenal responses to strenuous exercise, which also occur in late gestation [20]. Since physical conditioning enhances insulin sensitivity [89], chronic exercise may be useful to promote glycogen storage and to maintain normal glucose tolerance [98, 195].

FIGURE 6.4

Hypothetical effects of pregnancy, acute maternal exercise, and maternal physical conditioning on maternal carbohydrate (CHO) utilization, maternal glycemic status, fetal glucose utilization, and fetal growth. (+) denotes positive relationships; (−) denotes negative relationships. (Adapted from Wolfe, L. A. and M. F. Mottola. Aerobic exercise in pregnancy: an update. Can. J. Appl. Physiol. 18:119–147, 1993.)

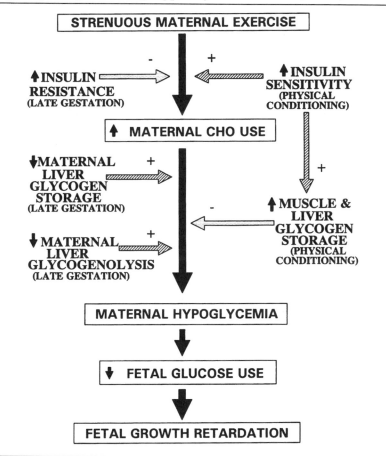

The hypothesis of reduced glucose availability to maternal skeletal muscle is further supported by measurements of respiratory gas exchange and blood lactate data from maximal or near-maximal exercise tests in healthy pregnant women. In this regard, several laboratories have reported lower peak RER values in late pregnancy than are obtained postpartum [9, 107, 118, 197]. Furthermore, lower blood lactate concentrations have also been reported during or following strenuous exercise in late pregnancy [20, 39, 117, 197]. Dilution of lactate in an expanded maternal blood volume [117] or fetal utilization of lactate as a metabolic fuel [24] could contribute to lower lactate levels. However, a significant correlation between peak RER values and peak postexercise lactate concentrations was observed by Wolfe et al. [197] during serial exercise tests during pregnancy and the postpartum period. These findings support the hypothesis that glucose availability to contracting maternal skeletal muscle is decreased, resulting in reduced maternal anaerobic working capacity.

The effects of strenuous maternal exercise on fetal fuel metabolism are also controversial. Both in humans [200] and in laboratory animals [131, 175], glucose uptake by maternal skeletal muscle is increased following acute strenuous exercise in late gestation. Treadway and Young [175] also reported that glucose uptake by the fetus was reduced by 40% following a 50-minute treadmill run in sedentary pregnant rats, suggesting that glucose uptake by the fetus is significantly compromised. In contrast, Mottola et al. [131] did not observe reduced fetal glucose uptake following treadmill running in trained pregnant rats. Their findings suggested that training may have spared glucose for conceptus consumption by promoting use of alternate fuel sources (e.g., lactate, free fatty acids) by nonexercising tissues. Clearly additional research is needed to determine the effects of both acute and chronic exercise on maternal-fetal fuel homeostasis.

Maternal-Fetal Temperature Regulation
Maternal heat exposure during specific stages of pregnancy is teratogenic for conceptual growth and development in various animal species [63, 188] and in pregnant women exposed to heat stress in the first trimester of pregnancy [121]. These teratogenic defects may result from a reversal in the fetal-maternal temperature gradient for heat exchange, whereby the flow of heat is now from mother to fetus [130].

It is not known what role maternal exercise plays in regulating body temperature, but some of the adaptations to pregnancy may enhance thermoregulation during maternal exercise. Clapp [34] suggested that a slight decrease in maternal core temperature at the onset of exercise may be due to the return of cool pooled blood from the periphery. In addition, he suggested that a downward shift in the sweating threshold allows evaporative heat loss at lower body core temperatures, that increased skin blood flow in pregnancy enhances heat transfer from the maternal core to the skin, and that an increase in minute ventilation during pregnancy may augment heat loss from the respiratory tract [34]. Furthermore, the absence of heat stress (accumulation of stress protein 72i) in the fetal tissues of trained (60–70% $\dot{V}O_2$max) pregnant rats exercised throughout gestation [129] supports the hypothesis that pregnancy-induced changes in thermoregulation may help protect the fetus from thermal stress during maternal exercise.

McMurray and Katz [116] have hypothesized that exercise in water may be more beneficial than exercise on land because water may facilitate heat loss and thermoregulation during pregnancy. However, Mottola et al. [130] reported that water temperature must be considered when exercise during immersion is suggested for controlling thermoregulation during gestation. Maternal exercise in warm water in rats (37.6±0.1°C) elevated maternal body core temperature by 2.3±0.1°C above resting values, with an increase in fetal abnormalities, compared with the same exercise intensity in thermoneutral water (34.6±0.4°C). They concluded that cool water may regulate maternal body temperature during swimming and that exercise in warm water should be avoided during pregnancy because of potential teratogenic effects.

Although it would seem that pregnancy may provide thermoregulation during exercise, there does seem to be a temperature threshold, above which, teratogenic alterations in the conceptus may occur. Because of this, it may be prudent to avoid strenuous maternal exercise and hot environments in the first trimester, when severe increases in body temperature would produce the most teratogenic problems and when pregnancy-induced protective thermal mechanisms may not be fully functional. Further research in this area is necessary.

EFFECTS OF CHRONIC MATERNAL EXERCISE ON PREGNANCY OUTCOME

As discussed in several earlier reviews [106, 193, 194, 196], much evidence supports a dose-response relationship between the quantity and quality of maternal exercise and maternal-fetal well-being. Moderate exercise improves maternal physical fitness and enhances maternal metabolic and cardiopulmonary capacities. Such exercise may also help to prevent various health problems associated with chronic physical activity (e.g., excessive weight pain, impaired glucose tolerance, poor posture, low back pain, greater susceptibility to anxiety or depression, poor body image). Conversely, the major risks of maternal overexertion include intrauterine growth retardation, altered fetal development, and shortened gestation [12, 44, 193, 194]. Thus, it would appear that the most important benefits of chronic exercise are maternal, whereas the risks apply primarily to fetal well-being.

The apparent dissociation between maternal benefits and fetal risks of chronic maternal exercise suggests that separate fetal and maternal dose-response curves may exist (Figure 6.5). The exact shapes of or interrelationship between the maternal and fetal dose-response curves for exercise need to be clarified to provide valid guidelines for occupational and recreational physical activity during pregnancy. For example, improvements in maternal metabolic and cardiopulmonary capacities may have fetoprotective effects by reducing the risk of maternal-fetal competition for metabolic substances, blood flow, and oxygen delivery. More information is also needed on the nature and extent of both placental and fetal adaptations to various levels of chronic maternal exercise. The effects of

FIGURE 6.5

Hypothetical dose-response relationships between the quantity and quality of maternal exercise on maternal and fetal well-being. (Adapted from Wolfe, L. A., P. Hall, K. A. Webb, L. Goodman, M. Monga, and M. J. McGrath. Prescription of aerobic exercise in pregnancy. Sports Med. 8:273–301, 1989.)

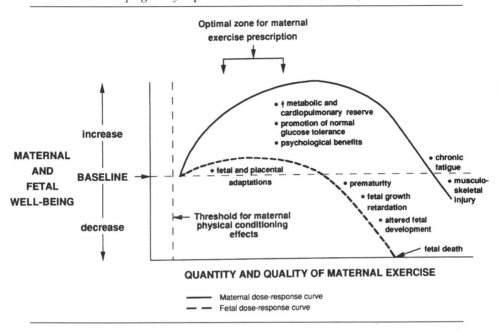

strenuous aerobic conditioning on fetal well-being have not been clarified, and such exercise may amplify maternal benefits and fetal risk simultaneously. Finally, the effects of nutritional, environmental, and psychological stresses as well as other confounding factors also need clarification.

Recent studies of chronic exercise in pregnancy fall into three main areas. First, studies of laboratory animals allow the use of tightly controlled experimental designs and mechanistic/invasive approaches that are usually not possible in studies of human subjects. Epidemiologic studies of pregnancy outcome in relation to occupational work provide an overview of the interrelationship between work activity, associated lifestyle factors, and pregnancy outcome. Finally, longitudinal physical conditioning studies are useful to confirm the maternal-fetal effects of carefully monitored and supervised exercise regimes in human subjects.

Animal Research

The literature reporting the effects of chronic exercise on pregnancy outcome in laboratory animals has previously been reviewed by Wolfe et al. [193]. The following section will consider recent animal experimentation that was not discussed in our previous review [193].

Studies reporting the effects of chronic maternal exercise on pregnancy outcome using the rat model have continued to show varying results. Courant and Barr [54] reported that newborn body weight and number per litter were unchanged in prepregnancy-trained (30 m·min⁻¹, 0° grade, 120 minutes treadmill running) maternal animals that continued running throughout pregnancy. When litter size was culled to 8 per dam, no difference in offspring growth occurred when mothers returned to exercise at 2 days postpartum and continued to exercise until day 14. These results agree with those of Mottola et al. [127] who also found no change in newborn (within 24 hours after birth) weight, organ weights, or skeletal muscle development in trained animals (prepregnancy-trained—30 m·min⁻¹, 10° incline, 120 min·day⁻¹) that ran 5 days·wk⁻¹ during pregnancy. In addition, Rodgers et al. [160] found no change in the oxidative, glycolytic, or contractile activities in skeletal muscle of offspring 28 days postpartum from animals prepregnancy-trained (26.8 m·min⁻¹, 1 hr·day⁻¹, 5 days·wk⁻¹) that continued exercise throughout pregnancy. Primary myocardial cell cultures isolated from 3- to 5-day-old neonates of dams swim-exercised at conception, 6 days·wk⁻¹ in 37°C water until birth, showed attenuation of ethanol toxicity and temporal protection from ethanol-induced damage [25]. Elevated cellular calcium content in these cell cultures may have played a role in the protective maternal-exercise effect [26], however the mechanism for this effect remains to be determined.

In contrast, Picarro et al. [147] found a decrease in newborn (within 24 hours after birth) body weight and no difference in number of offspring born to animals running on a treadmill at 70%, 80%, and 90% of $\dot{V}O_2$ max, compared with animals exercising at 60% $\dot{V}O_2$ max and sedentary control animals. These pregnant animals were not prepregnancy-trained and began exercise at conception. It appears that high-intensity maternal exercise (70% or greater) with no prepregnancy training in exercising rats may place undue stress on the fetal environment. Future studies of pregnant rats should include prepregnancy familiarization with the apparatus and exercise protocol before the animals are mated.

Although most of the data cited above from the offspring of chronically exercised rats are encouraging, these results must be interpreted cautiously because postnatal life outside the maternal environment may confound the effects of maternal exercise that has occurred during prenatal growth and development. When fetal assessment is actually done in exercising pregnant rats (between days 17 and 21, term is approximately 21 days), the more recent literature remains controversial.

Regular voluntary wheel exercise (before and during pregnancy) had no ill effects on fetal number per litter, number of resorptions, or fetal weight on day 17 of gestation [95]. The pregnant exercising rats voluntarily reduced exercise by 35% from prepregnant values, and succinate dehydrogenase/ SDH levels measured in the maternal skeletal muscle did not differ from those of sedentary control animals. This may indicate that the intensity of the voluntary exercise was too mild to elicit physiological adaptations or a training response, and may explain why no alterations were seen in fetal outcome.

In studies where SDH levels in the maternal skeletal muscle have increased as a result of a training response to treadmill running, the effect of chronic maternal exercise on fetal outcome is uncertain. Acute exercise decreases uteroplacental blood flow as a dose-response [94] when blood is rerouted to the working muscles of the mother. Jones et al. [93] examined the effects of long-term treadmill training on the attenuation of this diminished uteroplacental blood flow during acute exercise. The results suggested that training does not attenuate the reduction in uterine blood flow; in spite of the decrease in uterine blood flow, fetal outcomes of trained animals and sedentary controls did not differ. Using the same exercise intensity (30 m·min^{-1}, 10° incline, 1 hr·day^{-1}, 5 days·wk^{-1}) Mottola and Christopher [128] found heavier fetuses in the trained group. These authors also found that chronic prepregnancy training and then abrupt cessation of exercise at conception, followed by sedentary life throughout pregnancy, decreased fetal body weight. Forcing a trained animal to stop exercise at conception may place undue stress on the maternal system, which may affect fetal outcome [128].

When fetal glucose uptake was examined in trained rats following acute exercise, the amount of glucose taken up by the fetus and placenta was not different from that in sedentary control animals without food and water for the same time period [131]. Fetal outcome was not different in the trained group; however, placental weight was lower than in sedentary controls [131]. In a similar study, prepregnant trained animals ran from days 2 to 18 of gestation inclusive, and exercise increased maternal body core temperature on average 0.6°C [129]. Fetal body weight and placental weight were lower in the trained animals than in sedentary controls. Fetal tissues were probed for heat shock protein (SP) 72i (accumulation of which would suggest fetal cells were exposed to heat stress). The results showed no difference in accumulation of SP 72i in fetal heart, hind limb, or placenta, compared with sedentary controls [129]. This suggests that exercise of this intensity did not elevate maternal body temperature enough to cause a heat stress response in the fetus, yet fetal growth was affected by the maternal exercise.

The above studies indicate that factors other than a diminished uteroplacental blood flow [94], an increase in maternal body temperature [129], or availability of maternal blood glucose [131] may affect fetal or placental growth in trained animals. The discrepancy in the literature is difficult to explain; however, protective mechanisms caused by training of the maternal system may reach a threshold beyond which fetal alterations in growth may occur. However, the smaller fetuses and placentas found in trained animals may not necessarily be problematic, because developmental abnormalities, although sought [129, 131], have not been found.

Developmental abnormalities have been reported when maternal exercise in warm water (37.6 ± 0.1°C) elevated maternal body temperature by 2.3 ± 0.1°C above resting values in trained animals, compared with the same exercise intensity in cool water (34.6 ± 0.4°C) [130]. Fifty-eight percent of the abnormal fetuses and 60% of the resorption sites were found in the warm water-swimming animals. Results suggested that cool water may regulate maternal body temperature during swimming exercise and that swimming in warm water, even by trained individuals, should be avoided during gestation, because of potential teratogenic effects [130]. Other developmental abnormalities, such as a retardation of skeletal ossification in fetuses of rats trained prior to pregnancy at 40% $\dot{V}O_2$max, continuing the exercise daily up to and including day 19 of gestation [177], have been reported. Daily exercise during pregnancy may be too strenuous, even in trained animals at lower exercise intensities, causing fetal developmental abnormalities to occur. Additional research is necessary to determine fetal developmental affects from chronic maternal exercise.

The effects of chronic maternal exercise on fetal outcome in other animal species have not been recently published. Although the pregnant sheep model is ideal for studying changes in the maternal and fetal environment, chronic exercise studies are not available because of problems associated with prepregnancy training, expense, or chronic catheter maintenance. Rats appear to be the most utilized animal model for training effects on fetal outcome; however, it is difficult to mimic the upright posture of the pregnant human, and this represents one of the difficulties associated with using animal model results to predict findings in human subjects. The rat model may be best used to understand underlying mechanisms in the physiological alterations associated with training and pregnancy and the ultimate effect on fetal growth and development.

Occupational Effects on Pregnancy Outcome
Studies of birth outcome and maternal occupation and employment have been conducted to determine the risk of adverse pregnancy outcome. These studies are conflicting and difficult to compare because many do not control for confounding variables related to lifestyle that influence pregnancy outcome. Some major determinants of lifestyle that may affect prematurity are socioeconomic status (based on occupation, income, and education), race, prenatal care, employment and work, social drugs (smoking, alcohol, etc.), maternal nutrition, psychosocial stress [133], and obstetric history [55]. Other confounding factors may include occupational toxins, maternal age, gravity, prepregnancy body weight [167], height, blood pressure, fitness level, and lifestyle leisure activities. In addition, there are differences in populations (number, geographic location), sample collection, defining job activity, and statistical analyses [193].

Keeping the above factors in mind, the following studies will be highlighted. An increased risk for spontaneous abortion (< 28 weeks gestation) was found in women exposed to various levels of physical stress during employment, particularly lifting heavy weights more than 15 times per day, other physical effort, standing more than 8 hours per day, working 46 or more hours per week, changing shift work, and those reporting exposure to noise, cold, and vibration [115]. Stillbirth rates were also increased with physical effort, standing more than 8 hours per day, and exposure to vibration [115]. In contrast, Nurminen et al. [134] found no relation between an increase in physical load (lifting and carrying objects over 5 kg) and threatened abortion. However, work involving more standing increased the risk, and an association was found between maternal physical load and offspring structural malformations [134].

The risk of preterm birth ($\leq$ 37 weeks gestation) was increased in women employed in the U.S. Army who had the highest physical activity levels [155]. Similarly, women who lift heavy weights in their occupation and women who work shift work may have a higher risk for retarded fetal growth and preterm birth [6]. Women who lifted weights above 12 kg more than 50 times per week increased the risk of preterm birth, but did not increase the risk of fetal death [3]. Women in jobs characterized by high physical exertion (based on job title) had a higher rate of preterm (more than 3 weeks early) and low-birth-weight delivery (under 2500 g) [84]. In contrast, Mottola and Wolfe [132] found no change in birth outcome in women, regardless of self-reported fitness levels or occupation.

Most studies caution against high workload, heavy lifting, and physical stress, such as long hours of standing, exposure to noise, vibration, and shift work. With more women entering the work force, research controlling for confounding variables must be conducted to understand the long-term health implications for the working mother and her offspring.

Human Physical Conditioning Studies
The most direct method of evaluating chronic physical activity effects on pregnancy outcome is to conduct controlled prospective studies of human subjects. Optimal design characteristics for this type of study include the following: large study sample; random assignment of subjects to experimental (exercising) and control (sedentary) groups; careful medical screening of subjects before entry to the study; individualized exercise prescription and monitoring of exercise performed; accurate assessment of changes in physical fitness during the experimental period; ongoing medical monitoring; and evaluation of confounding effects (changes in nutrition, physical activity outside the exercise program) that could affect the experimental results [44, 193].

Most completed studies have used medical records compiled at labor and delivery to provide data. Available information usually includes gestational age at birth, length of labor and its three substages, type of delivery (e.g., vaginal, cesarian), infant birth weight and gender, evidence of fetal distress (e.g., meconium-stained amniotic fluid, fetal bradycardia), use of medications (e.g., analgesics, anesthetics, oxytocic drugs), and other perinatal complications [21]. Additional information had been obtained in some studies on neonatal morphometrics [42]. Useful morphometric indices include head circumference, length, ponderal index, adiposity/ lean body mass via the skinfold technique, placental weight, and feto-placental weight ratio [29, 42, 58]. In addition to comparison with a sedentary control group, it is also very helpful to compare birth outcome data from exercising subjects with epidemiologic data from the population under study [5].

As reviewed previously [193], numerous investigations have attempted to determine the effects of physical conditioning on pregnancy outcome. Many of these studies have included cross-sectional evaluations of birth outcomes in successful athletes [69, 201], studies of the relationships between maternal physical fitness [152, 153], case studies of physically active women [87, 178], and investigations with retrospective [91, 111] or uncontrolled prospective designs [52, 79]. Finally, a number of controlled prospective studies have used study samples that are too small to detect statistical differences in the birth outcomes of active and inactive subjects [27, 51, 57, 166, 198]. The fundamental design flaws in these studies reduce their usefulness in characterizing the relationships between chronic physical activity and measures of pregnancy outcome [193].

An overview of major controlled perspective physical conditioning studies appears in Table 6.5. As might be expected, such studies are few in number since they are labor-intensive, expensive and require the coopera-tive efforts of obstetricians, fitness specialists and statistical consultants to provide valid results. The following section provides an integrated discussion of these studies and their relationship to other physiological studies of physical conditioning in pregnancy.

The earliest of these investigations was published by Clapp and Dickstein [37]. The authors interviewed a total of 336 antepartal obstetric patients to obtain information on their normal physical activity levels and intentions to participate in regular exercise during pregnancy. Those who participated in regular endurance exercise (aerobic dance, running, cross-country skiing) were reinterviewed between 28 and 34 weeks, to document their actual levels of physical activity during pregnancy. Those who moved from the area or who developed significant obstetric complications were excluded from data analysis. Physically active subjects (n=76) were assigned to three groups in accordance with their habitual levels of activity before becoming pregnant: high activity (n=15), moderate activity (n=36), and minimal activity (n=25). Approximately 60% of these active subjects voluntarily discontinued regular exercise prior to the 28th week of gestation. These subjects gained more weight (2.2 kg) than sedentary control subjects, but infant birth weight and gestational age at delivery were similar to mean values in the control group. Conversely, physically active subjects who exercised beyond the 28th week delivered significantly earlier

(−8 days), gained less weight (−4.6 kg), and delivered lighter infants (−500 g) than active women who discontinued exercise.

Subsequent studies by Clapp and associates [42, 43] of pregnant recreational athletes provided new data that help to explain the findings of Clapp and Dickstein [37] cited above. In this regard, Clapp and Capeless [42] examined neonatal morphometrics of the infants of recreational runners and aerobic dancers who continued to exercise at or above 50% of preconceptual levels. Findings were compared with those of the infants of a control group matched for maternal age, pregravid weight, parity, and socioeconomic status, who discontinued exercise before the end of the first trimester. Infants of the women who remained active had significantly lower birth weights (−310 g), ponderal indexes (−0.24), and fetoplacental weight ratios (−0.7), but skeletal measures (head circumference, crown-heel length) were similar to those of the control group. Indices of neonatal fat mass explained 70% of the difference in birth weight between groups. Specific findings included significantly lower values for two-site skinfold thicknesses (−1.5 mm), estimated percentage body fat (−5.0%), and estimated fat mass (220 g). Thus, it appears that lower fetal adiposity accounts for a significant proportion of the difference in birth weight of active women who continued to exercise throughout the third trimester and those who ceased participation in late gestation. The mean birth weight of the infants of women who ceased exercise participation was somewhat higher than average (≈ 3690 g), whereas the birth weights of infants of women who continued to exercise were only marginally lower than average (≈ 3380 g).

A recent study by Clapp and Rizk [43] also examined the effects of exercise participation in pregnancy on placental growth in 18 recreational athletes (9 aerobic dancers, 4 runners, and 5 swimmers) who continued to exercise strenuously throughout the second trimester. Findings were compared with those of 16 matched controls. Placental volume, measured by an ultrasonographic technique, was significantly greater in the recreational athletes than in controls at 16, 20, and 24 weeks gestation. Follow-up analysis of neonatal morphometrics indicated that highest birth weights and placental weights were observed in women (n=7) who remained active throughout midpregnancy and decreased their activity levels in late pregnancy. Values for birth weight and placental weight tended to be lower than control values in women who maintained or increased their exercise levels in late gestation. These results suggest that placental growth may be stimulated by hypoxic stress associated with strenuous exercise participation continued through midgestation. However, continued participation in high-volume antigravitational exercise in late gestation may limit placental volume and limit fetal substrate delivery.

Two other recent investigations examined early pregnancy outcome [40] and the onset, time course, and outcome of labor [41], respectively, in

TABLE 6.5
Summary of Controlled Studies of Maternal Physical Conditioning and Pregnancy Outcome

Authors	Sample Size		Duration of Conditioning	Conditioning Program	Birth Outcome Results (EG vs. CG)					
	EG Exercised Group	CG Control Group			Maternal Weight Gain	Length of Gestation	Labor Duration	Problems	Infant Birth Weight (g)	APGAR 1 APGAR 5
Clapp and Dickstein [37]	47 (II) 29 (III)	152 (I)	discontinued by 28th week (II) → term (III)	Running, aerobic dance, x-country ski > 50% age-adjusted HR ≥ 30 minutes ≥ 3X/week	(II) ↑ 2.2 kg (III) ↓ 4.6 kg	(II) ↔ (III) ↓ 8 days	NA NA	↔ ↔	(II) ↔ (III) ↓ 500 g	NA NA
Kulpa et al. [104]	38	47	throughout pregnancy	Various aerobic activities, ≈ 75% age-predicted HR max ≈ 15–20 min-utes > 1X/week	↓ (2.9 kg) multigravid EG vs multigravid CG	↔	↓ 2nd stage primigravid EG vs primigravid CG	↔ multiparous ↓ meds	↔	↔
Hall and Kaufmann [78]	82 low 309 medium 61 high	393	Entry → term	Muscle and aerobic conditioning, HR ≤ 140 beats/min ≈ 45 minutes ≈ 3X/week	NA	↔	↔, ↓ in multi-paras	↓ C-section	↑ 150 g	↑, ↑

Study										
Clapp and Capeless [42]	77	55	EG: throughout pregnancy CG: prepregnancy	Running, aerobic dance ≥ 50% of preconceptual activity ≥ 30 minutes ≥ 3X/week	↓ 2.9 kg	↔	NA	NA	↓ 310 g	↔
Clapp [41]	87	44	EG: throughout pregnancy CG: prepregnancy discontinued by end of TM 1	Running, aerobic dance > 50% max capacity ≈ 30 minutes ≈ 3X/week	NA	↓ 5 days	↓ active labor & stage 1	↓ less obstetric intervention	↓ 400 g	↑
Beckmann and Beckmann [15]	50	50	8.6 weeks → term	Calisthenics, 1 hr 2X/week	↓ 1.5 kg	↔	↓ stage 1 & 2	↓ meds ↑ spontaneous vaginal delivery	↔	↔
Brenner et al. [21]	54	36	Tm2 → Tm3	Cycle ergometer HR target ≈ 14–25 minutes ≈ 3X/week	↑ 1.7 kg	↔	↔	↔	↔	↔
Sternfeld et al. [174]	161 total			Aerobic exercise	NA	↔	↔	↔	↔	↔

NA = data not available; ↓ = EG lower; ↔ = no difference; ↑ = EG higher; EG = exercise group; CG = control group; HR = heart rate; Tm = trimester.

recreational athletes who remained active during pregnancy. The former study by Clapp [40] examined the incidence of spontaneous abortion in 47 runners, 40 aerobic dancers, and 28 physically fit controls who ceased strenuous exercise participation prior to conception. The incidence of spontaneous abortion was 17% in the runners, 18% in the aerobic dancers, and 25% in the controls. These results suggested that the incidence of early pregnancy wastage is not increased by continued exercise participation during pregnancy by recreational athletes. In another study by Clapp (41], labor characteristics were compared in 87 recreational athletes who continued exercise participation (> 50% of preconceptual level) throughout pregnancy and 44 recreational athletes who discontinued participation before the end of the first trimester. The incidence of preterm labor (prior to 263 days) was the same (9%) in both groups. However, the average onset of labor was significantly earlier (−5 days) in the group who remained active. Other differences between the active and inactive groups included a lower incidence of abdominal and vaginal surgical delivery, a shorter mean duration of the active stages of labor, and reduced incidence of indicators of fetal distress (26 verses 50%). As in other reports from this research group [37, 42, 43], birth weight was also significantly lower in the group who remained physically active (3369 verses 3776 g).

Several other investigations have reported findings that differ significantly from those of Clapp and associates concerning aerobic-type physical conditioning and infant birth weight. For example, Kulpa et al. [104] studied the pregnancy outcomes of a large group of women (n=141) with low-risk pregnancies. Subjects were first tested (Bruce treadmill test) to measure their aerobic fitness during the first trimester and were then given individualized prescriptions (heart rate target, 75% of maximum) for aerobic exercise. The exercise modalities included walking, jogging, swimming, cycling, cross-country skiing, aerobics, and racquetball, and subjects kept records of actual exercise performed. Follow-up tests of aerobic fitness were conducted during the third trimester (Åstrand-type cycle ergometer test) and postpartum (Bruce treadmill test). Dropouts (n=20), noncompliant subjects (n=2), and those who aborted spontaneously (n=8) were excluded from final data analysis. Also, subjects with significant perinatal complications (n=2) were assigned to a "nonqualifying" group. The remaining subjects were then assigned either to an exercise group (17 primigravidas, 21 multigravidas) or a control group (20 primigravidas, 27 multigravidas). The latter had exercised no more than once per week for 15–20 minutes at the target heart rate. Changes in aerobic working capacity (max METs) between first trimester and postpartum treadmill tests were significantly greater in the exercised group. All subject groups gained acceptable amounts of weight. However, multigravid exercising subjects gained significantly less weight than multigravid controls (12.5 kg versus 15.4 kg). A trend also existed toward a shorter active phase of the second stage of labor in primigravid exercisers versus primigravid controls. Exercise had no apparent effect on either neonatal morbidity or the incidence of obstetric complications. There were no significant differences between groups in gestational age at delivery, Apgar scores at birth, or birth weight. A noteworthy feature of this study is that all subjects were given nutritional counseling to ensure that caloric intake satisfied the additional energy demands of both pregnancy and exercise.

Hall and Kaufmann [78] studied birth outcome data from the clinical records of 845 women receiving obstetric care in private practices in Florida. Women without contraindications to exercise were asked to participate in supervised, individually prescribed exercise classes conducted 3 days·wk⁻¹ throughout pregnancy. These classes included a 5-minute aerobic warmup, approximately 45 minutes of muscular conditioning exercise, and a period of cycling (duration not specified) at a maternal heart rate ≤ 140 beats·min⁻¹. At the end of the study the subjects were assigned to one of the following groups in accordance with the number of sessions attended during pregnancy: control group (0–10 sessions, n=393), low-exercise group (11–20 sessions, n=82), medium-exercise group (21–59 sessions, n=309), high-exercise group (60–99 sessions, n=61). Specific findings included significantly higher 1- and 5-minute Apgar scores in the high-exercise group versus other groups and a nonsignificant data trend (p=0.06) toward lower birth weights in the control group versus high-exercise group. The need for cesarian section decreased with greater exercise participation. Finally, the mean length of hospital stay was highest in the control group and lowest in the high exercise group.

Another important study is that of Lokey et al. [105], who used a statistical meta-analysis to the pooled data from prospective studies conducted prior to 1989 that examined the effects of regular aerobic-type exercise on conventional pregnancy outcome variables. This approach helps to circumvent design problems of individual studies, including small sample sizes or failure to also study a nonexercising control group. The final analyses were applied to 18 studies, which employed 26 exercising groups (total subjects, 1357) and 11 control groups (total subjects, 957). These studies included the major investigations of Clapp and Dickstein [37], Kulpa et al [104], and Hall and Kaufmann [78] described above. The results indicated that the experimental subjects exercised an average of 3.3 days·wk⁻¹ for 43 min·day⁻¹ at a target heart rate between 140 and 152 beats·min⁻¹. No significant differences were found between exercising and nonexercising groups for maternal weight gain (12.9 versus 14.2 kg), gestational age at birth (39.8 versus 39.9 wk), length of labor (10.1 versus 7.3 hr), infant birth weight (3.4 versus 3.5 kg), or 5-minute Apgar scores (8.8 versus 8.4). Thus, it appears that moderate aerobic conditioning does not significantly alter conventional indexes of labor and pregnancy outcome.

Two other recent studies also support the hypothesis that moderate

aerobic conditioning does not jeopardize fetal development or complicate labor. Sternfeld et al. [174] studied the effects of varying levels of
exercise participation prior to conception and during each trimester on
pregnancy outcome data obtained from the medical records of 161 women.
Subjects were divided into the following exercise participation groups for
each time period: I—involvement in aerobic exercise excluding vigorous
walking for $\geq$ 3 days·wk^{-1}, > 20 min·day^{-1}; II—same as group I, but including
vigorous walking: III—regular involvement in aerobic exercise < 3
days·wk^{-1}, < 20 min·day^{-1}; IV—no regular involvement in aerobic exercise.
No significant effects were observed for exercise participation before
pregnancy or at any time during pregnancy on gestational age at birth,
birth weight, spontaneous versus induced labor, length of labor, mode of
delivery, 1- and 5-minute Apgar scores, or frequency of maternal/fetal
labor complications.

Wolfe and associates [21, 22, 192, 194, 197] studied the effects of chronic
weight-supported exercise (upright cycling) on conventional pregnancy
outcome variables and maternal-fetal responses to graded exercise in 54
healthy, previously sedentary women. A nonexercising control group
(n=36) with similar characteristics was also studied. All subjects entered the
study at the beginning of the second trimester. Experimental subjects
participated in a progressive individually prescribed exercise regimen
during the second and third trimester and detrained postpartum. Classes
were supervised by qualified prenatal fitness instructors and included a
warmup, periods of muscular conditioning and stationary cycling, and a
cooldown period. Subjects were also given advice on good nutrition during
pregnancy. The target heart rate for stationary cycling was approximately
140–150 beats·min^{-1}. Cycling duration was increased from 14 to 25
min·session^{-1} during the second trimester and was held constant during the
third trimester. All subjects were tested using a graded submaximal cycling
protocol on entry to the study, at the end of the second and third
trimesters, and 3–4 months postpartum. Pregnancy outcome data were
obtained from medical records compiled during labor and delivery.
Physiological studies provided evidence for improvements in aerobic
working capacity and the work rate at the onset of blood lactate
accumulation during graded exercise between study entry and third-
trimester testing [197]. Surprisingly, exercising subjects gained slightly
more weight, and skinfold thicknesses increased to a significantly greater
extent during the course of the exercise program [197]. Parallel studies of
blood biochemistry (plasma insulin, glucose) [195] suggested that this was
due at least in part to exercise-induced attenuation of insulin resistance
that develops during the pregnancy as a result of the antiinsulin effects of
gestational hormones. Pregnancy outcomes were favorable in both groups,
and no significant differences existed for gestational age at birth (39.9
versus 39.5 wk), infant birth weight (3539 versus 3592 g), 1- and 5-minute
Apgar scores, or the frequency of labor complications in the exercised

versus the control group. A nonsignificant data trend also existed for a shorter duration of labor in the exercised group.

Only one major study has examined the effects of muscular strength training by itself on labor and pregnancy outcomes. Beckmann and Beckmann [15] examined the effects of an antepartal muscular conditioning regimen on the labor outcomes of 50 healthy primiparous women. Data obtained from the subjects' medical records were compared with those of 50 nonexercising pregnant controls with similar characteristics. The exercise program was conducted twice per week for one hour, and each subject participated for a minimum of 12 weeks. Classes included a warmup and cooldown, specific exercises to strengthen the upper and lower limbs and abdominal region, as well as Kegel exercises to strengthen the perineal muscles. Mean values were similar with regard to infant birth weight and length, gestational age at delivery and both 1- and 5-minute Apgar scores. The exercised group gained significantly less weight (11.8 versus 13.3 kg) and had shorter first and second stages of labor. Significant trends also existed toward less need for oxytocin-augmented delivery and a greater likelihood of spontaneous vaginal delivery.

SUMMARY AND CONCLUSIONS

A significant body of experimental evidence supports the general concept that dose-response relationships exist between the quantity and quality of maternal exercise and both maternal and fetal well-being. However, the maternal and fetal dose-response curves appear to differ significantly from one another. In particular, strenuous aerobic conditioning may be more beneficial than moderate activity in enhancing maternal metabolic and cardiopulmonary capacities (i.e., aerobic fitness), but fetal risks of strenuous conditioning appear to be much greater than with moderate activity. Specific findings that support this general hypothesis include the following:

1. Studies involving both animal models [32, 33, 82, 93, 94, 108] and human subjects [125, 126, 157] have reported that uterine blood flow decreases during acute strenuous maternal exercise. The magnitude of this reduction appears to be directly correlated with the exercise intensity and duration [108]. In humans, exercise posture [125] and pregnancy complications [125, 126, 157] also appear to be important determinants of uterine blood flow during exercise. Reduced uterine blood flow may be compensated by blood flow redistribution favoring the cotyledons versus myometrium [56], exercise-induced hemoconcentration [77], and increased fetal arteriovenous oxygen extraction [110]. Studies of exercising laboratory animals further suggest that fetal PO_2 is only moderately reduced [32, 68, 109, 137].

2. The most common FHR response to maternal dynamic exercise is an increase of approximately 5–25 beats·min^{-1} with a gradual return to preexercise baseline during postexercise recovery [10, 38, 45, 60, 179, 191, 192]. The degree of FHR elevation appears to depend on the modality, intensity, and duration of maternal exercise [45, 92] as well as gestational age [38, 45, 192]. The best explanation for FHR elevation is a fetal sympathoadrenal response to exercise-induced fetal hypoxia [45, 50, 59, 108, 137, 182], although factors such as increased fetal temperature [181], changes in fetal arousal levels [96], or maternal-fetal transfer of catecholamines [122, 169] may also contribute to this response.

3. Fetal bradycardia is occasionally observed in association with acute bouts of maternal aerobic exercise in healthy women experiencing normal pregnancies [28, 192]. Such responses occur more frequently in association with maximal than moderate submaximal aerobic exercise, and the most common time of occurrence is in the immediate postexercise recovery period [28, 192]. Postexercise FHR deceleration is probably a reflex vagal response to acute hypoxia [139, 142] associated with maternal hypotension and reduced uterine blood flow during recovery from strenuous exercise [192]. Such responses are usually moderate and transient and are not usually associated with reduced FHR variability or significant perinatal mortality and morbidity [28, 192]. However, exercise-induced FHR abnormalities also appear to be more prevalent in women with uteroplacental insufficiency [23, 85, 151, 153, 170, 173]. Fetal bradycardia is a normal protective response to acute hypoxia, aimed at preservation of blood flow and oxygen delivery to the fetal brain, heart, and other vital organs [48, 49, 142].

4. Several laboratories have reported maternal hypoglycemic responses to strenuous aerobic-type exercise in late gestation [20, 39, 148]. Factors that may contribute to such responses include increases in fetal glucose uptake with advancing gestation, increased carbohydrate utilization by contracting maternal skeletal muscle [19, 149, 150], decreased maternal liver glycogen stores [128], or reduced catecholamine-mediated liver glycogenolysis in late pregnancy [20]. The influence of such postexercise maternal hypoglycemic responses on fetal glucose availability and uptake remain to be clarified.

5. Although more research is definitely needed, available information supports the concept that rises in core temperature in response to strenuous exercise are attenuated as a result of a reduced sweating threshold and augmented skin blood flow [34]. These adaptations are reported to appear in early pregnancy and may be useful in preventing teratogenic effects associated with chronic thermal stress [63, 188].

6. Recent studies using the exercising rat model have produced conflicting results concerning the effects of chronic maternal exercise on fetal development [25, 26, 54, 95, 127, 147, 160]. These inconsistencies may

be due to variations in the modality, intensity, duration, frequency, and time of the application of the exercise stimulus (i.e., dose-response effects). Other confounding variables may include psychological stress related to the use of forced exercise, the degree of thermal stress, and nutritional factors [193].

7. Studies of the effects of maternal occupational work on pregnancy outcome have produced conflicting results, probably because of the difficulties in controlling the effects of confounding variables such as maternal age, nutrition, drug use, psychological factors, and other environmental factors [55, 133, 167]. Some evidence suggests that involvement in heavy lifting [3, 115], shift work, activities involving prolonged standing [115, 134], and chronic exposure to noise or vibration [115] may increase the risk of prematurity or fetal growth retardation.

8. Data from controlled prospective physical conditioning studies [21, 78, 104, 105, 174] support the hypothesis that moderate aerobic conditioning of healthy well-nourished women can improve maternal physical fitness without increasing the risk of premature labor, fetal growth retardation, or altered fetal development. Such exercise may also be useful in preventing gestational glucose intolerance [98, 154, 195] and preserving maternal energy stores in late gestation [30, 197]. Some evidence suggests that such conditioning may help facilitate labor in primiparous women [21, 104].

9. Studies of continued participation in strenuous exercise during pregnancy by recreational athletes [37, 40–43] indicate that the length of gestation is slightly reduced and infant birth weight is lower in women who continue such exercise during the third trimester. The main cause of diminished birth weight appears to be reduced adiposity. Conversely, continued exercise participation until midgestation may augment placental vascular volume and may promote maternal weight gain.

10. Although further study is needed, existing information supports the hypothesis that properly performed static or high-resistance exercise does not jeopardize fetal well-being [113, 191] or alter pregnancy outcome [15, 78].

RECOMMENDATIONS FOR FUTURE STUDY

Considerable progress has been made during the past decade in providing reliable information on the interactive effects of pregnancy and exercise. However, since both pregnancy and exercise are extremely complex biological processes, many important theoretical and practical questions remain to be answered, and this remains an important and extremely challenging area for future study. Recognizing this, an N.I.H. working subcommittee was formed in 1991 to evaluate the existing knowledge base and to provide specific recommendations for future study [44]. The findings of this working subcommittee and those of the present review are in close agreement and support the urgent need for additional study in the following areas:

1. More information is needed on both maternal and fetoplacental metabolic, endocrine, cardiorespiratory, and thermal adaptations to acute and chronic exercise in healthy human subjects. In particular, physiological mechanisms that are fetoprotective need to be identified and quantified to provide a clear understanding of the normal level of maternal-fetal adaptive reserve.

2. Large-scale controlled prospective studies are still required to accurately describe the dose-response relationships between various types (e.g., static, dynamic, intermittent) and modalities (e.g., walking, swimming, weight training) of prenatal recreational and occupational physical activity and valid measures of labor and pregnancy outcome. The latter should include measures of maternal energy balance, detailed evaluation of fetal growth and development, effects on labor characteristics and fetal well-being during the neonatal period, the time course of recovery from labor, postnatal growth and development, and maternal psychosocial well-being. Studies of occupational physical activity should pay particular attention to the identification of the confounding influences of psychological, nutritional, postural, and environmental stresses that may alter the normal dose-response relationships between chronic physical activity and pregnancy outcome.

3. Very little information currently exists on the effects of postnatal physical activity on the time course and extent of postpartum recovery and the process of lactation.

4. The validity of various animal models (e.g., rat, sheep, hamster) to predict physiological responses and pregnancy outcome in human subjects needs to be critically examined. This should include evaluation of species differences in the function of specific physiological processes (e.g., cardiorespiratory function, fuel metabolism, thermoregulation, reproductive functions), identification of exercise modalities and intensities that are analogous to those encountered by human subjects, and the ability to control for confounding factors (e.g., psychological effects of forced exercise) that may not be operative in the human model.

5. The effects of maternal aging, environmental factors (e.g., heat exposure, altitude, pollution, noise), lifestyle factors (nutrition, smoking, alcohol intake), and maternal-fetal disease states on exercise/pregnancy relationships need to be examined. This should include the study of maternal and fetal well-being during exercise in the presence of

these conditions. The value of chronic maternal exercise in preventing or treating various gestational conditions (e.g., pregnancy-induced hypertension, gestational diabetes, gestational low back pain) should also be studied in detail.

ACKNOWLEDGMENTS

The following agencies have given financial support for exercise/pregnancy research at Queen's University and the University of Western Ontario: Health and Welfare (Canada), Canadian Fitness and Lifestyle Research Institute, Ontario Ministry of Tourism and Recreation, Ontario Ministry of Health, Ontario Thoracic Society, and the Natural Sciences and Engineering Research Council of Canada.

Thanks are also extended to Michele C. Amey for word processing and editing the final manuscript.

REFERENCES

1. Abitbol, M. M., A. G. Monheit, J. Poje, and M. A. Baker. Nonstress test and maternal position. *Obstet. Gynecol.* 68:310–316, 1986.
2. Acker, H. Chemoreceptor and baroreceptor function with respect to fetal heart rate variability. W. Kunzel (ed). *Fetal Heart Rate Monitoring.* New York: Springer-Verlag, 1985, pp. 223–233.
3. Ahlborg, G., L. Bodin, and C. Hogstedt. Heavy lifting during pregnancy—A hazard to the fetus? A prospective study. *Int. J. Epidemiol.* 19:90–97, 1990.
4. American College of Obstetricians and Gynecologists. Pregnancy and the postnatal period. *ACOG Home Exercise Programs.* Washington, D.C.: American College of Obstetricians and Gynecologists, 1985.
5. Arbuckle, T. E., R. Wilkins, and G. J. Sherman. Birth weight percentiles by gestational age in Canada. *Obstet. Gynecol.* 81:39–48, 1993.
6. Armstrong, B. G., A. D. Nolin, and A. D. McDonald. Work in pregnancy and birth weight for gestational age. *Br. J. Indust. Med.* 46:196–199, 1989.
7. Artal, R., L. D. Platt, M. Sperling, R. K. Kammula, J. Jilik, and R. Nakamuro. Exercise in pregnancy 1. Maternal cardiovascular and metabolic responses in normal pregnancy. *Am. J. Obstet. Gynecol.* 140:123–127, 1981.
8. Artal, R., Y. Romem, R. H. Paul, and R. Wiswell. Fetal bradycardia induced by maternal exercise. *Lancet* 2:258–260, 1984.
9. Artal, R., R. Wiswell, Y. Romem, and F. Dorey. Pulmonary responses to exercise in pregnancy. *Am. J. Obstet. Gynecol.* 154:378–383, 1986.
10. Artal, R., S. Rutherford, Y. Romem, R. K. Kammula, F. J. Dorey, and R. A. Wiswell. Fetal heart rate responses to maternal exercise. *Am. J. Obstet. Gynecol.* 155:729–733, 1986.
11. Artal-Mittlemark, R., and M. D. Posner. Fetal responses to maternal exercise. R. Artal-Mittlemark, R. A. Wiswell, and B. L. Drinkwater (eds.) *Exercise in Pregnancy,* ed. 2. Baltimore: Williams & Wilkins, 1991, pp. 213–224.
12. Artal-Mittlemark, R., F. Dorey, and T. H. Kirschbaum. Effect of maternal exercise on pregnancy outcome. R. Artal-Mittlemark, R. A. Wiswell, and B. L. Drinkwater (eds). *Exercise in Pregnancy,* ed. 2, Baltimore: Williams & Wilkins, 1991, pp. 228–229.
13. Ball, R. H., and J. T. Parer. The physiological mechanisms of variable decelerations. *Am. J. Obstet. Gynecol.* 166:1683–1689, 1992.

14. Baumann, H., A. Huch and R. Huch. Doppler sonographic evaluation of exercise-induced blood flow velocity and wave form changes in fetal, uteroplacental and large maternal vessels in pregnant women. *J. Perinat. Med.* 17:279–287, 1989.
15. Beckmann, C. R. B., and C. A. Beckmann. Effect of a structured antepartum exercise program on pregnancy and labor outcome in primiparas. *J. Reprod. Med.* 35: 704–709, 1990.
16. Bocking, A. D., R. Gagnon, S. E. White, J. Homan, K. M. Milne, and B. S. Richardson. Circulatory responses to prolonged hypoxemia in fetal sheep. *Am. J. Obstet. Gynecol.* 159:1418–1424, 1988.
17. Boddy, K., G. S. Dawes, R. Fisher, S. Pinter, and J. S. Robinson. Foetal respiratory movements, electrocortical and cardiovascular responses to hypoxaemia and hypercapnea in sheep. *J. Physiol. (London)* 243:599–618, 1974.
18. Bonds, D. R., and M. Delivoria-Papadopoulos. Exercise during pregnancy-potential fetal and placental metabolic effects. *Ann. Clin. Lab. Sci.* 15:91–99, 1985.
19. Bonen, A., and M. H. Tan. Dissociation between insulin binding and glucose utilization after intense exercise in mouse skeletal muscle. *Horm. Metab. Res.* 21:172–178, 1989.
20. Bonen, A., P. Campagna, L. Gilchrist, D. C. Young, and P. Beresford. Substrate and endocrine responses during exercise at selected stages of pregnancy. *J. Appl. Physiol.* 73:134–142, 1992.
21. Brenner, I. K. M., M. Monga, K. Webb, M. McGrath, and L. Wolfe. Controlled prospective study of aerobic conditioning effects on pregnancy outcome. (Abstr.) *Med. Sci. Sports Exerc.* 23:S169, 1991.
22. Brenner, I. K. M., L. A. Wolfe, M. Monga, G. A. Dumas, and M. J. McGrath. Effects of maternal exercise and physical conditioning on fetal well-being. *Proceedings of the International Conference on Physical Activity, Fitness and Health.* May 10–13, Toronto, 1992.
23. Brotanek, V., and C. Sureau. Exercise test as a physiologic form of antepartum stress test. *Int. J. Gynaecol. Obstet.* 23:327–333, 1985.
24. Burd, L. I., M. D. Jones, M. A. Simmons, E. L. Makowski, G. Meschia, and F. C. Battaglia. Placental production and foetal utilisation of lactate and pyruvate. *Nature* 254:710–711, 1975.
25. Butler, A. W., R. P. Farrar, M. A. Smith, and D. Acosta. Attenuation of ethanol toxicity in primary myocardial cell cultures from offspring of swim-trained pregnant rats. *Toxic. in Vitro* 1:39–44, 1987.
26. Butler, A. W., M. A. Smith, R. P. Farrar, and D. Acosta. The effects of ethanol on cellular calcium content in primary myocardial cell cultures from offspring of sedentary and swim-trained pregnant rats. *Biochem. Biophys. Res. Comm.* 142:496–500, 1987.
27. Carr, S. R., M. W. Carpenter, R. Terry, A. Lengle, and B. Haydon. Obstetrical outcome in aerobically trained women (abstract). *Am. J. Obstet. Gynecol.* 166:380, 1992.
28. Carpenter, M. W., S. P. Sady, B. Hoegsberg, M. A. Sady, B. Haydon, et al. Fetal response to maternal exertion. *JAMA* 259:3006–3009, 1988.
29. Catalano, P. M., E. D. Tyzbir, S. R. Allen, J. H. McBean, and T. L. McAuliffe. Evaluation of fetal growth by estimation of neonatal body composition. *Obstet. Gynecol.* 79:46–50, 1992.
30. Catalano, P. M., N. M. Roman, E. D. Tyzbir, A. O. Merritt, P. Driscoll, and S. B. Amini. Weight gain in women with gestational diabetes. *Obstet. Gynecol.* 81:523–528, 1993.
31. Catanzarite, V. A. *Fetal Monitor Interpretation.* Baltimore: Williams & Wilkins, 1987.
32. Chandler, K. D., and A. W. Bell. Effects of maternal exercise on fetal and maternal respiration and nutrient metabolism in the pregnant ewe. *J. Dev. Physiol.* 3:161–176, 1981.
33. Chandler, K. D., B. J. Leury, A. R. Bird, and A. W. Bell. Effects of undernutrition and exercise during late pregnancy on uterine, fetal and uteroplacental metabolism in the ewe. *Br. J. Nutr.* 53:625–635, 1985.
34. Clapp, J. F. III., The changing thermal response to endurance exercise during pregnancy. *Am. J. Obstet. Gynecol.* 165:1684–1689, 1991.
35. Clapp, J. F. III, and E. L. Capeless. The changing glycemic response to exercise during pregnancy. *Am. J. Obstet. Gynecol.* 165:1678–1683, 1991.

36. Clapp, J. F. III. Acute exercise stress in the pregnant ewe. *Am. J. Obstet. Gynecol.* 136:489–494, 1980.
37. Clapp, J. F. III, and S. Dickstein. Endurance exercise and pregnancy outcome. *Med. Sci. Sports Exerc.* 16:556–562, 1984.
38. Clapp, J. F. III. Fetal heart rate response to running in midpregnancy and late pregnancy. *Am. J. Obstet. Gynecol.* 153:251–252, 1985.
39. Clapp, J. F. III, M. Wesley, and R. H. Sleamaker. Thermoregulatory and metabolic responses to jogging prior to and during pregnancy. *Med. Sci. Sports Exerc.* 19:124–130, 1987.
40. Clapp, J. F. III. The effects of maternal exercise in early pregnancy outcome. *Am. J. Obstet. Gynecol.* 161:1453–1457, 1989.
41. Clapp, J. F. III. The course of labour after endurance exercise during pregnancy. *Am. J. Obstet. Gynecol.* 163:1799–1805, 1990.
42. Clapp, J. F. III, and E. L. Capeless. Neonatal morphometrics after endurance exercise during pregnancy. *Am. J. Obstet. Gynecol.* 163:1805–1811, 1990.
43. Clapp, J. F. III, and K. H. Rizk. Effect of recreational exercise on midtrimester placental growth. *Am. J. Obstet. Gynecol.* 167:1518–1521, 1992.
44. Clapp, J. F. III, R. Rokey, J. L. Treadway, M. W. Carpenter, R. M. Artal, and C. Warrnes. Exercise in pregnancy. *Med. Sci. Sports Exerc.* 24:S294–S300, 1992.
45. Clapp, J. F. III, K. D. Little, and E. L. Capeless. The fetal heart rate response to sustained recreational exercise. *Am. J. Obstet. Gynecol.* 168:198–206, 1993.
46. Cohen, W. R., G. J. Piasecki, and B. T. Jackson. Plasma catecholamines during hypoxemia in the fetal lamb. *Am. J. Physiol.* 243:R520–R525, 1982.
47. Cohen, W. R., G. J. Piasecki, H. E. Cohn, J. B. Young, and B. T. Jackson. Adrenal secretion of catecholamines during hypoxaemia in fetal lambs. *Endocrinology.* 114:383–390, 1984.
48. Cohn, H. E., E. J. Sacks, M. A. Heymann, and A. M. Rudolph. Cardiovascular responses to hypoxia and acidemia in fetal lambs. *Am. J. Obstet. Gynecol.* 120:817–824, 1974.
49. Cohn, H. F., G. J. Piasecki, and B. T. Jackson. The effect of fetal heart rate on cardiovascular function during hypoxemia. *Am. J. Obstet. Gynecol.* 138:1190–1199, 1980.
50. Cohper, D. E., and C. P. Huber. Heart rate response of the human fetus to induced maternal hypoxia. *Am. J. Obstet. Gynecol.* 98:320–335, 1967.
51. Collings, C. A., L. B. Curet, and J. P. Mullin. Maternal and fetal responses to a maternal aerobic exercise program. *Am. J. Obstet. Gynecol.* 145:702–707, 1983.
52. Collings, C. A., and L. B. Curet. Fetal heart rate response to maternal exercise. *Am. J. Obstet. Gynecol.* 151:498–501, 1985.
53. Conners, G., C. Hunse, L. Carmichael, R. Natale, and B. Richardson. The role of carbon dioxide in the generation of human fetal breathing movements. *Am. J. Obstet. Gynecol.* 158:322–327, 1988.
54. Courant, G. T., and S. I. Barr. Exercise during rat pregnancy and lactation: maternal effects and offspring growth. *Physiol. Behav.* 47:427–433, 1990.
55. Creasy, R. K. Lifestyle influence on prematurity. *J. Dev. Physiol.* 15:15–20, 1991.
56. Curet, L. B., J. A. Orr, J. H. G. Rankin, and T. Ungerer. Effect of exercise on cardiac output and redistribution of uterine blood flow in pregnant ewes. *J. Appl. Physiol.* 40:725–728, 1976.
57. Dale, E., K. M. Mullinax, and D. H. Bryan. Exercise during pregnancy: Effects on the fetus. *Can. J. Appl. Sport Sci.* 7:98–103, 1982.
58. Dauncy, M. J., G. Gandy, and D. Gairdner. Assessment of total body fat in infancy from skinfold thickness measurements. *Arch. Dis. Child* 52:223–227, 1977.
59. Dawes, G. S., S. L. B. Duncan, B. V. Lewis, C. L. Merlet, J. B. Owen-Thomas, and J. T. Reeves. Hypoxaemia and aortic chemoreceptor function in foetal lambs. *J. Physiol.* 201:105–116, 1969.
60. Dressendorfer, R. H., and R. C. Goodlin. Fetal heart rate response to maternal exercise testing. *Physician Sportsmed.* 8:91–94, 1980.

61. Durak, E. P., L. Jovanovic-Peterson, and C. M. Peterson. Comparative evaluation of uterine response to exercise on five aerobic machines. *Am. J. Obstet. Gynecol.* 162:754–756, 1990.

62. Eden, R. D., L. S. Seifert, J. Frese-Gallo, V. Bartasius, and W. N. Spellery. Effect of gestational age on baseline fetal heart rate during the third trimester of pregnancy. *J. Reprod. Med.* 32:285–286, 1987.

63. Edwards, M. J. Hyperthermia as a teratogen: a review of experimental studies and their clinical significance. *Teratogenesis Carcinog. Mutagen.* 6:563–582, 1986.

64. Edwards, M. J. Congenital defects in guinea pigs following induced hyperthermia during gestation. *Arch. Pathol.* 84:42–48, 1967.

65. Edwards, M. J. Congenital defects in guinea pigs: prenatal retardation of brain growth of guinea pigs following hyperthermia during gestation. *Teratology* 2:329–366, 1969.

66. Edwards, M. J. The experimental production of arthrogryposis multiplex congenita in guinea pigs by maternal hyperthemia during gestation. *J. Pathol.* 104:221–234, 1981.

67. Edwards, M. J., R. C. Penny, and I. Zevnik. A brain deficit in new-born guinea pigs following prenatal hyperthermia. *Brain Res.* 28:341–345, 1971.

68. Emmanouilides, G. C., C. J. Hobel, K. Yashiro, and G. Klyman. Fetal responses to maternal exercise in the sheep. *Am. J. Obstet. Gynecol.* 112:130–137, 1972.

69. Erdelyi, G. J. Gynecological survey of female athletes. *J. Sports Med. Phys. Fitness* 2:174–179, 1962.

70. Fisher, N. L., and D. W. Smith. Occipital encephalocele and early gestational hyperthermia. *Pediatrics* 68:480–483, 1981.

71. Fisher, D. J., M. A. Heymann, and A. M. Rudolph. Fetal myocardial oxygen and carbohydrate consumption during acutely induced hypoxemia. *Am. J. Physiol.* 242:H657–H661, 1982.

72. Freeman, R. K., and T. J. Garite. *Fetal Heart Rate Monitoring.* Baltimore: Williams & Wilkins, 1981, pp. 9–28.

73. Gettinger, A., A. B. Roberts, and S. Campbell. Comparison between subjective and ultrasound assessments of fetal movements. *Br. Med. J.* 2:88–90, 1978.

74. Gimovsky, M. L., and S. N. Caritis. Diagnosis and management of hypoxic fetal heart rate patterns. *Clin. Perinatol.* 9:313–324, 1982.

75. Goodrich, S. M., and J. E. Wood. Peripheral venous distensibility and velocity of venous blood flow during pregnancy and during oral contraceptive therapy. *Am. J. Obstet. Gynecol.* 90:740–744, 1964.

76. Goodrich, S. M., and J. E. Wood. The effect of estradiol 17-beta on peripheral venous distensibility and velocity of venous blood flow. *Am. J. Obstet. Gynecol.* 96:407–412, 1966.

77. Greenleaf, J. E., V. A. Convertino, R. W. Stremel, E. M. Bernauer, W. C. Adams, and S. R. Vignau. Plasma (Na^+), (CA^{2+}), and volume shifts and thermoregulation during exercise in men. *J. Appl. Physiol.* 43:1026–1032, 1977.

78. Hall, D. C., and D. A. Kaufmann. Effects of aerobic and strengh conditioning on pregnancy outcomes. *Am. J. Obstet. Gynecol.* 157:1199–1203, 1987.

79. Hauth, J. C., L. C. Gilstrap III, and K. Widmer. Fetal heart rate reactivity before and after maternal jogging during the third trimester. *Obstet. Gynecol.* 142:545–547, 1982.

80. Hay, W. W., and J. W. Sparks. Placental, fetal, and neonatal carbohydrate metabolism. *Clin. Obstet. Gynaecol.* 28:473–483, 1985.

81. Heymann, M. A. Fetal hemodynamic alterations during advancing gestation. W. Kunzel (ed). *Fetal Heart Rate Monitoring: Clinical Practice and Pathophysiology.* New York: Springer-Verlag, 1985, pp. 66–69.

82. Hohimer, A. R., J. M. Bissonnett, J. Metcalfe, and T. A. McKean. Effect of exercise on uterine blood flow in the pregnant pygmy goat. *Am. J. Physiol.* 246:H207–H212, 1984.

83. Hollingsworth, D. R. Maternal metabolism in normal pregnancy and pregnancy complicated by diabetes mellitus. *Clin. Obstet. Gynaecol.* 28:457–472, 1985.

84. Homer, C. J., S. Beresford, S. A. James, E. Siegel, and S. Wilcox. Work-related physical exertion and risk of preterm, low birthweight delivery. *Paediat. Perinat. Epidemiol.* 4:161–174, 1990.

85. Hon, E. H., and R. Wohlgemuth. The electronic evaluation of fetal heart rate. *Am. J. Obstet. Gynecol.* 81:361–371, 1961.

86. Hudlicka, O. Regulation of muscle blood flow. *Clin. Physiol.* 5:201–229, 1985.

87. Hutchinson, P. L., K. J. Cureton, and P. B. Sparling. Metabolic and circulatory responses to running during pregnancy. *Physician Sportsmed.* 9:55–58, 61, 1981.

88. Ibarra-Pollo, A. A., E. Guiloff, and G. Gomez-Rogers. Fetal heart rate throughout pregnancy. *Am. J. Obstet. Gynecol.* 113:814–818, 1972.

89. Ivy, J. L. The insulin-like effect of muscle contraction. *Exerc. Sport Sci. Rev.* 15:29–51, 1987.

90. James, E. L., J. R. Raye, O. Greshom, L. L. Makowski, G. Meschia, and F. C. Battaglia. Fetal oxygen consumption, carbon dioxide production, and glucose uptake in a chronic sheep preparation. *Pediatrics* 50:361–367, 1972.

91. Jarrett J. C., and W. N. Spellacy. Jogging during pregnancy: an improved outcome? *Obstet. Gynecol.* 61:705–709, 1983.

92. Jones, M. D., Jr., R. E. Sheldon, L. L. Peeters, G. Meschia, F. C. Battaglia, and E. L. Makowski. Fetal cerebral oxygen consumption at different levels of oxygenation. *J. Appl. Physiol.* 43:1080–1084, 1977.

93. Jones, M. T., K. I. Norton, D. R. Dengel, and R. B. Armstrong. Effects of training on reproductive tissue blood flow in exercising pregnant rats. *J. Appl. Physiol.* 69:2097–2103, 1990.

94. Jones, M. T., R. E. Rawson, S. Riplog, and D. Robertshaw. Oxygen consumption and uterine blood flow in exercising pregnant sheep. *Med. Sci. Sports Exerc.* 23:S169, 1991.

95. Jones, M. T., K. I. Norton, D. M. Black, R. E. Graham, and R. B. Armstrong. Effect of regular voluntary exercise on resting cardiovascular responses in SHR and WKY pregnant rats. *J. Appl. Physiol.* 73:713–720, 1992.

96. Jost, R. G., E. J. Quilligan, S-Y Yeh, and G. G. Anderson. Intrauterine encephalogram of the sheep fetus. *Am. J. Obstet. Gynecol.* 114:535–539, 1972.

97. Jovanovic, L., A. Kessler, and C. M. Peterson. Human maternal and fetal response to graded exercise. *J. Appl. Physiol.* 58:1719–1722, 1985.

98. Jovanovic-Peterson, L., E. P. Durak,, and C. M. Peterson. Randomized trial of diet versus diet plus cardiovascular conditioning on glucose levels in gestational diabetes. *Am. J. Obstet. Gynecol.* 161:415–419, 1989.

99. Katz, V. L., R. McMurray, M. J. Berry, and R. C. Cefalo. Fetal and uterine responses to immersion and exercise. *Obstet. Gynecol.* 72:225–230, 1988.

100. Katz, V. L., R. McMurray, W. E. Goodwin, and R. C. Cefalo. Non-weight bearing exercise during pregnancy on land and during immersion: a comparative study. *Am. J. Perinatol.* 7:281–284, 1990.

101. Keegan, K. A. The nonstress test. *Clin. Obstet. Gynecol.* 30:921–935, 1987.

102. Kilham, L., and V. H. Ferm. Exencephaly in fetal hamsters following exposure to hyperthermia. *Teratology* 14:323–326, 1976.

103. Knuttgen, H. G., and K. Emerson. Physiological response to pregnancy at rest and during exercise. *J. Appl. Physiol.* 36:549–553, 1974.

104. Kulpa, P. J., B. M. White, and R. Visscher. Aerobic exercise in pregnancy. *Am. J. Obstet. Gynecol.* 156:1395–1403, 1987.

105. Lokey, E. A., Z. V. Tran, C. L. Wells, B. C. Meyers, and A. C. Tran. Effects of physical exercise on pregnancy outcomes: a meta-analytic review. *Med. Sci. Sports Exerc.* 22:1234–1239, 1991.

106. Lotgering, F. K. Maternal and fetal responses to exercise during pregnancy. *Physiol. Rev.* 61:1–36, 1985.

107. Lotgering, F. K., M. B. Van Doorne, P. C. Struijk, J. Pool, and H. C. S. Wallenberg. Maximal aerobic exercise in pregnant women: heart rate, O_2 consumption, CO_2 production and ventilation. *J. Appl. Physiol.* 70:1016–1023, 1991.

108. Lotgering, F. K., R. D. Gilbert, and L. D. Longo. Exercise responses in pregnant sheep: oxygen consumption, uterine blood flow and blood volume. *J. Appl. Physiol. (Respir. Environ. Exerc. Physiol.)* 55: 834–841, 1983.

109. Lotgering, F. K., R. D. Gilbert, and L. D. Longo. Exercise responses in pregnant sheep: blood gases, temperatures and fetal cardiovascular system. *J. Appl. Physiol. (Respir. Environ. Exerc. Physiol.)* 55: 842–850, 1983.

110. Lotgering, F. K., and L. D. Longo. Exercise and pregnancy. How much is too much? *Contemp. OB/GYN* 23(Jan):63–77, 1984.

111. Lutter, J. M., V. Lee, and S. Cushman. Fetal outcome of women who ran while pregnant, A preliminary report. *The Melopomene Report.* 3(October):6–8, 1984.

112. Maršál, K., O. Lofgren, and G. Gennser. Fetal breathing movements and maternal exercise. *Acta Obstet. Gynecol. Scand.* 58:197–201, 1979.

113. Maršál, K., G. Gennser, and O. Lofgren. Effects on fetal breathing movements of maternal challenges. *Acta. Obstet. Gynecol. Scand.* 58:335–342, 1979.

114. Martin, C. B. Pharmacological aspects of fetal heart rate regulation during hypoxia. W. Kunzel (ed). *Fetal Heart Rate Monitoring: Clinical Practice and Pathophysiology.* New York: Springer-Verlag, 1985, pp. 170–184.

115. McDonald, A. D., J. C. McDonald, B. Armstrong, N. M. Cherry, R. Cote, et al. Fetal death and work in pregnancy. *Br. J. Ind. Med.* 45:148–157, 1988.

116. McMurray, R. G., and V. L. Katz. Thermoregulation in pregnancy: implications for exercise. *Sports Med.* 10:146–158, 1990.

117. McMurray, R. G., V. L. Katz, M. J. Berry, and R. C. Cephalo. The effect of pregnancy on metabolic responses during rest, immersion and aerobic exercise in the water. *Am. J. Obstet. Gynecol.* 158:481–486, 1988.

118. McMurray, R. G., A. C. Hackney, V. L. Katz, M. Gall, and W. J. Watson. Pregnancy-induced changes in the maximal physiological response during swimming. *J. Appl. Physiol.* 71:1454–1459, 1991.

119. McMurray, R. G., M. F. Mottola, L. Wolfe, R. Artal, L. Millar, and J. M. Pivarnik. Recent advances in understanding maternal and fetal responses to exercise. *Med. Sci. Sports Exerc.* 25:1305–1321, 1993.

120. Meis, P. J., J. R. Ureda, M. Swain, R. T. Kelly, M. Penry, and P. Sharp. Variable decelerations during nonstress tests are not a sign of fetal compromise. *Am. J. Obstet. Gynecol.* 154:586–590, 1986.

121. Milunsky, A., M. Ulcickas, K. J. Rothman, W. Willett, S. S. Jick, and H. Jick. Maternal heat exposure and neural tube defects. *JAMA* 268:882–885, 1991.

122. Morgan, C. D., M. Sandler, and M. Panigel. Placental transfer of catecholamines in vitro and in vivo. *Am. J. Obstet. Gynecol.* 112:1068–1075, 1972.

123. Moore, D. H., J. C. Jarrett II, and P. J. Bendick. Exercise induced flow changes in uterine artery blood flow as measured by Doppler ultrasound in pregnant subjects. *Am. J. Perinatol.* 5:94–97, 1988.

124. Moore, K. L. *The Developing Human: Clinically Oriented Embryology,* ed 4. Toronto: W. B. Saunders, 1988, pp. 286–333.

125. Morris, N., S. B. Osborn, H. P. Wright, and A. Hart. Effective uterine blood flow during exercise in normal and pre-eclamptic pregnancies. *Lancet* 2:481–484, 1956.

126. Morrow, R. J., J. W. K. Ritchie, and S. B. Bull. Fetal and maternal hemodynamic responses to exercise in pregnancy assessed by Doppler ultrasonography. *Am. J. Obstet. Gynecol.* 160:138–140, 1989.

127. Mottola, M. F., K. M. Bagnall, and A. N. Belcastro. Effects of strenuous maternal exercise on fetal organ weights and skeletal muscle development in rats. *J. Dev. Physiol.* 11:111–115, 1989.

128. Mottola, M. F., and P. D. Christopher. Effects of maternal exercise on liver and skeletal muscle glycogen storage in pregnant rats. *J. Appl. Physiol.* 71:1015–1019, 1991.

129. Mottola, M. F., K. McKenzie, C. L. Schachter, J. Mezzapelli, J. Vanheest, and R. M. Tanguay. Accumulation of stress protein 72i in fetuses of trained pregnant rats. (abstr.) *Physiologist.* 34:175, 1992.

130. Mottola, M. F., H. M. Fitzgerald, N. C. Wilson, and A. W. Taylor. Effect of water

temperature on exercise-induced maternal hyperthermia on fetal development in rats. *Int. J. Sports Med.* 14:248–251, 1993.

131. Mottola, M. F., J. Mezzapelli, C. L. Schachter, and K. McKenzie. Training effects on maternal and fetal glucose uptake following acute exercise in the rat. *Med. Sci. Sports Exerc.* 25:841–846, 1993.

132. Mottola, M. F., and L. A. Wolfe. Active living and pregnancy. *Proceedings of the International Conference on Physical Activity, Fitness and Health,* Chpt. 18. Champaign, IL: Human Kinetics Publishers, 1994.

133. Newton, R. W., and L. P. Hunt. Psychosocial stress in pregnancy and its relation to low birth weight. *Br. Med. J.* 288:1191–1194, 1984.

134. Nurminen, T., S. Lusa, J. Ilmarinen, and K. Kurppa. Physical work load, fetal development and course of pregnancy. *Scand. J. Work. Environ. Health* 15:404–414, 1989.

135. Nuwayhid, B., C. R. Brinkmann III, C. Su, J. A. Bevan, and N. S. Assali. Development of autonomic control of fetal circulation. *Am. J. Physiol.* 228:337–344, 1975.

136. Orr, J., T. Ungerer, J. Will, K. Wernicker, and L. B. Curet. Effect of exercise stress in carotid, uterine, and iliac blood flow in pregnant and non-pregnant ewes. *Am. J. Obstet. Gynecol.* 114:213–217, 1972.

137. Palmer, S. M., G. K. Oates, J. A. Champion, D. A. Fisher, and C. K. Hobel. Catecholamine physiology in the ovine fetus. III. Maternal and fetal response to acute maternal exercise. *Am. J. Obstet. Gynecol.* 149:426–434, 1984.

138. Paolone, A. M., M. Shangold, P. Dennis, J. Minnitti, and S. Weiner. Fetal heart rate measurement during maternal exercise-avoidance of artifact. *Med. Sci. Sports Exerc.* 19:605–609, 1987.

139. Parer, J. T. Effect of acute maternal hypoxia on fetal oxygenation and the umbilical circulation in the sheep. *Eur. J. Obstet. Gynecol. Reprod. Biol.* 10:125–136, 1980.

140. Parer, J. T. *Handbook of Fetal Heart Rate Monitoring.* Toronto: W. B. Saunders, 1983.

141. Parer, J. T. The influence of β-adrenergic activity on fetal heart rate and the umbilical circulation during hypoxia in fetal sheep. *Am. J. Obstet. Gynecol.* 147:592–597, 1983.

142. Parer, J. T. Fetal heart rate. R. K. Creasy, and R. Resnick (eds). *Maternal-Fetal Medicine: Principles and Practice.* Toronto: W. B. Saunders, 1989, pp. 314–343.

143. Parer, J. T., and E. G. Livingston. What is fetal distress? *Am. J. Obstet. Gynecol.* 162:1421–1427, 1990.

144. Patrick, J., and R. Gagnon. Fetal breathing and body movement. R. K. Creasy and R. Resnik (eds). *Maternal-Fetal Medicine: Principles and Practice,* ed 2. Toronto: W. B. Saunders, 1989, pp. 271–272.

145. Pernoll, M. L., J. Metcalfe, and M. Paul. Fetal cardiac response to maternal exercise. L. D. Lange and D. D. Reneau (eds). *Fetal and Newborn Cardiovascular Physiology: Fetal and Newborn Circulation.* New York: Garland, 1978, pp. 389–398.

146. Pernoll, M. L., J. Metcalfe, P. A. Kovack, R. Wachtel, and M. J. Durham. Ventilation at rest and exercise in pregnancy and postpartum. *Respir. Physiol.* 25:295–310, 1975.

147. Piccaro, I. C., G. X. Turecki, T. L. Barros-Neto, A. K. Russo, A. C. Silva, and J. Tarasantchi. Effect of exercise training during pregnancy: maternal and fetal responses of the rat. *Braz. J. Med. Biol. Res.* 22:1535–1538, 1989.

148. Platt, L. D., R. Artal, J. Semel, L. Sipos, and R. K. Kammula. Exercise in pregnancy II. Fetal responses. *Obstet. Gynecol.* 147:487–491, 1983.

149. Ploug, T., H. Galbo, J. Vinten, M. Jorgensen, and E. A. Richter. Kinetics of glucose transport in rat muscle: effects of insulin and contractions. *Am. J. Physiol.* 252:E12–E20, 1987.

150. Ploug, T., H. Galbo, T. Ohkuwa, J. Tranum-Jensen, and J. Vinten. Kinetics of glucose transport in rat skeletal muscle membrane vesicles: effects of insulin and contractions. *Am. J. Physiol.* 262:E700–E711, 1992.

151. Pokorny, J., and J. Rous. The effects of mother's work on foetal heart sounds. J. Horsky

and Z. K. Stembara (eds). *Intrauterine Dangers to the Fetus.* Amsterdam: Exerpta Medica, 1967, pp. 354–357.

152. Pomerance, J. J., L. Gluck, and V. A. Lynch. Physical fitness in pregnancy: its effects on pregnancy outcome. *Am. J. Obstet. Gynecol.* 119:867–876, 1974.

153. Pomerance, J. J., L. Gluck, and V. A. Lynch. Maternal exercise as a screening test for uteroplacental insufficiency. *Obstet. Gynecol.* 44:383–387, 1974.

154. Pritchard, J. A., P. C. MacDonald, and N. F. Gant. *Williams Obstetrics,* ed 17. Norwalk, CT: Appleton-Century-Crofts, 1985, pp. 529, 598–601.

155. Ramirez, G., R. M. Grimes, J. F. Annegers, B. R. Davis, and C. H. Slater. Occupational physical activity and other risk factors for preterm birth among US army primigravidas. *Am. J. Public Health* 80:728–729, 1990.

156. Rauramo, I. Effect of short-term physical exercise on fetal heart rate and uterine activity in normal and abnormal pregnancies. *Ann. Chir. Gynaecol.* 76:274–279, 1987.

157. Rauramo, I., and M. Forss. Effect of exercise on placental blood flow in pregnancies complicated by hypertension, diabetes or intrahepatic cholestasis. *Acta Obstet. Gynecol. Scand.* 67:15–20, 1988.

158. Rauramo, I., and M. Forss. Effect of exercise on maternal hemodynamics and placental blood flow in healthy women. *Acta Obstet. Gynecol. Scand.* 67:21–25, 1988.

159. Renou, P., W. Newman, and C. Wood. Autonomic control of fetal heart rate. *Am. J. Obstet. Gynecol.* 105:949–953, 1969.

160. Rodgers, C. D., M. F. Mottola, K. Corbett, and A. W. Taylor. Skeletal muscle metabolism in the offspring of trained rats. *J. Sports Med. Phys. Fitness* 31:389–95, 1991.

161. Rowell, L. B., and D. S. O'Leary. Reflex control of the circulation during exercise: chemoreflexes and mechanoreflexes. *J. Appl. Physiol.* 69:407–418, 1990.

162. Ruissen, C., W. Jager, M. V. Drongelen, and H. Hoogland. The influence of maternal exercise on the pulsatility index of the umbilical artery blood velocity waveform. *Eur. J. Obstet. Gynecol. Reprod. Biol.* 37:1–6, 1990.

163. Sady, S. P., M. W. Carpenter, P. P. Thompson, M. A. Sady, B. Maydon, and D. R. Coustan. Cardiovascular response to cycle exercise during and after pregnancy. *J. Appl. Physiol.* 66:336–341, 1989.

164. Shenker, L., C. Astle, K. Reed, and C. Anderson. Embryonic heart rate before the seventh week of pregnancy. *J. Reprod. Med.* 31:333–335, 1986.

165. Shinebourne, E. A., E. K. Vapaavuori, R. L. Williams, M. A. Heymann, and A. M. Rudolph. Development of baroreflex activity in unanesthetized fetal and neonatal lambs. *Circ. Res.* 31:710–718, 1972.

166. Sibley, L., R. O. Ruhling, J. Cameron-Foster, C. Christensen, and T. Bolen. Swimming and physical fitness during pregnancy. *J. Nurse-Midwifery.* 26:3–12, 1981.

167. Simpson, J. L. Are physical activity and employment related to preterm birth and low birth weight? *Am. J. Obstet. Gynecol.* 168:1231–1238, 1993.

168. Smith, C. V., J. P. Phelen, and R. H. Paul. A prospective analysis of the influence of gestational age on the baseline fetal heart rate and reactivity in a low-risk population. *Am. J. Obstet. Gynecol.* 153:780–782, 1985.

169. Sodha, R. J., M. Proegler, and H. Schneider. Transfer and metabolism on norepinephrine studied from maternal-to-fetal and fetal-to-maternal sides in the in vitro perfused human placental lobe. *Am. J. Obstet. Gynecol.* 148:474–481, 1984.

170. Soiva, K., A. Salmi, M. Grönroos, and T. Peltonen. Physical working capacity during pregnancy and effect of physical work tests on foetal heart rate. *Ann. Chir. Gynaecol. Fenn.* 53:187–196, 1964.

171. Sørensen, K. E., and K. Børlum. Heart function in response to short-term maternal exercise. *Br. J. Obstet. Gynaecol.* 93:310–313, 1986.

172. Steegers, E. A. P., G. Buunk, R. A. Binkhorst, H. W. Jongsma, P. F. F. Wijn, and P. R. Hein. The influence of maternal exercise on the uteroplacental vascular bed resistance and the fetal heart rate during normal pregnancy. *Eur. J. Obstet. Gynecol. Reprod. Biol.* 27:21–26, 1988.

173. Štembera, Z. K., and J. Hodr. The "exercise test" as an early diagnostic aid for foetal distress. J. Horsky and Z. K. Stembera (eds). *Intrauterine Dangers to the Fetus*. Amsterdam: Exerpta Medica, 1967, pp. 349–353.

174. Sternfeld, B., S. Sidney, and B. Eskenazi. Patterns of exercise during pregnancy and effects on pregnancy outcome. *Med. Sci. Sports Exerc.* 24:S170, 1992.

175. Treadway, J. L., and J. C. Young. Decreased glucose uptake by the fetus after maternal exercise. *Med. Sci. Sports Exerc.* 21:140–145, 1989.

176. Tucker, S. M. *Fetal Monitoring and Fetal Assessment in High Risk Pregnancy*. Saint Louis: C. V. Mosby, 1978.

177. Uriu-Hare, J. Y., C. L. Keen, E. A. Applegate, and J. S. Stern. The influence of moderate exercise in diabetic and normal pregnancy on maternal and fetal outcome in the rat. *Life Sci.* 45:647–654, 1989.

178. Uzendoski, A. M., R. W. Latin, K. E. Berg, and S. Moshier. Physiological response to aerobic exercise during pregnancy and post-partum. *J. Sports Med. Phys. Fitness* 30:77–82, 1990.

179. Van Doorn, M. B., F. K. Lotgering, P. C. Struijk, J. Pool, and H. C. S. Wallenberg. Maternal and fetal cardiovascular responses to strenuous bicycle exercise. *Am. J. Obstet. Gynecol.* 166:854–859, 1992.

180. Veille, J., A. R. Hohimer, K. Burry, and L. Speroff. The effect of exercise on uterine activity in the last eight weeks of pregnancy. *Am. J. Obstet. Gynecol.* 151:727–730, 1985.

181. Walker, D., A. Walker, and C. Wood. Temperature of the human fetus. *J. Obstet. Gynecol. Br. Commonw.* 76:503–511, 1969.

182. Walker, A., L. Maddern, E. Day, P. Renou, J. Talbot, and C. Wood. Fetal scalp tissue oxygen tension measurements in relation to maternal dermal oxygen tension and fetal heart rate. *J. Obstet. Gynaecol. Br. Commonw.* 78:1–12, 1971.

183. Walker, A. M., J. Cannata, M. H. Dowling, B. Ritchie, and J. E. Maloney. Sympathetic and parasympathetic control of heart rate in unanesthetized fetal and newborn lambs. *Biol. Neonate* 33:135–143, 1978.

184. Walker, A. M., J. P. Cannata, M. H. Dowling, B. Ritchie, and J. E. Maloney. Age-dependent pattern of autonomic heart rate control during hypoxia in fetal and newborn lambs. *Biol. Neonate* 35:198–208, 1979.

185. Walker, A. M., J. P. Cannata, B. Ritchie, and J. E. Maloney. Hypotension in fetal and newborn lambs: different patterns of reflex heart rate control revealed by autonomic blockade. *Biol. Neonate* 44:358–365, 1983.

186. Walker, D. W. Peripheral and central chemoreceptors in the fetus and newborn. *Annu. Rev. Physiol.* 46:687–703, 1984.

187. Walsh, S. Z., W. W. Meyer, and J. Lind. *The Human Fetal and Neonatal Circulation Function and Structure*. Springfield, IL: Charles C. Thomas, 1974, pp. 5–72.

188. Warkany, J. Teratogen updata: hyperthermia. *Teratology* 33:365–371, 1986.

189. Watson, W. J., V. L. Katz, A. C. Hackney, M. M. Gall, and R. G. McMurray. Fetal responses to maximal swimming and cycling exercise during pregnancy. *Obstet. Gynecol.* 77:382–386, 1991.

190. Wilkening, R. B., and G. Meschia. Fetal oxygen uptake, oxygenation, and acid-base balance as a function of uterine blood flow. *Am. J. Physiol.* 244:H749–H755, 1983.

191. Webb, K., L. Wolfe, S. Lowe-Wylde, and M. Monga. A comparison of fetal heart rate (FHR) reponses to maternal static and dynamic exercise (abstract). *Med. Sci. Sports Exerc.* 23:S169, 1991.

192. Webb, K. P., L. A. Wolfe, P. Hall, J. E. Tranmer, and M. J. McGrath. Fetal heart rate (FHR) responses to maternal exercise and physical conditioning. (Abstract) *Med. Sci. Sports Exerc.* 21:532, 1989.

193. Wolfe, L. A., P. J. Ohtake, M. F. Mottola, and M. J. McGrath. Physiological interactions between pregnancy and aerobic exercise. *Exerc. Sports Sci. Rev.* 17:295–351, 1989.

194. Wolfe, L. A., P. Hall, K. A. Webb, L. Goodman, M. Monga, and M. J. McGrath.

Prescription of aerobic exercise in pregnancy. *Sports Med.* 8:273–301, 1989.

195. Wolfe, L. A., A. Bonen, R. M. C. Walker, and M. J. McGrath. Glycemic responses to graded exercise in pregnancy. (abstr.). *Med. Sci. Sports Exerc.* 25:S73, 1993.

196. Wolfe, L. A., and M. F. Mottola. Aerobic exercise in pregnancy: an update. *Can. J. Appl. Physiol.* 18:119–147, 1993.

197. Wolfe, L. A., R. M. C. Walker, A. Bonen, and M. J. McGrath. Respiratory adaptations to acute and chronic exercise in pregnancy. *J. Appl. Physiol.* (in press).

198. Wong, S. C., and D. C. McKenzie. Cardiorespiratory fitness during pregnancy and its effect on outcome. *Int. J. Sports Med.* 8:79–83, 1987.

199. Wood, P. L., and H. G. Dobbie. *Electronic Fetal Heart Rate Monitoring: A Practical Guide.* London: Macmillan, 1989, pp. 1–6.

200. Young, J. C., and J. L. Treadway. The effect of prior exercise on oral glucose tolerance in late gestational women. *Eur. J. Appl. Physiol.* 64:430–433, 1992.

201. Zaharieva, E. Olympic participation by women. Effects on pregnancy and child birth. *JAMA* 221:992–995, 1972.

202. Zuspan, F. P., L. A. Ciblis, and S. V. Rose. Myometrial and cardiovascular responses to alterations in plasma epinephrine and norepinephrine. *Am. J. Obstet. Gynecol.* 84:841–851, 1962.

7
Physical Fitness and Cognitive Functioning in Aging

WOJTEK J. CHODZKO-ZAJKO, Ph.D.
KATHLEEN A. MOORE, M.S.

In this paper we review the literature that has examined the nature and strength of the relation between physical fitness and cognitive performance in old age. We consider both cross-sectional studies, which have investigated differences in cognitive performance between discrete groups of high- and low- fit older adults, and training studies, which have examined the effect of exercise training regimens on cognitive performance. We do not consider the acute or short-term effects of a single bout of physical activity on cognitive performance. These data have been reviewed elsewhere [98] and are beyond the scope of this manuscript. Studies that examine the acute effects of a single bout of exercise stress are discussed only when they contribute directly to our understanding of general principles underlying the relationship between physical fitness and cognitive performance.

DEFINITION AND DELIMITATION OF KEY CONCEPTS

COGNITION. Definitions of cognition and cognitive processing vary considerably across psychological disciplines. Thus the concept of cognition as defined by a social psychologist need not coincide with the operational definition of cognition adopted by an experimental or cognitive psychologist. In this review we restrict ourselves to an experimental psychological interpretation of cognition focusing on the underlying operations used in the processing of information by the central nervous system. These processes include memory, attention, perception, vigilance, and problem solving as well as reaction time, movement time, digit symbol substitution, and many others. (Interested readers are referred to Eysenck [37] and Barsalou [4] for a discussion of the development of cognitive psychology as a dominant paradigm in experimental psychology.)

Extant theoretical models of cognition and aging are of limited clinical utility. Indeed the vast majority of research in the area of cognition, physical activity, and aging has focused on interactions between activity and cognition in relatively healthy, nonclinical populations. Accordingly, this review focuses primarily on research studies examining the activity-cognition relation in nonclinical populations. Discussions about the assessment and management of clinical dementia are beyond the scope of this paper.

AGE AND AGING. At first glance it may seem unnecessary to define or delimit either of the terms "age" or "aging." For the vast majority of lay people, "age" is defined simply as the number of years, months, or days that have elapsed since a particular point in time, usually birth. In much the same manner, the "aging process" is also usually defined with reference to the passage of time, or more specifically, the passage of calendar time. However, a cursory examination of the gerontology literature reveals that the above interpretations are incomplete and that more complex definitions of both "age" and "aging" are necessary if we are to increase our understanding of the biological processes accompanying senescence. In this review we will adopt both "chronological" and "biological" interpretations of age and aging.

"Chronological age" generally refers to the length of time an individual or object has existed, and its measurement is largely independent of biological, social, and/or psychological factors. Conversely, the concept of "biological age" attempts to characterize stages of senescence in terms of discrete biological rather than chronological processes. Thus research designs emphasizing chronological age tend to focus on elements of calendar time (years, decades, etc.) as the principal unit of analysis; whereas, biological age–oriented research focuses on senescent changes in biological or physiological processes and their effect on subsequent behavior.

A central tenet underlying much of the research in the area of physical fitness, cognition, and aging is the notion that physically fit individuals may be biologically younger than less-fit individuals of the same chronological age. From this point of view, research studies that examine the relationship between age, physical fitness, and behavior necessarily focus on both chronological and biological interpretations of aging.

PHYSICAL FITNESS. Many researchers have examined the relationship between physical fitness and cognitive performance in advancing age. Unfortunately little consensus has emerged with respect to either how to define physical fitness or how best to measure it. For the most part, studies that have examined the relationship between physical fitness and cognition have tended to focus on cardiovascular (aerobic) components of fitness rather than anaerobic fitness. Aerobic fitness is usually defined as an individual's capacity to perform continuous, repetitive physical work involving the major muscle groups of the body.

In cross-sectional studies, subject pools are usually divided into discrete high- and low-fitness groups, and differences in cognitive processing between these groups are examined. Fitness differences between the groups may be determined directly, by objective laboratory or field tests of physiological performance, or inferred indirectly, by selecting groups that vary with respect to their physical activity levels(e.g., masters athletes vs. sedentary controls). There are advantages and disadvantages associated with both direct and indirect approaches to the quantification of fitness [20]. The definition of physical fitness adopted in this review is both broad and nonspecific. As one might expect, the adoption of such a broad criterion reduces our ability to generalize about the relationship between physical fitness and cognitive performance. However, it is our belief that such a strategy is necessary, since it most accurately reflects a complex literature in which there is little agreement about how best to define physical fitness and ancillary constructs such as physical health and wellness [20, 85].

In addition to examining differences in cognitive performance between discrete high- and low-fitness groups, researchers have also examined the effects of exercise training on cognitive performance. In these designs, exercise training is manipulated as the independent variable. Training has usually, but not always, been defined in terms of aerobic rather than anaerobic exercise. Except where stated, throughout this review, exercise training will refer to structured physical activity of sufficient frequency, intensity, and duration to bring about reliable changes in cardiovascular performance. For the most part, such training regimens involve walking, jogging, bicycling, and/or swimming programs of at least 3–4 months duration, meeting several times a week for a minimum of thirty minutes of continuous aerobic exercise.

AGING AND COGNITION

Before discussing any intervening effect of physical fitness on the relationship between cognitive performance and advancing age, it is important to first consider age-related changes in cognition in general. Despite a widespread perception that cognitive performance necessarily deteriorates with advancing age, not all aspects of cognitive function decline at a similar rate with advancing age. Elderly individuals often experience profound deficits in some aspects of cognitive functioning, while at the same time experiencing little or no loss of functioning in others.

Recent research has demonstrated that our understanding of age-related changes in cognitive performance can be enhanced by an evaluation of the processing requirements of specific cognitive tasks [42, 43, 76]. Building upon earlier work by, among others, Kahneman [51], Posner and Snyder [68], and Shiffrin and Schneider [82, 84], Hasher and Zacks [42] have proposed a model in which cognitive processes can be viewed as being distributed along an automatic-to-effortful processing continuum. In this scheme, effortful cognitive processes are conceived of as those requiring the allocation of considerable attentional resources for their successful performance, whereas automatic cognitive processes are thought to be only minimally dependent upon attentional resources (In Figure 7.1 we present a schematic that illustrates how different cognitive processes can be distributed along an automatic-to-effortful processing continuum).

Capacity theories of attention are frequently invoked to explain the discrepancies observed between cognitive tasks with advancing age [13, 19]. In general, these theories propose that aging is associated with a reduction in the processing resources available for the execution of cognitive tasks. Since effortful processing tasks such as free-recall memory depend upon the availability of sufficient attentional resources for their successful completion, these tasks are disproportionately compromised by age-related declines in attentional capacity. Automatic processes, on the other hand, can be performed without conscious attention and are thus relatively immune to declines in attentional capacity [42].

In addition to helping to explain differences in age effects between effortful and automatic tasks, capacity models of aging also predict that age-related declines in cognitive performance should be greater for tasks requiring the rapid processing of information than for tasks that can be performed at a self-paced rate [13]. Behavioral slowing is sometimes characterized as the single most ubiquitous phenomenon accompanying advancing age [76]. While the precise mechanism responsible for the slowing of behavior is not fully understood, it is widely accepted that age-related decrements in the speed of performance occur as a result of central processing limitations rather than peripheral factors such as decreased sensory acuity or compromised musculoskeletal integrity [13, 93]. Since

FIGURE 7.1
Cognitive processing demand continuum.

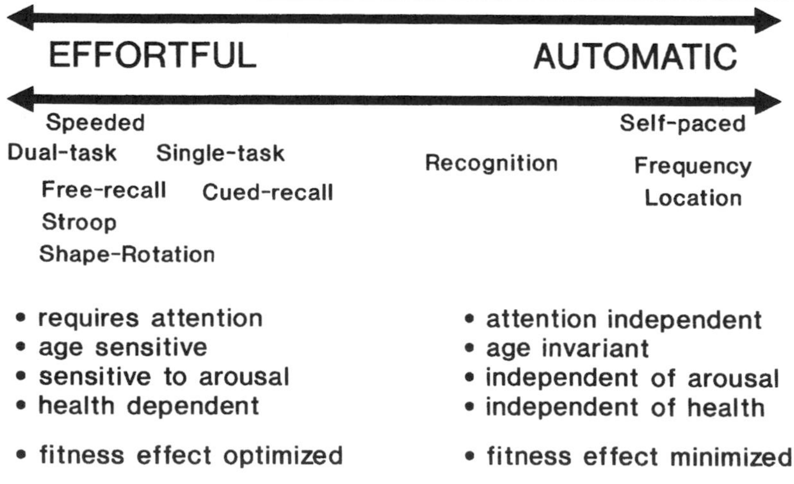

EFFORTFUL		AUTOMATIC
Speeded		Self-paced
Dual-task Single-task	Recognition	Frequency
Free-recall Cued-recall		Location
Stroop		
Shape-Rotation		

• requires attention	• attention independent
• age sensitive	• age invariant
• sensitive to arousal	• independent of arousal
• health dependent	• independent of health
• fitness effect optimized	• fitness effect minimized

reaction time tasks require both vigilance and the rapid selection of an appropriate response, two attentionally demanding processes, individuals with reduced attentional capacity are at a disadvantage in performing these tasks.

In summary, cognition is not a unitary phenomenon, and broad generalizations about the effect of age on cognition should be avoided. Age-related changes in cognitive performance appear to be maximized for tasks that require rapid and/or attentionally demanding processing, and minimized for tasks that are more automatic or which can be performed at a self-paced rate.

PHYSICAL FITNESS, COGNITION AND AGING: THE KEY QUESTIONS

Although both processing resources and cognitive performance inevitably and inescapably decline with advancing age, there are often considerable differences between subjects with respect to both the rate and extent of this decline. In recent years extensive attention has focused on the identification of various factors that may potentially alter the rate and extent of cognitive decline in aging. Of key interest to the present discussion is the notion that high levels of fitness may be associated with less-pronounced cognitive decline in old age. (For earlier reviews see [3, 19, 30, 89, 90, 92, 95].

Researchers in this area have focused on three fundamental questions:

1. Do high-fit older adults exhibit superior cognitive performance when compared with less-fit individuals of the same chronological age?
2. Can relatively short term exercise training bring about meaningful cognitive changes in previously sedentary older adults?
3. By what mechanisms does physical fitness influence cognitive performance in old age?

Our review examines the evidence pertaining to each of the above questions. We begin with a discussion of cross-sectional differences in cognitive performance between discrete high- and low-fit groups.

DOES PHYSICAL FITNESS INFLUENCE COGNITIVE DECLINE IN OLD AGE?

Ill-Health, Disease and Cognitive Performance

Gerontologists have speculated that ill-health and disease may result in an acceleration of degenerative processes in advancing age (see [7, 14] for a review of research in this area). Impaired cognitive processing is associated with numerous disease states. For example, patients with Parkinson's disease perform less well than age-matched controls on complex reaction time tasks [48], as do individuals suffering from clinical depression [101], schizophrenia [45], and manic-depressive psychosis [46].

In addition to the association between behavioral disorders and cognition, similar relationships have also been observed in cardiovascular and circulatory pathology. In an early study, Reitan [70] demonstrated that individuals with either hypertension or cardiovascular disease perform less well than age-matched healthy controls on a variety of cognitive and perceptual-motor tasks. The association between cardiovascular health and cognitive decline appears to be robust and has been extensively replicated [31, 41, 48, 58, 59, 80, 87, 103].

Taken as a whole, these studies suggest that a wide variety of disease states may be associated with a disruption in cognitive performance and that these disruptions may be more pronounced in older adult populations [7].

Good Health, Physical Fitness and Cognitive Performance
In addition to the studies linking ill-health and cognition, other investigators have speculated that exceptionally good health may be associated with enhanced performance on selected aspects of cognitive functioning. Earliest evidence for a link between health status and cognitive functioning emerged from a series of cross-sectional studies that compared cognitive performances of athletes and nonathletes [15, 17, 18, 55, 65, 105]. In these studies health and physical fitness were seldom measured directly, rather fitness differences were inferred to exist between the discrete athletic and nonathletic comparison groups. In general, modest but reliable differences in processing speed were observed between athletes and nonathletes.

Identification of differences in processing speed between athletes and nonathletes is insufficient evidence to conclude that there is an association between fitness and cognition in the population as a whole [89]. Psychomotor speed and fast reaction times are necessary components for success in many athletic events. It is likely that individuals with genetically endowed propensities in these areas are disproportionately represented in athletic subgroups. Furthermore, since the early athlete vs. nonathlete research focused almost exclusively on college-age subjects, caution is warranted before extending the results of these studies to older adults.

It was not until the mid-seventies that the first studies were specifically designed to test the hypothesis that physical fitness, per se, was associated with enhanced cognitive performance in older individuals. In a classic study, Spirduso [88] compared simple and choice reaction times of young (approximately 20 yr) and older (over 60 years) regular exercisers and nonexercisers. She found that older racquetball players were significantly faster on both simple and choice reaction time tasks than age-matched sedentary controls. Indeed the older exercisers performed the cognitive tasks at a level comparable to individuals more than thirty years their junior.

This basic finding that physical fitness is associated with an enhancement in cognitive processing speed has been replicated many times since Spirduso's initial study [2, 5, 20, 22, 28, 36, 50, 67, 71, 83, 96]. The association between physical fitness and cognitive performance appears to generalize to a variety of aerobic exercise activities including racquetball [71, 88, 91], walking and jogging [2, 5, 71], swimming [44], and other aerobic activity [71, 83], and is sufficiently robust to be detected by several different methods of assessing fitness, including self-report inventories [2, 5, 22, 50, 67, 71, 83, 96] as well as more traditional laboratory tests of physiological fitness and aerobic capacity [20–22, 29, 36, 64, 83].

Factors Influencing the Magnitude of the Relationship between Physical Fitness and Cognitive Performance
In recent years, considerable attention has focused on the nature of the tasks selected for the evaluation of cognitive performance in physical fitness research [19, 44, 92, 95]. An important experimental question has been whether certain cognitive tasks are more sensitive to physical fitness effects than others. Numerous factors can influence the magnitude of age effects in cognition research [19, 44, 92]. These include task-dependent factors such as speed of processing, task-complexity, and stimulus-response compatibility, as well as subject-dependent factors such as, practice, motivation, compensatory behaviors, age, and level of fitness. Each of the above factors can influence the outcome of an experimental investigation of the relation between physical fitness and cognitive performance. We briefly discuss each of the above factors and their implications for physical fitness research.

FIGURE 7.2
Task and subject-dependent factors influencing fitness-cognition relationship.

TASK DEPENDENT FACTORS:

• Speed of Processing	increases fitness effect
• Task Complexity	increases fitness effect
• S-R Compatibility	decreases fitness effect

SUBJECT DEPENDENT FACTORS:

• Practice	decreases fitness effect
• Motivation/arousal	unclear
• Compensatory Strategies	decreases fitness effect
• Chronological Age	unclear
• Level of Fitness	unclear

Task-dependent Factors Influencing the Relationship between Physical Fitness and Cognitive Performance

SPEED OF PROCESSING. As mentioned above, behavioral slowing is one of the most frequently replicated findings in experimental aging research [76]. Reaction time and movement time experiments reveal that older adults are almost always slower to respond than younger individuals [92, 102]. In addition to discriminating between young and older adults, speed of behavior tasks appears to be highly sensitive to differences in physical fitness. A large number of reaction-time studies report significant differences between high- and low-fit older adults [5, 20, 22, 29, 36, 50, 64, 67, 71, 83, 96], with only a few exceptions [16, 78]. These findings suggest that when cognitive performance is evaluated by tasks in which processing speed is the principal dependent measure, the relationship between physical fitness and cognitive performance is robust.

TASK COMPLEXITY. In contrast to findings linking physical fitness and performance on speeded tasks, less is known about the relationship between physical fitness and performance on more complex tasks in which qualitative rather than temporal aspects of cognition are evaluated (e.g., memory, problem solving, sustained attention, dual task performance). While some studies have shown reliable fitness effects on selected measures of fluid intelligence [28, 32, 97], working memory [28, 60], and abstract reasoning [64], almost as many studies have been unable to demonstrate fitness effects for crystallized intelligence [32], fluid intelligence [28, 95], frequency, location, and recognition memory [21], as well as abstract reasoning [64].

A number of researchers have proposed that much of the confusion that permeates the literature in this area can be resolved if closer attention is paid to the demand level of the tasks selected for the evaluation of cognitive performance [19, 44]. Chodzko-Zajko [19] has suggested that tasks that require novel and/or complex cognitive processing are likely to be more strongly related to physical fitness than more simple or over-learned tasks. Several recent studies lend support to this hypothesis. Stones and Kozma [95, 96] report two studies in which young and older adults were divided into physically active and physically inactive subgroups and asked to perform a series of tapping tasks that differed greatly in both familiarity and task complexity. Of greatest interest to the present discussion was the observation that the beneficial effects of physical activity were most pronounced for the tasks requiring the greatest attentional demand. The authors state that one interpretation of their findings might be that "tasks requiring effortful processing may be more sensitive to the tonic effects of exercise" [95]. Similar conclusions were drawn by Chodzko-Zajko et al. [21], who examined the influence of cardiovascular fitness on automatic and effortful memory. In this study, middle-aged and older adults were divided into discrete fitness groups. Significant differences were found between high- and low-fitness groups on an attentionally demanding free-recall memory test, but no differences were found for frequency and location memory. Frequency and location memory are generally considered to be highly automatized cognitive processes that make only minimal demands on attentional resources. The authors concluded that the relationship between physical fitness and cognition is task- specific and that the prophylactic effects of physical fitness on effortful memory need not necessarily extend to cognitive tasks requiring less effortful processing.

Several other studies have found task-specificity effects on the relationship between physical fitness and cognitive performance [32, 36, 44, 96]. In an important recent study, Hawkins, Kramer, and Capaldi [44] found a relationship between fitness and cognition for complex dual-task performance but not for several less demanding cognitive tasks. Consistent with the findings described above, Hawkins et al. concluded that attentional demand may be important in differentiating between tasks that show positive fitness effects and those that do not.

In summary, there is increasingly strong support for the hypothesis that processing demand is an important factor in determining the magnitude of the relationship between physical fitness and cognitive performance. When cognitive tasks are selected that require considerable attentional demand, physical fitness effects are likely to be robust; fitness effects are likely to be smaller or nonexistent for less effortful cognitive tasks. Due to the considerable variability between tasks, most researchers have chosen to evaluate cognition by using a battery of cognitive tasks that can assess a broad range of processing abilities. It is doubtful that any single cognitive task can be identified as the optimal means for assessing cognition in fitness research. Rather, future research is likely to continue to depend upon multivariate batteries for the assessment of cognition.

STIMULUS-RESPONSE COMPATIBILITY. Stimulus-response (S-R) compatibility refers to the extent to which a stimulus appears to be both natural and logical [92]. For example, right-handed responses are more compatible with stimuli located on the right side of a stimulus array than with those occurring on the left. In a series of elegant experiments, Spirduso and her colleagues have demonstrated convincingly that S-R incompatibility not only increases reaction time as a whole, but also increases reaction time differences between young and older subjects [56]. With respect to the effects of fitness, Stones and Kozma [96] found that chronic exercise was more strongly related to atypical movements than to overlearned familiar movements. Their conclusion was that less compatible responses require greater central processing and are consequently more likely to demonstrate significant fitness effects.

Subject-dependent Factors Influencing the Relationship between Physical Fitness and Cognitive Performance

PRACTICE. Extended practice reduces the magnitude of age effects in motor and cognitive performance research [62,75]. When older adults are given ample time to practice novel tasks, performance differences between young and older subjects are often substantially reduced [92]. Although older persons appear to benefit more from extended practice than younger individuals [104], age differences do not appear to be completely eliminated by practice [79].

The relationship that practice on a cognitive task has to its sensitivity to physical fitness is unclear. Stones and Kozma [96] found that fitness effects were greatest for novel, relatively unpracticed tasks and smaller for overlearned, highly practiced movements. This finding appears to be consistent with Hasher and Zacks' [42, 43] theory of automaticity. The theory states that extended practice decreases the demand level of an experimental task, thereby reducing the magnitude of the performance decrement with both advancing age and deteriorating fitness. Regardless of the mechanism by which practice influences cognitive performance, care must be taken to ensure that adequate practice is given to subjects when assessing cognitive performance in the laboratory. (See Spirduso [90, 92] for a discussion of practice effects in physical fitness research.)

MOTIVATION AND AROUSAL. Although level of motivation and arousal indisputably play an important role in the successful execution of cognitive tasks, there is no reason to believe that age-related declines in cognitive performance can be attributed to motivational factors [52]. Some evidence suggests that many older adults are at least as motivated, if not more motivated, than college students, when asked to perform a variety of cognitive processing tasks [52]. With respect to physical fitness research, we have been able to find no evidence to suggest that high-fit subjects differ in motivation or arousal level from less-fit contemporaries. Thus it seems unlikely that cognitive performance differences between high- and low-fit groups can be attributed to differential levels of arousal and/or motivation.

COMPENSATORY STRATEGIES. Welford [102] has suggested that many older adults are able to minimize the consequences of age-related declines in central processing resources by adopting compensatory strategies such as anticipation, trading speed for accuracy, and adopting conservative response criteria. One example of the effective use of compensatory strategies is provided by Salthouse [75], who showed that older typists were able to maintain typing speed by anticipating forthcoming characters more efficiently than younger individuals. It seems likely that many older adults are able to maintain adequate levels of functioning in spite of quite profound declines in underlying capacity by adopting stereotypic, over-learned strategies that maximize available resources [72].

With respect to the implications for physical fitness research, it is often difficult to predict the extent to which fitness differences between subjects will manifest themselves in observable differences in cognitive performance. Many of the sensory and motor systems underlying cognitive performance appear to have sufficient redundancy built into them that adequate performance can sometimes be maintained by compensatory adjustments, in spite of quite profound decreases in sensory acuity, muscle strength, and/or central processing resources [102]. The evidence presented above suggests that compensatory behaviors are most likely to be effective for overlearned familiar tasks and less advantageous for novel or especially complex tasks.

CHRONOLOGICAL AGE. Some controversy pertains to the extent to which the beneficial effects of physical fitness on cognitive performance can be shown to apply across the life span [95]. More simply put, does physical fitness have an influence on cognitive performance regardless of age, or do the effects of fitness on cognition only become apparent as people grow older?

Stones and Kozma [95] have suggested that at least two theoretical models can be invoked to explain the relationship between physical fitness, cognitive performance, and age. In their tonic and overpractice effect model (TOPE), they propose that the effects of chronological age and lifestyle factors on cognitive performance are essentially independent. A key prediction of this model is that physical fitness should benefit cognitive performance regardless of age.

In contrast, their moderator model suggests that regular physical activity influences cognitive performance by altering the rate at which an individual ages. According to the model, physical fitness should not affect cognitive performance for young adults because these individuals still have sufficient attentional capacity to perform most cognitive tasks without noticeable impairment. However, as available attentional resources decline with age, the effect of factors such as physical fitness, health, and disease is augmented. Thus the moderator model predicts an age by fitness interaction for cognitive performance, whereas the TOPE model does not.

Enough well-controlled experimental studies have yet to be carried out to reject either of the above hypotheses. While statistically significant age by fitness interactions have been found in a number of studies [16, 29, 50, 71, 83, 88], there are at least as many investigations in which the magnitude of the fitness effect does not appear to vary as a function of age. A number of methodological problems contribute to our inability to resolve this important question. First, it is difficult to operationally define criteria for the division of young and older subjects into discrete high- and low-fitness groups. For example, relatively high-fit elderly individuals often have absolute oxygen consumption values that do not differ from, or are even lower than, those observed in younger adults characterized as low-fit. Since researchers do not agree on the criteria for assigning subjects to high- and low-fitness groups, the comparison of age by fitness interactions across studies is problematic. A second but related problem pertains to the wide variation in cognitive tasks selected for the evaluation of cognitive performance. Since physical fitness effects on cognition are highly task specific, it is almost impossible to make meaningful comparisons across studies unless identical cognitive tasks are selected.

In summary, it is presently difficult to definitively conclude whether or not the magnitude of the relationship between physical fitness and cognitive performance varies reliably across the life span. Credible evidence has been amassed in support of both the age-dependent and age-independent hypotheses. Future research is needed, which can focus specifically on the resolution of this intriguing question.

LEVEL OF FITNESS. On first glance, one of the most obvious subject-related factors influencing the cross-sectional relationship between physical fitness and cognitive performance ought to be the magnitude of the fitness differences between high- and low-fit groups. It would seem logical that the larger the differences in fitness between groups, the greater should be the differences in cognitive performance. Unfortunately there is almost no credible evidence against which to test such a "dose-dependent" relationship. Because of the wide variation in methodological approaches to the assessment of both physical fitness and cognitive performance, meaningful meta-analyses cannot be performed to examine the strength of the fitness-cognition relationship across studies. To date it has not been established whether there is any minimum threshold necessary for the emergence of beneficial effects of fitness on cognition. Indeed, it is quite possible that the magnitude of the required fitness effect might vary from task to task as a function of the demand level of the task selected for the evaluation of cognitive performance [19, 44]. Extensive additional research is needed before definitive statements can be made about any minimum threshold of physical fitness necessary for the emergence of reliable cognitive differences between subjects.

Not only is it unclear how large physical fitness differences must be to detect cognitive differences between subjects, there is also some debate about how best to measure physical fitness in cognition research [20]. The most common approach has been to measure maximal oxygen uptake (VO_2max) in response to an exercise stress test. There are a number of objections to the exclusive reliance on such measures for the evaluation of fitness in elderly populations [20]. Sidney and Shephard [85] have shown that both direct and indirect measurement of VO_2max can be problematic in older adults. As many as 30% of subjects over 60 years of age are unable to attain the "oxygen plateau" required for the direct determination of VO_2max. Similarly, indirect estimation of VO_2max from submaximal values has been shown to underestimate direct measures by as much as 25%. Sidney and Shephard conclude that valid measures of maximal oxygen consumption can be obtained in only approximately two-thirds of the elderly population.

A further objection to the reliance of exercise-stress test data for the evaluation of fitness is that large numbers of elderly subjects cannot meet the relatively stringent medical criteria required for participation in even submaximal exercise tests [1]. Thus, most studies that rely on stress tests to determine fitness have been restricted to a relatively healthy subset of the elderly population. The exclusive dependence on exercise-based testing for the evaluation of physical fitness has effectively excluded more infirm subjects from participation in research, and thus has limited the extent to which findings can be generalized to the elderly population as a whole.

Cognizant of the shortcomings associated with VO_2max, several researchers have attempted to develop more complex multivariate fitness scores to use in cognition research [20, 28, 95,]. In general, composite measures of fitness are more sensitive to cognitive performance than any single measure in isolation. For example, Chodzko-Zajko and Ringel [20] developed a multivariate fitness criterion, the index of physiological status (IPS), which was derived from a number of resting cardiovascular, hemodynamic, pulmonary, and anthropometric parameters. In a study of 70 older males, the IPS was found to be more strongly correlated with complex reaction time ($r = -.40$) than was VO_2max ($r = -.13$).

The above findings suggest that although numerous studies have demonstrated an association between physical fitness and cognitive performance, there is little consensus about how best to measure fitness in the laboratory. Clearly there are shortcomings associated with exclusive reliance on maximal oxygen consumption as the measure of fitness. However, to date no agreement has been reached on an acceptable alternative.

Summary:Cross-Sectional Studies
A growing body of evidence suggests that physically fit older adults often process cognitive information more efficiently than less-fit individuals of the same chronological age. However, the relationship between physical fitness and cognition is highly task-dependent. Physical fitness effects are most likely to be observed in tasks that require rapid or effortful cognitive processing and are less likely to occur in self-paced or automatic processing tasks. Because numerous task and subject-related factors can influence the relationship between fitness and cognition, extreme caution is warranted before making generalizations about the influence of fitness on cognitive performance.

CAN RELATIVELY SHORT TERM EXERCISE TRAINING BRING ABOUT MEANINGFUL IMPROVEMENTS IN COGNITIVE PERFORMANCE IN PREVIOUSLY SEDENTARY OLDER ADULTS?

The identification of significant differences in cognitive performance between discrete high- and low-fitness groups is insufficient evidence to conclude that exercise or physical activity caused these differences. The interpretation of positive fitness effects in cross-sectional studies is complicated by such factors as self-selection bias [44] and practice effects [92]. To circumvent these problems, researchers have attempted to assess the effect of exercise training on cognition more directly by training previously sedentary individuals and examining changes in cognitive performance in response to the treatment [10–12, 28, 32, 34, 35, 40, 44, 57, 66, 99].

Two early studies in young adults first suggested that relatively short term (3–4 months) exercise training may result in improvement in cognitive performance [40, 99]. However, the lack of an appropriate control group made the interpretation of these studies problematic. More recently, Elsayed, Ismail, and Young [32] examined the effect of 4 months of jogging and calisthenics on cognitive performance in 70 healthy men (age 24–68 years). Cognition was measured using a battery of fluid and crystallized intelligence tests. Significant pre-to-post improvements were found for the fluid but not for the crystallized intelligence tests. Elsayed et al. suggested that the effects of exercise training on cognition are task-specific and restricted to novel (fluid) rather than familiar (crystallized) tests of intellectual functioning. Unfortunately, this study also failed to include a nonexercise control group, making it impossible to determine whether improvements were due to training or practice effects (see also [44]).

In the first well-controlled training study of exercise and cognition, Dustman et al. [28] randomly assigned 43 sedentary adults to aerobic exercise (n = 13), strength and flexibility (n = 15), or nonexercise control (n = 15) groups and assessed the effect of 4 months of training on a battery of cognitive tests. Increases in aerobic capacity, relative to the control group, were observed for both exercise groups, although the changes were larger in the aerobic exercise (27%) group than in the strength/flexibility group (11%). With respect to cognition, significant pre-to-post changes were observed in the aerobic exercise group for some cognitive tasks but not for others. Specifically, improvements were observed for Critical Flicker Fusion, the Digit Symbol Substitution scale of the Wechsler Adult Intelligence Scale, Simple Reaction Time, and the Stroop task, whereas no changes were seen for Choice Reaction Time, Culture Fair IQ, or Digit Span. In contrast, the strength training and sedentary control groups showed little or no cognitive improvement. Dustman and his colleagues concluded that short-term aerobic training is associated with significant improvement in selected aspects of cognitive functioning.

A number of subsequent investigations have attempted to replicate Dustman et al.'s finding of beneficial effects of exercise on cognitive performance. [10–12, 34, 35, 44, 57, 66]. In a series of elegant experiments, Blumenthal et al. subjected middle-aged and older adults to 4–8 months of aerobic exercise, strength training, yoga, or sedentary living and examined pre-to-post changes in a variety of cognitive parameters [10–12, 34, 57].

In their first study, Blumenthal and Madden [10] randomly assigned 28 middle-aged males (age 30–58 years) to either 4 months of aerobic exercise (n = 13) or 4 months of strength training (n = 15). Cognitive performance was evaluated using the Sternberg Memory Search paradigm [94]. The study found that both groups improved significantly on the memory search task; however, only the aerobic exercise group increased in aerobic capacity. The authors concluded that the improvements in cognitive performance were independent of changes in aerobic capacity and that there was no evidence in support of the hypothesis that aerobic exercise enhances cognitive performance.

A number of criticisms have been raised to the above study. First, the relative youth of the subjects (30–58 years) may have reduced the likelihood of observing training effects on cognitive performance. Second, the absence of a sedentary control group made interpretations of pre-to-post changes problematic. And third, the subjects were already relatively high-fit at the beginning of the study, resulting in much smaller improvements in aerobic capacity (15%) than in the Dustman et al. [28] study (27%).

In an attempt to control for some of the above factors, Blumenthal et al. extended their research to include an older sample of subjects (60–83 years) and a wider range of activities, including aerobic exercise and yoga, as well as a sedentary waiting-list control group. A number of studies have now been published from this data set, including two 3- to 4-month training studies [11, 34], an 8-month cross-over study [57], and a 14-month investigation [12]. In addition to standard memory search and word comparison tasks, cognitive performance was also evaluated using a dual-task paradigm in which subjects were asked to complete the above memory search and word comparison tests while simultaneously performing an auditory processing task. The selection of the dual-task criterion for the evaluation of cognitive performance is important because these tasks are extremely attentionally demanding, and they should have maximized the likelihood of detecting significant exercise training effects (see Fig. 7.1). Despite significant increases in aerobic capacity (11.6%), there were no training effects for any of the cognitive performance measures assessed. The authors concluded that they found no evidence to support the hypothesis that short-term aerobic exercise results in beneficial changes in cognitive performance.

The nonsignificant findings of Blumenthal et al. are supported by the results of another well-controlled training study [66]. Panton et al. [66] randomly assigned 49 older adults (age 70–79 into aerobic exercise (n = 17), strength-training (n = 20), and sedentary control groups (n = 12) and assessed changes in reaction time in response to the various treatments. Despite substantial improvements in aerobic capacity (20%), no effects of aerobic training on cognitive parameters were observed.

Taken in combination, the Panton and Blumenthal studies appeared to have shifted the weight of the evidence to favor the conclusion that short-term exercise training has no effect on cognitive performance. However an important recent study necessitates a reevaluation of this conclusion. Hawkins et al. [44] assessed the effect of exercise training on cognitive performance, using cognitive measures similar to those selected by Blumenthal et al. Thirty-six older adults were randomly assigned to 10 weeks of aerobic exercise (n = 18) or sedentary control regimens (n = 18). Cognitive performance was assessed using both single and dual-task procedures. While neither group changed with respect to single-task performance, significant changes in dual-task performance were observed for the exercise, but not the control, group. These findings are at variance with the Blumenthal et al. studies, which did not find changes in either single- or dual-task performance [11, 12, 34, 57]. In an attempt to explain the discrepancies between their study and those of the Blumenthal group, Hawkins et al. noted that their dual-task paradigm was associated with significantly greater temporal demand. They suggest that this difference in time pressure caused their cognitive measures to be more attentionally demanding and thus more sensitive to the effects of exercise training. It is important to note that Hawkins et al. assessed exercise training effects by changes in resting heart rate and not by improvements in maximal oxygen consumption. This makes it impossible to compare the magnitude of the training effect in the Hawkins study to the Blumenthal, Panton et al., and Dustman et al. studies.

An important issue in interpretation of the exercise training data pertains to the duration of the exercise treatment. In general, researchers have opted for training programs of between 4 and 8 months duration, presumably because these are the minimum durations required to obtain reliable training effects for most cardiovascular parameters. However, it is unclear why these durations should be considered sufficient for the manifestation of meaningful changes in cognitive behavior. Many of the physiological mechanisms that have been proposed to explain the relationship between physical fitness and cognition involve relatively long term chronic adaptations that are likely to take considerably longer than 8 months before their effects are observed. (Several direct and indirect mechanisms are discussed in the final section of this review.) The absence of significant training effects on cognition in short-term exercise training studies should not be taken as evidence to rule out a causal relation between exercise training and cognition. Rather, these studies demonstrate that cardiovascular changes observed in response to exercise training do not necessarily coincide with cognitive changes. The possibility of an indeterminate time lag between cardiovascular changes and more central cognitive changes has not been tested. Interventions over many years may well achieve quite different results from the short-term training studies. Extended longitudinal studies are needed to examine the effect of lifelong physical activity on age-related cognitive decline.

Summary: Training Studies
No clear picture has emerged with respect to the effect of exercise on cognitive performance. Two well-controlled studies have successfully demonstrated improvement in cognitive performance following training,

while three studies have not. There is some reason to believe that the magnitude of the improvement in aerobic capacity, as well as the demand-level of the cognitive task, may be important in determining the presence or absence of training effects. However, when changes in cognitive performance have been observed following short-term exercise training, the magnitude of these changes has always been small. At present there is no compelling evidence to suggest that short-term exercise training results in clinically significant improvements in cognition.

BY WHAT MECHANISM DOES PHYSICAL FITNESS INFLUENCE COGNITIVE PERFORMANCE?

Despite the wealth of studies that have examined the relation between physical fitness and cognitive performance, surprisingly little is known about the mechanisms by which exercise or physical activity might influence cognition. In her influential 1980 review article, Spirduso [89] speculated that regular physical activity might influence cognitive processing by (*a*) altering cerebral circulation or (*b*) promoting neurotrophic changes, such as nerve cell regeneration or neurotransmitter repletion. Spirduso noted that the evidence in support of either of the above hypotheses was entirely circumstantial and that there had been no direct tests of either mechanism. More than a decade has passed since Spirduso's review, and we are still a long way from being able to make definitive statements about the mechanism or mechanisms by which physical fitness might influence cognitive performance [19]. Nonetheless, some progress has been made in a number of areas. We will summarize the research evidence in support of several direct and indirect mechanisms by which exercise/physical activity has been proposed to influence cognitive processing.

Cerebral Circulation Hypothesis

It has been proposed that chronic exercise maintains cerebrovascular integrity by enhancing oxygen transportation to the brain [28, 89]. Several lines of evidence support the hypothesis that impaired cerebral circulation may have adverse consequences for cognitive performance. In an early study, McFarland [58] demonstrated that the cognitive declines observed in elderly subjects were similar to those seen in younger individuals under conditions of hypoxia. A subsequent study demonstrated small but significant improvements in cognitive performance following hyperbaric oxygen supplementation [6]. Recently, Kennedy et al. [53] studied the effects of prolonged hypoxia in eight young adults who spent 40 days in a decompression chamber. Hypoxia was found to be associated with significant cognitive impairment on a variety of cognitive tasks.

Research in clinical populations has also supported an association between cerebrovascular circulation and cognitive performance. The increased incidence of cardiovascular disease with age has been estimated to result in an almost 50% decline in cerebral blood flow by age 50 [54]. Individuals with cardiovascular pathology have impaired cognitive performance relative to healthy controls [47, 59]. However, some evidence suggests that the effects of circulatory impairment may be stronger for speeded than for non-speeded cognitive tasks [48].

In a recent experimental study, Rogers, Meyer, and Mortel [74] classified 90 elderly volunteers into three discrete activity groups, (*a*) currently working, (*b*) retired high-activity, and (*c*) retired low-activity. Cerebral blood flow was measured by the radioactive Xe inhalation method, and cognitive performance was assessed using a standardized cognitive screening examination. Individuals in the retired low-activity group had lower cerebral blood flow, and these changes were associated with significant decrements in cognitive performance. Rogers et al. concluded that individuals who retire and lead a sedentary lifestyle are at increased risk of cerebrovascular disease with associated cognitive impairment. Furthermore, they proposed that regular participation in physical activity can minimize cognitive decline by sustaining optimal cerebral perfusion. Unfortunately, Rogers et al. neither manipulated exercise behavior nor measured physical fitness directly, and thus care should be taken in extrapolating their results to the physical fitness and exercise science literature.

In summary, some circumstantial evidence suggests that impaired cerebrovascular circulation is associated with accelerated cognitive decline. However, the effect of either physical fitness or short-term exercise training on this relationship has yet to be subjected to experimental test.

Neurotrophic Stimulation Hypothesis
Aging is associated with degenerative changes throughout much of the central nervous system [25, 27]. Included among these changes are disruptions in neurotransmitter synthesis and degradation [73], as well as structural alterations to neuronal cell bodies and axons [63]. Both of the above can result in significant neurologic impairment as well as cellular necrosis and death. It has long been suggested that prolonged activity may be associated with an amelioration of the severity of neural degeneration with advancing age [100].

Understandably much of the research in this area has focused on the animal model. Prolonged physical activity is associated with increased brain weight in both primates [38] and rats [69], and movement-enriched environments are associated with increased capillary growth [8] as well as an increased number of dendritic connections [24]. It is presently unclear at what age physical activity effects on neurological structure and function are greatest. Black, Isaacs, and Greenough [9] have argued that enriched movement experiences may be most beneficial for young animals to the extent that it enables them to optimize neural development, resulting in a more substantial "neural reserve" that can be drawn upon in old age (see also [90]).

Research in humans has also shown that significant neural changes accompany advancing age. Both generalized and site-specific [49, 81] morphological changes have been described in the older population, as have alterations in neurotransmitter synthesis and degradation [61]. It has been proposed that exposure to chronic exercise stress may have beneficial effects on individuals' reactivity to acute psychological stressors [26]. However, for the most part, the relation between physical activity, aging, and central nervous system integrity has yet to be subjected to experimental test.

In an recent study, Sothmann and his colleagues [86] examined the effects of physical fitness on plasma catecholamine responses to cognitive stress in middle-aged adults. The authors were able to demonstrate a relationship between physical fitness and sympathetic reactivity to a complex verbal reasoning task. These data suggest that physical fitness may be associated with altered neurochemical responses to selected cognitive tasks; however, since these findings were based exclusively on data from younger adults, there is a real need to replicate this study in an older population.

In summary, evidence from animal models suggests that physical activity may be associated with a diminution of age-related degenerative changes in several neurological parameters. While there are theoretical reasons to believe that similar processes may be operating in humans, there is a shortage of empirical data in this area, and further research is needed before definitive conclusions can be drawn.

Neural Efficiency Hypothesis

Both the cerebral circulation and the neurotrophic stimulation hypotheses propose direct mechanisms by which physical activity might influence cognitive performance. These hypotheses are not mutually exclusive, and there is no reason why both mechanisms might not be operating simultaneously. In addition to these mechanisms, another class of explanations has attempted to explain the relation between physical fitness and cognition in aging in terms of the efficiency with which information is processed by the central nervous system.

A number of researchers have examined electroencephalographic (EEG) data in an attempt to determine whether physical fitness influences cognitive processing in old age [2, 29, 33]. EEG data do not provide us with a direct mechanism by which fitness may influence cognitive performance, since electrophysiological recordings simply reflect the activity of underlying neural systems. They do, however, provide us with an indirect window through which valuable information can be obtained about the functioning of the central nervous system.

Advancing age is associated with predictable changes in both raw and computer-averaged electrophysiological responses. For example, older adults exhibit decreased EEG alpha frequencies, when compared with younger subjects [39]. Similarly, auditory, visual, and somatosensory averaged evoked potentials (AEPs) also demonstrate reliable changes with advancing age [30]. Dustman has proposed that these changes reflect a slower, less efficient nervous system with advancing age.

A question of interest to the present discussion is whether physical fitness and/or exercise training can be shown to delay the onset of age-related changes in electrophysiological parameters. Dustman, Emmerson, Ruhling, et al. [29] studied electrophysiological responses of young (20–31 years) and older (50–62 years) adults who were divided into high- and low-fitness groups in accordance with their maximal oxygen consumption. Age and fitness effects were observed for a variety of EEG parameters including somatosensory evoked potentials, visual evoked potentials, and cortical coupling. Cognitive performance was better for young men than for older men, and for high-fit than low-fit subjects. The authors concluded that physical fitness was associated with more efficient CNS processing. This finding was generally consistent with an earlier study [33], which found that age-related changes in P300 latency were minimized in a high-fit group of older adults, compared with less healthy individuals of the same chronological age.

In summary, some evidence suggests that high-levels of fitness may be associated with a reduction in the magnitude of the age-related changes in selected electrophysiological parameters. High-fit individuals appear to process cognitive information faster and more efficiently than less-fit individuals of the same chronological age. However, there have been no well-controlled studies of the effects of exercise training on EEG responses, and it is unclear to what extent fitness differences can be modified by short-term exercise training.

Recent advances in computerized axial tomography and other imaging techniques have exciting implications for research in this area [23]. The application of these procedures to physical fitness and cognition research is likely to increase our understanding of the underlying mechanisms by which physiological changes influence cognitive behavior in aging.

Summary: Potential Mechanisms for the Fitness-Cognition Relationship
A number of mechanisms have been proposed to explain the relationship between physical fitness and cognitive performance in old age. Some evidence suggests that high-fit adults process information in the central nervous system faster and more efficiently than less-fit individuals of the same chronological age. This increase in efficiency may be secondary to improvements in cerebral circulation, nerve cell regeneration, and/or changes in neurotransmitter synthesis and degradation. To date, research in this area has been almost exclusively cross-sectional, and there is a real need to extend these findings in well-controlled training studies.

CONCLUSIONS

Age-related decrements in cognitive performance are now well established. However, cognition is not a unitary phenomenon, and there are wide variations between cognitive tasks with respect to the magnitude of changes observed with advancing age. Age-related changes in cognitive performance appear to be maximized for tasks that require rapid and/or attentionally demanding processing and minimized for tasks that are more automatic or can be performed at a self-paced rate.

Although both processing resources and cognitive performance inevitably and inescapably decline with advancing age, there are often considerable differences between subjects with respect to both the rate and extent of this decline. In recent years, extensive attention has focused on the notion that high levels of fitness may be associated with less pronounced cognitive decline in old age. Substantial evidence now supports the hypothesis that physically fit older adults often process cognitive information more efficiently than less-fit individuals of the same chronological age. However, the relationship between physical fitness and cognition is highly task dependent. Physical fitness effects are most likely to be observed with tasks that require rapid or effortful cognitive processing and are less likely to occur with self-paced or automatic processing tasks. Because numerous task and subject-related factors can influence the relationship between fitness and cognition, extreme caution is warranted before making generalizations about the influence of physical fitness on cognitive performance.

Despite a cross-sectional association between fitness and cognitive performance, the effect of exercise training on cognitive performance is not clear. Two well-controlled studies have successfully demonstrated improvement in cognitive performance following training, while three studies have not. Some evidence suggests that the magnitude of the improvement in aerobic capacity, as well as the demand-level of the cognitive task, may be important in determining the presence or absence of training effects. However, when changes in cognitive performance have been observed following exercise training, the magnitude of these changes has always been small. At present there is no compelling reason to believe that short-term exercise training results in clinically significant improvements in cognition.

A number of mechanisms have been proposed to explain the relationship between physical fitness and cognitive performance in old age. Some evidence suggests that high-fit adults process information in the central nervous system faster and more efficiently than less-fit individuals of the same chronological age. This increase in efficiency may be secondary to improvements in cerebral circulation, nerve cell regeneration, and/or changes in neurotransmitter synthesis and degradation. To date, research in this area has been almost exclusively cross-sectional, and there is a real need to extend these findings in well-controlled training studies.

REFERENCES

1. American College of Sports Medicine. *Resource Manual for Guidelines for Exercise Testing and Prescription: Second Edition.* Philadelphia: Lea & Febiger, 1993
2. Arito, H., and M. Oguri. Contingent negative variation and reaction time of physically-trained subjects in simple and discriminative tasks. *Ind. Health* 28:97–106,1990.
3. Barsalou, L. W. *Cognitive Psychology: An Overview for Cognitive Scientists.* Hillsdale, NJ: Lawrence Erlbaum, 1992.
4. Bashore, T. R. Age, physical fitness, and mental processing speed. *Annu. Rev. Gerontol. Geriatr.* 9:121–144, 1989.
5. Baylor, A. M., and W. W. Spirduso. Systematic aerobic exercise and components of reaction time in older women. *J. Gerontol.* 43:121–126, 1988.
6. Ben-Yishai, Y., and L. Diller. Changing of atmospheric environment to improve mental and behavioral function. *N.Y. State J. Med.* 12:2877–2880, 1973.
7. Birren, J.E., A. M. Woods, and M. V. Williams. Behavioral slowing with age: causes, organization, and consequences. L. W. Poon (ed). *Aging in the 1980s: Psychological Issues.* Washington, D.C.: APA, 1980, pp. 293–308.
8. Black, J. E., W. T. Greenough, B. J. Anderson, and K. R. Isaacs. Environment and the aging brain *Can. J. Psychol.* 41:111–130, 1987.
9. Black, J. E., K. R. Isaacs, and W. T. Greenough. Usual versus successful aging: some notes on experiential factors. *Neurobiol. Aging* 12:325–328, 1991.
10. Blumenthal, J. A., and D. J. Madden. Effects of aerobic exercise training, age, and physical fitness on memory- search performance. *Psychol. Aging* 3:280–285, 1988.
11. Blumenthal, J. A., C. F. Emery, D. J. Madden, et al. Cardiovascular and behavioral effects of aerobic exercise training in healthy older men and women. *J. Gerontol.* 44:147–157, 1989.
12. Blumenthal, J. A., C. F. Emery, D. J. Madden, et al. Long-term effects of exercise on psychological functioning in older men and women. *J. Gerontol.* 46:352–361,1991.
13. Botwinick, J. *Aging and Behavior.* New York: Springer-Verlag, 1985, pp. 229–248.
14. Botwinick, J., and J. E. Birren. Cognitive processes: mental abilities and psychomotor responses in aged men. J. E. Birren, R.N. Butler, S. W. Greenhouse, L. Sokoloff, and M. R. Yarrow (eds). *Human Aging: A Biological and Behavioral Study.* Washington, D.C.: U.S. Government Printing Office, 1963, pp. 143–156.
15. Botwinick, J., and L. W. Thompson. Age differences in reaction time: An artifact? *Gerontologist* 8:25–28, 1968.
16. Bunce, D. J., P. B. Warr, and T. Cochrane. Attention gaps in choice responding as a function of age and physical fitness. Paper presented at the 1992 Atlanta conference on Aging and Cognition, 1992.
17. Burley, L. R. A study of the reaction time of physically trained men. *Res. Q.* 15:232–239, 1944.
18. Burpee, R. H., and W. Stroll. Measuring reaction time of athletes. *Res. Q.* 7:110–118, 1936.
19. Chodzko-Zajko, W. J. Physical fitness, cognitive performance and aging. *Med. Sci. Sports Exerc.* 23:868–872, 1991.
20. Chodzko-Zajko, W. J., and Ringel, R. L. Physical fitness measures and sensory and motor performance in aging. *Exp. Gerontol.* 22:317–328, 1987.
21. Chodzko-Zajko, W. J., P. B. Schuler, J. S. Solomon, B. Heinl, and N. Ellis. The influence of age and physical fitness on automatic and effortful cognitive processing. *Int. J. Aging Hum. Dev.* 35(4):265–285, 1992.
22. Clarkson-Smith, L., and A. A. Hartley. Relationships between physical exercise and cognitive abilities in older adults. *Psychol. Aging* 4:183–189, 1989.
23. Cohen, G. D. *The Brain in Human Aging.* New York: Springer, 1988, pp 3–76.
24. Cottman, C. W. Synaptic plasticity, neurotrophic factors, and transplantation in the aged brain. E. L. Schneider and J. W. Rowe (eds). *Handbook of the Biology of Aging: Third Edition.* New York: Van Nostrand Rinehold, 1990, pp. 255–274.

25. Cottman, C. W., and V. R. Holets. Structural changes at synapses with age: plasticity and regeneration. C. E. Finch and E. L. Schneider (eds). *Handbook of the Biology of Aging: Second Edition*. New York: Van Nostrand Rinehold, 1985, pp. 617–644.

26. Dienstbier, R. A. Arousal and physiological toughness: implications for mental and physical health. *Psychol. Rev.* 96:84–100, 1989.

27. Duara, R., E. D. London, and S. I. Rapoport. Changes in structure and energy metabolism of the aging brain. C. E. Finch and E. L. Schneider (eds). *Handbook of the Biology of Aging: Second Edition*. New York: Van Nostrand Rinehold, 1985, pp. 595–618.

28. Dustman, R. E., R. O. Ruhling, E. M. Russell, et al. Aerobic exercise training and improved neuropsychological function of older individuals. *Neurobiol. Aging* 5:35–42, 1984.

29. Dustman, R. E., R. Y. Emmerson, R. O. Ruhling, et al. Age and fitness effects on EEG, ERPs, visual sensitivity, and cognition. *Neurobiol. Aging* 11:193–200, 1990.

30. Dustman, R. E., R. Y. Emmerson, and D. E. Shearer. Electrophysiology and aging: slowing, inhibition, and aerobic fitness. M. L. Howe, M. J. Stones, and C. J. Brainerd (eds). *Cognitive and Behavioral Performance Factors in Atypical Aging*. New York: Springer-Verlag, 1990, pp. 103–149.

31. Elias, M. F., M. A. Robbins, N. R. Schultz, and T. W. Pierce. Is blood pressure an important variable in research on aging and neuropsychological test performance? *J. Gerontol.* 45:128–135, 1990.

32. Elsayed, M., A. H. Ismail, and R. J. Young. Intellectual differences of adult men related to age and physical fitness before and after an exercise program. *J. Gerontol.* 35:383–387, 1980.

33. Emmerson, R. Y., R. E. Dustman, D. E. Shearer. P3 latency and symbol digit performance correlations in aging. *Exp. Aging Res.* 15:151–159, 1990.

34. Emery, C. F., and J. A. Blumenthal. Perceived changes among participants in an exercise program for older adults. *Gerontologist* 30:516–521, 1990.

35. Emery, C. F., and M. Gatz. Psychological and cognitive effects of an exercise program for community-residing older adults. *Gerontologist* 30:184–188, 1990.

36. Era, P., J. Kokela, and E. Heikkinen. Reaction and movement times in men of different ages. *Percept. Mot. Skills* 63:111–130, 1986.

37. Eysenck, M. W. *Cognitive Psychology: An International Review*. Chichester, England: John Wiley and Sons, 1990.

38. Floeter, M. K., and Greenough, W. T. Cerebellar plasticity: modification of Purkinje cell structure by differential rearing in monkeys. *Science* 206:227–229, 1979.

39. Gaches, J. Etudes statistique sur les traces "alpha largement developee" en function de l'age. *Presse Med.* 68:1620–1622, 1960.

40. Gibson, D., P. V. Karpovich, and P. D. Gollnick. *Effect of Training on Reflex and Reaction Time*. Research Report DA-49–007–MD–889, Office of the Surgeon General, 1961.

41. Haas, A., and H. A. Rusk. Respiratory function in hemiplegic patients. Paper presented at the American Congress of Rehabilitation Medicine, Philadelphia, PA, 1965.

42. Hasher, L., and R. T. Zacks. Automatic and effortful processes in memory. *J. Exp. Psychol. [Gen.]* 108:356–388, 1979.

43. Hasher, L. and R. T. Zacks. Working memory, comprehension, and aging: a review and a new view. *Psychol. Learn. Motiv.* 22:193–225, 1988.

44. Hawkins H, A. F. Kramer, and D. Capaldi. Aging, exercise, and attention. *Psychol. Aging* 7:643–653, 1992.

45. Hemsley, D. R., and D. V. Hawks. Speed of response and associative errors in schizophrenia. *Br. J. Soc. Clin. Psychol.* 13:293–303, 1974.

46. Hemsley, D. R., and H. C. Phillips. Models of mania: an individual case study. *Br. J. Psychiatry* 127:78–85, 1975.

47. Herrschaft, H., and U. Kunze. Correlation between the clinical picture of the EEG and cerebral blood flow after partial occlusion of the middle cerebral artery in man. *J. Neurol.* 215:191–201, 1977.

48. Hicks, L. H., and J. E. Birren. Aging, brain damage, and psychomotor slowing. *Psychol. Bull.* 74:377–396, 1970.

49. Horvath, T. B., and K. L. Davis. Central nervous system disorders in aging. E. L. Schneider and J. W. Rowe (eds). *Handbook of the Biology of Aging: Third Edition.* New York: Van Nostrand Rinehold, 1990, pp. 306–329.

50. Hultsch, D. F., M. Hammer, and B. J. Small. Age differences in cognitive performance in later life: relationships to self-reported health and activity lifestyle. *J. Gerontol.* 48:1–11, 1993.

51. Kahneman, D. *Attention and Effort.* Englewood Cliffs, NJ: Prentice Hall, 1973.

52. Kausler, D. H. Motivation, human aging, and cognitive performance. J. E. Birren and K. W. Schaie (eds). *The Handbook of Psychology and Aging: Third Edition.* San Diego: Academic Press, 1990, pp. 171–183.

53. Kennedy, R. S., W. P. Dunlap, L. E. Banderet, M. G. Smith, and C. S. Houston. Cognitive performance in a simulated climb of Mount Everest: Operation Everest II. *Aviat. Space Environ. Med.* 60:99–104, 1989.

54. Kety, S. S. Human cerebral blood flow and oxygen consumption as related to aging. *J. Chron. Dis.* 3:478, 1956.

55. Knapp, B. N. Simple reaction times of selected top-class sportsmen and research students. *Res. Q.* 32:409–411, 1961.

56. Light, K. E., and W. W. Spirduso. Effects of adult aging on the movement complexity factor of response programming. *J. Gerontol.* 45:107–109, 1989.

57. Madden, D. J., J. A. Blumenthal, P. A. Allen, and C. F. Emery. Improving aerobic capacity for healthy older adults does not necessarily lead to improved cognitive performance. *Psychol. Aging* 4:307–320, 1989.

58. McFarland, R. A. Experimental evidence of the relationship between aging and oxygen want: in search of a theory of aging. *Ergonomics* 6:339–366, 1963.

59. Meyer, J. S., K. M. A. Welch, J. L. Titus, et al. Neurotransmitter failure in cerebral infraction and dementia. R. D. Terry and S. Gershon (eds). *Neurobiology of Aging.* New York: Raven Press, 1976.

60. Milligan, W. L., D. A. Powell, C. Herley, and E. Furchtgott. A comparison of physical health and psychosocial variables as predictors of reaction time and serial learning performance in elderly men. *J. Gerontol.* 39:704–710, 1984.

61. Morgan, D. G., and P. C. May. Age-related changes in synaptic neurochemistry. E. L. Schneider and J. W. Rowe (eds). *Handbook of the Biology of Aging: Third Edition.* New York: Van Nostrand Rinehold, 1990, pp. 219–254.

62. Murrell, F. H. The effect of extensive practice on age differences in reaction time. *J. Gerontol.* 25:268–274, 1970.

63. Norwood, T. H., J. R. Smith, C. H. Stein. Aging at the cellular level: the human fibroblastlike cell model. E. L. Schneider and J. W. Rowe (eds). *Handbook of the Biology of Aging: Third Edition.* New York: Van Nostrand Rinehold, 1990, pp.131–156.

64. Offenbach, S. I., W. J. Chodzko-Zajko, and R. L. Ringel. The relationship between physiological status, cognition, and age in adult men. *Bull. Psychon. Soc.* 28:112–114, 1990.

65. Olsen, E. A. Relationship between psychological capacities and success in college athletics. *Res. Q.* 27:79–89, 1956.

66. Panton, L. B., J. E. Graves, M. L. Pollock, J. M. Hagberg, and W. Chen. Effect of aerobic resistance training on fractionated reaction time and speed of movement. *J. Gerontol.* 45:26–31, 1990.

67. Perlmutter, M., and L. Nyquist. Relationships between self-reported physical and mental health and intelligence performance across adulthood. *J. Gerontol* 45:145–155, 1990.

68. Posner, M. I., and C. R. R. Snyder. Attention and cognitive control. R. L. Solso (ed). *Information Processing and Cognition.* Hillsdale, N.J.: Lawrence Erlbaum, 1975, pp. 317–342.

69. Pysh, J. J., and G. M. Weiss. Exercise during development induces an increase in Purkinje cell dendritic tree size. *Science* 206:230–231, 1979.

70. Reitan, R. N. Intellectual and affective changes in essential hypertension. *Am. J. Psychiatry* 110:817–824, 1954.

71. Rikli, R., and S. Busch. Motor performance of women as a function of age and physical activity level. *J. Gerontol.* 41:645–649, 1986.
72. Ringel, R. L., and W. J. Chodzko-Zajko. Age, health and the speech process. H. K. Ulatowska (ed). *Aging and Communication.* New York: Thieme, 1988, pp. 95–107.
73. Rogers, J., and F. E. Blume. Neurotransmitter metabolism and function in the aging central nervous system. C. E. Finch, and E. L. Schneider (eds). *Handbook of the Biology of Aging: Second Edition.* New York: Van Nostrand Rinehold, 1985, pp. 645–691.
74. Rogers, R. L., J. S. Meyers, and K. F. Mortel. After reaching retirement age physical activity sustains cerebral perfusion and cognition. *J. Am. Geriat. Soc.* 38:123–128, 1990.
75. Salthouse, T. A. Effects of age and skill in typing. *J. Exp. Psychol. [Gen.]* 113:345–371, 1984.
76. Salthouse, T. A. Speed of behavior and its implications for cognition. J. E. Birren and K. W. Schaie (eds.) *Handbook of the Psychology of Aging.* New York: Van Nostrand Rinehold, 1985.
77. Salthouse, T. A. *Theoretical Perspectives on Cognitive Aging.* Hillsdale, N.J.: Lawrence Erlbaum, 1991.
78. Salthouse, T. A., D. H. Kausler, and J. S. Saults. Age, self-assessed health status, and cognition. *J. Gerontol.* 45:156–160, 1990.
79. Salthouse, T. A., and B. L. Somberg. Skilled performance: Effects of adult age and experience on elementary processes. *J. Exp. Psychol. [Gen.]* 111:176–207, 1982.
80. Sands, L. P., and W. Meredith. Blood pressure and intellectual functioning in late midlife. *J. Gerontol. [Psychol. Sci.]* 47:P81–P84, 1992.
81. Sapolsky, R. M. The adrenocortical axis. E. L. Schneider and J. W. Rowe (eds). *Handbook of the Biology of Aging: Third Edition.* New York: Van Nostrand Rinehold, 1990, pp. 330–348.
82. Schneider, W., and R. N. Shiffrin. Controlled and automatic information processing: I. Detection, search and attention. *Psychol. Rev.* 84:1–66, 1977.
83. Shay, K. A., and D. L. Roth. Association between aerobic fitness and visuospatial performance in healthy older adults. *Psychol. Aging.* 7:15–24, 1992.
84. Shiffrin, R. N., and W. Schneider. Controlled and automatic information processing: II. Perceptual learning, automatic attending and a general theory. *Psychol. Rev.* 84:127–190, 1977.
85. Sidney, K. H., and R. J. Shephard. Maximum and submaximum exercise tests in men and women in the seventh, eight, and ninth decades of life. *J. Appl. Physiol.* 43:280–287, 1977.
86. Sothmann, M. S., T. S. Horn, B. A. Hart, A. B. Gustafson. Comparison of discrete cardiovascular groups on plasma catecholamine and selected behavioral responses to psychological stress. *Psychophysiology* 24:47–54, 1987.
87. Spieth, W. Slowness of task performance and cardiovascular diseases. A. T. Welford, and J. E. Birren (eds). *Behavior, Aging, and the Nervous System.* Springfield, IL: Charles C. Thomas, 1965.
88. Spirduso, W. W. Reaction and movement time as a function of age and physical activity level. *J. Gerontol.* 30:435–440, 1975.
89. Spirduso, W. W. Physical fitness, aging, and psychomotor speed: a review. *J. Gerontol.* 35:850–865, 1980.
90. Spirduso, W. W. *Pysical Dimensions of Aging.* Champaign, IL: Human Kinetics, In Press.
91. Spriduso, W. W., and P. Clifford. Neuromuscular speed and consistency of performance as a function of age, physical activity level, and type of physical activity. *J. Gerontol.* 33:26–30, 1978.
92. Spirduso, W. W., and P. G. MacRae. Motor performance and aging. J. E. Birren and K. W. Schaie (eds). *The Handbook of Psychology and Aging: Third Edition.* San Diego: Academic Press, 1990, pp. 184–197.
93. Stelmach, G. E., N. L. Coggin, and A. Garcia-Colera. Movement specification time with age. *Exp. Aging Res.* 13:39–46, 1987.
94. Sternberg, S. Memory scanning: mental processes revealed by reaction time experiments. *Am. Sci.* 57:421–457, 1969.

95. Stones, M. J., and A. Kozma. Physical activity, age, and cognitive/motor performance. M. L. Howe, and C. J. Brainerd (eds). *Cognitive Development in Adulthood: Progress in Cognitive Development Research.* New York: Springer-Verlag, 1988, pp. 273–321.

96. Stones, M. J., and A. Kozma. Age, exercise and coding performance. *Psychol. Aging* 4:190–194, 1989.

97. Suominen-Troyer, S. S., K. J. Davis, A. H. Ismail, and G. Salvendy. Impact of physical fitness on strategy development in decision-making tasks. *Percept. Mot. Skills* 62:71–77, 1986.

98. Tomporowski, P. D., and N. R. Ellis. Effects of exercise on cognitive processes: a review. *Psychol. Bull.* 99:338–346, 1986.

99. Tweit, A. H., P. D. Gollnick, and G. R. Hurn. Effects of a training program on total body reaction time of individuals of low fitness. *Res. Q.* 34:508–513, 1963.

100. Vogt, C., and O. Vogt. Aging of nerve cells. *Nature* 58:304, 1956.

101. Weckowicz, T. E., R. W. Nutter, D. G. Cruise, and K. A. Yonge. Speed in test performance in relation to depressive illness and age. *J. Can. Psychiatr. Assoc.* 17:241–250, 1972.

102. Welford, A. T. Motor skills and aging. J. A. Mortimer, F. J. Pirozzolo, and G. J. Maletta (eds). *The Aging Motor System.* New York: Praeger, 1982.

103. Wilke, F. L., C. Eisdorfer, and J. B. Nowlin. Memory and blood pressure in the aged. *Exp. Aging Res.* 2:3–16, 1976.

104. Williams, H. G. Aging and eye-hand coordination. C. Bard, M Fluery, and L. Hay (eds). *Development of Eye-Hand Coordination Across the Lifespan.* Columbia, SC: University of South Carolina Press, 1990, pp. 327–357.

105. Youngen, L. A. A comparison of reaction and movement times of women athletes and nonathletes. *Res. Q.* 30:349–355, 1959.

8
Thermoregulatory Thermogenesis in Humans during Cold Stress

IRA JACOBS, Dr. Med. Sc.
LUCIE MARTINEAU, Ph.D.
ANDRÉ L. VALLERAND, Ph.D.

Given that a large proportion of our country's geography lies at latitudes where cold exposure is a fact of life, strategies for survival and/or rescue of victims exposed to potentially lethal intensities or durations of cold exposure concern us. There should be no debate that the best way to ensure survival is to insulate the human from cold; clothing/textile sciences have developed such technology to a high degree. There are emergencies, however, when such insulation is not available or eventually becomes ineffective. The battle for survival then becomes one between the physiological ability to generate heat and the rate at which heat is lost to the environment. In such situations, like cold water immersion or more prolonged cold air exposure, the extent of our physiological ability to insulate body heat (i.e., vasoconstriction) is rapidly exploited. The only remaining key to avoiding or delaying hypothermia thus depends on increasing heat production.

For those wondering why a review about physiological responses to cold is presented in this book, which is primarily concerned with physical exertion, we presume that it is because of our focus on skeletal muscle energy metabolism. The same tissue that is responsible for bone movement and force generation also "shivers" when humans are cold. This shivering by skeletal muscle is by far the predominant source, in humans, of the heat production with which our body attempts to offset its heat loss to the cold environment and thereby maintain stable and warm internal temperatures.

Our interest in related research was initially stimulated a decade ago when pondering the feasibility of delaying hypothermia by stimulating metabolic heat production with exogenous stimuli. After an initial literature review, we realized that there was a significant body of literature concerned with the biophysics of human heat loss/gain, but very little empirical evidence describing the substrates used to fuel shivering in humans and the effects of manipulating substrate availability on human temperature regulation during cold exposure. We therefore thought it crucial to carry out fundamental studies of energy metabolism in cold-stressed humans, to have sufficient information available to subsequently propose potential strategies for increasing metabolic heat production.

Our initial studies were concerned with documenting the change in rates of specific macronutrient oxidation that fuel the increase in resting metabolic rate elicited by shivering, which we will refer to as thermoregulatory thermogenesis (TT). More recently, we have investigated the potential to elicit "supramaximal" increases in shivering thermogenesis via administration of exogenous stimuli. This review is limited to describing these and related studies. The reader is referred to other excellent reviews for other aspects of human physiological responses to cold stress [16, 17, 24, 50, 66, 106, 130].

COMPONENTS AND MECHANISMS OF THERMOGENESIS

Components of Daily Thermogenesis

Before reviewing various components and mechanisms of TT, it is important to clarify the four components of daily energy expenditure or metabolic rate (M) [102]. Resting metabolic rate (RMR), about 70% of the daily expenditure (Table 8.1), represents the energy expended in a resting postabsorptive state and in comfortable ambient conditions. Exercise-induced thermogenesis (EIT) is the additional energy expenditure associated with spontaneous physical activity in free-living conditions, reflecting the energy costs of weight-bearing activities such as standing, walking, and exercising. At about 20% of the daily M, EIT plays a smaller but still important role in the overall energy balance. EIT could be as high as about 2000 kcal (8368 kJ) in marathoners [41]. The thermic effect of food (TEF; also known as diet-induced thermogenesis) is related to food energy intake and the proportion of energy derived from carbohydrates, fats, and proteins. TEF can increase daily heat production by about 10% in subjects fed a regular mixed diet [57, 58, 102]. TEF consists of two components, obligatory and facultative thermogeneses. Obligatory thermogenesis (formerly known as the specific dynamic action of foods) is related to the absorption, breakdown, and storing of ingested nutrients, whereas facultative thermogenesis is related to the activation of the sympathetic nervous system [57, 58, 102]. The remaining component of M is TT.

In the absence of thermal stress, TT is virtually 0% of the daily M. During cold stress, however, total M rises, and TT can account for a significant fraction of the daily energy expenditure. Table 8.1 exemplifies these changes. Assume the total daily M at thermal neutrality is 2500 kcal (10,460 kJ; Table 8.1); thus RMR amounts to 1750 kcal (7,322 kJ or ≈ 0.250 liter·min^{-1} $\dot{V}O_2$). If we assume that an individual is sedentary but continuously cold-stressed, energy expenditure increases to 2.5 times RMR [109,114] or 4375 kcal (2.5×1750 kcal= 4375 kcal or 18,305 kJ), and TT, or the cold-induced thermogenesis, is equal to that amount less RMR, or 2625

TABLE 8.1
Components of Thermogenesis (M)

Components	% of Daily M at Thermal Neutrality	% of Daily M in Cold
Resting metabolic rate (RMR)	≈70% (1750 kcal)	≈34% (1750 kcal)
Thermic effect of food (TEF)		
Obligatory M		
Facultative M		
	≈10% (250)	≈ 5% (250)
Exercise-induced M	≈20% (500)	≈10% (500)
Thermoregulatory M		
Shivering M		
Nonshivering M		
	≈ 0%	≈51% (2625)
	100% (or 2500 kcal)	100% (or 5125 kcal)

kcal (4375–1750= 2625 kcal or 10,983 kJ). Since TEF and EIT could well be the same in the cold as in thermal neutrality, total M in the cold is now 5125 kcal (21,443 kJ) and TT can account for ≈50% of the daily M in the cold. The intent of this example is simply to show that TT is not a negligible component of M in the cold, when extrapolated to 24 hr such as in survival conditions.

Mechanisms of Thermoregulatory Thermogenesis: Shivering

Thermoregulatory thermogenesis can be subdivided into shivering and nonshivering components [3]. As discussed earlier, there is a close relationship between $\dot{V}O_2$ and shivering activity. In some species, such as sheep, cold exposure increases M sevenfold, almost entirely by shivering [10]. In cold-exposed cattle where M was increased by 40%, hindlimb $\dot{V}O_2$ increased by 400% [8]. Some previous reviews suggested that in humans all thermoregulatory thermogenesis is derived from muscular contractions [37, 98]. Shivering is a form of involuntary rhythmic contractions of skeletal muscle, where no useful work is performed. Shivering is activated by acetylcholine and involves cellular processes similar to those occurring in other forms of muscle contraction [50, 51]. The conversion of chemical energy to mechanical work, including shivering, is inefficient and results in the release of about 75% of the energy as heat [86].

Previous reviews of shivering (e.g., [44, 98]) have not included information about the relative intensity with which skeletal muscle shivers. By simultaneously monitoring the surface electromyographical activity (EMG) of several muscle groups during cold exposure, we know that shivering occurs after less than five minutes of cold exposure in nonobese individuals and that the intensity of shivering increases over time [104]. Muscles of the trunk region typically begin to shiver sooner, and at a higher intensity, than those of the limbs [9, 104]. To estimate the intensity of muscle contraction during shivering, the EMG has been expressed relative to the EMG and external forces generated during maximal and submaximal contractions of the same muscles prior to cold exposure [9]. Based on the regression of force: EMG, the calculated intensity of muscle contraction during maximal levels of shivering is low, ranging up to 15–20% of a maximum voluntary contraction [9]. The fact that so many muscle groups are recruited during shivering, albeit at low intensities, results in increases in energy demand to fuel this muscular activity. As a result, metabolic rate typically increases by up to five times normal resting rates during shivering [38].

Mechanisms of Thermoregulatory Thermogenesis: Nonshivering
Heat is a by-product of most metabolic processes, not only muscle fiber contraction. For example, TEF was described above as a component of daily M, where heat is indeed produced without muscular contraction [57, 58, 102]. In the cold, TT in humans can still increase, even when shivering is inhibited by curare [56]. Mechanisms for TT, unrelated to shivering, could include ion pumping (e.g., sodium/potassium pumps [45]), and futile metabolic cycles [120] like the glucose cycle (glucose↔glucose-6-phosphate), the fructose-6-phosphate cycle (fructose-6-phosphate↔fructose 1,6-diphosphate), and the triglyceride–fatty acid cycle (lipolysis↔lipogenesis [29]). Futile metabolic cycles allow the energy stored in food reserves to be simply converted to heat in various tissues [120]. For example, it has been suggested that the fructose-6-phosphate cycle serves to prewarm flight muscles in insects [80]. There is a high concentration of sodium/potassium pumps in human skeletal muscle and it was estimated that 4–20% of the RMR can be attributed to sodium/potassium transport [19, 31]. If mechanisms unrelated to shivering have a significant effect on TT in humans, and in which tissues, are questions that have not yet been clarified.

A thermogenic tissue that may have been overlooked in the cold is the vascular smooth muscle. It has been suggested that the norepinephrine-induced increase in thermogenesis in resting skeletal muscle can be partly explained by vasoconstriction in the perfused hindlimb [18, 30]. Since norepinephrine, vasopressin, and angiotensin II each stimulate vasoconstriction and VO_2 and since both of these responses are blocked by vasodilators, it was suggested that the vascular system plays a key role in the regulation of resting muscle thermogenesis. This raises the possibility that part of the O_2 consumed is due to work performed by cells contributing to vasoconstriction [18, 20]. This concept becomes even more relevant in the cold, since it has been shown that the sensitivity to norepinephrine of the arterial bed of the hypothermic pig increases tenfold, compared with euthermia, strongly suggesting a greater role for the vascular system heat production in the cold [15, 96]. Research is required to determine the importance of vascular smooth muscle thermogenesis in cold-exposed humans.

Brown adipose tissue (BAT) is another interesting thermogenic tissue. BAT is a highly thermogenic tissue that produces heat because its mitochondria can become loosely coupled so that substrates can be oxidized at a rate not controlled by ATPases. Therefore, in the uncoupled state, BAT mainly produces heat at a high rate that is out of proportion to ATP yield (for review see [51]). This is due to the existence in BAT of a unique high-conductance proton pathway and an uncoupling protein. Currently, there is debate, not about whether BAT is present in humans [63, 64, 97, 99], but whether BAT has a role at all in daily human thermogenesis. Some authors think its contribution to energy expenditure is negligible, whereas others have suggested that because of its high oxidative capacity, a small quantity of BAT that is not readily detected in a larger mass of white adipose tissue could have a noticeable impact on energy expenditure, possibly in the range of about 10% of the daily energy turnover [99, 100]. Noting that only 40% of the epinephrine-induced increase in whole body heat production was taking place in skeletal muscle, it was suggested that adipose tissue could contribute to this facultative thermogenesis [97].

Although the liver is responsible for about 40% of RMR [8], its increase in VO_2 during cold exposure is rather small. Furthermore, during severe cold stress liver VO_2 is not increased but reduced due to reductions in blood flow [3]. The importance of the liver during cold exposure does not seem to lie as a heat source, but rather in converting extra nutrients to a form suitable for utilization by peripheral heat-generating tissues [103].

This section has described some of the components of energy expenditure that are responsible for the increased TT during cold exposure. Quantification of the specific energy substrates that fuel TT in humans remains, however, rather obscure. This topic is the focus of the next section.

SUBSTRATE SOURCES FOR THERMOREGULATORY THERMOGENESIS

The direct relationship between shivering and the increases in oxygen consumption and heat production is well established [16], but less effort has been expended on elucidating the proportion of the increased TT in humans that is due to the oxidation of specific macronutrient substrates (i.e., carbohydrate, fat, protein). We therefore conducted a study to determine the oxidation rates of these substrates during acute cold exposure [109]. Male fasting subjects rested in air for 2 hr at 29°C on one occasion and at 10°C on another occasion. Substrate utilization was calculated using indirect calorimetry and the nonprotein respiratory exchange ratio, which was derived from the respiratory exchange ratio and the urinary urea nitrogen output. Cold exposure increased the 2-hr energy expenditure 2.5-fold, compared with the warm; the rates of carbohydrate and lipid oxidation were significantly increased to 5.9 and 1.6 times, respectively, the rates observed in the warm. No significant cold-induced change in protein oxidation was calculated. This study [109] demonstrated that in contrast with the warm air exposure, where lipid oxidation accounted for the greater relative contribution to total energy expenditure (59% vs. 18% for lipid and carbohydrate, respectively), shivering increased carbohydrate oxidation so that it accounted for 51% of total energy expenditure, while the relative contribution of lipid oxidation was reduced to 39% of total energy expenditure.

Figure 8.1 shows that shivering during cold water immersion also increases lipid and carbohydrate oxidation rates by factors similar to those reported above for cold air, so that 50% of metabolic heat produced during cold water immersion is due to carbohydrate oxidation [71, 72].

Circulating Substrates

These studies showed that both carbohydrates and lipids fuel the energy demand for shivering, but they do not identify the form or source of substrate that is oxidized, e.g., circulating vs. intramuscular stores for carbohydrates, or free fatty acids (FFA) vs. triglycerides for lipid, etc. Experiments with rats and dogs showed that cold stress increased glucose turnover, glucose tolerance, glucose uptake, and oxidation in animals [22,

FIGURE 8.1

Oxidation rate of carbohydrate and lipids during cold water immersion at 18°C. Data are expressed as means ± SE (n = 11) and were calculated from the average $\dot{V}O_2$ and RER during each 15-min period. † Significantly different from previous 15-min value (P<0.05).

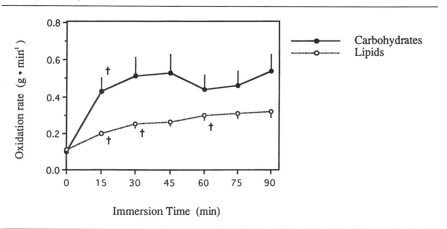

76, 115]. Other studies showed that lipolysis, lipid oxidation, and free fatty acid turnover were also increased during cold exposure in animals [47, 83, 87, 89, 103]. There was also evidence that shivering thermogenesis in cold-exposed animals is a glycogenolytic process; cold-induced increases in heat production were accompanied by intramuscular glycogen utilization in hypothermic birds [33, 82], mammals [39, 77], and rodents [62, 67]. Minaire et al. [77] estimated from isotopic tracer techniques that muscle glycogen provided about 15% of the overall energy supply in cold-exposed dogs. Results of studies with mice and pigeons [67, 82] suggested that intramuscular glycogen per se was a limiting factor for survival during hypothermic stress.

Reports about the net changes in blood metabolite and hormone concentrations after cold exposure indicated that FFA, glycerol, and catecholamine concentrations were increased and glucose concentration was decreased (e.g.,[43, 52, 94]). The potential implications of changes in blood substrates on body temperature regulation in humans were attested to by studies associating hypothermia and hypoglycemia [35, 60, 78]. Molnar and Read [78] reported that hypoglycemia was associated with more rapid decreases in rectal temperature in cold-water immersed subjects. Very recently the glucose clamp technique was used in humans immersed in cold water and demonstrated that TT was reduced and cooling was more rapid when glucose concentration was clamped at hypoglycemic concentrations (Mekjavic, I., personal communication, May 1993).

Vallerand et al. [108] administered a standard intravenous glucose tolerance test to subjects resting for 3 hours in cold air (10°C) and on another occasion at 29°C. This was the first study to document that cold air exposure significantly increases the rate of glucose uptake from the circulation. This same study also showed that this more rapid rate of disappearance of glucose from the circulation occurs with a lower blood insulin concentration. This finding may not necessarily be due to a cold-specific effect, since insulin sensitivity of muscle is increased by any acute exercise [53, 132], not only shivering [115].

To similarly address lipid metabolism, we carried out a study in which an intravenous fat tolerance test (IVFTT) was administered to cold-stressed subjects [110]. The purpose of this study was to determine if plasma triglycerides provided fatty acids for oxidation during prolonged cold air exposure. The IVFTT was administered to male subjects after they had been resting for two hours, at 29°C on one day and 10°C on another day. The IVFTT consisted of the rapid infusion (within 90 sec) of 1 ml·kg^{-1} of exogenous triglycerides in the form of 10% Intralipid. Blood samples were taken before and repeatedly for another 40 min while the subject remained resting at the specific temperature. Although cold exposure increased lipid oxidation rates by 70%, fat tolerance was not affected. These results were interpreted as indicating that white adipose and possibly intramuscular triglycerides, but not plasma triglycerides, are the preferred sources of fatty acids for oxidation in cold-stressed humans [110].

In another series of experiments, the circulating FFA of immersed subjects was manipulated by having the subjects ingest nicotinic acid in the form of niacin pills prior to and during the water immersion [72, 73]. The effect of the nicotinic acid is to block lipolysis, and this effect was demonstrated by the observation that the plasma FFA and glycerol concentrations were dramatically reduced prior to, and during, the water immersion. M was virtually unaffected; the proportion of the total heat production that could be attributed to fat oxidation was significantly reduced, but there was compensation by simply increasing carbohydrate oxidation.

Muscle Glycogen Utilization

Our investigations show that in resting subjects, exposed to either cold air or cold water, carbohydrates and fat contribute approximately equally to heat production [71, 109]. From a strategic point of view, this finding seems unfortunate because the body's availability of carbohydrates is quite limited compared with the abundant fat and protein stores. We were already aware of the well-established positive relationship between muscle glycogen concentration and endurance exercise performance of skeletal muscle [11]. We therefore speculated that there may be a similar detrimental effect caused by depleted muscle glycogen stores on another form of muscle contraction, i.e., shivering and the associated TT. The first question was whether muscle glycogen is one of the stores from which glucose is derived for oxidation during shivering. We therefore carried out a descriptive study that demonstrated that skeletal muscle glycogen concentration is decreased during cold water immersion in both a lower body muscle, the vastus lateralis [70], and in an upper body muscle, the deltoid [69]. Twenty-one subjects were immersed in stirred 18°C water for 66±7 (SD) min, and biopsies were obtained from the thigh musculature before and after immersion. The average increase in metabolic rate was 3.5 times resting values, and each of the subjects had lower glycogen concentrations after the immersion (Fig. 8.2). Analyses were performed on whole muscle homogenates as well as on specific muscle fiber types. Glycogen depletion occurred to a similar degree in both fast-twitch and slow-twitch muscle fiber types (Fig. 8.3). The relatively small degree of glycogen depletion that was observed, however, was similar to that reported for rats [62] and suggests that intramuscular glycogen is unlikely to be completely depleted before hypothermia occurs, thus glycogen is probably not as critical for humans as it is for mice [67] and pigeons [82]. The rate of glycogen utilization during shivering, however, was much greater than would be expected from physical exercise of a similar duration and causing a similar increase in metabolic rate [74, 92]. Experiments with cold-exposed dogs [68] showed that cold exposure causes greater sympathoad-

FIGURE 8.2

*Individual and mean values (n = 21) for muscle glycogen levels before and after water immersion at 18°C. *Significantly different from preimmersion value (P<0.01). From Martineau and Jacobs (70).*

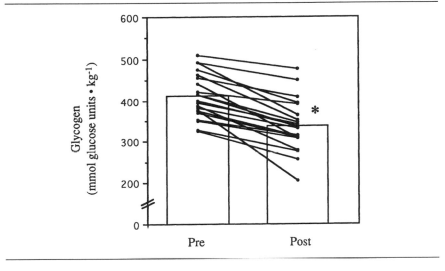

renal system activity than is observed in dogs exercising at the same metabolic rate. Thus, the relatively high rate of glycogen depletion for the measured metabolic rates in our water immersion studies is probably explained by the large increases in catecholamine secretion (slight increase for epinephrine, but >10–fold increases for norepinephrine) typically observed with cold water immersion in humans [52, 69, 73].

In all of our related studies, our subjects invariably show a decrease in glycogen concentration after cold water immersion [70–73]. The reader is referred, however, to the only other published study that documents human muscle glycogen concentration changes after cold water immersion [131]; the results of that study contrast with our own. Young et al. [131] reported that glycogen concentration did not change in their subjects, who were also immersed in 18°C water, for up to three hours. It is difficult to explain this discrepancy, although we suspect that at least part of the reason is that our subjects were leaner (11% vs. 17% of body mass as fat). We suspect this because of the inverse relationship in our water immersion studies between body fat content and the rate of glycogen utilization [69]. Moreover, leaner individuals are known to have greater increases in metabolic rate than an individual of higher body fat content for the same cold stress [59, 130] and for the same change in mean skin temperature [104]. Our own observations would also suggest that the greater the cold stress is, the greater is the proportion of energy derived from carbohydrate oxidation during shivering. This is exemplified in Figure 8.4, which shows

FIGURE 8.3

Frequency distribution of the optical density of periodic acid–Schiff stain of slow-twitch (ST) and fast-twitch (FT) muscle fibers before and after cold water immersion at 18°C in seminude subjects (n = 13). The frequency is expressed as a relative cumulative frequency. There is a direct relationship between optical density of the stain in a fiber and its muscle glycogen concentration. The graph shows that there is a slightly greater frequency of ST fibers with lower optical densities after immersion, and no difference for the FT fibers. The difference between fiber types in this regard is not considered significant.

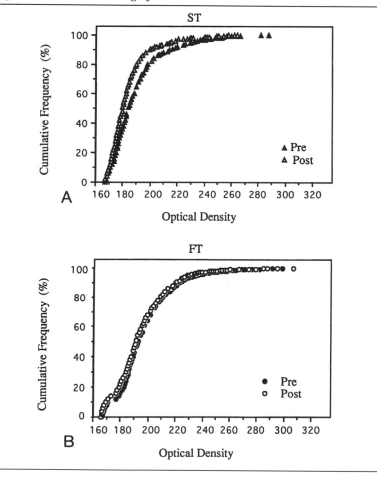

that a greater proportion of heat production during water immersion was derived from carbohydrate oxidation than from lipid oxidation in subjects who were leaner and therefore were only immersed for about 40 min before their rectal temperature reached 35.5°C; in the other subjects, who were all immersed for 90 min without reaching the rectal temperature

FIGURE 8.4

Total heat production (mean ± SE) during immersion in a group who were only immersed for an average of 42 min (IT42) before their rectal temperatures reached 35.5°C, and another group (IT90) who were immersed for 90 min with rectal temperature remaining above 35°C. Heat production was calculated from the RER and V̇O₂ values. The calculated percentage contribution of fat (lower part of the bar) and carbohydrate (upper part of the bar) to the total heat production is also shown. LBM is lean body mass. *Significant within group difference (P<0.05). †Significantly different from previous 30–min period mean value (P<0.001).

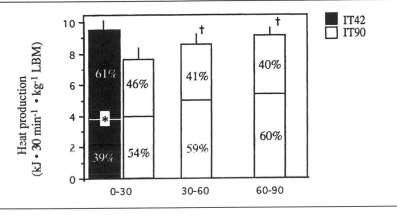

criterion for halting the experiment, there was no difference between the amount of heat derived from carbohydrate or lipid oxidation.

Glycogen and Exercise in the Cold

The rate of oxygen consumption is increased during light exercise in the cold, compared with the same exercise performed at a comfortable ambient temperature. This additional cost has been attributed to the increased metabolic demand of shivering [16, 26, 50]. We speculated that the increased substrate utilization required to fuel the cumulative effect of both shivering and exercise on oxygen uptake in the cold would include muscle glycogen. A study was therefore carried out to test the hypothesis that more glycogen would be depleted during light exercise in the cold [54]. Male subjects were divided into light- and moderate-intensity exercise groups, matched for aerobic fitness. Both groups exercised on a cycle ergometer in cold air, in a balanced order fashion, for 30 min at 9°C on one day and at 21°C on another day. They lay quietly for 30 min at the temperature prior to beginning exercise. The light-intensity group exercised at 55 W and a V̇O₂ of about 1 liter·min⁻¹; the moderate intensity group exercised at 103 W and a V̇O₂ of about 1.7 liter·min⁻¹. Figure 8.5 supports our hypothesis, because in the light-intensity group significantly more glycogen was utilized at 9°C than at 21°C. In the moderate-intensity group

FIGURE 8.5

*Change in thigh muscle glycogen concentration after 30 min of light- or moderate-intensity exercise at 21°C and 9°C. The change was greater in the cold, but only for the light-intensity exercise. *Significant difference (P<0.05) between cold and warm trials.*

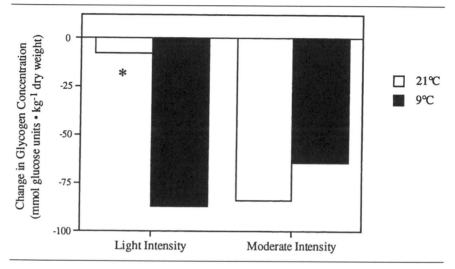

there was no difference between trials, and this is consistent with the abolition of shivering with increasing exercise intensity as the heat produced by exercise replaces the heat generated by shivering [49, 87, 101]. The implications of these findings are perhaps more meaningful when these findings are put into the context of the well-established relationship between muscle glycogen concentration and endurance exercise performance [11]. Our results suggest that a critically low glycogen concentration is probably reached significantly more rapidly in an exercising muscle if the individual is being cooled during exercise or has been shivering or cooled prior to commencing exercise.

Glycogen Availability and Thermogenesis

As discussed earlier, some animal studies suggested that muscle glycogen stores may limit cold tolerance and that elevated muscle glycogen stores may increase cold tolerance in mice and pigeons [67, 81, 82]. Having determined that intramuscular glycogen is one of the carbohydrate stores used to fuel shivering in humans, experiments were conducted to clarify whether alterations of muscle glycogen availability would affect temperature regulation [71]. Subjects were immersed in 18°C water on three occasions, in each case after well-established dietary and exercise procedures were used to elicit either low, normal, or high glycogen levels in large skeletal muscle groups. The $\dot{V}O_2$ increased progressively and similarly during the water immersion to 3.7 times preimmersion rates, equivalent to an energy expenditure of about 28 % of these subjects' $\dot{V}O_2$max on a cycle ergometer. The respiratory exchange ratio, as expected, was significantly lower during the low-glycogen trial, and this caused the calculated M to be significantly lower for this trial, compared with the other two trials (Fig. 8.6). This effect was also associated with a significantly more rapid rate of decrease of rectal temperature (Fig. 8.6) during the low-glycogen trial, compared with the other two trials. Thus the reduced availability of muscle glycogen was associated with a more rapid body cooling rate in humans. There was a significant amount of glycogen remaining in the muscle tissue at the end of the immersion in the low-glycogen condition, contrasting with the near total glycogen exhaustion observed in cold-stressed animals [67, 82]. "It is therefore probable that metabolic heat production is limited in association with, rather than because of, reduced glycogen availability" [71].

Higher than normal glycogen levels did not change the thermoregulatory response to cold water immersion [71]. Although the high glycogen levels did not cause increased TT, nor did they slow the rate of cooling, beginning the immersion with such high glycogen concentrations would probably mean that more time would be required before a "critically" low glycogen concentration is reached which might impair TT. Such is the case with mice [67]. Energy expenditure in cold-stressed small rodents can reach 80% of their exercise $\dot{V}O_2$max [21], whereas in humans we rarely see shivering metabolic rates in excess of 40% $\dot{V}O_2$max. As is the case with physical exercise, the relative intensity of energy expenditure elicited by cold stress probably determines whether or not increases in muscle glycogen availability will be beneficial to cold resistance.

Preferred Fuel

For reasons that are still unclear, carbohydrates seem to be a somewhat preferred substrate during shivering thermogenesis. There are similarities to hard physical exertion in that the musculature is not able to maintain the same intensity of exertion when carbohydrate stores are depleted, i.e., a shift to a greater reliance on fat oxidation to fuel muscle contraction is not sufficient for the musculature to be able to maintain a high level of exertion, just as core temperature could not be maintained as well when carbohydrate stores were depleted [71].

BIOCHEMICAL ENHANCEMENT OF THERMOREGULATORY THERMOGENESIS

Besides the new knowledge yielded by the studies described above about the influence of cold on energy metabolism, substrate utilization, and mechanisms and sites of TT, there are also practical applications of this work. One such application is to use this knowledge to enhance M in the

FIGURE 8.6

A. *Changes in rectal temperature (T_{re}) during cold water immersion at 18°C in subjects with low, normal, or high glycogen levels in large muscle groups. Data are expressed as means ±SE (n= 6). †Significantly different from mean value of normal condition. ‡Significantly different from mean value of high condition. The arrows indicate the first value significantly different from preimmersion value. From Martineau (69).*

B. *Total heat production (mean ± SE) during the first 30 min of immersion in eight seminude subjects with low, normal, or high glycogen levels in large muscle groups. The calculated percentage contribution of fat (lower part of the bar) and carbohydrate (upper part of the bar) to the total heat production is also shown. †, ‡Significantly different from mean value of normal and high conditions, respectively. §Significant within trial difference between carbohydate and fat (P<0.05).*

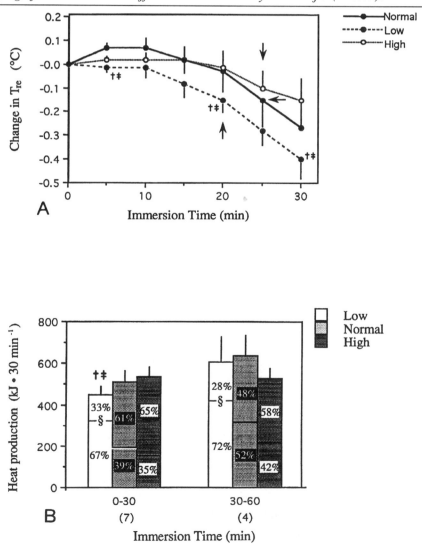

cold, thereby reducing the body's heat debt and generating warmer body temperatures, and thus improving cold tolerance. This *hypermetabolic* approach contrasts with the *hypometabolic* response that is also sometimes observed in cold-adapted humans, where heat production and heat losses are both reduced in an effort to conserve energy [12, 88, 130]. It is important to clarify this concept, which is summarized in the heat balance equation described below. The heat balance equation summarizes whole body heat exchanges by incorporating heat production (or heat gains) and all heat losses (all terms in $W \cdot m^{-2}$; [105, 119]):

$$\dot{S}=\dot{M}-(R+\dot{C})-\dot{E}_{persp}-\dot{C}_{resp}-\dot{E}_{resp}$$

where M is the metabolic rate, R+C is the rate of dry heat exchange, E_{persp} is the evaporative heat loss rate from the skin, C_{resp} and E_{resp} are the rates of convective and evaporative heat loss by the respiratory tract, and S is the rate of heat debt (determined as the balance of heat gains and heat losses). A negative S ($W \cdot m^{-2}$) signifies a negative heat storage or a positive heat debt.

Integrated over time, S (converted to kJ or kcal) will eventually correspond to a drop in core temperature (T_c). Both S and the change in T_c have been used as indices of cold tolerance or resistance, although S is inherently more robust, since it is based on more parameters than just T_c alone. Therefore, heat balance is much more informative than a simple profile of the time-course of changes in T_c, which has sometimes been shown to vary out of proportion to the heat debt [116, 117]. A graphic example of the problem inherent in using T_c as an index of cold tolerance is that some hypothermia victims have been found conversant and others comatose at the same T_c of 32°C [25].

Because of our high capacity for heat loss and poor resistance to cold, it is not surprising that numerous experiments have attempted to enhance man's tolerance to cold. Various diets, different exercise regimens, repeated exposures to cold air or cold water [88, 105, 101, 130], as well as the administration of various hormones and pharmacological agents have all been used [107, 111, 114]. The use of a pharmacological approach with thermogenic agents is attractive, primarily because of the potential for effecting an acute and rapid response.

Animal Studies
During the study of endocrine responses to the cold, it was discovered that the administration of several hormones (for various periods of time) could markedly delay the onset of hypothermia. Such hormones include catecholamines, thyroxine, the combination of thyroxine and cortisol, and growth hormone (for review see [66, 95]). Although very useful for our understanding of cold-induced thermogenesis, these hormones have little direct application to our needs because of health risks and/or the duration

of treatment required to cause an increase in M. There are, however, a wide variety of pharmacological agents that are effective in delaying the onset of hypothermia in animals.

Dinitrophenol is an extremely potent thermogenic agent because of its uncoupling effect on oxidative phosphorylation [42]. Unfortunately, this uncoupling effect is generalized to virtually all tissues. The thermogenic effect of dinitrophenol is further enhanced in the presence of thyroxine [34], but an application to humans is not apparent for the reasons described in the preceding paragraph.

Caffeine, the most well known methylxanthine, is an established thermogenic agent at comfortable ambient temperatures [1, 65]. When administered in the cold, it significantly reduced the drop in T_{re} in animals and delayed the onset of hypothermia [32, 36]. Another effective xanthine is theophylline. During the last decade, Wang has repeatedly shown that a significantly warmer T_{re} is associated with the thermogenic effect of an acute administration of theophylline in rats [122–124]. Other potent agents in the cold include amphetamines, CNS stimulants [129], which, with or without epinephrine [85], markedly increase M and produce significantly warmer T_{re} in the cold, compared with a placebo. It certainly appears as though sympathomimetics and methylxanthines are two classes of pharmacological agents that are likely to be beneficial in cold-exposed humans.

Human Studies

As early as 1942, Scheurer reported that the ingestion of caffeine by men exposed to a cool ambient temperature reduced the decrease in mean skin temperature ($\overline{T}_{sk}$) [93]. Similarly, LeBlanc [65] found that caffeine ingestion before retiring for the night in a cool environment, significantly increased $\dot{V}O_2$ and provided a warmer $\overline{T}_{sk}$, but did not influence T_{re}. Others reported that caffeine ingestion tends to exaggerate the drop in $\overline{T}_{sk}$ in cold air [40, 75] or that it caused a significant increase in M in cold water [26]; but in these cases there was no measurable effect on T_{re}. One postimmersion rewarming study found that caffeine ingestion could significantly attenuate the T_{re} afterdrop, a phenomenon that was associated with slight increases in norepinephrine, epinephrine, and heart rate; VO_2 was not reported [2].

Following up on his animal work, Wang et al. reported that the drop in T_{re} in cold-exposed individuals can be reduced with the prior ingestion of theophylline with/without energy substrates. This was demonstrated in acute cold air studies performed either at rest or during intermittent exercise [125–127]. It was suggested that, as in animals, the effectiveness of theophylline in enhancing cold tolerance, as defined by the drop in T_{re}, was due to an increased energy substrate mobilization, a factor thought to be limiting for TT and thus cold tolerance [121–123, 125]. The corresponding metabolic data in humans are, however, not convincing. The marked improvements in T_{re} attributed to the theophylline treatments were not accompanied by any significant changes in M [125–127]. In our own investigation, RMR was significantly increased by 21% prior to a cold water immersion (15°C) after a combined theophylline and acute feeding treatment, compared with the feeding treatment alone; this effect did not persist during the water immersion [55]. It was decided to reinvestigate the concept linking energy substrate mobilization, TT, and cold tolerance, since it is important to the understanding of energy metabolism in the cold and the potential for biochemical enhancement of cold tolerance.

Can Energy Substrate Mobilization Alter Cold-induced Thermogenesis?
After proper familiarization to ensure good reproducibility of thermal and metabolic responses between cold tests [110], we exposed fasting seminude (jogging shorts only) subjects to 5°C (wind of 1 m·sec^{-1}) for three hours on three occasions at weekly intervals: following the ingestion of either a noncaloric placebo, pure carbohydrates (CHO) containing 340 kcal (1422 kJ), or a 340 kcal commercially available chocolate bar (Cold Buster) purported to improve cold tolerance [119]. Results showed that there were no differences across all three trials with respect to T_{re}, T_{sk}, M, and the heat debt (minute by minute mathematical balance of heat production minus all heat losses) (Fig. 8.7; [119]). Further, ingesting either the isocaloric pure CHO or the chocolate bar did increase CHO oxidation, as expected, but entirely at the expense of lipid oxidation, with no change in M [119]. In light of results of other related studies [126], we were surprised by the lack of effect on M. We therefore retested the energy mobilization theory in another study performed at a somewhat milder temperature (10°C) with different subjects; identical results were obtained [118].

Our studies were initially done on subjects resting in the cold. In these studies M rose to about 2.5–3.5 times resting M [118, 119]. Wang et al. suggested in some studies [126, 127] but not all [125], that a higher M, such as that seen during intermittent exercise, is required to fully exploit the energy-mobilizing effect of ingesting substrates and/or xanthines on cold thermogenesis and cold tolerance. We therefore carried out another study in which M was raised by about 3.4 times and by as much as 6.7 times resting values during an intermittent rest/exercise protocol, similar to the protocol of Wang et al. [126, 127]. The ingestion of a food supplement containing energy substrates and theobromine had no influence on M, T_{re}, T_{sk}, and heat debt [112]. As reported above, the food supplement increased CHO oxidation, but this was offset by a decreased rate of lipid oxidation [112].

We questioned whether the dose of substrates we employed was too small to influence substrate mobilization and M. In trials where beneficial effects on cold tolerance were reported, only about 300 kcal (1255 kJ) were administered [125–127]. We recently completed a study in which subjects ingested as much as 710 kcal (2970 kJ) in an effort to maximize substrate

FIGURE 8.7

*Influence of ingestion of pure carbohydrate (100% CHO) or chocolate bar (Cold Buster) on T_{re} profile (**A**) and heat debt (**B**) during 3-hr exposure at rest to 5°C, 1 m·sec⁻¹ wind. Data are mean ± SE.*

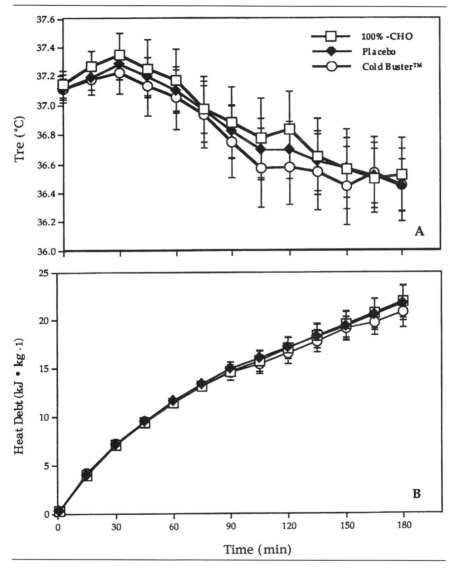

mobilization in the cold [113]. This energy content had no beneficial effect on any measured thermal physiology parameters, even though it did increase CHO *mobilization* and oxidation at the expense of lipid *mobilization* and oxidation. Energy substrate *utilization* is crucial to fuel M in the cold [111], but our data do not support the contention that M is limited by insufficient energy substrate *mobilization* in humans, and we suggest that other factors are required to enhance thermoregulatory thermogenesis, which in turn could reduce the heat debt and thus ameliorate cold resistance. Relevant experiments with sympathomimetics are described in the next section.

Ephedrine/Xanthines Mixtures in the Cold
Recent studies have firmly established that certain β–adrenergic agonists, such as ephedrine (E), and xanthines (X), such as caffeine (C) and theophylline (T), significantly increase resting M in humans exposed to comfortable ambient temperatures, either on a short- or long-term basis [5, 6, 27, 28]. These experiments demonstrated the efficacy and safety of these antiobesity compounds at comfortable ambient conditions. Whether mixtures of E/X can enhance thermoregulatory thermogenesis and cold tolerance, and by which mechanisms, was examined in two separate studies.

In one study, the ingestion of E/C (1 mg·kg^{-1}/2.5 mg·kg^{-1}) in the cold significantly increased the overall M by 19%, compared with the same subjects receiving the placebo (Fig. 8.8, [114]). This increase in M was mainly fueled by a significantly greater increase in CHO oxidation in comparison with the placebo. There were no changes in lipid or protein oxidation rates. This enhanced TT was associated with significantly smaller drops in (and thus warmer) T_{re} and $\bar{T}_{sk}$, a significantly reduced body heat debt, and slightly higher blood catecholamine levels.

In another study of E/X, the ingestion of E/C/T (44, 60, 100 mg,

FIGURE 8.8

Influence of ephedrine/caffeine ingestion on average heat production in cold-exposed subjects.

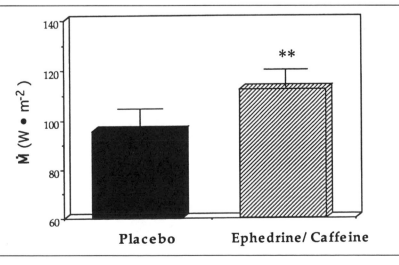

FIGURE 8.9

Influence of ephedrine/caffeine/theophylline ingestion on heat production (A) and heat debt (B) in cold-exposed subjects.

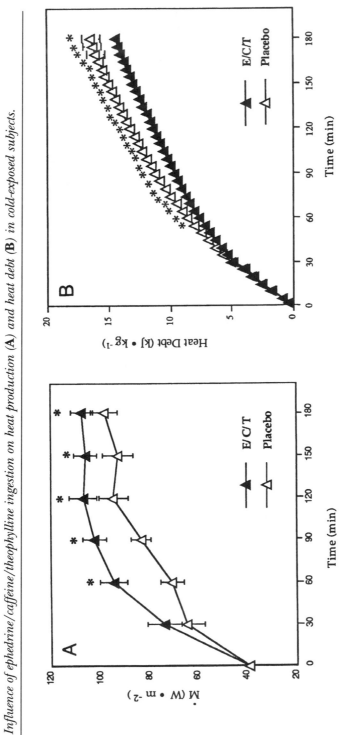

respectively) significantly increased M by 17% during the 3 hours in the cold, in contrast to the placebo condition (Fig. 8.9; [107]). This was achieved through a significantly greater lipid oxidation and a slightly greater carbohydrate oxidation. This enhanced TT was directly related to a significantly smaller heat debt (Fig. 8.9), slightly warmer T_{re}, and significantly warmer T_{sk}.

The exact mechanism of cellular action of E/X in the enhancement of TT is still uncertain, but it is likely that it includes an increased sympathomimetic effect. On the one hand, E is an adrenergic agonist that stimulates both ß and α receptors and can increase plasma catecholamine levels and M [28, 48]. Like norepinephrine and epinephrine, stimulation of $ß_1$-, $ß_2$- and $ß_3$-adrenergic receptor can increase M [13, 61]. On the other hand, X such as C and T act either by inhibition of phosphodiesterase activity, by antagonistic effects of adenosine receptors, or by a translocation of intracellular calcium [90]. By combining these actions, E/X compounds could thus increase liver and skeletal muscle glycogenolysis, white adipose tissue lipolysis, and the activation of the sympathetic nervous system [5, 6, 27, 28, 48, 90, 114]. An increase in either CHO or lipid oxidation would probably depend on the actual dosage of E and X used.

It is still not clear which particular tissue is responsible for the E/X-induced increase in TT. It could well take place in skeletal muscle, which is the major site of heat production during both shivering [66, 114] and the E-induced thermogenesis at comfortable ambient temperature [6]. Since E/X increase heat production without muscular contractions at comfortable ambient temperatures [27] and since E/X increase cold-induced thermogenesis without any evidence of greater shivering (subjective data not shown), it is thus possible that E/X act via mechanisms unrelated to shivering, either at the level of striated muscle or smooth muscle in the vascular bed, as described in an earlier section of this review [20]. This suggestion has received support from Hetteriacchi [46] who has shown that ephedrine increases thermogenesis in the perfused hindlimb by stimulating α-adrenergic receptors that control vasoconstriction in this tissue. Whether the E/X-induced increase in TT is due to vascular smooth muscle thermogenesis can only be answered after further research.

The results of our studies of E/X mixtures in the cold demonstrate that these treatments significantly enhance TT, produce warmer body temperatures, and reduce the heat debt (Figs. 8.8, 8.9). When compared with other studies of thermogenic agents (Table 8.2), the improvements in important thermophysiological parameters such as the changes in M, dry heat loss (R+C), heat debt (S), as well as ΔT_{re} and $\Delta \bar{T}_{sk}$ appear more favourable with E/X than with the others. Table 8.2 also highlights the value of a heat balance analysis and that it should be performed more often, since the heat debt certainly appears to be a more robust index of cold resistance than T_{re} alone. In conclusion, ephedrine/xanthines mixtures are a safe and effective pharmacological means of enhancing cold-induced thermoregu-

TABLE 8.2

Influence of Different Compounds on Important Thermoregulation Parameters in the Cold

	M	R + C	S	ΔT_{re}	$\Delta \bar{T}_{sk}$
Ephedrine-caffeine-theophylline (Vallerand et al. 1993)	↑ 17%	↑ 4%	↓ 12%	↓ 24%	↓ 8%
Ephedrine-caffeine (Vallerand et al. 1989)	↑ 19%	↑ 5%	↓ 14%	↓ 41%	↓ 11%
Theophylline-rest (Wang et al. 1986)	↔	—	—	↓ 56%	—
Theophylline+substrates-rest (Wang et al. 1986)	↑ 3%	—	—	↓ 56%	—
Theophylline-exercise (Wang et al. 1987)	↑ 3%	—	—	↓ 33%	—
Theophylline+substrates-exercise (Wang et al. 1987)	↑ 7%	—	—	↓ 55%	—
Cold Buster (Vallerand et al. 1992)	↔	↔	↔	↔	↔
Caffeine (LeBlanc 1987)	↑ 7%	—	—	↔	↓ 7%
Caffeine-rest (McNaughton et al. 1990)	↑ 16%	—	—	↔	↑ 16%
Caffeine-exercise (Graham et al. 1991)	↔	—	—	↔	↑ 7%
Caffeine-exercise (Doubt et al. 1991)	↑ 16%	—	—	↔	↓ 3%

Comparisons with a placebo (%): ↑ increase; ↓ decrease: ↔ no change; — not available. M: metabolism; R + C: dry heat loss; S: heat debt; ΔT_{re}: change in T_{re}; $\Delta \bar{T}_{sk}$: change in $\bar{T}_{sk}$.

latory thermogenesis and delaying the onset of hypothermia in humans. Further work is required to determine the effectiveness of these agents for longer cold exposures and at deeper levels of hypothermia.

FACTORS LIMITING THERMOREGULATORY THERMOGENESIS

There are reports that TT can reach as high as 50% of $\dot{V}O_2$max in humans [38]. But why is metabolic rate so limited during shivering, even at the risk of death from hypothermia?

It has been suggested that at least two important factors limit maximum O_2 consumption in humans: blood O_2 transport and a peripheral factor comprising O_2 transfer and mitochondrial O_2 utilization [23]. Pendergast [84] concluded that for exercising humans, who were also cooling in cold water, oxygen transport and peripheral oxygen utilization impairments caused by the cold stress limited work capacity. With regard to temperature regulation in cold-stressed rodents, Wang concluded that it was neither the exhaustion of respiratory-cardiovascular functions for gas transport [121] nor the saturation of oxidative capacity [128], but energy substrate mobilization that limited TT [121, 122]. Our own research, described earlier, does not support this substrate mobilization hypothesis, which may be more applicable to smaller animals with a less favorable surface area to mass ratio or to situations in which specific energy stores are depleted in humans [112, 113]. This does not imply that the supply of energy substrates to the thermogenic machinery and central nervous system (CNS) is not important. As an example, hypoglycemia in the hypothermic hamster impairs CNS functions and results in cardiovascular or respiratory failure, whereas glucose infusion increased their survival time 5-fold [91]. In cold-exposed humans, hypoglycemia ($\approx$2.5 mmol. liter^{-1}) suppresses shivering and accelerates the drop in T_{re} [35, 60 Mekjavic, personal communication 1993]. It is interesting to note that the opposite, provoking hyperglycemia, does not improve TT [112, 113, 118, 119].

We suggest that in humans there are other factors required to enhance TT, which in turn could reduce the heat debt and facilitate maintenance of body temperatures during cold stress. One such factor could well be the muscle mass available for shivering thermogenesis. This concept is supported by the report of Bell et al. [9] that peripheral muscles have a smaller role in shivering thermogenesis than trunk muscles, thus reducing effectively the available muscle mass in humans.

The sympathoadrenal system can also modulate TT. Both norepinephrine and epinephrine are key thermogenic hormones [4, 5]. Astrup et al. [7] have also provided evidence for an epinephrine-induced thermogenesis in skeletal muscles and a norepinephrine-induced thermogenesis unrelated to skeletal muscle in humans, suggesting that the sympathoadrenal system plays a physiological role in the daily energy balance (7,100). Also, several studies have shown that pharmacological agents that increase facultative or thermoregulatory thermogenesis have been associated with increments in plasma catecholamine levels, although this relationship requires further study, particularly in the cold [5, 27, 114].

Finally, corticotropin-releasing factor (CRF) could have an impact on TT, but it has not yet been applied in this regard to human subjects. CRF acts within the CNS to activate the sympathetic nervous system and the sympathoadrenal outflow and to increase VO_2 and plasma catecholamines [14, 79]. Further, it has been suggested that CRF could enhance shivering thermogenesis by increasing muscular activity [79], an interesting hypothesis that merits further research.

CONCLUSIONS

Is it feasible to stimulate increases in metabolism that are of sufficient magnitude that hypothermia is significantly delayed or avoided in acutely cold-stressed humans? This is the question that has been addressed by the research presented and interpreted in this chapter. More fundamental knowledge about the effects of cold stress on the mechanisms of human TT is needed before the question can be answered with certainty.

In our attempt to consolidate relevant knowledge about the question posed above, we have reviewed the role and mechanisms of thermoregulatory thermogenesis during cold stress in humans. The mechanisms by which shivering and nonshivering thermogeneses can be activated, as well as their proposed sites of action, have been presented. Research has been discussed concerning the role of specific circulating and intramuscular energy substrates in fueling thermoregulatory thermogenesis. We have also discussed the potential for dietary/pharmacological interventions to enhance cold tolerance and whether energy substrate mobilization limits thermoregulatory thermogenesis. This review included discussion of some other factors that may also be limiting for thermoregulatory thermogenesis. In this context, the metabolic and thermal implications of using thermogenic antiobesity agents, such as sympathomimetics and methylxanthines, were considered.

A dilemma facing scientists engaged in this research is the justified constraint of ethical considerations about the discomfort caused by cold stress and the health risks associated with inducing actual hypothermia in humans. Thus, there are few controlled studies, including our own, that document healthy human metabolic responses to severe hypothermia. This problem is further exacerbated because there are few, if any, good animal models of human TT in the cold.

Our strategy has been to attempt to first clarify the importance of specific macronutrients and the magnitude of their contribution to TT, and then to use this knowledge to evaluate and/or develop substances that might acutely enhance TT in humans.

Efforts in both areas remain incomplete, and we invite others to join us in applying more elaborate techniques to fill some of the knowledge gaps identified above.

ACKNOWLEDGMENTS

The authors gratefully acknowledge the technical assistance of the staff of the Environmental Physiology Section at the Defence and Civil Institute of Environmental Medicine. We are particularly grateful to Ms. I. Schmegner for her technical and editorial assistance.

REFERENCES

1. Acheson K. J., B. Zahorska-Markiewicz, P. Pittet, K. Anantharaman, and E. Jéquier. Caffeine and coffee: their influence on metabolic rate and substrate utilization in normal weight and obese individuals. *Am. J. Clin. Nutr.* 33:989–997,1980.
2. Ahlers, S., R. Hesslink, S. Lewis, and J. Thomas. Caffeine Attenuates the Afterdrop in

Rectal Temperature after Mild Cooling. Bethesda: Naval Medical Research Institute, 1990 (NMRI 90–110).

3. Alexander, G. Cold thermogenesis. D. Robertshaw (ed). *International Review of Physiology. Environmental Physiology III, Volume 20.* Baltimore: University Park Press, 1979, pp. 43–155.

4. Astrup, A., J. Bulow, N. Christensen, J. Madsen, and F. Quaade. Facultative thermogenesis induced by carbohydrate: a skeletal muscle component mediated by epinephrine. *Am. J. Physiol.* 250:E226–E229, 1986.

5. Astrup, A., B. Buemann, N. J. Christensen, S. Toubro, G. Thorbek, et al. The effect of ephedrine/caffeine mixture on energy expenditure and body composition in obese women. *Metabolism* 41:686–688, 1992.

6. Astrup, A., J. Bulow, J. Madsen, and N. J. Christensen. Contribution of BAT and skeletal muscle to thermogenesis induced by ephedrine in man. *Am. J. Physiol.* 248:E507–E515, 1985.

7. Astrup, A., L. Simonsen, J. Bülow, J. Madsen, and N. J. Christensen. Epinephrine mediates facultative carbohydrate-induced thermogenesis in human skeletal muscle. *Am. J. Physiol.* 257:E340–E345, 1989.

8. Bell, A., P. Clarke, and G. Thompson. Changes in the metabolism of the shivering hind leg of the young ox during several days of continuous cold exposure. *Q. J. Exp. Physiol.* 60:267–284, 1975.

9. Bell, D. G., P. Tikuisis, and I. Jacobs. Relative intensity of muscular contraction during shivering. *J. Appl. Physiol.* 72:2336–2342, 1992.

10. Bennett, J. W. The maximum metabolic response of sheep to cold: effects of rectal temperature, shearing, feed consumption, body posture and body weights. *Aust. J. Agric. Res.* 23:1045–1054, 1973.

11. Bergström, J., L. Hermansen, E. Hultman, and B. Saltin. Diet, muscle glycogen and physical performance. *Acta Physiol. Scand.* 7:140–150, 1967.

12. Bittel, J. Heat debt as an index for cold adaptation in men. *J. Appl. Physiol.* 62:1627–1634, 1987.

13. Blaak, E. E., M. A. Van Baak, K. P. G. Kempen, and W. H. M. Saris. Role of alpha and beta-adrenoceptors in sympathetically mediated thermogenesis. *Am. J. Physiol.* 264:E11–E17, 1993.

14. Brown, M., L. Fisher, J. River, J. Spiess, C. River, and W. Vale. Corticotropin-releasing factor: effects on the sympathetic nervous system and oxygen consumption. *Life Sci.* 30:207–210, 1981.

15. Bruttig, S., and D. Roberts. *Cold Induced Changes in Arterial Sensitivity.* Natick, MA: U.S. Army Institute of Environmental Medicine, 1991 (Technical Report T11–91).

16. Burton, A. C., and O. C. Edholm. *Man in a Cold Environment.* London: Arnold, 1955.

17. Buskirk, E. R. Cold stress: a selective review. L. Folinsbee, J. Wagner, J. Borgia, et al. (eds). *Individual Human Adaptations.* New York: Academic Press, 1978, pp. 249–266.

18. Clark, M. G., S. Rattigan, and E. Q. Colquhoun. Hypertension in obesity may reflect a homeostatic thermogenic response. *Life Sci.* 48:939–947, 1991.

19. Clausen, T., van Hardeveld, C., and M. Everts. Significance of cation transport in control of energy metabolism and thermogenesis. *Physiol. Rev.* 71:733–774, 1991.

20. Colquhoun E. Q., and M. G. Clark. Open question: has thermogenesis in muscle been overlooked and misinterpreted? *News Physiol. Sci.* 6:256–259, 1991.

21. Conley, K. E., E. R. Weibel, C. R. Taylor, and H. Hoppeler. Aerobic capacity estimated by exercise vs. cold exposure: endurance training effects in rats. *Respir. Physiol.* 62:273–280, 1985.

22. Depocas, F., and R. Masironi. Glucose as fuel for thermogenesis. *Am. J. Physiol.* 199:1051–1058, 1960.

23. di Prampero, P. E., and G. Ferretti. Factors limiting maximal oxygen consumption in humans. *Respir. Physiol.* 80:113–128, 1990.

24. Doubt, T. Physiology of exercise in the cold. *Sports Med.* 11:367–381, 1991.

25. Doubt, T., and T. Francis. Hazards of cold water. J. S. Torg et al. (eds). *Current Therapy in Sports Medicine.* Philadelphia: B. C. Decker, 1990, pp. 150–155.

26. Doubt, T. J., and S. S. Hsieh. Additive effects of caffeine and cold water during submaximal leg exercise. *Med. Sci. Sports Exerc.* 23:435–442, 1991.

27. Dulloo, A. G., and D. S. Miller. The thermogenic properties of ephedrine methylxanthine mixtures: human studies. *Int. J. Obes.* 10:467–481, 1986.

28. Dullo, A. G., J. Seydoux, and L. Girardier. Dietary and pharmacological effectiveness of thermogenic stimulation in obesity treatment. Y. Oomura et al. (eds). *Progress in Obesity Research.* London: J. Libbey, 1990, pp. 135–144.

29. Elia, M., C. Zed, G. Neale, and G. Livesey. The energy cost of triglyceride-fatty acid recycling in nonobese subjects after an overnight fast and four days of starvation. *Metabolism* 36:251–255, 1987.

30. Eldershaw, T., E. Colquhoun, K. Dora, Z. Peng, and M. Clark. Pungent principles of ginger *(Zingiber officinale)* are thermogenic in the perfused rat hindlimb. *Int. J. Obes.* 16:755–763, 1992.

31. Else, P. Oxygen consumption and sodium pump thermogenesis in a developing mammal. *Am J. Physiol.* 261:R1575–R1578, 1991.

32. Estler, C. J., H. P. T. Ammon, and C. Herzog. Swimming capacity of mice after prolonged treatment with psychostimulants. I. Effect of caffeine on swimming performance and cold stress. *Psychopharmacology* 58:161–166, 1978.

33. Freeman, B. M. Some aspects of thermoregulation in the adult Japanese quail *(Coturnix coturnix jaonica).* *Comp. Biochem. Physiol.* 34:871–881, 1970.

34. Frommel, E., and F. Valette. De l'influence de la thyroxine sur la temperature dinitrée du cobaye. *Arch. Sci. (Geneva)* 3:54–56, 1950.

35. Gale E., T. Bennett, J. H. Green, and I. A. Macdonald. Hypoglycemia, hypothermia and shivering in man. *Clin. Sci.* 61:463–469, 1981.

36. Gennari, G. The effect of caffeine on passive hypothermia in experimental cooling. *Rendic Ist San Pubb. Roma* 2:515–522, 1940.

37. Glickman, N., H. Mitchell, R. Keeton, and E. Lambert. Shivering and heat production in men exposed to intense cold. *J. Appl. Physiol.* 22:1–8, 1967.

38. Golden, F., I. Hampton, G. Hervey, and A. Knibbs. Shivering intensity in humans during immersion in cold water. *J. Physiol. (London)* 290:48P, 1979.

39. Górski, J., A. Kuryliszyn, and U. Wereszczynska. Effect of acute cold exposure on the mobilization of intramuscular glycogen and triglycerides in the rat. *Acta Physiol. Pol.* 32:755–759, 1981.

40. Graham T. E., P. Sathasivam, and K. W. McNaughton. Influence of cold, exercise and caffeine on catecholamines and metabolism in men. *J. Appl. Physiol.* 70:2052–2058, 1991.

41. Hagerman, F. C. Energy metabolism and fuel utilization. *Med. Sci. Sports Exerc.* 24:S309–S314, 1992.

42. Hall, V. E., F. P. Attardo, and J. H. Perryman. Influence of dinitrophenol on body temperature threshold for thermal polypnea. *Proc. Soc. Exp. Biol.* 69:413–415, 1948.

43. Hanson, P. G., and R. E. Johnson. Variations of plasma ketones and free fatty acids during acute cold exposure in man. *J. Appl. Physiol.* 20:56–60, 1965.

44. Hemingway, A. Shivering. *Physiol. Rev.* 43:397–422, 1963.

45. Herpin, P., B. McBride, and H. Bayley. Effect of cold exposure on energy metabolism in the young pig. *Can. J. Physiol. Pharmacol.* 65:236–245, 1987.

46. Hettiarachi, M., E. Colquhoun, J. Ye, S. Rattigan, and M. Clark. Norephedrine (phenylpropanolamine) stimulates oxygen consumption and lactate production in the perfused rat hindlimb. *Int. J. Obes.* 15:37–43, 1991.

47. Himms-Hagen, J. Lipid metabolism during cold exposure and cold acclimation. *Lipids* 7:310–320, 1972.

48. Hoffman B. B., and R. J. Lefkowitz. Catecholamines and sympathomimetic drugs. A. G.

Bilman, T. W. Rall, and A. S. Nies (eds). *The Pharmacological Basis of Therapeutics.* New York: Pergamon, 1990, p. 187.

49. Hong, S., and E. R. Nadel. Thermogenic control during exercise in a cold environment. *J. Appl. Physiol.* 47:1084–1089, 1979.

50. Horvath, S. M. Exercise in a cold environment. D. Miller (ed). *Exercise and Sport Sciences Reviews, Vol. 9.* Philadelphia: Franklin Institute Press, 1982, pp. 221–263.

51. Horwitz, B. A. Biochemical mechanisms and control of cold-induced cellular thermogenesis in placental mammals. L. Wang (ed). *Advances in Comparative and Environmental Physiology.* Heidelberg: Springer Verlag, 1989, pp. 83–116.

52. Hurley, B. F., and E. M. Haymes. The effects of rest and exercise in the cold on substrate mobilization and utilization. *Aviat. Space Environ. Med.* 53:1193–1197, 1982.

53. Ivy, J., and J. Holloszy. Persistent increase in glucose uptake by rat skeletal muscle following exercise. *Am. J. Physiol.* 241:C200–C203, 1981.

54. Jacobs, I., T. Romet, and D. Kerrigan-Brown. Muscle glycogen depletion during exercise at 9°C and 21°C. *Eur. J. Appl. Physiol.* 54:35–39, 1985.

55. Jacobs, I., I. C. H. Wang, T. Romet, M. Kavanagh, and J. Frim. Effects of theophylline ingestion on thermoregulation during 15°C water immersion. *Undersea Biomed. Res.* In review.

56. Jensen, K., A. Rabøl, and K. Winkler. Total body and splanchnic thermogenesis in curarized man during a short exposure to cold. *Acta Anaesth. Scand.* 24:339–344, 1980.

57. Jéquier, E. Thermogenesis and its role in energy metabolism. *Bibl. Nutr. Dieta* 39:6–12, 1986.

58. Jéquier, E. Energy metabolism in human obesity. *Soz. Praventivmed.* 34:58–62, 1989.

59. Keatinge, W. R. The effects of subcutaneous fat and of previous exposure to cold on the body temperature, peripheral blood flow, and metabolic rate of men in cold water. *J. Physiol. (London)* 153:166–178, 1960.

60. Kedis, L. H., and J. B. Field. Hypothermia: a clue to hypoglycemia. *N. Engl. J. Med.* 271:785–787, 1964.

61. Kurpad, A., R. Kulkarni, D. Ridriguez, and P. Shetty. Characteristics of norepinephrine stimulated thermogenesis in undernourished subjects. *J. Biosci.* 17:293–303, 1992.

62. Larkin, L., B. Horwitz, and R. McDonald. Effect of cold on serum substrate and glycogen concentration in young and old Fisher 344 rats. *Exp. Gerontol.* 27:179–190, 1992.

63. Lean, M., W. James, G. Jennings, and P. Trayhurn. Brown adipose tissue in patients with phaeochromocytoma. *Int. J. Obes.* 10:219–227, 1986.

64. Lean, M., W. James, G. Jennings, and P. Trayhurn. Brown adipose tissue uncoupling protein content in human infants, children and adults. *Clin. Sci.* 71:291–297, 1986.

65. LeBlanc, J. Various influences on the response to sleeping in the cold. *Proceedings of the 27th DRG Seminar on Sleep and Its Implications for the Military.* Lyon, France: NATO Report DS/A/DR(88)47, 1987, pp. 35–43.

66. LeBlanc, J. *Man in the Cold.* Springfield, IL.: Charles C. Thomas, 1975.

67. LeBlanc, J., and A. Labrie. Glycogen and non specific adaptation to cold. *J. Appl. Physiol.* 51:1428–1432, 1981.

68. Lucas, A., A. Therminarias, and M. Tanche. Plasma catecholamines in dogs during cold exposure and muscular exercise at the same level of energy expenditure. *J. Physiol. (Paris)* 78:231–234, 1982.

69. Martineau, L. *Substrate Availability and Temperature Regulation during Cold Water Immersion in Humans.* Ph.D. Thesis. Toronto: University of Toronto, 1990.

70. Martineau, L., and I. Jacobs. Muscle glycogen utilization during shivering thermogenesis in humans. *J. Appl. Physiol.* 65:2046–2050, 1988.

71. Martineau, L., and I. Jacobs. Muscle glycogen availability and temperature regulation in humans. *J. Appl. Physiol.* 66:72–78, 1989.

72. Martineau, L., and I. Jacobs. Free fatty acid availability and temperature regulation in cold water. *J. Appl. Physiol.* 67:2466–2472, 1989.

73. Martineau, L., and I. Jacobs. Effects of muscle glycogen and plasma FFA availability on human metabolic responses in cold water. *J. Appl. Physiol.* 71:1331–1339, 1991.

74. McLellan, T., and I. Jacobs. Muscle glycogen utilization and the expression of relative exercise intensity. *Int. J. Sports Med.* 12:21–26, 1991.

75. McNaughton K. W., P. Sathasivam, A. L. Vallerand, and T. E. Graham. Influence of caffeine on metabolic responses of men at rest in 28 and 5°C. *J. Appl. Physiol.* 68:1889–1895, 1990.

76. Minaire, Y., J. Forichon, J. Jomain, and G. Dallevet. Independence of the circulating insulin levels of the increased glucose turnover in shivering dogs. *Experientia* 37:745–747, 1981.

77. Minaire, Y., A. Pernod, J. C. Vincent-Falquet, and M. Mottaz. Comparison of carbohydrate utilization in running and shivering dogs. *Horm. Metab. Res.* 5:80–83:1973.

78. Molnar, G. W., and R. C. Read. Hypoglycemia and body temperature. *JAMA* 227:916–921, 1974.

79. Nakamori, T., A. Morimoto, K. Morimoto, N. Tan, and N. Murakami. Effects of α– and ß–adrenergic antagonists on rise in body temperature induced by psychological stress in rats. *Am. J. Physiol.* 264:R156–R161, 1993.

80. Newsholme, E., and C. Start. *Regulation in Metabolism.* New York: J. Wiley & Sons, 1973, pp. 88–145.

81. Parker, G. H., and J. C. George. Effect of in vivo cold exposure on intracellular glycogen reserves in the "starling type" avian pectoralis. *Life Sci.* 15:1415–1423, 1975.

82. Parker, G. H., and J. C. George. Glycogen utilization by the white fibres in the pigeon pectoralis as main energy process during shivering thermogenesis. *Comp. Biochem. Physiol.* 50:433–437, 1975.

83. Paul, P., and W. L. Holmes. Free fatty acid metabolism during stress: exercise, acute cold exposure and anaphylactic shock. *Lipids* 8:142–150, 1973.

84. Pendergast, D. R. The effect of body cooling on oxygen transport during exercise. *Med. Sci. Sports Exerc.* 20:S171–S176, 1988.

85. Pick E. F., and S. Feitelberg. Thermogenetic action of adrenalin and benzedrine on the brain. *Arch. Int. Pharmacodyn.* 77:219–225, 1948.

86. Prusiner, S., and M. Poe. Thermodynamic considerations of mammalian heat production. O. Lindberg (ed). *Brown Adipose Tissue.* New York: Elsevier, 1970, pp. 263–283.

87. Pugh, L. G. C. E. Cold stress and muscular exercise, with special reference to accidental hypothermia. *Br. Med. J.* 2:333–337, 1967.

88. Radomski, M. W., and C. Boutelier. Hormone response of normal and intermittent cold-preadapted humans to continuous cold. *J. Appl. Physiol.* 53:610–616, 1982.

89. Radomski, M. W., and T. Orme. Response of liporotein lipase in various tissues to cold exposure. *Am. J. Physiol.* 220:1852–1856, 1971.

90. Rall, T. W. Drugs used in the treatment of asthma. The methylxanthines, chromolyn sodium and other agents. A. G. Bilman, T. W. Rall, A. S. Nies (eds). *The Pharmacological Basis of Therapeutics.* New York: Pergamon, 1990, p. 618.

91. Resch, G. E., and X. J. Musacchia. A role for glucose in hypothermic hamsters. *Am. J. Physiol.* 231:1729–1734, 1976.

92. Saltin, B., and J. Karlsson. Muscle glycogen utilization during work of different intensities. B. Pernow and B. Saltin (eds). *Muscle Metabolism during Exercise.* New York: Plenum, 1971, pp. 289–299.

93. Scheurer, O., and W. Hugo. Beeinflussung der hauttetemperaturen durch herzund Gefabmittel. *Muench. Med. Wochenschr.* 89:907–911, 1942.

94. Seitz, H. J., W. Krone, H. Wike, and W. Tarnowski. Rapid rise in plasma glucagon induced by acute cold exposure in man and rat. *Pflügers Arch.* 389:115–120, 1981.

95. Sellers, E. A. Hormones in the regulation of body temperatures. E. Schönbaum and P. Lomax (eds). *The Pharmacology of Thermoregulation.* Basel: Karger, 1972, pp. 57–71.

96. Shiota, M., and S. Masumi. Effect of norepinephrine on consumption of oxygen in perfused skeletal muscle from cold-exposed rats. *Am J. Physiol.* 254:E482–E489, 1988.

97. Simonsen, L., J. Bülow, J. Madsen, and N. H. Christensen. Thermogenic response to epinephrine in the forearm and abdominal subcutaneous adipose tissue. *Am J. Physiol.* 263:E850–E855, 1992.

98. Sowood, P. J. *Shivering; A Review.* Farnborough, UK: Royal Air Force Inst. Aviat. Med., 1984 (IAM Rep. 636).

99. Stock, M. Thermogenesis and brown fat: relevance to human obesity. *Infusionstherapie* 16:282–284, 1989.

100. Stock, M. Thermogenesis and energy balance. *Int. J. Obes.* 16 (Suppl. 2):S13–S16, 1992.

101. Strømme, S., K. L. Andersen, R. W. Elsner. Metabolic and thermal responses to muscular exertion in the cold. *J. Appl. Physiol.* 18:756–763, 1963.

102. Tappy, L., and E. Jéquier. The components of energy expenditure in human obesity. *Acta Clin. Belg.* 47 (Suppl. 14):13–17, 1992.

103. Thompson, G. E. Physiological effect of cold exposure. D. Robertshaw (ed). *International Review of Physiology II, vol. 15.* Baltimore: University Press, 1977, pp. 29–69.

104. Tikuisis, P., D. G. Bell, and I. Jacobs. Shivering onset, metabolic response, and convective heat transfer during cold air exposure. *J. Appl. Physiol.* 70:1996–2002, 1991.

105. Tikuisis, P., D. McCracken, and M. Radomski. Heat debt during cold air exposure before and after cold water immersions. *J. Appl. Physiol.* 71:60–68, 1991.

106. Toner, M., and W. D. McArdle. Physiological adjustments of man to the cold. K. B. Pandolf, M. N. Sawka, and R. R. Gonzalez (eds). *Human Performance Physiology and Environmental Medicine at Terrestrial Extremes.* Indianapolis: Benchmark Press, 1988, p. 400.

107. Vallerand, A. L. Effects of ephedrine/xanthines on thermogenesis and cold tolerance. *Int. J. Obes.* (Suppl 1):S53–S56, 1993.

108. Vallerand, A. L., J. Frim, and M. F. Kavanagh. Plasma glucose and insulin responses to oral and intravenous glucose in cold-exposed men. *J. Appl. Physiol.* 65:2395–2399, 1988.

109. Vallerand, A. L., and I. Jacobs. Rates of energy substrates utilization during human cold exposure. *Eur. J. Appl. Physiol.* 58:873–878, 1989.

110. Vallerand, A. L., and I. Jacobs. Influence of cold exposure on plasma triglyceride clearance in humans. *Metabolism* 39:1211–1218, 1990.

111. Vallerand, A. L., and I. Jacobs. Energy metabolism during cold exposure. *Int. J. Sports Med.* 13(Suppl 1):S191–S193, 1992.

112. Vallerand, A. L., and I. Jacobs. *Interaction of a Food Supplement, Intermittent Exercise and Cold Exposure on Heat Balance.* North York, Ontario: Defence & Civil Institute of Environmental Medicine, 1993 (Report Number 93–19).

113. Vallerand, A. L., and I. Jacobs. *Effects of a High-Energy Food Supplement on Cold-induced Thermogenesis.* North York, Ontario: Defence & Civil Institute of Environmental Medicine Report Number 93–36, 1993.

114. Vallerand, A. L., I. Jacobs, and M. F. Kavanagh. Mechanism of enhanced cold tolerance by an ephedrine-caffeine mixture in humans. *J. Appl. Physiol.* 67:438–444, 1989.

115. Vallerand, A. L., F. Pérusse, and L. J. Bukowiecki. Cold exposure potentiates the effect of insulin on in vivo glucose uptake. *Am J. Physiol.* (253) *(Endocrinol. Metab. 8)*:E575–E581, 1987.

116. Vallerand, A. L., G. Savourey, and J. Bittel. Determination of heat debt in the cold: partitional calorimetry vs. conventional methods. *J. Appl. Physiol.* 72:1380–1385, 1992.

117. Vallerand, A. L., G. Savourey, A.-M. Hannique, and J. Bittel. How should body heat storage be determined in humans: by thermometry or calorimetry? *Eur. J. Appl. Physiol.* 65:286–294, 1992.

118. Vallerand A. L., I. F. Schmegner, and I. Jacobs. *Influence of the Cold Buster Sports Bar on Heat Debt, Mobilization and Oxidation of Energy Substrates.* North York, Ontario: Defence & Civil Institute of Environmental Medicine, (Report Number 92–60) 1992.

119. Vallerand, A. L., P. Tikuisis, M. B. Ducharme, and I. Jacobs. Is energy substrate mobilization a limiting factor for cold thermogenesis? *Eur. J. Appl. Physiol.* 67:239–244, 1993.

120. Wajngot, A., V. Chandramouli, W. Schumann, K. Kumaran, S. Efendic, and B. Landau.

Testing of the assumptions made in estimating the extent of futile cycling. *Am J. Physiol.* 256:E668–E675, 1989.

121. Wang, L. C. H. Factors limiting maximum cold-induced heat production. *Life Sci.* 23:2089–2098, 1978.

122. Wang, L. C. H. Effects of feeding on aminophylline induced supra-maximal thermogenesis. *Life Sci.* 29:2459–2466, 1981.

123. Wang, L. C. H., and E. C. Anholt. Elicitation of supramaximal thermogenesis by aminophylline in the rat. *J. Appl. Physiol.* 53:16–20, 1982.

124. Wang, L. C. H., and T. F. Lee. Enhancement of maximal thermogenesis by reducing endogenous adenosine activity in the rat. *J. Appl. Physiol.* 68:580–585, 1990.

125. Wang, L. C. H., S. F. P. Man, and A. N. Belcastro. Improving cold tolerance in men: Effects of substrates and aminophylline. K. Cooper, P. Lomax, E. Schönbaum, and W. Veale (eds). *Homeostasis and Thermal Stress.* Basel: Karger, 1986, pp. 22–26.

126. Wang, L. C. H., S. F. P. Man, and A. N. Belcastro. Metabolic and hormonal responses in theophylline-increased cold resistance in males. *J. Appl. Physiol.* 63:589–596, 1987.

127. Wang, L. C. H., S. F. P. Man, A. N. Belcastro, and J. C. Westly. Single, optimal oral dosage of theophylline for improving cold resistance in man. P. Lomax, and E. Schönbaum (eds). *Thermoregulation: Research and Clinical Applications.* Basel: Karger, 1989, pp. 54–58.

128. Wang, L. C. H., and R. E. Peter. Metabolic and respiratory response during Helox-induced hypothermia in the white rat. *Am J. Physiol* 229:890–895, 1975.

129. Weihe, W. H. The effect of temperature on the action of drugs. E. Schönbaum and P. Lomax (eds). *The Pharmacology of Thermoregulation.* Basel: Karger, 1973, pp. 155–169.

130. Young, A. J. Human adaptation to cold. K. B. Pandolf, M. N. Sawka, and R. R. Gonzalez (eds). *Human Performance Physiology and Environmental Medicine at Terrestrial Extremes.* Indianapolis: Benchmark Press, 1988, pp. 401–434.

131. Young, A. J., S. R. Muza, M. Sawka, P. Neufer, J. Bogart, and K. Pandolf. Thermoregulation during cold water immersion is unimpaired by low muscle glycogen levels. *J. Appl. Physiol.* 66:1809–1816, 1989.

132. Zorzano, A., T. W. Balon, M. N. Goodman, and N. B. Ruderman. Glycogen depletion and increased insulin sensitivity and responsiveness in muscle after exercise. *Am J. Physiol.* 251:E664–E669, 1986.

9
Endurance Exercise in Aging Humans: Effects on Energy Metabolism

ERIC T. POEHLMAN, Ph.D.
PAUL J. ARCIERO, Ph.D.
MICHAEL I. GORAN, Ph.D.

The overall objective of this chapter is to review new information regarding the adaptive changes in energy metabolism in response to endurance exercise in older individuals. More specifically, we review studies that have examined biological and environmental factors involved in the regulation of energy requirements, energy intake, energy expenditure, and body composition in older men and women, since it is ultimately the net balance between energy intake and energy expenditure that regulates energy balance in humans.

Our first specific objective in this chapter is to review the effects of age on the components of energy balance in humans. This includes a review of age-associated changes in (a) resting metabolic rate, (b) the thermic effect of a meal, (c) physical activity, (d) total energy expenditure, and (e) energy intake. Our second objective is to examine the effects of endurance exercise on the aforementioned components. Finally, we review the results of studies that examined the effects of age and physical activity on insulin-like growth factor-1 and sympathetic nervous system activity, two hormonal systems implicated in the regulation of energy expenditure and body composition. The reader is referred to earlier reviews that examined the effects of age on energy metabolism [74, 79, 80, 85, 88].

RESTING METABOLIC RATE (RMR) AND AGING

Resting metabolic rate (RMR) represents the largest component (50–80%) of total energy expenditure in older adults [78, 79] and thus is quantitatively very important in the regulation of energy balance and body composition. One of the most consistent physiological changes that occurs with age is the well-documented decline in RMR. Cross-sectional [12, 106, 126–128, 137, 145] and longitudinal investigations [54, 107, 138] have reported a decline in RMR with age, which coincides with the decline in fat-free mass [32, 34, 76]. More recent investigations have confirmed these findings [31, 37, 81, 87, 90, 92, 140]. More recent studies [81, 87] have suggested a curvilinear decline in RMR with advancing age, in which the decline is accelerated beyond the middle-age and postmenopausal years.

Determinants of the Decline in Resting Metabolic Rate in Aging Humans
Several studies have attributed the age-related decline in RMR primarily to the loss of fat-free mass [54, 90, 137, 138], whereas others have suggested that other physiological variables may contribute to the lower RMR in the elderly [37, 81, 140]. In the Baltimore Longitudinal Study [137, 138], cross-sectional and longitudinal designs showed that the loss of muscle mass in healthy men, as measured by 24-hr creatinine excretion, fully accounted for the age-related decline in RMR. It has been postulated that the rate of decline in RMR with age approximates the rate of loss of fat-free mass. For example, both Forbes and Reina [34] and Novak [76] reported a 3% decline in fat-free mass per decade, similar to the 3.22% decline found by Keys et al. [54] and the 3.7% decline reported by Tzankoff and Norris [138]. This rate of decline is somewhat higher, however, than the 1.2% decline in RMR per decade reported in a group of 115 men studied five times during a 17-yr period between the ages of 50 and 67 yr [54]. Surprisingly, these authors reported that this group of older men experienced little or no change in body mass and composition, which probably partially explained the small decline in RMR.

There is uncertainty whether other physiological factors may also contribute to the age-related reduction of RMR. Recently, Fukagawa et al. [37] examined the relationship between fat-free mass and RMR in young men (18–33 yr), older men (69–89 yr), and older women (67–75 yr). They found that absolute RMR was significantly lower in older men (1.04 kcal·min^{-1}) and older women (0.84 kcal·min^{-1}) than in younger men (1.24 kcal·min^{-1}), and the lower RMR persisted even after adjusting for differences in fat-free mass. However, RMR did not differ between older men and older women after controlling for differences in fat-free mass. The authors concluded that differences in fat-free mass between younger and older individuals cannot fully account for the lower RMR in older individuals, thus suggesting that aging is associated with an alteration in the metabolic activity of lean tissue contained in the fat-free mass component.

Vaughn et al. [140] recently measured 24-hr energy expenditure and its components (e.g., basal metabolic rate and sleeping metabolic rate) in younger and older individuals in a room calorimeter. They found that basic metabolic rate was significantly lower in both groups of older subjects than in younger subjects, even after adjustment for differences in fat-free mass, fat mass, and gender. Collectively, these studies suggest that age and alterations in body composition are independent predictors of the decline in RMR, but they cannot fully account for the decrement.

We have performed a series of experiments to examine other possible modulators of the fall in RMR in older men and women. In the first of these studies, Poehlman et al. [81] examined whether differences in maximal aerobic capacity ($\dot{V}O_2$ max), daily energy intake, and plasma concentrations of thyroid hormones in a large group of 300 healthy males (17–78 yr) could explain the reduction in RMR with age, independent of changes in fat-free mass. Our results showed a curvilinear decline in RMR with age, in which the reduction in RMR was accelerated in males after 40 yr. Furthermore, fat-free mass could not fully account for the lower RMR in men over 40 yr. It was only after statistically controlling for differences in fat-free mass, fat mass, and maximal aerobic capacity that the association between RMR and age became nonsignificant. Variations in antecedent dietary practices and plasma thyroid hormones were not independent predictors of the decline in RMR. The results of this study suggested an influence of $\dot{V}O_2$max, independent of the decline in fat-free mass, on the decline in RMR in healthy males. Although the mechanism for the influence of $\dot{V}O_2$max on RMR cannot be defined at this point, it is conceivable that $\dot{V}O_2$max is a biological marker for several energy-consuming processes that may diminish as individuals age and become less physically active.

In a subsequent study, Poehlman et al. [96] examined whether a decrease in erythrocyte Na-K pump activity contributes to a portion of the decline in RMR after adjusting for the loss of fat-free mass with advancing age. Specifically, erythrocyte Na-K pump rate and rate constant were determined from plasma and erythrocyte Na and K concentrations using flame photometry after incubation with and without ouabain in 27 younger (17–39 yr) and 25 older (56–76 yr) males. We found that a lower RMR persisted in older (1.14 ± 0.12 kcal·min^{-1}) than in younger men (1.21 ± 0.12 kcal·min^{-1}, P<0.05) after controlling for differences in fat-free mass. No age differences were found, however, between older (1.17 ± 0.13 kcal·min^{-1}) and younger men (1.20 ± 0.13 kcal·min^{-1}) after adjusting for both fat-free mass and erythrocyte Na-K pump rate constant. These results suggest an independent, but small contribution of changes in Na-K pump activity to the age-related decline in RMR.

In a related study in females, Poehlman et al. [87] considered the association of several metabolic and lifestyle variables as modulators of the decline in resting metabolic rate and fat-free mass in 183 healthy females (18–81 yr). We found a nonsignificant decline (0.6% per decade) in RMR in females 18–50 yr, whereas a significant decline (4.0% per decade) was observed in females 51–81 yr (Fig. 9.1). These rates of decline in RMR compared favorably with the results of others [31]. However, in contrast to our previous study in males [81], no age effect on RMR was found after controlling for the effects of fat-free mass. This finding was not surprising since the age-related decline in fat-free mass with age closely paralleled the decline in RMR (Fig. 9.2).

When the decline in RMR was compared in males and females, we found that the decline in RMR in males occurred at an earlier age ($\approx$40 yr) than in females ($\approx$50 yr), and the decline beyond the middle-age years was

FIGURE 9.1

Curvilinear decline in resting metabolic rate (RMR) with age in 183 females.

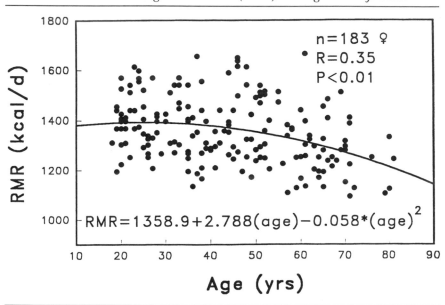

FIGURE 9.2

Curvilinear decline in fat-free weight with age in 183 females.

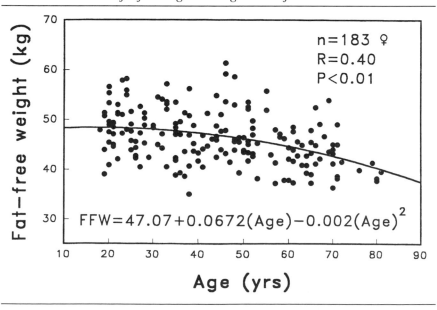

steeper in males (-11 kcal·day·$^{-1}$year^{-1}) than females (-5.5 kcal·day^{-1}year^{-1}). In conclusion, these findings suggest that gender is an important parameter to consider when examining the pattern, as well as the rate of decline in RMR with advancing age. Taken together, in agreement with earlier studies, we have shown that changes in body composition are the most important predictors of the decline in RMR with advancing age. Furthermore $\dot{V}O_2$max and Na-K pump activity also appear to be small independent determinants of the fall in RMR with age in men. In women, however, we were only able to identify the decline in fat-free mass as the single determinant of the decline in RMR with age.

Resting Metabolic Rate, Menopausal Status, and Body Composition
Menopausal status influences RMR and thus must be taken into account or controlled in experimental studies that examine the influence of environmental factors regulating RMR. For example, RMR is higher in premenopausal females during the luteal phase of the menstrual cycle than in the follicular phase [8, 29, 144]. It has even been proposed that the higher incidence of overweight observed in females with advancing age may be partially due to the loss of an increase in RMR experienced during the luteal phase (postovulatory) [29]. It has been suggested that the decrement in RMR experienced from the pre- to postmenopausal years may result in an energy conservation that approaches 15,000–20,000 kcal·yr^{-1} [29]. The transition from the pre- to postmenopausal years has also been associated with increased body weight gain [149] and deleterious changes in body composition [87]. We have recently shown that the lower RMR in postmenopausal women, relative to premenopausal women, was primarily due to deleterious changes in body composition and a decline in aerobic fitness [1]. Poehlman et al. [87] showed a nonsignificant decline in both RMR and FFM in healthy women up to age 50 yr, whereas after 50 years of age, a dramatic decline in these variables was noted (Figs. 9.1 and 9.2). The suggestion is that the estrogen-deficient state may partially contribute to alterations in energy expenditure and body composition. Interestingly, Arciero et al. [3] showed that menopausal status was a significant and independent factor contributing to a lower RMR among older women (> 50 years old). Recently, Gardner and Poehlman [39] showed a significant decline in leisure-time physical activity and fat-free mass in postmenopausal women, relative to the premenopausal years. The implication is that physical activity may play an important role, particularly in postmenopausal women, in offsetting a gain in body fat and in preserving fat-free mass. From their data, Gardner and Poehlman [39] predicted that the percentage body fat of healthy older women can be lowered by 0.16–0.35% for every 100 kcal·day^{-1} increase in physical activity, independent of age, mass, body mass index, and subcutaneous fat.

Kohrt et al. [55] recently examined the association of age and physical activity on body composition and fat distribution in endurance-trained and sedentary, younger and older women. The average difference in fat mass between younger and older sedentary women was 12.2 kg, but it was only 5.5 kg in the trained women. Moreover, differences in skinfold thicknesses at central upper body sites (e.g., subscapular and pectoralis) between the sedentary younger and older women averaged 86%, compared with only 39% in the trained women. These findings suggest that chronic participation in endurance exercise during menopause may reduce the accumulation of body fat, especially in the upper truncal regions, thus lowering the risk of developing cardiovascular and metabolic disorders [20, 149]. Wells et al. [146], showed that pre-, peri-, and postmenopausal master women endurance runners (mean=42 km·week^{-1}) (35–70 yr) had similar measures of cardiorespiratory fitness after accounting for differences in age and training status.

Collectively, these initial cross-sectional studies point toward an accelerated decline in resting metabolic rate and body composition during the postmenopausal years that may be blunted by increasing the level of physical activity. However, systematic longitudinal studies are needed to examine changes in total energy expenditure, its components, and body composition during the transition from the pre- to postmenopausal years. These studies should also consider the impact of hormone replacement therapy on alterations in body composition and energy expenditure.

Prediction of Resting Metabolic Rate in Older Individuals
Because of the limitations involved in accurately measuring energy intake in older individuals [45, 51, 79], it has been recommended that energy needs be estimated by measuring daily energy expenditure in healthy individuals [45, 51, 79, 80, 152]. RMR has served as the basis upon which estimates of total energy needs have been developed [152]. However, many of the prediction equations of RMR in older individuals have been derived from data extrapolated from younger individuals [48, 77] or are based on smaller sample sizes in the older age ranges [35, 48, 70, 77, 152] and have not been tested for accuracy using cross-validation procedures.

These issues have recently been addressed by our laboratory [2, 3], in which age- and gender-specific equations to predict RMR in clinical and field-testing settings using easily measured variables were developed. We showed that a measure of body mass, leisure-time activity, age, and chest skinfold predicted RMR in older males, within a standard error of estimate of ± 42 kcal/d. These four variables yielded the following prediction equation:

$$[\text{RMR (kcal/d)} = 9.7(\text{mass, kg}) - 6.1 \text{ (chest skinfold, mm)} - 1.8 \text{ (age, yr)} + 0.1 \text{ (activity questionnaire, kcal/d)} + 1060)]$$

In older women, measures of body mass, height, and menopausal status were found to best predict RMR within a standard error of estimate of ± 66 kcal/d, yielding the prediction equation:

$$[RMR\ (kcal/d) = 7.8\ (mass,\ kg) + 4.7\ (height,\ cm) - 39.5\ (menopausal$$
$$status;\ 1\text{--}3) + 143.5)]$$

These equations were derived from a population of healthy Caucasian men and women ≤ 81 yr and thus may not be applicable to other racial groups or the "oldest old" (>80 yr) population. However, these studies represented an initial attempt to more accurately predict RMR in older individuals, from data specifically obtained in this population.

Resting Metabolic Rate, Aging, and Physical Activity
Physical activity, especially in the form of endurance exercise, exerts a significant influence on energy intake [45, 86, 150, 151] and energy expenditure and is thus an important regulatory component of the energy balance equation. Both cross-sectional and exercise intervention studies have examined the influence of chronic physical training on RMR in younger individuals and report that RMR per kilogram of fat-free mass is increased by endurance training [56, 58, 91, 93 135, 148], although not universally found by others [7, 11, 49, 57, 69]. The reader is referred to earlier reviews that have addressed the influence of exercise training on younger individuals and methodological considerations that may help explain discrepant results among studies [78, 85, 88, 94]. Less information is available regarding the effects of physical activity and/or endurance training on RMR in elderly individuals. Nearly 40 years ago, Shock [126] first alluded to the possibility that physical activity may influence RMR in older individuals. At the time, Shock observed that RMR declined at a slower rate in older individuals who were more physically active in community life than in those who were institutionalized.

In one of the earliest longitudinal studies, involving 16 elite runners followed up 20 or more years later, Dill et al. [21] showed that the average decline in fat-free mass was estimated to be only 1% per decade, and RMR expressed per body surface area declined only 7.8% from the fifth to the eighth decade of life. These results should be interpreted in light of the fact that fat-free mass and body fat were not directly measured, but estimated, based on observations of runners at a later time with similar exercise training habits.

Previous cross-sectional investigations have shown that endurance-trained older men have a higher RMR than sedentary older men, independent of differences in fat-free mass and percentage body fat. For example, Lundholm et al. [64] observed that a higher RMR in 10 well-conditioned older men than in 10 sedentary older men, even after adjusting for differences in fat-free mass and body fat between the two groups. More recently, a series of experiments have examined whether physical activity attenuates the age-related decline in RMR independent of changes in body composition. Poehlman et al. [90] showed that a group of older men (≥ 59 years) who had been running an average of 55.5 ± 5.5 km per week for 15.4 ± 4.2 years had a 6% greater RMR (measured at least 36 hr after the last exercise bout) than a group of sedentary older men, independent of differences in fat-free mass. In a subsequent exercise intervention study, Poehlman and Danforth [83] endurance trained 19 older individuals [13 males and 6 females] on a cycle ergometer three times per week for 8 weeks, while maintaining the volunteers in energy balance. These investigators reported that RMR increased by 10% following endurance training, in the absence of changes in fat-free mass. Furthermore, the increase in RMR was associated with a higher rate of norepinephrine appearance into the circulation and with increased food intake. These findings suggest that an increase in RMR is found when an increase in energy expenditure is matched with a proportionate increase in food intake to maintain energy balance. Moreover, the increased RMR may be mediated by enhanced sympathetic nervous system activity. These findings suggest that a state of "increased energy flux" (e.g., increased energy intake matched to an increased level of energy expenditure) increases RMR in older individuals.

Recently, Poehlman et al. [86] examined the effects of two levels of endurance training (light and moderate intensity) on RMR in 6 healthy older men and one older woman under controlled in-patient clinical conditions. In this study, RMR was measured after (*a*) a 10-day inpatient control period (no exercise); (*b*) a 10-day light exercise period (150 kcal per session, 3 times/week); and (*c*) a 10-day moderate exercise period (300 kcal per session, 3 times/week). No significant change in RMR was found after the control (1.03 ± 0.12 kcal/min) and light exercise periods (1.04 ± 0.12 kcal/min); however, RMR increased 9% (1.13 ± 0.14 kcal/min) after moderate endurance training, despite no measurable changes in body composition (Fig. 9.3). These results possibly suggest that a threshold of energy expenditure generated by endurance exercise may be necessary to enhance RMR and subsequent food intake in elderly persons.

THERMIC EFFECT OF A MEAL, PHYSICAL ACTIVITY, AND AGING

The thermic effect of a meal is the increase in energy expenditure following food ingestion, which is due to the energy cost of digestion, transportation, and storage of nutrients. To date, only a few studies have examined the influence of age and physical activity on the thermic effect of a meal (TEM), and all of these are cross-sectional in design. The limited number of studies may be due to methodological considerations involving the length of the measurement (1–6 hr) and the limited contribution of TEM (10%) to total 24-hr energy expenditure, in comparison to RMR and the energy expenditure associated with physical activity.

In the 1950s, Tuttle et al. [136] first examined the thermic response to a protein meal in eight younger men (20–30 years) and six older men (72–84 years) during a 4.5-hr postprandial period. They found that the total area under the postprandial response curve over basal oxygen consumption

FIGURE 9.3

Changes in RMR (kcal/min) during baseline, light exercise, and moderate exercise. RMR is similar between baseline and light exercise conditions, but significantly increased (P<0.01) during moderate exercise. Bars are the mean ± SEM.

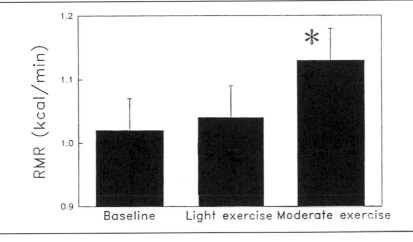

levels was similar in the younger (9.7%) and older (11.9%) men, despite the older men experiencing a blunted initial thermic response to the meal in the first 2 hr. This earlier study demonstrated that older men do not have a decrease in the thermic effect of a protein meal challenge, compared with younger men.

Not until the 1980s was the influence of age on TEM again considered. Morgan and York [71] measured the thermic response for 3 hr following administration of two mixed meals containing 480 kcal and 950 kcal in a group of younger (24 ± 0.7 yr of age) and older (71 ± 1.4 yr of age) men. Although the thermic response was positively related to the size of the meal in both groups, the older men had a significantly lower thermic response than the younger group, despite the fact that both meal challenges consisted of a relatively greater proportion of the daily food intake of the older men. The investigators hypothesized that the blunted thermogenic response in the older individuals is due to a chronic adaptation to a lower food intake in an attempt to maintain body energy stores. Golay et al. [42] observed a 25% lower thermic response to glucose ingestion as well as a decreased postprandial glucose oxidation rate in older (38–68 yr) than in younger (18–39 yr) volunteers. Bloesch et al. [10] measured TEM for 3 hours following a 75-g oral glucose load in 12 older (61 ± 3 yr) and 12 younger (25 ± 1 yr) men and showed a 15% lower thermogenic response in the older compared to the younger. These findings were recently corroborated and extended by Schwartz et al. [123], who showed that a lower thermic response to a meal in the elderly was associated with reduced sympathetic nervous system activity. These preliminary findings favor the interpretation that the lower TEM in older individuals may represent an energy conservation mechanism that contributes to their lower energy needs and propensity to accumulate body fat. In contrast, Fukagawa et al. [36] found no difference among younger men, older men, and older women in their thermic response to a protein meal challenge measured during a 6-hour postprandial period.

Influence of Physical Activity on Thermic Effect of a Meal

Because it is common for food intake to be consumed in close proximity to physical exercise, it is of interest to examine the relationship between acute and chronic exercise with meal ingestion. Schutz et al. [120] measured TEM in seven older men (68.8 ± 3 yr) at rest and during acute exercise following meals containing varying amounts of protein. The authors noted a dose-dependent response in which the higher the protein content of the meal, the greater the thermic response. Interestingly, however, TEM in combination with the exercise bout did not differ from the thermic response followed by rest. These findings do not support a potentiating caloric benefit of exercise on TEM when exercise is performed in close proximity to food ingestion by older individuals.

Two lines of evidence have recently shown that the level of physical activity may be an important modulator of TEM in older individuals. Lundholm et al. [64] examined TEM for 3 hours in 10 endurance-trained and 10 sedentary older men after ingestion of a 500 kcal liquid meal of mixed dietary composition. They found a greater TEM in the trained older men than in the untrained, whereas no differences in plasma catecholamines were noted between the groups. These findings suggested that the enhanced thermic response to a meal in older trained men was not mediated by circulating catecholamines, but by some other energy-consuming processes that remain to be identified. We have recently measured TEM for 3 hours in four separate groups of healthy men: 10 sedentary younger, 10 active younger, 7 sedentary older, and 9 active older men [92]. A mixed liquid meal with an energy content of 10 kcal·kg FFM $^{-1}$ was administered to each volunteer. The results showed no age-related differences in the thermic response to a meal challenge, although the physically active older and younger men had a significantly greater thermic effect of a meal than their age-matched sedentary counterparts. Collectively, these studies provide preliminary evidence for a potentiating effect of a physically active lifestyle on TEM in older individuals.

TOTAL ENERGY EXPENDITURE IN THE ELDERLY

This section reviews data on the age-related changes in total energy expenditure and the associated implications for the determination of energy requirements in the elderly.

Vaughan et al. [140] examined age-related differences in 24-hr energy expenditure by comparing data collected in 38 elderly men and women (71 ± 6 yr; 71.2 ± 13.5 kg) and 64 younger men and women (24 ± 4 yr; 84.5 ± 23.1 kg) living in a room calorimeter. On an absolute basis, 24-hr sedentary energy expenditure was significantly lower by 13% in the elderly (2155 ± 352 kcal·min^{-1}, vs. 1870 ± 285 kcal·min^{-1}). There was no significant difference in sedentary 24-hr energy expenditure between younger and older subjects after adjustment for differences in fat-free mass, fat mass, and gender. These date suggested that the age-related reduction in 24-hr sedentary energy expenditure is primarily explained by age-related differences in body composition.

Studies in metabolic chambers [140] offer the opportunity to quantify total energy expenditure under controlled and artificial sedentary living conditions. The recent availability of the doubly labeled water technique allows accurate quantification of total energy expenditure over extended time periods (typically 7–14 days) under free-living conditions in an unobtrusive and noninvasive manner. Since doubly labeled water is a relatively new technique for use in humans, there have only been three published studies in elderly humans to date [44, 45, 105].

The doubly labeled water technique was first introduced by Lifson et al. in the 1950s [60] as an isotopic technique for measuring carbon dioxide production rate in small animals and was originally validated in adult humans by Schoeller et al. [117, 119] and subsequently by others [19, 101, 124, 147]. As reviewed elsewhere [97, 104, 113, 115, 116), the technique has an accuracy of 5–10% relative to long-term indirect calorimetry. Speakman et al. [129] recently provided revised equations for doubly labeled water, which improved the accuracy of previously performed validation studies to approximately 3%. The theoretical precision of the doubly labeled water technique is 3–5% [17, 43, 118]. However, the experimental reliability in young, free-living males is ±12%, because of fluctuations in physical activity levels of individuals over time [43]. Under more controlled sedentary living conditions, the experimental reproducibility of the technique is ±8%, closer to theoretical estimates [46].

The doubly labeled water technique is based on the fact that deuterium-labeled water is lost from the body in the usual routes of water loss (urine, sweat, evaporative losses), whereas oxygen-18-labeled water is lost from the body in the usual routes of water loss and also via carbon dioxide production, through the carbonic anhydrase equilibrium [60]. The difference in the rate of loss of these two isotopes is therefore a function of the rate at which the body produces carbon dioxide. The assumptions of the doubly labeled water technique [60–62, 75] and the equations for calculating CO_2 production are reviewed elsewhere [98, 129].

There are advantages and disadvantages of the doubly labeled water technique, as outlined in Table 9.1. One of the major strengths of this technique is that it can be used to estimate the cost of energy expenditure during nonexercising time when used in combination with the measure-

TABLE 9.1
Advantages and Disadvantages of the Doubly Labeled Water Technique

Advantages	Disadvantages
Noninvasive and unobtrusive	Availability and expense of oxygen-18 ($\approx$\$900 for a 70-kg adult)
Measurement under free-living conditions	Reliance on isotope ratio mass spectrometry for analysis of samples
Measurements over extended time periods (7–14 days)	A direct measure of CO_2 production and not energy expenditure
Can be used to estimate activity energy expenditure when combined with measurement of resting metabolic rate	Not suitable for epidemiological studies

ment of RMR by indirect calorimetry [45]. This is of particular importance since accurate quantification of this component of daily energy expenditure has traditionally proven difficult, especially under free-living conditions. Other methods that have previously been used to estimate the daily energy cost of physical activity (e.g., activity diaries, motion sensors, heart rate monitoring) have been difficult to apply because they either require a high degree of dependence on the research subject, are too inaccurate, and/or the invasive nature of the technique applied does not exclude the possibility of a behavioral change in usual activity during the measurement period.

The disadvantages of the doubly labeled water technique make it unsuitable for large-scale epidemiologic studies. Since the doubly labeled water technique is a direct measure of CO_2 production, additional information on macronutrient oxidation during the study period is required to convert CO_2 production to O_2 consumption before energy expenditure can be calculated. Unfortunately, this issue is mistakenly associated as the major limitation of the doubly labeled water technique. During a period of energy balance, the food quotient of the diet, obtained from published population-specific data [24, 153] or calculated from dietary information [9] is used to derive O_2 consumption from CO_2 production. Even with the complete absence of information on the food quotient, the maximum error in deriving energy expenditure from carbon dioxide production rate is only 3–5% [24].

In our preliminary studies [45] of free-living total energy expenditure in healthy older subjects (7 men, 68 ± 6 yr, 77.1 ± 7.4 kg; 6 women, 64 ± 5 yr, 65.2 ± 7.8 kg), we found a high degree of interindividual variation in total energy expenditure (range 1856–3200 kcal·min^{-1}; coefficient of variation ± 18.2%). This was due primarily to interindividual variation in physical activity (range, 187–1235 kcal·min^{-1}; coefficient of variation ± 63.7%), which contributed 10–43% of total energy expenditure. Variation in total energy expenditure was most significantly related to $\dot{V}O_2$max (r=0.79), and this relationship was independent of differences in fat-free mass (Fig. 9.4). We are unsure whether the basis of this relationship is an increased total energy expenditure associated with a physically active lifestyle, leading to a higher $\dot{V}O_2$max, or alternatively, the individuals with a higher $\dot{V}O_2$max may be engaging in physical activities more frequently and intensely because of the higher work capacity. The practical implication of this finding is that $\dot{V}O_2$max should be considered a useful physiological marker for total energy expenditure and therefore a useful variable for the determination of energy requirements in healthy elderly persons.

Despite wide interindividual variation, the energy expenditure associated with physical activity could be accurately predicted from the leisure-time activity as estimated by a questionnaire [45]. This was surprising, given the relatively simple task of estimating leisure-time activity from a structured interview [133]. These results essentially validated this questionnaire as an estimate of the energy expended in leisure time, although these findings need to be repeated in a larger sample size.

Roberts et al. [105] have also used the doubly labeled water technique to measure daily energy expenditure in elderly men. Total energy expendi-

FIGURE 9.4

Partial correlation between total energy expenditure and $\dot{V}O_2$max after adjustment for fat-free mass. TEE is total energy expenditure measured over 10 days using doubly labeled water; $\dot{V}O_2$max is maximal aerobic capacity from a cycle ergometer test to exhaustion. For both variables, the residuals are the difference between the observed value and that predicted from its correlation with fat-free mass. Male subjects indicated by filled symbols, and female subjects by open symbols.

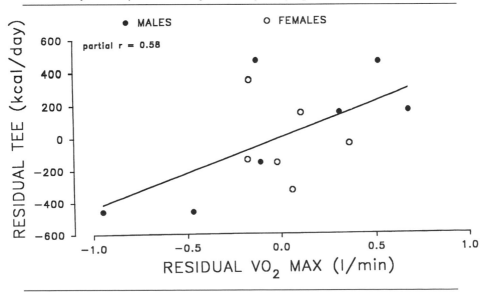

ture in 15 elderly men (69 ± 2 yr; 75.5 ± 2.5 kg) was 2,498 ± 100 kcal·d^{-1}. They found that daily energy expenditure values in the elderly were significantly higher than the RDAs for energy. These authors concluded that current RDAs for energy may significantly underestimate usual energy requirements in older men.

ENERGY REQUIREMENTS IN THE ELDERLY

Ideally, energy requirements are defined as the energy intake required to support optimal physiological function and physical activity. According to the 1985 World Health organization (WHO) report on protein and energy requirements [152], energy requirements in nonpregnant, nonlactating, and nongrowing persons are defined as the energy intake needed to match energy expenditure and should be based on measurements of energy expenditure rather than determination of energy intake. Energy requirements have traditionally been examined in the context of malnourishment, or to assess population energy requirements in developing countries. Clearly, there is a need to provide well-founded recommendations for dietary energy, not only in developing countries, but in developed countries where overnourishment (i.e., obesity) is a growing concern.

The establishment of guidelines, however, for individual energy requirements has been a problematic issue, primarily due to (*a*) reliance on the questionable nature of energy intake data; (*b*) limitations of the factorial approach to predict energy needs as multiples of resting/basal energy requirements; and (*c*) the failure to recognize the heterogeneity of the population with respect to age, body composition, and physical activity, which are important modulators of energy needs.

How energy intake data relates to energy requirements remains dubious, mainly because of the difficulty in measuring energy intake under free-living conditions. The technique of self-recording energy intake is too dependent on the motivation level and cooperation of subjects. In addition, the very act of recording energy intake may actually alter ingestive behavior, even in compliant volunteers. These methodological weaknesses have been highlighted by several studies that suggest that self-reporting energy intake is consistently underestimated, when compared with measures of total energy expenditure [6, 45, 59, 99, 114]. Our studies show that healthy older subjects underreported energy intake by 20% [45], and this effect was more pronounced in females (30% underreporting) than in males (12% underreporting). A further concern of the reliance on existing energy intake data for determining requirements is that preexisting data bases on energy intake may not be relevant to the modified lifestyle of the 1990s, particularly because of changes in physical activity patterns over the last few decades, and to increased reliance on labor-saving devices (e.g., central heating, cars) by adults [100].

An alternative method to estimate energy needs has been to rely on estimating total daily energy expenditure using a factorial approach, which uses multiples of resting energy expenditure. James et al. [51] defined the energy requirements of the elderly at approximately 1.51 times basal metabolic rate, based on subjective assessment of the activity pattern of an individual and a factorial-type calculation based on the energy costs of the various activities performed. The factorial approach, however, does not take into account two components of daily energy expenditure that contribute to individual variation: (*a*) the thermic effect of feeding, which contributes approximately 10–15% of daily energy expenditure [78, 92] and (*b*) the energy cost of nonspecific, spontaneous activity (fidgeting), which is highly variable between subjects and contributes as much as 500–700 kcal·d^{-1} in young adults, even when they are confined to a room calorimeter [102, 121]. Thus, the factorial approach in which RMR is multiplied by a constant activity factor is based on an inappropriate mathematical model for total energy expenditure, since total energy expenditure has at least three compartments (resting, physical activity, and thermic response to feeding). We have recently reviewed data from our laboratory and others to show that resting metabolic rate explains less than 50% of individual variation in total energy expenditure [14]. Stated another way, the ratio of total energy expenditure to resting energy expenditure (the activity factor) is highly variable even in the healthy elderly population [44], in which activity energy expenditure is not confounded by occupationally related energy expenditure (range of activity factor, 1.25–2.11; mean 1.51 ± 0.27). These data suggest that factors in addition to RMR need to be identified to further explain individual variation in total energy expenditure and thus more accurately predict individual energy requirements.

The doubly labeled water technique can provide a valuable tool to determine energy requirements in selected populations. Because the technique however does not lend itself to epidemiologic studies, a preferred approach is to identify biological markers of total energy expenditure, using the doubly labeled water as the "gold standard," and, thereafter develop a model enabling energy requirements to be predicted from easily measured parameters. We have used this approach in our preliminary studies to develop alternative models for estimating total energy expenditure and energy requirements to maintain body composition (Table 9.2). $\dot{V}O_2$max and leisure-time activity by questionnaire in combination explained 86% of the biological variation in total energy expenditure. Also, leisure-time activity by questionnaire in combination with RMR explained 83% of the biological variation in total energy expenditure. The limitation of these two equations is that they are based on a small group of subjects and thus need to be replicated in a larger sample of healthy older individuals. The development of equations for estimating total energy expenditure in healthy elderly people will be based on much

TABLE 9.2
Preliminary Alternative Models for Estimating Total Energy Expenditure in Healthy Elderly Persons

Equation	Total Energy Expenditure (kcal/day) =	SEE (kcal/day)	Total R^2
1	(391*$\dot{V}O_2$ max) + (0.79*LTA) + 1363	± 217	0.86
2	(1.29*LTA) + (0.98*RMR) + 387	± 242	0.83

$\dot{V}O_2$ max is maximal aerobic capacity (liters/ min), LTA is leisure time activity kcal/ day) from a 12-month recall questionnaire, and RMR is resting metabolic rate (kcal/day).

larger data bases and possibly the collection of data from several laboratories. In addition, any new equations will have to be cross-validated in independent samples. To have practical benefit, new equations for estimating energy requirements should take into account the heterogeneity of the elderly population with specific regard to body composition and physical activity level.

Effect of Exercise on Total Energy Expenditure in the Elderly
One of the goals of an exercise program is to maximize daily energy expenditure, which should theoretically result in improvements in insulin sensitivity, reduction in blood pressure, and normalization of body composition. In a recent experiment, we examined the effect of 8 weeks of endurance training on total free-living energy expenditure in the elderly [44]. Our main question was whether elderly subjects become more or less physically active during the nonexercising portion of the day in response to short-term endurance training. This is an important consideration, since the energy expenditure associated with physical activity is the most variable component of daily energy expenditure. The daily energy expenditure associated with physical activity has been shown to vary from 138 to 685 kcal/day in younger subjects confined to a calorimeter [102] and from 187 to 1,235 kcal·d^{-1} in healthy free-living elderly persons [45]. Furthermore, physical activity energy expenditure accounts for most individual variation in daily energy expenditure in younger individuals [43]. Thus, it is conceivable that an adaptation in the energy expenditure associated with physical activity can affect the overall change in total energy expenditure and body composition in response to training in older individuals, although this question has not been systematically examined.

We therefore submitted 11 healthy older individuals (56–78 yr; 5 females and 6 males) to an 8-week endurance training program. The training program involved cycling three times per week, beginning at a net energy expenditure of 150 kcal per session at 60% of $\dot{V}O_2$max in week 1, increasing to an expenditure of 300 kcal per exercise session three times per week at 85% of $\dot{V}O_2$max by week 8 [44]. The difference in energy expenditure components during the last 10 days of training, relative to the 10 days prior to beginning training, are summarized on Fig. 9.5. These data show that there was no significant increase in total daily energy expenditure (2408 ± 478 to 2474 ± 497 kcal·d^{-1}), despite an increase in energy expenditure due to (*a*) a significant increase in RMR (1596 ± 214 to 1763 ± 170 kcal/day) and (*b*) the average daily energy cost of the endurance training (equivalent to 150 kcal·d^{-1} when averaged over the 10-day doubly labeled water study period). Thus, the energy expenditure of physical activity, during nonexercising time was significantly reduced (571 ± 386 vs 340 ± 452 kcal·d^{-1}) during the last 10 days of endurance training, compared with pretraining levels.

The absence of an increase in total energy expenditure in this study suggests a compensatory "energy-conserving" reduction in spontaneous physical activity and/or a reduction in voluntary physical activities during the 10-day measurement period. Decreases in spontaneous physical activity have been shown to occur in response to strenuous physical activity in animal studies [130, 134]. It is conceivable that the level of exercise during the last

FIGURE 9.5
Adaptive changes in the components of total energy expenditure after 8 weeks of endurance training in healthy elderly persons. A summary of the components of total energy expenditure (TEE) in the "average" elderly person before and during the last 10 days of vigorous endurance training. TEE measured over 10 days under free living conditions with doubly labeled water; resting metabolic rate (RMR) measured upon wakening by respiratory gas analysis; thermic effect of a meal (TEM) assumed to be 10% of TEE; TRAINING is the daily energy cost of the structured activity when averaged over the 10-day doubly labeled water study period (i.e., 5 sessions of 300 kcal over 10 days); the energy expenditure of physical activity (EEPA) derived from the difference between TEE and RMR after adjusting for the thermic response to feeding and the energy cost of the structured activity.

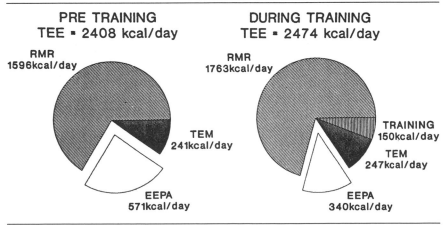

PRE TRAINING
TEE ▪ 2408 kcal/day

RMR
1596kcal/day

TEM
241kcal/day

EEPA
571kcal/day

DURING TRAINING
TEE ▪ 2474 kcal/day

RMR
1763kcal/day

TRAINING
150kcal/day

TEM
247kcal/day

EEPA
340kcal/day

week of training (3 hours per week at 85% of $\dot{V}O_2$max) was too vigorous and thus fatigued the elderly participants during the remainder of the day. Another possibility was that the exercise program was too short for individuals to adapt to the increased energy demands, and a long-term exercise program may yield increases in daily energy expenditure. Nonetheless, from a clinical perspective, our results could be interpreted to indicate that vigorous endurance exercise should not be recommended to the elderly as the most efficient exercise prescription because of its blunting effect on physical activity during nonexercising time. Furthermore, it can no longer be assumed that participation in high-intensity endurance exercise will result in a net increase in daily energy expenditure in elderly persons.

Our findings, however, should not be interpreted to indicate that all levels of endurance training will not increase total daily energy expenditure. Exercise prescriptions of lower intensity and varying durations should be examined to verify their influence on total energy expenditure, its components, and cardiovascular risk factors, since it is conceivable that a lower level of endurance training may increase the energy expenditure of physical activity, as well as total daily energy expenditure.

ENERGY INTAKE AND AGING

The decline in energy and macronutrient intake with advancing age is a consistent finding [23, 47, 65, 66, 110] in the scientific literature. Recent longitudinal data collected over a 6-year time period reported a decline of 307 kcal·d⁻¹y⁻¹ in older females and a 395 kcal·d⁻¹y⁻¹ decline in older males [40]. Furthermore, it is estimated that 30% of community-dwelling older persons have diets deficient in at least one major nutrient [72]. Ryan et al. [110], using a national household survey of food consumption practices of individuals 65 years of age and older, found that a large proportion of noninstitutionalized elderly Americans consume diets that fail to meet dietary standards. More specifically, approximately 40% of persons 65 years of age and older had mean energy intakes below two-thirds the recommended daily allowance. In general, the methodology used to assess habitual energy intake in the elderly has relied upon 24-hr recall, 3- and/or 7-day food diaries, or food frequency questionnaires. A recent study in our laboratory [44] suggested a significant underreporting of energy intake by as much as 30% in older individuals, compared with measurement of daily energy expenditure, as assessed from doubly labeled water. If the underreporting of energy intake is a consistent finding in older persons, it is possible that the age-related decline in energy intake is less than previously reported.

Energy Intake, Aging, and Physical Activity
A more complete understanding of the role of exercise and its influence on energy balance requires a rudimentary examination of the relationship

between energy intake and physical activity. Voorrips et al. [142] compared two groups of elderly women with different patterns of daily physical activity for dietary intake and nutritional status. Interestingly, the nutrient intake of both groups showed little differences. If these individuals were in energy balance, the absence of significant differences in energy intake between the active (1643 ± 333 kcal·d^{-1}; n=25) and inactive women (1761 ± 381 kcal·d^{-1} kcal·d^{-1}; n=23) suggests an underreporting of energy intake in the physically active women. Other studies have found a 7% greater energy intake in physically active males than in inactive males, but no difference was found between active and inactive females [68].

We have previously postulated that the energy expenditure associated with physical activity may be one physiological signal involved in the regulation of energy balance [86]. Unfortunately, the influence of physical activity on voluntary food intake has proven to be a difficult area to examine because of limitations in experimental designs and the myriad of physiological and psychological factors that influence food intake and exercise behavior. Most studies that have examined the relationship between physical activity and energy intake have been performed in younger individuals. For example, in exercise training experiments, energy intake has been reported to be unaffected in both lean [67] and obese individuals [22]. However, the net increase in the energy expenditure of physical activity in these studies was small (100 kcal/d) and of short duration. Furthermore, volunteers either recorded their own food intakes and/or were aware of the study's hypothesis. The meticulous studies of Woo and Pi-Sunyer [150, 151] showed that young, lean women maintained energy balance by increasing food intake in response to moderate physical activity, whereas obese women did not match intake to the increase in energy expenditure. Until recently, no studies have systematically examined the interrelationships between physical activity and spontaneous energy intake in older persons.

We have recently examined the effects of two levels of endurance training (light and moderate exercise) on covertly monitored voluntary energy intake under controlled living conditions [86]. Energy intake was measured by covert assessment in a clinical research environment during (*a*) a 10-day inpatient control period (no exercise), (*b*) a 10-day light exercise period (150 kcal per session, 3 times/wk), and (*c*) a 10-day moderate exercise period (300 kcal per session, 3 times/wk). No significant change in energy intake was found between the control (2378 ± 130 kcal/d) and light exercise (2449 ± 161 kcal·d^{-1}) periods, whereas energy intake increased 17% ($P<0.01$) during moderate exercise (2785 ± 161 kcal·d^{-1}), compared with the control period. The relative macronutrient intake was not different among the three experimental conditions, suggesting that endurance training does not selectively influence the percentage of macronutrient intake in older persons. We interpret these findings to suggest that the normal processes that regulate energy intake in response to moderate exercise are fundamentally intact in nonobese older individuals. Identification of a threshold of energy expenditure that affects food intake may have nutritional relevance in the older population. Nutrient requirements of the elderly are considered to be at least equal to those of younger adults [74], and in some cases higher intakes of specific nutrients (i.e., protein and calcium) have been recommended [41, 139]. Because energy intake generally declines with age [23], intake of specific nutrients would also probably decline. Therefore, clinical interventions that stimulate energy expenditure and hence, energy intake while maintaining energy balance would enhance nutritional and cardiovascular health.

INSULIN-LIKE GROWTH FACTOR-1 AND AGING

We now focus on insulin-like growth factor-1 and norepinephrine. Specifically, we first consider the effects of aging on these hormones (or neurotransmitters) and their interaction with chronic exercise training.

The insulin-like growth factors, IGF-I and II, are small peptides that are structurally related to insulin. These hormones were first described on the basis of their stimulation of anabolic processes in cartilage [112]. Subsequent work has established their effects on growth of bone [13] and muscle cells [27]. The aforementioned work suggests that IGF-1 might play an important role in the maintenance as well as the formation of these tissues. Recently, there has been a great deal of interest in the role of IGF-1 in reversing several catabolic processes with advancing age. The hypothesis has been put forward that blunted secretion of IGF-1 and growth hormone in aging humans contributes to the decrease in muscle mass, accumulation of total body fat, and reduced muscular strength [52, 108].

In the absence of disease states that impair IGF-1 production, plasma IGF-1 concentration reflects the integrated secretion of growth hormone. Similar to a decline in growth hormone production with advancing age, it is commonly found that plasma levels of IGF-1 are reduced in aging men [109, 141] and women [109, 132]. Clemmons and Van Wyk examined IGF-1 in a cross-sectional study of 226 normal adults [16]. They observed a progressive decline in IGF-1 from age 20 through age 60. Levels of circulating IGF-1 measured in adults in their seventh decade were approximately half of those at age 20. Florini et al. [30] investigated the relationship between growth hormone secretion and IGF-1 levels as a function of age in healthy men. Because blood samples were taken over a 24-hr period, it was possible to analyze for relationships between average IGF-1 levels and growth hormone secretion. They found a significant correlation between IGF-1 level and 24-hr integrated growth hormone level and postulated that lower blood levels of IGF-1 in older men may be responsible for the age-related catabolic effects on muscle and bone. To our knowledge, however, no longitudinal studies have been performed to examine age-related changes in IGF-1 concentrations.

Insulin-like Growth Factor-1, Aging, and Physical Activity
It is presently unclear whether the decline in plasma levels of IGF-1 with advancing age reflects the effects of aging itself or the influences of changes in lifestyle. Several recent studies suggest that lifestyle and environmental factors interact with the aging process to modulate IGF-1. For example, short-term periods of energy deficit are associated with a reduction in IGF-1 [15], whereas short-term energy surplus is associated with an increase in IGF-1 [33]. The macronutrient composition of the diet, particularly dietary protein, influences plasma concentrations of IGF-1 [50]. Recently, several investigators have reported that adiposity is positively associated with IGF-1 [18, 109], since indices of obesity correlated highly with IGF-1, independent of age. In these prior studies, however, the possibility that increased adiposity reflected lower levels of physical activity was not considered.

Recent cross-sectional studies suggest that physical activity may be an independent modulator of plasma levels of IGF-1 in healthy individuals. Rudman [108] found that IGF-1 correlated positively with a questionnaire of daily physical activities in older free-living and institutionalized men. Kelly et al. [53] found a positive relationship between plasma levels of IGF-1 and predicted $\dot{V}O_2max$ in 134 individuals (r=0.47; P<0.01), and this relationship persisted in a group of postmenopausal women (r=50; P<0.01). Poehlman and Copeland [82] showed that serum levels of IGF-1 were 33% lower in older men than in younger men. Furthermore, measured $\dot{V}O_2max$ was found to be the best single predictor of serum levels of IGF-1 in these populations. We interpreted these findings to suggest that IGF-1 is influenced primarily by the level of physical activity rather than adiposity and age, per se.

We have recently performed an exercise intervention study to examine the effects of 8 weeks of endurance training on changes in IGF-1, IGF-1 binding protein-1 (IGFBP-1), IGFBP-3, and $\dot{V}O_2max$ in 10 older men and 8 older women [95]. As expected, endurance training increased $\dot{V}O_2max$ in males (14%) and females (14%), but females showed a smaller increase in IGF-1 (8%) than males (19%). The correlation between changes in $\dot{V}O_2max$ and IGF-1 was significant in males (r=0.79; P<0.02), but not in females (r=0.22; NS). No group changes were noted in IGFBP-1, the binding protein implicated in the regulation of glucose homeostasis, or the growth hormone–dependent IGFBP-3. However, individual changes between IGF-1 and IGFBP-3 showed a tendency to be related in males (r=0.48; P=0.15) but not in females (-0.21; NS; Fig. 9.6). Since circulating concentrations of IGF-1 in well-nourished individuals closely reflect growth hormone secretion, our results suggest that endurance training might influence the growth hormone/IGF-1-axis in a sexual dimorphic fashion. Furthermore, the trend for a significant relationship between changes in

FIGURE 9.6

Pearson product correlations between the absolute changes in IGF-1 and V̇O₂max in males (r=0.73; P<0.01) and females (r=0.17; NS) in response to endurance training. The regression equation for males is, change in IGF-1(ng·ml⁻¹) - 7.201 + 28.273 (V̇O₂max, liter·min⁻¹).

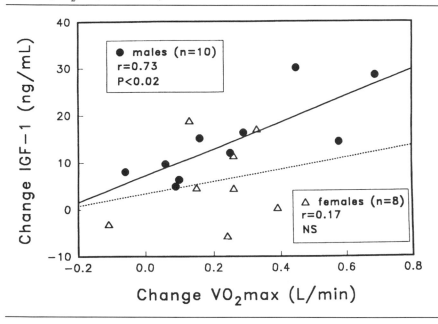

IGF-1 and IGFBP-3 in males, but not in females, suggests that the increase in IGF-1 may depend on growth hormone action in males but less so in females. Further studies should prolong the exercise training program and increase the sample size of men and women to more fully explore gender differences in IGF-1 and IGFBP-3 in response to chronic exercise. Collectively, these findings lend further support to the concept that some of the hormonal (e.g., the age-associated decline in IGF-1) and somatic (e.g., the associated decline in fitness) correlates of aging can be ameliorated by participation in an endurance training regimen.

SYMPATHETIC NERVOUS SYSTEM ACTIVITY AND AGING

The sympathoadrenal system is composed of the sympathetic nervous system and the adrenal medullae. Norepinephrine and epinephrine are the major neurohumoral messengers of the sympathoadrenal system in humans [63, 125], and they play key roles in the metabolic adaptation to stressors encountered in the external environment that serve to regulate physiological functions such as blood pressure, body temperature, and fuel metabolism within a narrow range.

It is now accepted that aging is associated with an increase in resting sympathetic nervous system activity, as estimated from plasma concentrations of norepinephrine [26, 28, 73]. Using tracer-labeled norepinephrine to estimate norepinephrine kinetics, the age-related increase in sympathetic tone has generally been attributed to an increase in plasma norepinephrine appearance [28, 89, 122]. Supiano et al. [131] have suggested, using compartmental analysis, that the increase in norepinephrine appearance in the elderly reflects an increase in extravascular release and not an increase in the processes that affect the transfer of norepinephrine into the circulation. That sympathetic nervous system activity increases with age is also supported by Wallin et al. [143], who observed that the number of impulses in sympathetic nerves to muscles increased with age. Although the results are still controversial, the heightened sympathetic tone has been reported to play a role in contributing to such medical complications as hypertension [25] and hyperlipidemia [111].

Sympathetic Nervous System Activity, Aging, and Physical Activity
It could be hypothesized that the age-related changes in the sympathetic nervous system are influenced by alterations in lifestyle that result in a decrease in physical activity and an increase in body fat rather than a true aging effect per se. Since each bout of exercise activates the sympathetic outflow to many organs, adaptive changes in older individuals might be predicted in the resting noradrenergic system as a result of long-term participation in physical activity. However, the effects of chronic physical activity on resting sympathetic tone has received little attention.

We have recently performed a cross-sectional study to examine the effects of age and level of physical activity on plasma norepinephrine kinetics in 67 younger and older healthy individuals well-characterized for their level of maximal aerobic fitness ($\dot{V}O_2$max) and body composition [89]. We found no significant differences between younger active and younger inactive men for plasma norepinephrine appearance or clearance into circulation. On the other hand, we found a higher rate of norepinephrine appearance in active older men than in inactive older men. This finding suggests that physically active older men have higher resting sympathetic tone because of an elevated rate of norepinephrine appearance. No effects of age or physical activity on norepinephrine clearance were found. These preliminary findings suggest that it is important to consider the habitual level of physical activity when evaluating sympathetic nervous system activity in healthy older men.

Because it is unclear whether introduction of physical activity in a previously inactive population influences sympathetic nervous system activity in older persons, we have recently performed exercise intervention studies to examine the impact of endurance training on norepinephrine kinetics, resting metabolic rate, and fatty acid oxidation. Specifically, we examined the effects of an 8-week endurance training program (cycling exercise) on RMR and norepinephrine kinetics in 13 males and 6 females. We found that training increased RMR by 10%, $\dot{V}O_2$max by 14%, and estimated energy intake by 12%, in the absence of changes in body composition. The increase in RMR was associated with a higher rate of norepinephrine appearance (r=0.57; P<0.05) and an increase in energy intake (r=0.56; P<0.05). Together, these factors accounted for 49% (r^2) of the variation of change in RMR. These findings suggest that the increase in RMR is partially mediated by an increased norepinephrine appearance rate and increased food intake in healthy older individuals. To our knowledge, only one other study has examined the influence of endurance training on RMR in older individuals, and they did not find a training effect on resting metabolic rate [69]. Perhaps the fact that the volunteers trained at a greater intensity in our study than in the training program of Meredith et al. may have contributed to the observed higher RMR, because higher training intensities have been shown to enhance metabolic rate [58].

The rate of free fatty acid mobilization from adipose tissue stores is generally considered to represent an important regulatory step controlling oxidative metabolism in working muscles, particularly during long-term exercise [38]. Sympathetic nervous system activity probably plays an important role, as catecholamines are important hormones influencing lipolysis in adult humans [4]. We recently examined the metabolic link between changes in norepinephrine kinetics and in vivo fat oxidation in response to endurance training in older individuals [84]. Fatty acid appearance (a measure of fatty acid availability) was determined from ^{14}C-palmitate infusion, and norepinephrine kinetics from infusion of ^{3}H-NE. We found that endurance training did not alter basal levels of free fatty acid appearance, but increased fat oxidation by 22%. Furthermore, the increase in norepinephrine appearance rate was associated with an increase in fat oxidation (r=0.69; P<0.01; Fig. 9.7) and resting metabolic rate (r=0.81; P<0.01). This study provides initial support for the involvement of a sympathetic component mediating changes in in vivo fat oxidation. Collectively, we would like to suggest the hypothesis that training-induced increases in sympathetic nervous system play a central role in shifting disposal of free fatty acids from nonoxidative to oxidative pathways and in increasing RMR in older individuals. A schematic diagram of this proposed hypothesis is depicted in Figure 9.8.

Two lines of evidence from the aforementioned studies suggest that regular endurance training may be of benefit in the regulation of energy balance with advancing age via its impact on resting metabolic rate and substrate utilization patterns. Ravussin et al. [103] has shown that a low resting metabolic rate after normalization for differences in body composition was associated with increased body weight. We have consistently found that endurance training increases RMR on the order of 8–10% in older

FIGURE 9.7

The relationship between change in fatty acid oxidation (as measured from ^{14}C palmitate infusion and indirect calorimetry) with the change in norepinephrine (NE) appearance in 17 older individuals.

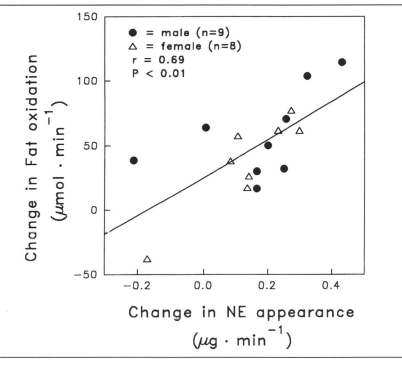

individuals, independent of changes in body composition [83, 86]. Second, a low ratio of fat oxidation to carbohydrate oxidation, as reflected in a higher 24-hr respiratory quotient [154], has been found to be an additional risk predisposing individuals to subsequent gain in body weight. Our results point toward a lowering of the fasting respiratory quotient and enhanced fatty acid oxidation in response to endurance training in older individuals.

SUMMARY

In summary, data suggest that the decline in RMR with advancing age is primarily related to the decline in fat-free mass. However, in addition to the erosion of fat-free mass, other factors such as Na-K pump activity, fat mass, maximal aerobic power, and menopausal status are important determinants influencing the decline in RMR in older individuals. Second, we provide revised prediction equations for RMR that are both gender- and sex-specific and use easily measured variables to facilitate their use in

FIGURE 9.8

A proposed hypothesis to link changes in energy expenditure, substrate utilization, and body composition in response to endurance training. The metabolic benefits of exercise are amplified when a large increase in total daily energy expenditure results from prolonged, low-intensity endurance exercise due to (a) the direct energy cost of the exercise; (b) an increase in resting metabolic rate (RMR) and a high level of nonexercising energy expenditure (NEEE). The net increase in daily energy expenditure will drive a higher rate of norepinephrine appearance into circulation and increased levels of fatty acid oxidation. This metabolic scenario will optimize the loss of body fat.

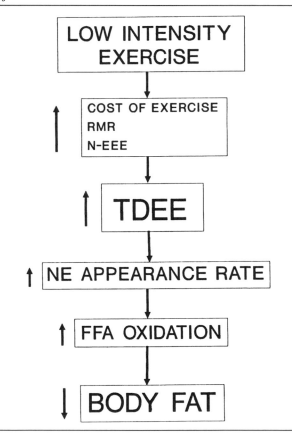

clinical and field settings. Third, preliminary studies suggest that older individuals may have a reduced energy expenditure following meal ingestion, although this is not a universal finding among investigators. Furthermore, several studies suggest that physically active older men exhibit higher thermic responses to a meal than sedentary older men. Data on total energy expenditure in free-living elderly persons are sparse.

However the available data suggest that there is large variation in total energy expenditure in the elderly population, caused primarily by differences in physical activity. The heterogeneity in physical activity makes estimation of individual energy requirements difficult. However, preliminary studies have suggested that measurement of $\dot{V}O_2$max and other activity indices may be useful markers for estimating energy requirements on an individual basis. Furthermore, attempting to "normalize" total energy expenditure in the elderly by prescribing physical activity is not as straightforward as it seems, due to exercise-induced compensatory reductions in physical activity during the remainder of the day. Levels of insulin-like growth factor-1 decline with advancing age. Preliminary evidence from cross-sectional and exercise intervention studies suggest that the lower serum levels of IGF-1 in older individuals may be partially due to diminished physical activity. Aging is associated with an increase in fasting levels of norepinephrine, primarily influenced by an elevated rate of norepinephrine into circulation; however, the clinical significance of the elevated sympathetic tone is unclear. Endurance training in older individuals has been found to increase basal levels of norepinephrine appearance into circulation, and this has been associated with an increased RMR and enhanced fat oxidation. Optimal exercise interventions need to be identified for the elderly, which maximally increase daily energy expenditure and offset metabolic deterioration with advancing age.

ACKNOWLEDGMENTS

Gratitude is expressed to all the volunteers that made this study possible. Special appreciation is extended to all colleagues at the University of Vermont and University of Maryland whose input and scientific exchange were instrumental in the conduct of this work. Dr. Eric T. Poehlman is supported by a grant from National Institute of Aging, (AG-07857), a Research Career and Development Award from the National Institute of Aging (KO4 AG00564), the American Association of Retired Persons Andrus Foundation (AARP), and a Biomedical Research Grant from the University of Vermont. Dr. M. I. Goran is supported by a grant from the American Diabetes Association, the National Institute of Child Health and Human Development, and the United States Department of Agriculture.

REFERENCES

1. Arciero, P. J., M. I. Goran, E. T. Poehlman. Resting metabolic rate is lower in females compared to males. *J. Appl. Physiol.* 75:2514–2520, 1993.
2. Arciero, P. J., M. I. Goran, A. W. Gardner, P. A. Ades, R. S. Tyzbir, and E. T. Poehlman. A practical equation to predict resting metabolic rate in older men. *Metabolism* 42:950–957, 1993.

3. Arciero, P. J., M. I. Goran, A. W. Gardner, P. A. Ades, R. S. Tyzbir, and E. T. Poehlman. A practical equation to predict resting metabolic rate in older females. *J. Am. Geriat. Soc.* 41:389–395, 1993.

4. Arner, P. Control of lipolysis and its relevance to development of obesity in man. *Diabetes Metab. Rev.* 4:507–515, 1988.

5. Bandini, L. G., and W. H. Dietz. Obesity in childhood and adolescence. *Growth Genet. Horm.* 7:6–9, 1991.

6. Bandini, L. G., D. A. Schoeller, H. N. Cyr, and W. H. Dietz. Validity of reported energy intake in obese and nonobese adolescents. *Am. J. Clin. Nutr.* 52:421–425, 1990.

7. Bingham, S. A., G. R. Goldberg, W. A. Coward, A. M. Prentice, and J. H. Cummings. The effect of exercise and improved fitness on basal metabolic rate. *Br. J. Nutr.* 61:155–173, 1989.

8. Bisdee, J. T., W. P. T. James, and M. A. Shaw. Changes in energy expenditure during the menstrual cycle. *Br. J. Nutr.* 61:187–199, 1989.

9. Black, A. E., A. M. Prentice, and W. A. Coward. Use of food quotients to predict respiratory quotients for the doubly- labelled water method of measuring energy expenditure. *Hum. Nutr. Clin. Nutr.* 40c:381–391, 1986.

10. Bloesch, D., Y. Schutz, E. Breitenstein, E. Jequier, and J. P. Felber. Thermogenic response to an oral glucose load in man: comparison between young and elderly subjects. *J. Am. Coll. Nutr.* 7:471–473, 1988.

11. Broeder, C. E., K. A. Burrhus, L. S. Svanevik, and J. H. Wilmore. The effects of aerobic fitness on resting metabolic rate. *Am. J. Clin. Nutr.* 55:795–801, 1992.

12. Calloway, D. H., and E. Zanni. Energy requirements and energy expenditure of elderly men. *Am. J. Clin. Nutr.* 33:2088–2092, 1980.

13. Canalis, E. The hormonal and local regulation of bone formation. *Endocrine Rev.* 3:62–77, 1983.

14. Carpenter, W. H., E. T. Poehlman, M. O'Connell, and M. I. Goran. A proposal for normalizing total energy expenditure based upon a meta-analysis. 1994. (In press).

15. Clemmons, D. R., A. Klibanski, L. E. Underwood, et al. Reduction of plasma immunoreactive somatomedin-C during fasting in humans. *J. Clin. Endocrinol.* 53:1247–1250, 1981.

16. Clemmons, D. R., and J. J. Van Wyk. Factors controlling blood concentrations of somatomedin C. *J. Clin. Endocrinol. Metab.* 13:113–143, 1984.

17. Cole, T. J., and W. A. Coward. Precision and accuracy of doubly labeled water energy expenditure by multipoint and two-point methods. *Am. J. Physiol.* 263:E965–E973, 1992.

18. Copeland, K. C., R. B. Colletti, J. D. Devlin, and T. L. McAuliffe. The relationship between insulin-like growth factor-1, adiposity and aging. *Metabolism* 39:584–587, 1990.

19. Coward, W. A., A. M. Prentice, P. R. Murgatroyd, et al. Measurement of CO_2 and water production rates in man using ^2H, ^{18}O-labelled H_2O; comparisons between calorimeter and isotope values. A. J. H. van Es (ed). *Human Energy Metabolism: Physical Activity and Energy Expenditure Measurements in Epidemiological Research Based upon Direct and Indirect Calorimetry.* Wageningen: Euro Nutrition Report 5; CIP-gegevens Koninklijke Bibliotheek, Den Haag, 1984, pp. 126–128.

20. Després, J-P., S. Moorjani, P. J. Lupien, A. Tremblay, A. Nadeau, and C. Bouchard. Regional distribution of body fat, plasma lipoproteins, and cardiovascular disease. *Arteriosclerosis* 10:497–511, 1990.

21. Dill, D. B., S. Robinson, and J. C. Ross. A longitudinal study of 16 champion runners. *J. Sports Med.* 7:4–27, 1967.

22. Durrant, M. L., J. P. Royston, and R. T. Wloch. Effect of exercise on energy intake and eating patterns in lean and obese humans. *Physiol. Behav.* 29:449–454, 1982.

23. Elahi, V. K., D. Elahi, R. Andres, J. D. Tobin, M. G. Butler, and A. H. Norris. A longitudinal study of nutritional intake in men. *J. Gerontol.* 38:162–180, 1983.

24. Elia, M. Energy equivalents of CO_2 and their importance in assessing energy expenditure when using tracer techniques. *Am. J. Physiol.* 260:E75–E88, 1991.

25. Esler, M., G. Jackman, A. Bobik, et al. Norepinephrine kinetics in essential hypertension.

Defective neuronal uptake of norepinephrine in some patients. *Hypertension* 3:149–156, 1981.

26. Esler, M., H. Skews, P. Leonard, G. Jackman, A. Bobik, and P. Korner. Age-dependence of norepinephrine kinetics in normal subjects. *Clin. Sci. Lond.* 60:217–219, 1981.

27. Ewton, D. Z., and J. R. Florini. Relative effects of somatomedins, multiplication-stimulating activity, and growth hormone on myoblasts and myotubes in culture. *Endocrinol.* 106:577–583, 1980.

28. Featherstone, J. A., R. C. Veith, D. Flatness, M. M. Murburg, E. C. Villacres, and J. B. Halter. Age and alpha-2 adrenergic regulation of plasma norepinephrine kinetics in human. *J. Gerontol.* 42:271–276, 1987.

29. Ferraro, R. S., A. M. Lillioja, A-M. Fontvieille, R. Rising, C. Bogardus, and E. Ravussin. Lower sedentary metabolic rate in women compared to men. *J. Clin. Invest.* 90:1–5, 1992.

30. Florini, J. R., P. N. Prinz, M. V. Vitello, and R. L. Hinz. Somatomedin-C levels in healthy young and older men: relationship to peak and 24-h integrated levels of growth hormone. *J. Gerontol.* 40:2–7, 1985.

31. Flynn, M. A., G. B. Nolph, A. S. Baker, W. M. Martin, and G. Krause. Total body potassium in aging humans: a longitudinal study. *Am. J. Clin. Nutr.* 50:713–717, 1989.

32. Forbes, G. B. The adult decline in lean body mass. *Hum. Biol.* 48:162–173, 1976.

33. Forbes, G. B., M. R. Brown, S. L. Welle, and L. E. Underwood. Hormonal response to overfeeding. *Am. J. Clin. Nutr.* 49:608–611, 1989.

34. Forbes, G. B., and J. C. Reina. Adult lean body mass declines with age: some longitudinal observations. *Metabolism* 19:653–663, 1970.

35. Fredrix, E. W. H. M., P. B. Soeters, I. M. Deerenberg, et al. Resting and sleeping energy expenditure in the elderly. *Eur. J. Clin. Nutr.* 44:741–747, 1990.

36. Fukagawa, N. K., L. G. Bandini, P. H. Lim, et al. Protein-induced changes in energy expenditure in young and older individuals. *Am. J. Physiol.* 260:E345–E352, 1991.

37. Fukagawa, N. A., L. G. Bandini, and J. B. Young. Effect of age on body composition and resting metabolic rate. *Am. J. Physiol.* 259:E233–E238, 1990.

38. Galbo, J. Hormonal and Metabolic Adaptation to Exercise. New York: Thieme-Stratton, 1983.

39. Gardner, A. W., and E. T. Poehlman. Physical activity is a significant predictor of body density in women. *Am. J. Clin. Nutr.* 57:8–14, 1993.

40. Garry, P. H., R. L. Rhyne, L. Halioua, and C. Nicholson. Changes in dietary patterns over a 6-year period in an elderly population. *Ann. N. Y. Acad. Sci.* S61:104–112, 1989.

41. Gersovitz, M., K. Motil, H. N. Munro, N. S. Scrimshaw, and V. R. Young. Human protein requirements: assessment of the adequacy of the current recommended dietary allowance for dietary protein in elderly men and women. *Am. J. Clin. Nutr.* 35:6–14, 1982.

42. Golay, A., Y. Schutz, C. Broquet, et al. Decreased thermogenic response to an oral glucose load in older subjects. *J. Am. Geriat. Soc.* 31:144–148, 1983.

43. Goran, M. I., W. H. Beer, E. T. Poehlman, R. R. Wolfe, and V. R. Young. Variation in total energy expenditure in young, healthy free living men. *Metabolism* 42:487–496, 1993.

44. Goran, M. I., and E. T. Poehlman. Endurance training does not enhance total energy expenditure in healthy older persons. *Am. J. Physiol.* 263:E950–E957, 1992.

45. Goran, M. I., and E. T. Poehlman. Total energy expenditure and energy requirements in healthy elderly persons. *Metabolism* 41:744–753, 1992.

46. Goran, M. I., E. T. Poehlman, and E. Danforth, Jr. Experimental reliability of the doubly labeled water technique. 1994. (In press)

47. Hallfrisch, J., D. Muller, D. Drinkwater, J. Tobin, and R. Andres. Continuing diet trends in men: the Baltimore longitudinal study of aging (1961–1987). *J. Gerontol.* 45:M186–M191, 1990.

48. Harris, J. A., and F. G. Benedict. *A Biometric Study of Basal Metabolism in Man.* Washington, D.C.: Carnegie Institution of Washington, (Carnegie Institute of Washington publication 279), 1919.

49. Hill, J. O., S. B. Heymsfield, C. B. McManus, and M. DiGirolamo. Meal size and the

thermic response to food in male subjects as a function of maximum aerobic capacity. *Metabolism* 33:743–749, 1984.

50. Isley, W. L., L. E. Underwood, and D. R. Clemmons. Changes in plasma somatomedin-C in response to ingestion of diets with variable protein and energy content. *JPEN* 8:407–411, 1984.

51. James, W. P. T., A. Ralph, and A. Ferro-Luzzi. Energy needs of the elderly: a new approach. H. N. Munro and D. E. Danford (eds). *Human Nutrition. A Comprehensive Treatise, vol. 6: Nutrition, Aging, and the Elderly.* New York: Plenum, 1989, pp. 129–151.

52. Kelijman M. Age-related alterations of the growth hormone/insulin like-growth-factor 1 axis. *J. Am. Geriatr. Soc.* 39:295–307, 1991.

53. Kelley, P. J., J. A. Eisman, M. C. Stuart, N. A. Pocock, P. N. Sambrook, and T. H. Gwinn. Somatomedin-C, physical fitness, and bone density. *J. Clin. Endocrinol. Metab.* 70:718–723, 1990.

54. Keys, A. H., H. L. Taylor, and F. Grande. Basal metabolism and age of adult man. *Metabolism* 22:579–587, 1973.

55. Kohrt, W. M., M. T. Malley, G. P. Dalsky, and J. O. Holloszy. Body composition of healthy sedentary and trained, young and old men and women. *Med. Sci. Sports Exerc.* 24:832–837, 1992.

56. Lawson, S., J. D. Webster, P. J. Pacy, and J. S. Garrow. Effect of a 10-week aerobic exercise programme on metabolic rate, body composition and fitness in lean sedentary females. *Br. J. Clin. Prac.* 41:684–688, 1987.

57. LeBlanc, J., P. Diamond, J. Cote, and A. Labrie. Hormonal factors in reduced postprandial heat production of exercise trained subjects. *J. Appl. Physiol.* 56:772–776, 1984.

58. Lennon, D., F. Nagle, F. Stratman, E. Shrago, and S. Dennis. Diet and exercise training effects on resting metabolic rate. *Int. J. Obesity* 9:39–47, 1985.

59. Lichtman, S. W., K. Pisarska, E. R. Berman, et al. Discrepancy between self-reported and actual caloric intake and exercise in obese subjects. *N. Engl. J. Med.* 327:1893–1898, 1992.

60. Lifson, N., G. B. Gordon, and R. McClintock. Measurement of total carbon dioxide production by means of $D_2{}^{18}O$. *J. Appl. Physiol.* 7:704–710, 1955.

61. Lifson, N., W. S. Little, D. G. Levitt, and R. M. Henderson. $D_2{}^{18}O$ (deuterium oxide) method for CO_2 output in small mammals and economic feasibility in man. *J. Appl. Physiol.* 39:657–664, 1975.

62. Lifson, N., and R. McClintock. Theory of use of the turnover rates of body water for measuring energy and material balance. *J. Theor. Biol.* 12:46–74, 1966.

63. Linares, O. A., and J. B. Halter. Sympathochromaffin system activity in the elderly. *J. Am. Geriat. Soc.* 35:448–453, 1987.

64. Lundholm, K., G. Holm, L. Lindmark, et al. Thermogenic effect of food in physically well-trained elderly men. *Eur. J. Appl. Physiol.* 55:486–492, 1986.

65. McGandy, R. B., C. H. Barrows, A. Spanias, A. Meredith, J. L. Stone, and A. H. Norris. Nutrient intakes and energy expenditure in men of different ages. *J. Gerontol.* 21:581–587, 1966.

66. McGandy, R. B., R. M. Russell, S. C. Hartz, et al. Nutritional status survey of healthy noninstitutionalized elderly: energy and nutrient intakes from three-day diet records and nutrient supplements. *Nutr. Res.* 6:785–798, 1986.

67. McGowan, C. R., L. H. Epstein, D. J. Kupfer, D. J. Bulik, and R. J. Robertson. The effect of exercise on non-restricted caloric intake in male joggers. *Appetite* 7:97–105, 1986.

68. Mensink, G. B. M., and L. Arab. Relationships between nutrient intake, nutritional status and activity levels in an elderly and in a younger population; a comparison of physically more active and more inactive people. *Zeitschrift Gerontol.* 22:16–25, 1989.

69. Meredith, C. N., W. R. Frontera, E. C. Fisher, et al. Peripheral effects of endurance training in young and older subjects. *J. Appl. Physiol.* 66:2844–2849, 1989.

70. Mifflin, M. D., S. T. St. Jeor, L. A. Hill, et al. A new predictive equation for resting energy expenditure in healthy individuals. *Am. J. Clin. Nutr.* 51:241–247, 1990.

71. Morgan, J. B., and D. A. York. Thermic effect of feeding in relation to energy balance in elderly men. *Ann. Nutr. Metab.* 27:71–77, 1983.

72. Morley, J. E. Nutritional status of the elderly. *Am J. Med.* 81:679–695, 1986.

73. Morrow, L. A., O. A. Linares, T. J. Hill, et al. Age differences in the plasma clearance mechanisms for epinephrine and norepinephrine in humans. *J. Clin. Endocrinol. Metab.* 65:508–511, 1987.

74. Munro, H. N., P. M. Suter, and R. M. Russell. Nutritional requirements of the elderly. *Annu. Rev. Nutr.* 7:23–49, 1987.

75. Nagy, K. A. CO_2 production in animals: analysis of potential errors in the doubly labeled water method. *Am. J. Physiol.* 238:R466–R473, 1980.

76. Novak, L. P. Aging, total body potassium, fat-free mass, and cell mass in males and females between ages 18 and 85 years. *J. Gerontol.* 27:438–443, 1972.

77. Owen, O. E., E. Kavle, R. S. Owen, et al. A reappraisal of the caloric requirements of women. *Am. J. Clin. Nutr.* 44:1–19, 1986.

78. Poehlman, E. T. A review: exercise and its influence on resting energy metabolism in man. *Med. Sci. Sports Exerc.* 21:515–525, 1989.

79. Poehlman, E. T. Energy expenditure and requirements in aging humans. *J. Nutr.* 122:2057–2065, 1992.

80. Poehlman, E. T. Regulation of energy expenditure in aging humans. *J. Am. Geriatr. Soc.* 41:552–559, 1993.

81. Poehlman, E. T., E. M. Berke, J. R. Joseph, A. W. Gardner, S. M. Katzman-Rooks, and M. I. Goran. Influence of aerobic capacity, body composition and thyroid hormones on the age-related decline in resting metabolic rate. *Metabolism* 41:915–921, 1992.

82. Poehlman, E. T., and K. C. Copeland. Influence of physical activity on insulin-like growth factor-1 in healthy younger and older men. *J. Clin. Endocrinol. Metab.* 71:1468–1473, 1990.

83. Poehlman, E. T., and E. Danforth, Jr. Endurance training increases metabolic rate and norepinephrine appearance rate in older individuals. *Am. J. Physiol.* 261:E233–E239, 1991.

84. Poehlman, E. T., A. W. Gardner, P. J. Arciero, M. I. Goran, and J. Calles-Escandon. Effects of endurance training on in-vivo measures of basal fatty acid metabolism and norepinephrine kinetics in older persons. *J. Appl. Physiol.* (under revision).

85. Poehlman, E. T., A. W. Gardner, and M. I. Goran. The impact of physical activity and cold exposure on food intake and energy expenditure in man. *J. Wilderness Med.* 1:265–278, 1990.

86. Poehlman, E. T., A. W. Gardner, and M. I. Goran. Influence of endurance training on energy intake, norepinephrine kinetics, and metabolic rate in older individuals. *Metabolism* 41:941–948, 1992.

87. Poehlman, E. T., M. I. Goran, A. W. Gardner, et al. Determinants of decline in resting metabolic rate in aging females. *Am. J. Physiol.* 264:E450–E455, 1993.

88. Poehlman, E. T., and E. S. Horton. Regulation of energy expenditure in aging humans. *Annu. Rev. Nutr.* 10:255–275, 1990.

89. Poehlman, E. T., T. McAuliffe, and E. Danforth, Jr. Effects of age and level of physical activity on plasma norepinephrine kinetics. *Am. J. Physiol.* 258:E256–E262, 1990.

90. Poehlman, E. T., T. McAuliffe, D. R. Van Houten, and E. Danforth, Jr. Influence of age and endurance training on metabolic rate and hormones in healthy men. *Am. J. Physiol.* 259:E66–E72, 1990.

91. Poehlman, E. T., C. L. Melby, and S. F. Badylak. Resting metabolic rate and postprandial thermogenesis in highly trained and untrained males. *Am. J. Clin. Nutr.* 47:793–798, 1988.

92. Poehlman, E. T., C. L. Melby, and S. F. Badylak. Relation of age and physical exercise status on metabolic rate in younger and older healthy men. *J. Gerontol.* 46:B54–B58, 1991.

93. Poehlman, E. T., C. L. Melby, S. F. Badylak, and J. Calles. Aerobic fitness and resting energy expenditure in young adult males. *Metabolism* 38:85–90, 1989.

94. Poehlman, E. T., C. L. Melby, and M. I. Goran. The impact of exercise and diet restriction on daily energy expenditure. *Sports Med.* 11:78–101, 1991.

95. Poehlman, E. T., C. J. Rosen, and K. C. Copeland. The influence of endurance training on insulin-like growth factor-1 in older individuals. *Metabolism.* (In press).
96. Poehlman, E. T., M. J. Toth, and G. D. Webb. Sodium-potassium pump activity contributes to the age-related decline in resting metabolic rate. *J. Clin. Endocrinol. Metab.* 76:1054–1059, 1993.
97. Prentice, A. M. Applications of the $^2H_2^{18}O$ method in free-living humans. *Proc. Nutr. Soc.* 47:258–269, 1988.
98. Prentice, A. M. (ed), *The Doubly-Labelled Water Method for Measuring Energy Expenditure: Technical Recommendations for Use in Humans. A Concensus Report by the IDECG Working Group.* Vienna: International Atomic Energy Agency, 1990.
99. Prentice, A. M., A. E. Black, W. A. Coward, et al. High levels of energy expenditure in obese women. *Br. Med. J.* 292:983–987, 1986.
100. Prentice, A. M., W. A. Coward, H. L. Davies, et al. Unexpectedly low levels of energy expenditure in healthy women. *Lancet:* 1419–1422, 1985.
101. Ravussin, E., I. Harper, R. Rising, and C. Bogardus. Energy expenditure by doubly labeled water: validation in lean and obese subjects. *Am. J. Physiol.* 261:E402–E409, 1991.
102. Ravussin, E., S. Lillioja, T. E. Anderson, L. Christin, and C. Bogardus. Determinants of 24-hour energy expenditure in man. Methods and results using a respiratory chamber. *J. Clin. Invest.* 78:1568–1578, 1986.
103. Ravussin, E., S. Lillioja, W. C. Knowler, et al. Reduced rate of energy expenditure as a risk factor for body weight gain. *N. Engl. J. Med.* 318:467–472, 1988.
104. Roberts, S. B. Use of the doubly labeled water method for measurement of energy expenditure, total body water, water intake, and metabolizable energy intake in humans and small animals. *Can. J. Physiol. Pharmacol.* 67:1190–1198, 1989.
105. Roberts, S. B., V. R. Young, P. Fuss, et al. What are the dietary energy needs of elderly adults? *Int. J. Obesity* 16:969–976, 1992.
106. Robertson, J. D., and D. D. Reid. Standards for the basal metabolism of normal people in Britain. *Lancet* 1:940–943, 1952.
107. Robinson, S., D. B. Dill, S. P. Tzankoff, J. A. Wagner, and R. D. Robinson. Longitudinal studies of aging in 37 men. *J. Appl. Physiol.* 38:263–267, 1975.
108. Rudman, D. Growth hormone, body composition, and aging. *J. Amer. Geriat. Soc.* 33:800–897, 1985.
109. Rudman, D., M. H. Kutner, C. M. Rogers, M. F. Lubin, G. A. Fleming, and R. P. Bain. Impaired growth hormone secretion in the adult population. Relation to age and adiposity. *J. Clin. Invest.* 67:1361–1369, 1981.
110. Ryan, A. S., L. D. Craig, and S. C. Finn. Nutrient intake and dietary patterns of older Americans: a national study. *J. Gerontol.* 47:M145–M150, 1992.
111. Sacks, F. M., and V. J. Dzau. Adrenergic effects on plasma lipoprotein metabolism. Speculation on mechanisms of action. *Am. J. Med.* 80(Suppl. 2A):71–81, 1986.
112. Salmon, W. D. Jr., and W. H. Daughaday. A hormonally controlled serum factor which stimulates sulfate incorporation of cartilage in vitro. *J. Lab. Clin. Med.* 49:825–836, 1957.
113. Schoeller, D. A. Measurement of energy expenditure in free-living humans by using doubly labeled water. *J. Nutr.* 118:1278–1289, 1988.
114. Schoeller, D. A. How accurate is self-reported dietary energy intake? *Nutr. Rev.* 48:373–379, 1990.
115. Schoeller, D. A., and C. R. Fjeld. Human energy metabolism: what have we learned from the doubly labeled water method. *Annu. Rev. Nutr.* 11:355–373, 1991.
116. Schoeller, D. A., and S. B. Racette. A review of field techniques for the assessment of energy expenditure. *J. Nutr.* 120 (Suppl.):1492–1495, 1990.
117. Schoeller, D. A., E. Ravussin, Y. Schutz, K. J. Acheson, P. Baertschi, and E. Jequier. Energy expenditure by doubly labeled water: validation in humans and proposed calculation. *Am. J. Physiol.* 250:R823–R830, 1986.
118. Schoeller, D. A., and P. B. Taylor. Precision of the doubly labelled water method using the two-point calculation. *Hum. Nutr. Clin. Nutr.* 41C:215–223, 1987.

119. Schoeller, D. A., and P. Webb. Five-day comparison of the doubly labeled water method with respiratory gas exchange. *Am. J. Clin. Nutr.* 40:153–158, 1984.

120. Schutz, Y., G. Bray, and S. Margen. Postprandial thermogenesis at rest and during exercise in elderly men ingesting two levels of protein. *J. Am. Coll. Nutr.* 6:497–506, 1987.

121. Schutz, Y., E. Ravussin, R. Diethelm, and E. Jequier. Spontaneous physical activity measured by radar in obese and control subjects studied in a respiration chamber. *Int. J. Obesity* 6:23–28, 1980.

122. Schwartz, R. S., L. F. Jaeger, and R. C. Veith. The importance of body composition to the increase in plasma norepinephrine appearance rate in elderly men. *J. Gerontol.* 42:546–551, 1987.

123. Schwartz, R. S., L. F. Jaeger, and R. C. Veith. The thermic effect of feeding in older men: the importance of the sympathetic nervous system. *Metabolism* 39:733–737, 1990.

124. Seale, J. L., W. V. Rumpler, J. M. Conway, and C. W. Miles. Comparison of doubly labeled water, intake-balance, and direct- and indirect-calorimetry methods for measuring energy expenditure in adult men. *Am. J. Clin. Nutr.* 52:66–71, 1990.

125. Shah, S. D., T. F. Tse., W. E. Clutter, and P. E. Cryer. The human sympathochromaffin system. *Am. J. Physiol.* 247:E380–E384, 1984.

126. Shock, N. W. Metabolism and age. *J. Chronic Dis.* 2:687–703, 1955.

127. Shock, N. W., D. M. Watkin, M. J. Yiengst, et al. Age differences in the water content of the body as related to basal oxygen consumption in males. *J. Gerontol.* 18:1–8, 1963.

128. Shock, N. W., and M. J. Yiengst. Age changes in basal respiratory measurements and metabolism in males. *J. Gerontol.* 10:31–50, 1955.

129. Speakman, J. R., K. S. Nair, and M. I. Goran. Revised equations for calculating CO_2 production from doubly labeled water in humans. *Am. J. Physiol.* 1993. (in press)

130. Stevenson, J. A. F., B. M. Box, V. Feleki, and J. R. Beaton. Bouts of exercise and food intake in the rat. *J. Appl. Physiol.* 21:118–122, 1966.

131. Supiano, M. A., O. A. Linares, M. J. Smith, and J. B. Halter. Age related differences in norepinephrine kinetics: effect of posture and sodium–restricted diet. *Am. J. Physiol.* 259:E422–E431, 1990.

132. Tan, K., and R. C. Baxter. Serum insulin like-growth factor 1 levels in adult diabetic patients: the effect of age. *J. Clin. Endocrinol Metab.* 63:651–655, 1986.

133. Taylor, H. L., D. R. Jacobs, B. Schucker, et al. Questionnaire for the assessment of leisure time physical activities. *J. Chronic. Dis.* 31:741–755, 1978.

134. Thomas, B. M., and A. T. Miller, Jr. Adaptation to forced exercise in the rat. *Am. J. Physiol.* 193:350–354, 1958.

135. Tremblay, A., E. Fontaine, E. T. Poehlman, D. Mitchell, L. Perron, and C. Bouchard. The effect of exercise-training on resting metabolic rate in lean and moderately obese individuals. *Int. J. Obesity* 10:511–517, 1986.

136. Tuttle, W. W., S. M. Horvath, L. F. Presson, and K. Daum. Specific dynamic action of protein in men past 60 years of age. *J. Appl. Physiol.* 5:631–634, 1953.

137. Tzankoff, S. P., and A. H. Norris. Effect of muscle mass decrease on age-related BMR changes. *J. Appl. Physiol.* 43:1001–1006, 1977.

138. Tzankoff, S. P., and A. H. Norris. Longitudinal changes in basal metabolism in man. *J. Appl. Physiol.* 45:536–539, 1978.

139. Uauy, R., N. S. Scrimshaw, and V. R. Young. Human protein requirements: nitrogen balance in response to graded levels of egg protein in elderly men and women. *Am. J. Clin. Nutr.* 32:779–785, 1985.

140. Vaughan, L., F. Zurlo, and E. Ravussin. Aging and energy expenditure. *Am. J. Clin. Nutr.* 53:821–825, 1991.

141. Vermeulen, A. Nyctohemeral growth hormone profiles in young and aged men: correlation with somatomedin-C levels. *J. Clin. Endocrinol. Metab.* 64:884–888, 1987.

142. Voorrips, L. E., W. A. van Staveren, and J. G. A. J. Hautvast. Are physically active elderly women in better nutritional condition than their sedentary peers? *Eur. J. Clin. Nutr.* 45:545–552, 1991.

143. Wallin, B. G., G. Sundlof, B. M. Eriksson, P. Dominiak, H. Grobecker, and L. E. Lindblad. Plasma noradrenaline correlates to sympathetic muscle nerve activity in normotensive man. *Acta. Physiol. Scand.* 111:69–73, 1981.

144. Webb, P. 24-hour energy expenditure and the menstrual cycle. *Am. J. Clin. Nutr.* 44:614–619, 1986.

145. Webb, P., and M. Heistand. Sleep metabolism and age. *J. Appl. Physiol.* 38:257–262, 1975.

146. Wells, C. L., M. A. Boorman, and D. M. Riggs. Effect of age and menopausal status on cardiorespiratory fitness in masters women runners. *Med. Sci. Sports Exerc.* 24:1147–1154.

147. Westerterp, K. R., F. Brouns, W. H. Saris, and F. T. Hoor. Comparison of doubly labeled water with respirometry at low- and high-activity levels. *J. Appl. Physiol.* 65:53–56, 1988.

148. Wilson, O. Field study of the effect of cold exposure and increased muscular activity upon metabolic rate and thyroid function in man. *FASEB Fed. Proc.* 25:1357–1362, 1966.

149. Wing, R. R., K. A. Matthews, L. H. Kuller, E. N. Meilahn, and P. L. Plantinga. Weight gain at the time of menopause. *Arch. Intern. Med.* 151:97–102, 1991.

150. Woo, R., and F. X. Pi-Sunyer. Effect of increased physical activity on voluntary intake in lean women. *Metabolism* 34:836–841, 1985.

151. Woo, R., J. S. Garrow, and F. X. Pi-Sunyer. Effect of exercise on spontaneous calorie intake in obesity. *Am. J. Clin. Nutr.* 36:470–477, 1982.

152. World Health Organization, *World Health Organization, Technical Report Series, Number 724. Energy and Protein Requirements.* Geneva: World Health Organization, 1985.

153. Wright, H., H. Guthrie, M. Wang, and V. Bernardo. The 1987–88 nationwide food consumption survey: an update of the nutrient intake of respondents. *Nutr. Today* 26:21–27, 1991.

154. Zurlo, F., S. Lilloja, A. Esposito-Del Puente, et al. Low ratio of fat to carbohydrate oxidation as predictor of weight gain: study of 24-h RQ. *Am. J. Physiol.* 259:E650–E657, 1990.

10
Growth Hormone Effects on Metabolism, Body Composition, Muscle Mass, and Strength

KEVIN E. YARASHESKI, Ph.D.

Growth hormone (GH) is essential for normal growth in developing mammals. Likewise, GH has diverse effects on carbohydrate and lipid metabolism, but this is not a primary focus here. Instead, this review focuses on the anthropometric, and especially the protein anabolic, consequences of exogenously administered GH. To accomplish this, some background information about the components of and the recent modifications to the classic GH/insulin like growth factor (IGF-I) axis hypothesis is presented. This includes the control of GH secretion, the roles of GH binding protein (GHBP) and IGF-I binding proteins (IGFBP) in regulating the metabolic and anthropometric effects of GH, and structural aspects of the IGF-I receptor. This information will assist in examining our initial experiences with the combined effects of GH treatment and resistance exercise on body composition, skeletal muscle protein metabolism, and muscle strength.

The recent availability of recombinant human GH has provided clinical investigators the opportunity to examine the prospect that GH treatment might enhance lean tissue or muscle protein accretion during anabolic conditions (e.g., growth, exercise) or suppress protein wasting associated with catabolic conditions (e.g., cachexia, surgery, aging). Early on in these trials, it has become clear that the traditional concepts that GH signals hepatic IGF-I (somatomedin-C) production and that serum IGF-I mediates the anabolic actions of GH were an oversimplification. Instead, it appears that the actions of GH are mediated by complex interactions among several hormones, their receptors, substrates, and serum binding proteins. In general, the anabolic or anticatabolic effects of GH treatment observed to date have not been extraordinary or consistent, possibly because GH has been administered in different doses and regimens to different populations under diverse conditions, and because we have an incomplete understanding of the interactions among all the components of the GH/IGF-I axis. After evaluating these studies, a hypothesis regarding the skeletal muscle protein anabolic effects of GH administration to individuals involved in resistance exercise training programs is presented.

OVERVIEW OF POSSIBLE APPLICATIONS FOR GROWTH HORMONE TREATMENT

Growth hormone modifies body composition through its effects on protein anabolism, carbohydrate tolerance, lipolysis, natriuresis, and bone and connective tissue turnover. These effects have been studied in vitro in a variety of cell types, in a variety of animal models, and in humans with assorted clinical conditions including short stature [32], GH deficiency [19, 26, 27, 44, 72, 100] or excess [90], cancer cachexia [116], surgery [6, 115], burns [58], nutrient restriction [22, 42, 77], glucocorticoid treatment [67, 84], chronic obstructive lung disease [92], obesity [105], senescence [98, 99, 122], impaired immune function [5], and in normal volunteers [8, 25, 35, 45, 46, 67, 87, 118, 120]. Without credible evidence, many believe that resistance exercise training supplemented with GH administration will result in "athletic gigantism." Despite the availability of recombinant human GH and the subsequent research activity, no unifying thesis regarding the effects of GH treatment on human muscle protein mass and function has evolved.

This is the result of the lack of a comprehensive and integrated understanding of the direct and indirect actions of GH and IGF-I, the properties of the expression products of the variant GH gene, or unrecognized cleavage products from alternate GH gene splicing. Also, the role of GH and IGF binding proteins, as well as other endocrine factors, in regulating the circulating concentrations and actions of GH and IGF-I needs to be clarified. Finally, the distribution of tissue GH and IGF receptors and the postreceptor binding events responsible for their metabolic actions require elucidation.

Additionally, the diverse nature of the models used to study GH actions include (*a*) differentiating and mature cell lines and tissues preincubated in vitro in the absence and presence of physiological or supraphysiological levels of GH and IGF-I, (*b*) hypophysectomized and intact animals of different species and age, (*c*) exposure to GH and IGF antisera or GH and IGF peptides, (*d*) GH-deficient children and adults, acromegalics, the elderly, and those with normal pituitary function. Although unequivocally necessary, these diverse approaches make it more difficult to condense the pertinent, and often conflicting, information about the actions and regulation of the GH-IGF-I axis. Despite this, several excellent reviews have appeared [30, 31, 69, 75, 76, 94, 106, 112, 113].

The ability of GH to modulate metabolism and body composition is best exemplified in (*a*) untreated acromegaly, where body weight, fat-free mass (FFM), and extracellular water content are increased, while body fat is reduced, and in (*b*) GH-deficient children, whose height, FFM, muscle strength, exercise capacity, extracellular fluid, and biochemical markers of bone turnover (i.e., serum osteocalcin) are all reduced, while their body fat content (especially central adiposity) is increased [19]. Interestingly, although they have larger than normal muscles, acromegalics do not have stronger than normal muscles [90]. In addition, FFM increased when GH was administered to (*a*) healthy sedentary young men in conjunction with a 12-wk progressive resistance exercise training program [118], (*b*) well-conditioned young men and women for 6 wk (methionyl-GH; 25), and (*c*) elderly (61–81 yr) men with low endogenous GH and IGF-I concentrations for 6 months [99]. Six months of GH therapy also moderately increased muscle mass and strength in GH-deficient adults [26]. In this regard, it is important to determine whether the GH-induced increase in FFM in exercising young or elderly adults results from an increase in muscle mass, and consequently, improved muscle strength and function.

Several anecdotal reports, some presented at a congressional hearing [63], have speculated that adolescent and adult strength athletes and bodybuilders can obtain GH (despite strict security and distribution regulations), are self-administering large doses of GH, and are experiencing dramatic increments in muscle mass and strength, as well as acromegalic side effects [23, 108, 114]. In fact, few placebo-controlled, double-blind investigations have tested these claims in physically active individuals with normal GH secretory function.

Resistance exercise training augments skeletal muscle strength and muscle cross-sectional area (hypertrophy) by enlarging type I, and in particular type II, muscle cell areas [50, 80, 117], but it is unclear whether these effects can be enhanced by GH supplementation. The increase in contractile protein must result from alterations in the rates of muscle protein synthesis and breakdown. For example, the rate of biceps and vastus lateralis muscle protein synthesis in young and elderly subjects increased rapidly during the initial phase (within 2 wk) of a progressive resistance exercise training program [18, 121]. In the elderly, this was not accompanied by an increase in the estimated rate of myofibrillar protein breakdown (urinary 3-methylhistidine excretion), suggesting that resistance exercise–induced muscle hypertrophy results, at least initially, from an increase in the rate of muscle protein synthesis. Whether GH supplementation enhances the exercise-induced increase in muscle protein synthesis in the elderly remains to be determined.

NEUROENDOCRINOLOGY OF ENDOGENOUS GROWTH HORMONE SECRETION

Growth hormone is the most abundant peptide hormone stored in the human anterior pituitary [112, 113]. Its intermittent, pulsatile secretory pattern is intricately regulated by neural control, metabolic and hormonal feedback mechanisms that involve brain neurotransmitters (acetylcholine, serotonin, and dopamine), hypothalamic peptides (growth hormone–releasing hormone [GHRH]), and somatostatin, as well as circulating levels of glucose, GH, IGF-I, and estrogens [97]. Growth hormone secretion may be augmented by sleep, psychogenic and physical stress, exercise, hypoglycemia, some amino acids, α-adrenergic and dopaminergic stimuli, while GH secretion may be inhibited by hyperglycemia, circulating IGF-I, ß-adrenergic agonists, and obesity [28]. Short-term (10–20 min) cycling exercise of sufficient intensity (≥ 5mM lactate) stimulates GH secretion (6–8 ng/ml) 15–40 min after exercise [40], but the metabolic effects that result from this GH surge are unclear. In addition, a novel series of GH-releasing secretagogues that potentiate the effects of GHRH have recently been described [14, 104]. This suggests that there may be other physiological releasing factors that operate through mechanisms not yet recognized.

COMPONENTS OF THE GROWTH HORMONE/ INSULIN-LIKE GROWTH FACTOR-I AXIS

GH RECEPTOR AND BINDING PROTEIN. Upon release into the circulation, GH binds to a membrane-bound receptor in target tissue, which elicits an intracellular signaling mechanism that has been partially described [43, 69]. In addition, circulating GH binds to a serum binding protein (GHBP) that (*a*) has been identified in the serum of humans and several animal species, (*b*) shares amino acid sequence homology with the extracellular domain of the rabbit GH receptor, (*c*) is absent or undetectable in patients with GH receptor deficiency (Laron dwarfs and African pigmies), (*d*) slows the clearance rate of circulating GH, and (*e*) modulates the interaction between GH and its tissue receptor. One model describing the physiological role of GHBP [66] suggests that GH binds to its cell surface receptor and increases GH receptor population and turnover rate, which increases the secretion of the binding protein either by shedding of the extracellular domain of the receptor or by increasing the synthesis rate of the binding protein. Circulating GH then complexes with the binding protein, which reduces the clearance rate of GH but prevents GH from interacting with its membrane receptor. This competition for circulating GH may reduce GH-receptor binding and the subsequent biological effect, and may partially explain the resistance to the anabolic effects of prolonged GH treatment reported in several clinical studies [64, 105, 118].

IGF BINDING PROTEINS. Once in the circulation, GH exerts some of its anabolic effects indirectly by stimulating the liver to produce and release IGF-I and II [28, 30, 69, 112]. In addition, IGF-I and its mRNA have been identified in almost all rat tissues, including muscle, heart, kidney, lung, uterus, ovary, bone, and cartilage [33, 89], suggesting that locally produced IGF-I may exert autocrine or paracrine cellular actions, but the mechanism by which these actions are mediated is not clear. A small amount (1–5%) of IGF-I circulates freely, but most of it circulates bound to a series of binding proteins (IGFBP 1–6; 106) that are also secreted by several cell types (including muscle; 85) in response to various physiological stimuli (e.g., GH, IGF, insulin, feeding/fasting) and can potentiate [38] or inhibit [73] IGF's proliferative actions on target tissues, by some unknown interaction with the IGF molecule or with the IGF-I cell surface receptor [9, 10, 20]. In vitro, potentiation of IGF-I action is associated with IGFBP-3 adherence to the bovine fibroblast cell surface, but the mechanism for this attachment is unclear because there is no known cell surface receptor for IGFBP-3 [24]. Regardless, structural and molecular modifications to the IGFBP-3 molecule seem to regulate capillary membrane permeability to IGF-I, and subsequently, IGF-I bioavailability, tissue specificity, affinity, and action.

Insulin-like growth factor BP-3 is the most abundant IGFBP found in human (adult) serum ($\approx$5nM). Most ($\approx$90%) IGFBP-3 is found in a large molecular weight ternary complex that is apparently inactive until structurally modified, perhaps by phosphorylation, glycosylation, or proteolytic dissociation of the α-subunit [9, 10]. The regulation of the biological effects of GH and IGF-I by the IGFBPs is currently an area of intensive investigation [106] that may help explain the variable metabolic effects reported during GH administration to different clinical populations [20].

IGF-I RECEPTOR. The IGF-I receptor complex is a membrane glycoprotein heterotetramer consisting of 2 α and 2 ß subunits linked by disulfide bonds. The α and ß subunit associations are necessary for effective signal transduction. The IGF-I receptor is structurally similar to the insulin receptor [111], and insulin cross-reacts with the IGF-I receptor to approximately the same extent that IGF-I cross-reacts with the insulin receptor [113]. In vivo, the insulin-like actions of IGF-I are approximately 10 times less effective than those of insulin. In fasting adults, however, IGF-I circulates in much higher concentrations (125–450 ng/ml) than insulin (0.3–1.0 ng/ml), but since most plasma IGF-I circulates bound to IGFBP-3, the actual, effective free hormone concentration is unknown. Insulin-like growth factor binding activates intracellular tyrosine-specific protein kinases located on the ß-subunit, which initiate phosphorylation of the ß-subunit [95] and presumably activate an additional IGF-I-specific signaling cascade. One preliminary report suggests that red and white rat muscles have similar IGF receptor populations, but tyrosine kinase activation by IGF-I binding may be 2–3 times greater in red than in white muscle [123]. Elucidation of the cellular events that follow GH and IGF-I receptor binding in humans will prove critical to our understanding of the diverse metabolic consequences of exogenous GH treatment.

INDIRECT METABOLIC ACTIONS OF GROWTH HORMONE

The primary indirect or IGF-I-mediated action of GH on body protein metabolism is believed to be the stimulation of protein synthesis resulting in skeletal and somatic growth; an effect mediated by both circulating and locally produced IGF-I [76, 113]. In this context, the synergy of GH and IGF-I may be explained by the dual effector theory of tissue growth, which predicts that GH promotes the differentiation of precursor cells and that subsequent multiplication of young differentiated cells requires circulating or local production of IGF-I [59]. Still, direct evidence coupling locally produced IGF-I with muscle hypertrophy in humans, either in response to exogenous GH or to muscle growth-promoting exercise, is lacking.

Several studies done in humans appear to confirm the IGF-I-mediated actions of GH, but contrasting mechanisms for the anabolic effect have been presented. When recombinant human GH was administered (100 µg/kg/day) for 8 days to healthy adult (18–36 yr) volunteers, plasma IGF-I increased (3-fold), the rate of nonoxidative disposal of leucine (i.e., whole body protein synthesis rate) was increased, the rate of leucine oxidation was reduced, and the rate of appearance of plasma leucine (i.e., whole body protein breakdown rate) was unchanged after an overnight fast and during the fed condition [67]. These anabolic effects of GH were capable of attenuating the catabolic effects of daily prednisone treatment (0.8 mg/kg/day). The possibility that the anabolic effects of GH were not indirectly mediated by IGF-I, and instead by the relative hyperinsulinemia associated with both GH and glucocorticoid treatment, was dismissed because the primary effect of insulin on amino acid metabolism, when amino acid availability is sufficient, is believed to be a reduction in proteolysis [47, 48]. However, when recombinant human IGF-I was administered by intravenous infusion into healthy adult (18–36 yr) volunteers for 8–28 hr, plasma IGF-I increased (to levels comparable to those in [67]); no change in the rate of whole body protein synthesis was observed in one study [84], while a decrease in the rate of whole body protein breakdown was observed in other studies [37, 109]. A decrease in the whole body protein breakdown rate has also been observed in fasted rats [70], while an increase in whole body protein synthesis was observed in fasted lambs during acute IGF-I administration [36]. Some of this disparity in protein kinetic information may be explained by the decline in plasma amino acid levels that typically occurs during IGF-I treatment. Also, during IGF-I infusion, insulin secretion, plasma insulin, and glucose concentrations decline [84, 109]. Thus, it is possible that some of the anabolic actions of GH are independent of IGF-I. Alternatively, current evidence confirms that IGF-I binding proteins (IGFBP 1–6) play an integral role in regulating the in vivo anabolic actions of GH and IGF-I [10, 20, 21] and that GH and IGF-I treatments affect circulating IGFBPs differently [77].

DIRECT METABOLIC ACTIONS OF GROWTH HORMONE

The direct actions of GH have been categorized into transient, acute insulin-like effects; and chronic, insulin-antagonistic or diabetogenic effects.

INSULIN-LIKE EFFECTS. The insulin-like effects are more readily demonstrable in vitro, especially in tissues removed from hypophysectomized animals or preincubated in the absence of GH. Under these conditions, GH acutely inhibits lipolysis in adipose tissue [12, 56], increases amino acid uptake into rat diaphragm muscle [75], and increases glucose uptake and oxidation in rat muscle and adipose tissue [12, 52]. In vivo, the acute insulin-like effects of GH are readily observed in hypophysectomized animals [4] and GH-deficient children [44], but are less reproducible in intact humans [2, 86] and were not observed when GH was infused into the human forearm while glucose uptake was measured using the arterial-venous balance technique [41, 45]. In general, the acute increase in muscle amino acid uptake occurs in young, hypophysectomized animals, requires supraphysiological levels of GH, and increases the activity of existing RNA [75, 76]. This appears to increase amino acid incorporation into contractile proteins of rat muscles (diaphragm, levator ani), but it is a transient phenomenon that lasts only minutes to a few hours, after which muscle becomes refractory to further GH stimulation [76]. Thus, it has been suggested that under normal physiological conditions, where tissues are primarily exposed to low levels of GH, the typical intermittent, transient GH secretory bursts may produce only minimal increments in amino acid incorporation into protein [75, 76].

Contrary to this suggestion, a 6-hr intravenous infusion of human methionyl-GH increased arterial GH concentration (to 15 ± 1 ng/ml), stimulated net amino acid uptake across the leg while reducing whole body leucine oxidation, and increased vastus lateralis myosin heavy chain mRNA levels without changing the arterial IGF-I concentration in normal young men starved for 10 days, followed by 10 days of hypercaloric intravenous feeding [42]. Thus, during this induced catabolic state, an isolated short-term GH infusion produced intracellular conditions suggestive of enhanced myofibrillar protein synthesis.

Similarly, the acute effects of an intrabrachial artery infusion of GH on forearm glucose and amino acid balance and kinetics (using [3H]phenylalanine and [14C]leucine tracers) were determined after 3 and 6 hr of GH infusion [45]. In this model, forearm venous GH concentration was 35 ± 6 ng/ml, forearm glucose uptake was unchanged, and net release of amino acids from forearm tissues was reduced. This was attributed to an increased rate of protein synthesis without a change in the rate of protein breakdown, but these observations were somewhat confounded by a large increase in forearm blood flow during the 6-hr GH infusion. In spite of this, these findings suggest that an abrupt increase in GH directly stimulates forearm and leg muscle protein synthesis. This did not require an increase in serum IGF-I and is opposite the antiproteolytic effect of insulin. Still, GH-mediated increase in muscle IGF-I production [88] could be responsible for the augmented rate of forearm or leg protein synthesis observed. Until the local production of IGF-I is assessed in normal humans under these conditions, the possibility exists that GH exerts acute effects on amino acid metabolism independent of IGF-I; a conclusion that (a) differs from that reached in studies where tissues refractoriness to continuous GH exposure was observed in hypophysectomized animals (reviewed above) and (b) is in opposition to the suggestion that the direct effects of GH on protein, carbohydrate, and lipid metabolism are of only minimal physiological significance [31, 94].

In addition, when GH and insulin were simultaneously infused into the brachial artery of healthy young (20 ± 1 yr) men for 6 hr, the forearm protein synthesis rate increased (as expected), but the rate of forearm protein breakdown was not reduced by the action of insulin [46]. This suggests that elevated GH and insulin concentrations do not provide an additive anabolic effect in excess of either GH or insulin alone and indicates that GH may blunt the ability of insulin to suppress proteolysis in the human forearm [46], similar to the antagonistic effect GH has on insulin's action on glucose metabolism.

INSULIN-ANTAGONISTIC EFFECTS. In general, prolonged GH exposure decreases glucose utilization and increases lipolysis in vitro. Decreased glucose uptake was observed in diaphragm muscle from hypophysectomized rats chronically treated with GH [52] and in diaphragm muscle from hypophysectomized rats incubated with GH [13], but this latter observation was not subsequently confirmed [3]. Incubation with GH reduced glucose oxidation and glucose conversion to lipid in adipose tissue from genetically GH-deficient mice [1] and in 3T3 adipocytes [101] after several hours, but human fat tissue incubated with GH exhibited no change in glucose oxidation, reduced glucose incorporation into triglycerides, and no increase in lipolysis [91]. A modest lipolytic effect of GH incubation was observed in adipose tissue from hypophysectomized and intact rats [55, 74]. While GH administration to intact rats increased lipolysis in adipose tissue incubated in vitro [102], it did not affect lipolysis in adipose tissue from hypophysectomized animals [52]. These modest, diverse effects on lipolysis have inspired the idea that GH simply potentiates the effects of more potent lipolytic agents (e.g., epinephrine; 54). Finally, the mechanism by which the lipolytic effects are mediated are not entirely clear but may be due to a direct inhibition of glucose metabolism by GH [57], a direct effect of GH on the adenylate cyclase–cyclic AMP–protein kinase system that activates a "hormone-sensitive lipase" [31], or an indirect effect of some unidentified intracellular protein synthesized in response to GH treatment [52, 53].

The diabetogenic effects of GH administration in humans are typified by higher circulating insulin levels and peripheral insulin resistance [29], but the origin of these effects has not been completely characterized following an intravenous bolus of GH, during a constant infusion of GH, or during a euglycemic-hyperinsulinemic clamp. Under these diverse conditions, GH increases circulating concentrations of nonesterified fatty acids, ß-hydroxybutyrate, and glycerol ≈2–3 hr after a GH pulse [87], increases lipid oxidation [8], and impairs insulin's ability to suppress hepatic glucose output and stimulate glucose uptake [96]. When 140 μg of GH was given as a single intravenous bolus to mimic an endogenous pulse, circulating GH concentration increased (to 21 ± 3 ng/ml) and forearm glucose uptake declined; this coincided with the peak increments in fatty acid, ß-hydroxybutyrate, and glycerol concentrations. This implies that substrate competition may have caused the elevated glucose and insulin levels and the peripheral insulin resistance induced by GH. However, this latter position has not been widely accepted, other possible mechanisms have been proposed, and as yet, no consensus theory has emerged [8, 15, 87, 96].

GROWTH HORMONE EFFECTS ON SKELETAL MUSCLE FUNCTION IN ANIMALS

Growth hormone was initially identified by the ability of crude pituitary extracts to promote growth [78] and increase body mass in the rat [39], and GH was subsequently found to be essential for normal skeletal muscle growth in hypophysectomized rats [103]. Initial studies reported small increments in muscle mass in rats treated with pituitary extracts [7, 93]. A subsequent study [11] found that quadriceps muscles from 6- to 9-month-old female rats treated with 500 μg GH/day for 21 days were 15–40% heavier but did not develop more twitch or tetanic tension, on a per unit muscle mass basis, than the quadriceps muscles taken from pair-fed untreated rats. The investigators suggested that GH-induced muscle enlargement was not the result of an increase in contractile protein, and therefore, provided no functional benefit to the larger muscles.

The role the GH/IGF-I axis plays in normal muscle growth has been examined, and it is interesting to note that compensatory hypertrophy of the soleus and plantaris muscles (synergist ablation model) can occur in hypophysectomized rats [49, 51], that IGF-I gene expression is activated in these compensatory hypertrophying muscles [34], and in at least one preliminary report, somatomedin-like activity was detected in extracts of compensatory hypertrophied rat soleus muscles [107]. However, 16 wk of resistance exercise training did not increase serum IGF-I levels in previously sedentary young men [118], fasting serum IGF-I levels were not elevated in experienced weight lifters with large muscle masses [120], and when experienced and novice weight lifters were given GH, serum IGF-I levels increased 2- to 3-fold, but no additional increase in muscle protein synthesis occurred [35, 118, 120]. These observations suggest that circulating IGF-I plays a minor role in inducing muscle growth during resistance exercise, but that muscle production of IGF-I may contribute to muscle hypertrophy. However, it is unclear whether IGF-I expression is enhanced in human muscles undergoing exercise-induced muscle hypertrophy.

The combined effects of GH treatment and muscle activity on rat muscle growth have been investigated. When soleus muscle atrophy was induced in young intact male Sprague-Dawley rats (125–135 g) during a 4-day space flight [71], GH administration ($\approx$556 µg/day) did not reduce the decline in muscle weight and muscle fiber cross-sectional area typically observed during space flight. This suggests that decrements in GH secretion during space flight play a minor role in regulating muscle protein mass in reduced gravity and that GH treatment does not counteract the muscle atrophy that occurs. In contrast, two preliminary reports suggest that intact and hypophysectomized hindlimb-suspended rats treated with a combination of GH (1 mg/kg) and short periods of ladder-climbing exercise experience less slow- and fast-muscle atrophy than hindlimb-suspended rats given either climbing exercise or GH alone [60, 79]. This combined effect of GH and increased muscle activity on rat muscle mass during suspension-induced muscle atrophy was not observed when the soleus and plantaris muscles of hypophysectomized young (100–125 g) male rats underwent compensatory hypertrophy (gastrocnemius tenotomy) with or without GH (1 mg GH/day) treatment [51]. Instead, compensatory hypertrophy increased muscle wet weight proportionally regardless of whether it was combined with daily GH or saline injections. Likewise, when hypophysecto-mized young male rats underwent unilateral denervation atrophy of the plantaris and soleus muscles and were then treated with GH [51], the increase in muscle weight was proportional in denervated and innervated contralateral muscles. These findings suggest that when GH treatment is combined with an increase or decrease in muscle activity, the increase in muscle size is in proportion to initial muscle size, regardless of whether the muscle was previously atrophied or has an intact nerve supply.

These findings have also been confirmed in the extensor digitorum longus (EDL) and soleus muscles of adult (16-wk-old) female rats receiving $\approx$1.5 mg GH/day for 4 wk following either ischemic necrosis of the EDL, denervation with subsequent reinnervation of the EDL and soleus, and denervation atrophy of the EDL and soleus [110]. These observations emphasize the apparent independence of muscle activity, neural innerva-tion, and GH in regulating muscle growth. Despite the autonomy of these growth-regulating processes, rat hindlimb muscles treated with GH while undergoing compensatory hypertrophy or reinnervation growth did not experience a synergistic effect on muscle weight from the two anabolic interventions. The reason for the discrepant results from unloading muscle atrophy experiments [60, 79] is unclear. Muscle force production was not assessed in any of these rat muscle studies, but on the basis of the proportional changes in muscle weight and the results of the earlier study [11], it might be predicted that compensatory muscle hypertrophy and reinnervation muscle growth combined with GH would not produce any greater tension/g muscle than in the corresponding saline-treated muscles. This implies that GH administration combined with exercise-induced muscle hypertrophy would not result in any further enhancement of muscle strength.

EFFECTS OF GROWTH HORMONE ON BODY COMPOSITION, ANABOLISM, AND MUSCLE FUNCTION

On the basis of its metabolic actions, the effects of GH on body protein mass (FFM), fat mass, and body water content are predictable, and best illustrated in the context of the different populations treated with GH.

GH-DEFICIENT ADULTS. When 22 (8 women, 14 men) GH-deficient adults (18–39 yr) were treated with GH ($\approx$20–30 µg/kg/day) for 4 months in a double-blind, placebo-controlled, crossover study [72], serum IGF-I increased (from 96 to 224 ng/ml), thigh muscle volume (computerized tomography image) increased (6%), thigh adipose tissue volume decreased (7%), and subscapular skinfold thickness decreased (16%). One patient withdrew from the study because of persistent edema in his hands and feet. Modest increments in quadriceps isometric muscle strength (8%) and physical work capacity (12%) were observed during GH replacement therapy. These changes in body composition and functional capacity were small, within the variability of the measurement techniques, and only imply that GH therapy is beneficial for GH-deficient adults. These findings must also be considered in light of the fact that these patients are supplemented with varying doses of several hormones in conjunction with GH (e.g., thyroxine, testosterone, estrogen, progesterone, glucocorticoids).

When 24 GH-deficient adults (8 women, 16 men; 21–51 yr) received GH replacement therapy ($\approx$35 µg/kg/day) during a 6-month randomized, double-blind, placebo-controlled trial [100], serum IGF-I increased (270%), lean body mass (LBM) measured using whole body potassium-40 counting increased (11%), and fat mass decreased (16%), while no changes in body composition were observed in the placebo group. In subsequent reports on the same patients [26, 27], total cross-sectional area of midthigh muscles and quadriceps muscle area increased (8 and 6%, respectively), but the peak voluntary isometric force production of only one muscle group (hip flexors) out of the nine tested, increased more (+1 standard deviation above the predicted mean) in the GH-treated group. In addition, maximum oxygen consumption and maximum power output on the cycle ergometer increased (17 and 12%, respectively), but whether this was due to the small increase in muscle mass or to changes in other determinants of maximum oxygen consumption (e.g., cardiac output, ventricular mass/dimensions, red cell mass, substrate availability) requires further study. On the basis of these nominal changes in muscle cross-sectional area and strength, it is premature to attribute the reported increases in LBM and physical work capacity to an increase in muscle mass, and the possibility that noncontractile protein content (e.g., connective tissue) was increased needs to be considered. Further, GH treatment increases potassium retention [64], and this may have artifactually increased the potassium-40 estimate of LBM. It is also noteworthy that most of the increase in LBM (4 kg of 6 kg increment) occurred within the first month of treatment, but continued GH treatment did not result in a progressive increase in LBM. Moreover, six GH recipients developed fluid retention, including swollen ankles and hands, which appeared to dissipate after 2–3 months but necessitated a reduction in dose or a diuretic agent. One GH recipient developed carpal tunnel compression, and 5 patients reported symptoms of arthralgia and myalgia. These are not trivial side effects, and they may limit the clinical use of GH, as well as render double-blind experimentation with GH problematic. These preliminary observations support the need for additional testing of the hypothesis that prolonged GH replacement therapy increases muscle mass and strength in GH-deficient adults.

Acromegaly, as well as treatment with GH and pituitary extracts, has been associated with increments in total body water [64, 118], which may be secondary to the increase in sodium, potassium, phosphorus, and calcium retention [65, 68, 83]. Of these, GH-induced sodium retention has been studied the most, and it is believed to result from an acute activation of the renin-angiotensin system and an increase in aldosterone secretion [65]. Apparently, prolonged GH treatment activates sodium reabsorption in the renal tubule, while the eventual increase in circulating IGF-I increases glomerular filtration rate and renal plasma flow [65]. In healthy individuals, the fluid and mineral retention presents only mild discomfort, but it may explain the peripheral edema, myalgia, and arthralgia reported by some GH recipients. The fluid retention rapidly increases body weight, which may be falsely interpreted as lean tissue growth, while the increase in glomerular filtration rate and renal plasma flow may increase urinary creatinine clearance and falsely elevate the estimate of muscle mass. The possibility that GH or IGF-I treatment may reduce the protein and muscle wasting and eventual kidney failure experienced by patients with chronic renal insufficiency is under investigation.

The observation that GH induces calcium and phosphorus retention [64] has inspired the hypothesis that GH or IGF-I treatment may benefit bone metabolism by enhancing bone formation and increasing bone mineral density [17, 83]. Under some in vitro conditions, GH appears to stimulate chondrogenesis and osteogenesis [82]. In intact adult dogs, bovine GH appears to increase bone formation, gut absorption of calcium, bone mineralization, and skeletal mass [62]. These effects are probably mediated by IGF-I because in vitro, IGF-I stimulates DNA and osteoblastic collagen synthesis in cultured bone cells [16]. However, when GH was administered (30–120 µg/kg/day) to elderly (>60 yr) men and women for 10 days [83], serum IGF-I, osteocalcin, and calcitriol concentrations increased, urinary calcium and hydroxyproline excretion increased, and urinary phosphorus excretion decreased. The ambiguity of the changes in markers of bone turnover during this short-term treatment period prohibited the conclusion that prolonged GH treatment would enhance bone formation in vivo. Instead, the possibility that GH treatment increases bone formation and resorption, without a resultant increase in net bone mass, needs to be evaluated.

OBESITY AND CALORIC RESTRICTION. Obesity is another condition in which the lipolytic and potential anabolic effects of GH therapy may prove beneficial. In a placebo-controlled random trial [105] of 20 (16 women, 4 men) obese subjects (20–54 yr; 30–67% over ideal body weight (IBW)) fed 75kJ and 1.2 g protein/kg IBW/day, 11 wk of methionyl-GH treatment (100 μg/kg IBW every other day) increased serum IGF-I (81%) and did not reduce body weight, accelerate the loss of body fat, or preserve FFM any better than in the placebo group. This suggests that the lipolytic effects of calorie restriction were not potentiated by GH treatment. During the first 33 days of GH treatment, nitrogen balance was more positive in the GH recipients, but this effect disappeared during the final 6 wk of treatment (Fig. 10.1). Consequently, FFM was not preserved, and muscle strength in the lower back and leg muscles, measured with a spring tensiometer, and maximal grip strength measured with a hand dynamometer increased comparably in the placebo (1–13%) and GH-treated (8–15%) groups. The rapid diminution in the nitrogen-sparing effect, the lack of greater muscle strength improvements with GH treatment, and the modest improvements in body composition and muscle performance observed suggest that muscle anabolism was not enhanced in these obese, calorie-restricted individuals, and the effectiveness of GH (given in the above dose regimen) in enhancing muscle anabolism in obesity requires further consideration.

Regardless of whether the initial nitrogen-sparing effect of GH treatment was due to an IGF-I-stimulated increase in protein synthesis or a reduction in proteolysis, within 1 month after initiating GH the subjects became resistant to the nitrogen-sparing effects of GH or IGF-I. Another study of young hypopituitary patients (9–27 yr) and adult patients (44–62 yr) with either Addison's disease, a melanoma, or obesity [64] reported a loss of the nitrogen-sparing effect of GH (2–4 mg/day) within 1 month, but after GH treatment was interrupted for 2 wk in the obese patient, the nitrogen-sparing effects were restored when GH was recommenced. The dissipation of the nitrogen-sparing effect that occurs with prolonged high-dose GH treatment may partially explain the small increments in FFM, muscle mass, and strength observed in other studies and raises questions about the appropriate dose and frequency of GH administration for optimal anabolic effects [81].

In a subsequent study [22], 6 normal, young adults (21–32 yr) were fed 83 kJ and 1 g protein/kg IBW/day for 2 wk, and the nitrogen-sparing effects of a 16-hr intravenous infusion of IGF-I (12 μg/kg IBW/hr) were compared with those of methionyl-GH injections (50 μg/kg IBW/day),

FIGURE 10.1

Daily urinary nitrogen balance (mean ± SE) in calorie-restricted, obese subjects receiving methionyl-GH (100 µg/kg IBW every other day; top panel) or saline (bottom panel) injections. Urinary nitrogen balance was significantly more positive in the GH recipients than in the saline recipients during the initial 33 days of treatment, but these effects on nitrogen retention did not persist for the remainder of the treatment period. (Reprinted with permission from Snyder, D. K., D. R. Clemmons, and L. E. Underwood. Treatment of obese, diet-restricted subjects with growth hormone for 11 weeks: effects on anabolism, lipolysis, and body composition. J. Clin. Endocrinol. Metab. 67:54–61, 1988.)

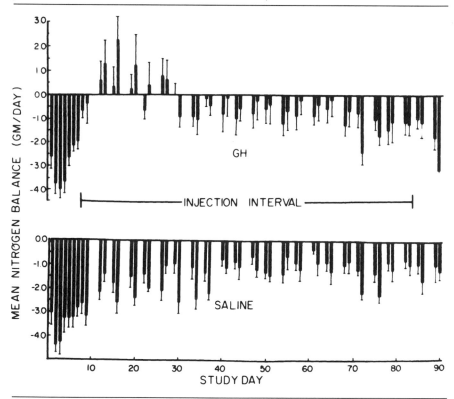

both administered during the final 6 days of calorie restriction. Under these conditions, IGF-I and GH improved nitrogen balance comparably (Fig. 10.2), but serum IGF-I levels during IGF-I treatment were 3-fold higher than during GH treatment, suggesting that GH is a more potent anabolic agent than IGF-I and that GH and IGF-I may promote anabolism through different mechanisms. Most importantly, a longer IGF-I treatment period is necessary to assess whether these subjects would become resistant to the observed short-term nitrogen-sparing effects of IGF-I treatment.

To address whether a combination of GH and IGF-I is more anabolic and

FIGURE 10.2

Urinary nitrogen balance (mean ± SE) in calorie-restricted, normal young adults treated for 6 days with either GH (black bar) or an IGF-I infusion (gray bar). Although IGF-I concentration was 3-fold higher during the IGF-I infusion, GH and IGF-I treatment resulted in similar, significant (P<0.001) improvements in nitrogen retention in comparison with the pretreatment period. (Reprinted with permission from Clemmons, D. R., A. Smith-Banks, and L. E. Underwood. Reversal of diet-induced catabolism by infusion of recombinant insulin-like growth factor-I in humans. J. Clin. Endocrinol. Metab. *75:234–238, 1992.)*

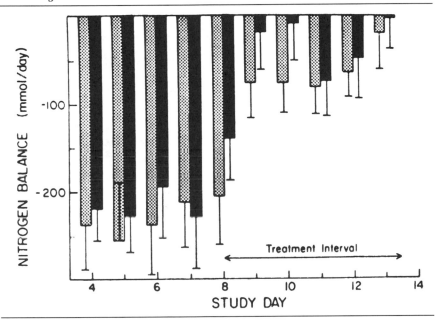

less hypoglycemic than IGF-I alone, 7 normal adults (22–47 yr) were fed 83 kJ and 1 g protein/kg IBW/day for 2 wk, and on the last 5 days of calorie restriction the subjects received either a 16-hr intravenous infusion of IGF-I (12 µg/kg IBW/hr) or a daily injection of GH (50 µg/kg IBW) in combination with the IGF-I infusion [77]. The GH plus IGF-I treatment resulted in greater circulating IGF-I levels, greater nitrogen and potassium retention, and an attenuated hypoglycemic response in comparison to treatment with IGF-I or GH individually (Fig. 10.3), confirming the idea that GH and IGF-I affect protein balance through different, yet somewhat permissive mechanisms. The permissive effect provided a larger nitrogen-sparing effect when GH treatment was combined with an IGF-I infusion, rather than when GH treatment induced endogenous IGF-I production, probably because the latter condition resulted in much lower circulating IGF-I levels. However, other regulators of the permissive effect must exist because, when comparable circulating IGF-I levels (1200–1800 ng/ml)

FIGURE 10.3

Urinary nitrogen balance (mean ± SD) in calorie-restricted normal young adults treated with a 16-hr continuous infusion of IGF-I (12 μg/kg IBW per hr) on days 8–12 (gray bars), or with an identical IGF-I infusion protocol combined with a single GH (50 μg/kg IBW) injection on days 8–12 (black bars). Nitrogen balance was significantly (P<0.01) more positive in the IGF-I plus GH group than in the IGF-I treated group on days 9–12. (Reprinted from Kupfer, S. R., L. E. Underwood, R. C. Baxter, and D. R. Clemmons. Enhancement of the anabolic effect of growth hormone and insulin-like growth factor I by use of both agents simultaneously. J. Clin. Invest. 91:391–396, 1993, by copyright permission of the American Society for Clinical Investigation.)

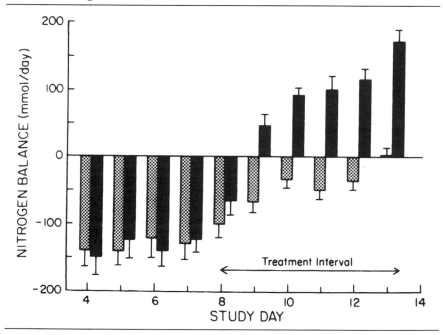

were achieved by IGF-I infusion and by GH treatment combined with IGF-I infusion, the nitrogen-sparing effect of the combined hormone treatment was greater.

The investigators suggested that the greater nitrogen and potassium retention with GH combined with IGF-I infusion reflected greater muscle protein and connective tissue accretion, but no direct measures of contractile protein growth or synthesis were made. Further, it is unclear whether these subjects would have become resistant to the nitrogen-sparing effects of combined GH and IGF-I treatment, as previously observed after 33 days of GH administration [105].

The permissive effects may have been regulated by the IGF binding proteins because GH plus IGF-I increased, while IGF-I reduced, the concentration of IGFBP-3 and the acid-labile subunit of the IGF binding protein complex. It was suggested that the induction of IGF binding proteins by GH plus IGF-I may have provided responsive tissues with a continuous exposure to IGF, which may have increased nitrogen retention more. However, IGF-I infusion also increased nitrogen retention, but the IGFBP-3 levels were reduced, thus dissociating nitrogen retention from changes in IGFBP-3. This implies that some optimal (yet unknown) free IGF-I:bound IGF-I ratio provides ideal tissue anabolism. More work is required before the anabolic effects of GH and IGF-I binding protein interactions are understood.

EXERCISE TRAINING. Few studies have examined whether GH administration enhances the anabolic effects of resistance exercise training and provides any additional muscle growth, strength, or improved physical performance. When young (22–33 yr), highly conditioned (resistance and aerobic trained) men and women were given 6 wk of methionyl-GH treatment (30–50 µg/kg, 3 days/wk) in a double-blind, placebo-controlled crossover study [25], serum IGF-1 increased (125%), FFM increased more (2.7 kg), and body fat mass decreased more (1.5 kg) than during the 6-wk placebo treatment period. The investigators provide partial evidence that the increase in FFM was not due to water retention, but whether it was the result of an accumulation of contractile protein, which might increase muscle strength, was not addressed.

This was considered in a study [120] in which the fractional rate of vastus lateralis muscle protein synthesis [119] and the whole body protein breakdown rate were determined using a constant intravenous infusion of [^{13}C]-leucine in 7 young (12 ± 2 yr) experienced male weight lifters before and after 14 days of GH treatment (40 µg/kg/day). In these well-trained lifters with a large but stabilized muscle mass, GH administration increased serum IGF-I concentration (160%), but did not increase the fractional rate of muscle protein synthesis or reduce the rate of whole body protein breakdown (Fig. 10.4). Likewise, in a double-blind placebo-controlled study [35], 18 healthy young (20–28 yr) male power athletes were given GH (≈35 µg/kg/day) during 6 wk of typical training (8–14 hr heavy resistance exercise per wk), and improvements in maximal concentric strength of the biceps and quadriceps muscles were not greater in the GH-treated group. Interestingly, serum IGFBP-3 concentration increased (20–40%) in the GH-treated group, supporting the idea that the binding protein prevents circulating IGF-I from mediating an anabolic effect. These observations suggest that resistance exercise–induced muscle hypertrophy may render the muscles unresponsive to the potential anabolic effects of exogenous GH administration, a finding similar to that reported in hypophysectomized rats undergoing compensatory hypertrophy combined with GH treatment [51]. This would suggest that the GH-induced increase in FFM

FIGURE 10.4

*Despite a significant (P<0.002) increase in serum IGF-I concentration (**A**), the fractional rate of vastus lateralis muscle protein synthesis (**B**), and the estimated rate of whole body protein breakdown (systemic leucine rate of appearance, (**C**) were unchanged in experienced weight lifters after 2 weeks of daily GH administration (40 μg/kg/day). (Reprinted with permission from Yarasheski, K. E., J. J. Zachwieja, T. J. Angelopoulos, and D. M. Bier. Short-term growth hormone treatment does not increase muscle protein synthesis in experienced weight lifters. J. Appl. Physiol. 74:3073–3076, 1993.)*

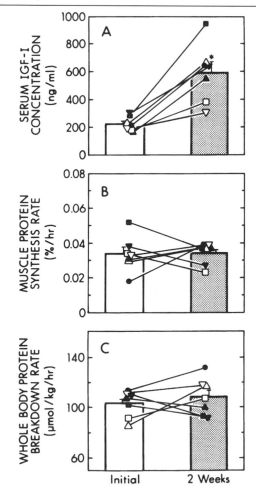

observed in well-trained individuals may not be attributed to an increase in muscle mass and that other FFM components (e.g., water, connective tissue, organ mass) need to be considered.

When 16 sedentary young (21–34 yr) men underwent a 12-wk supervised resistance exercise training program, while GH (40 μg/kg/day, 5 days/wk) or placebo injections were given in a double-blind placebo-controlled random trial [118], FFM, total body water (by deuterium dilution space), and whole body protein synthesis ([15N]-glycine kinetics) increased more in the GH recipients (Table 1). However, the fractional rate of skeletal muscle protein synthesis, torso and limb circumferences, concentric (1 repetition max.) and isokinetic (dynamometer) measures of muscle strength did not increase more in the GH recipients (Tables 10.2 & 10.3). These observations confirmed the anabolic effects of resistive exercise, but suggested that GH administration to these exercising young men did not further increase the rate of mixed muscle protein synthesis, and this was supported by the lack of a greater increase in muscle strength. The greater increase in whole body protein synthesis observed in the GH recipients could only be attributed to an increase in lean tissue other than skeletal muscle.

The possibility that a portion of the increase in lean tissue was connective

TABLE 10.1

Whole-Body Amino Acid and Protein Turnover

Rate	Leucine Kinetics, $\mu mol \cdot kg\,FFM^{-1} \cdot h^{-1}$		Protein Kinetics, g protein $\cdot kg\,FFM^{-1} \cdot day^{-1}$	
	Initial	*Final*	*Initial*	*Final*
	Exercise + placebo			
Intake	98 ± 6	102 ± 6	1.80 ± 0.04	1.80 ± 0.03
Turnover	194 ± 2	205 ± 6	5.4 ± 0.1	5.5 ± 0.1
Oxidation	63.3 ± 3.3	65.0 ± 5.3	$1.63 \pm 0.05^*$	1.62 ± 0.04
Synthesis	131 ± 4	140 ± 6	3.8 ± 0.1	3.9 ± 0.1
Breakdown	97 ± 6	104 ± 6	3.6 ± 0.1	3.7 ± 0.1
	Exercise + GH			
Intake	89 ± 6	86 ± 6	1.80 ± 0.04	1.80 ± 0.04
Turnover	172 ± 5	177 ± 4	5.0 ± 0.1	5.2 ± 0.2
Oxidation	61.4 ± 4.7	48.2 ± 5.0†	$1.66 \pm 0.10^*$	1.35 ± 0.08‡§
Synthesis	110 ± 5	128 ± 2	3.3 ± 0.1	3.8 ± 0.2‡§
Breakdown	83 ± 7	91 ± 6	3.2 ± 0.1	3.4 ± 0.2†

Values are mean ± SE. Leucine kinetics were measured during a 6-hr constant [1–13C]leucine infusion in the postprandial condition. Protein kinetics were measured with [15N]glycine during a 60 hr period while subjects consumed an isocaloric controlled protein diet.

*Total urinary nitrogen excretion × 6.25. Both tracers indicated that exercise plus GH reduced (P<0.05) whole-body amino acid oxidation. In the exercise plus GH group, whole body protein synthesis and breakdown (using [15N]glycine) increased above initial (P<0.01), and the increase in protein synthesis was greater than that in the exercise plus placebo group. Reprinted with permission from Yarasheski, K. E., J. A. Campbell, K. Smith, M. J. Rennie, J. O. Holloszy, and D. M. Bier. Effect of growth hormone and resistance exercise on muscle growth in young men. *Am. J. Physiol.* 262 (*Endocrinol. Metab.* 25): E261–E267, 1992.

TABLE 10.2
Muscle Strength Improvement

Exercise	Exercise + Placebo		Exercise + GH	
	Delta	% Change	Delta	% Change
Shoulder press	5.3 ± 0.5	53 ± 6	6.5 ± 0.9	60 ± 10
Bench press	6.1 ± 0.7	43 ± 6	6.2 ± 1.3	43 ± 11
Deltoids	4.4 ± 0.5	47 ± 7	4.5 ± 0.4	50 ± 6
Bicep curl	4.4 ± 0.3	36 ± 3	4.2 ± 0.6	33 ± 4
Latissimus	6.5 ± 0.4	59 ± 5	6.3 ± 0.5	60 ± 8
Arm cross	6.5 ± 0.4	73 ± 8	6.4 ± 0.5	66 ± 10
Knee extension	9.7 ± 0.9	63 ± 10	8.8 ± 1.2	65 ± 16
Leg press	4.9 ± 0.7	26 ± 4	4.8 ± 0.5	34 ± 5
Knee flexion	4.1 ± 0.4	47 ± 8	5.0 ± 0.8	71 ± 17
Average	5.8 ± 0.6	50 ± 4.8	5.9 ± 0.5	54 ± 4.7

Values are mean ± SE. Final strength score greater ($P<0.01$) than initial for all exercises in both groups. Delta scores represent absolute increase in number of 4.5-kg weights lifted. Average and individual delta and % change scores were not different between groups.
Reprinted with permission from Yarasheski, K. E., J. A. Campbell, K. Smith, M. J. Rennie, J. O. Holloszy, and D. M. Bier. Effect of growth hormone and resistance exercise on muscle growth in young men. *Am. J. Physiol.* 262 (*Endocrinol. Metab.* 25): E261–E267, 1992.

TABLE 10.3
Maximum Knee Extensor and Flexor Muscle Force Production

	Exercise + Placebo			Exercise + GH		
	Initial	Final	% Change	Initial	Final	% Change
Concentric						
Knee extensors	212 ± 13	248 ± 10†	17	191 ± 11	214 ± 9*	12
Knee flexors	137 ± 11	158 ± 7*	15	122 ± 12	143 ± 6*	17
Isometric						
Knee extensors	220 ± 13	252 ± 13†	14	198 ± 15	207 ± 7	4
Knee flexors	131 ± 8	158 ± 8†	20	127 ± 13	140 ± 16	10

Values are mean ± SE. Maximum force (N · m) determined using a Cybex dynamometer. Concentric force measured at 60°/sec angular velocity. Isometric force measured at 135° of knee extension. The maximum concentric force production of the knee flexor and extensor muscles increased in both groups ($P<0.05$), but these increments and the increments in maximum isometric force production were not greater in the exercise plus GH group.
Reprinted with permission from Yarasheski, K. E., J. A. Campbell, K. Smith, M. J. Rennie, J. O. Holloszy, and D. M. Bier. Effect of growth hormone and resistance exercise on muscle growth in young men. *Am. J. Physiol.* 262 (*Endocrinol. Metab.* 25): E261–E267, 1992.

tissue, fluid, or noncontractile protein was inferred from the observation that whole body protein synthesis (but not skeletal muscle protein synthesis) was increased in the GH recipients and from the observation that 2 of 9 GH recipients developed symptoms of carpal tunnel compression (and were removed from the study). In this regard, GH and IGF-I administration have been associated with connective tissue, as well as spleen, thymus, and kidney growth in hypophysectomized rats [61]. Further, the lack of a greater muscle anabolic effect of prolonged GH treatment combined with resistance training is in agreement with the early animal experiments [11, 51, 93] and the observation that the initial nitrogen-sparing effect of GH dissipates with prolonged GH treatment [64, 105]. Taken collectively, these studies suggest that resistance exercise training activates muscle protein anabolism near some limit, and supplementation with GH does not further enhance muscle protein synthesis, but other proteins may increase their synthesis rates. Therefore, on the basis of the available evidence, attempting to enhance muscle hypertrophy and function by supplementing resistance exercise with daily GH administration is not advocated.

AGING. Growth hormone secretion and serum IGF-I levels decline with advancing aging. These endocrine changes, termed the "somatopause," correlate with decrements in FFM, muscle mass and total body water and the increase in body fat associated with advancing age [98]. Growth hormone administration ($\approx$30 μg/kg; 3 days/wk) to 21 healthy older men (61–81 yr) increased FFM (whole body potassium-40, 9%), reduced body fat (14%), and increased bone density in the lumbar spine (1.6%), but improvements in muscle mass and strength were not assessed [99]. However, preliminary evidence [122] suggests that when GH supplementation was combined with 16 wk of progressive resistance exercise training in elderly (67 ± 1 yr) men, FFM increased more in the GH-treated group than in the resistance exercise training plus placebo group (4.9 ± 0.8 vs. 2.0 ± 0.6 kg). However, the additional increment in FFM did not appear to be muscle protein, because knee extensor and flexor muscle strength, measured on an isokinetic dynamometer, and concentric muscle strength (1 repetition maximum), measured on 9 upper and lower body Nautilus exercises, did not increase more in the GH recipients [122]. This does not rule out the possibility that GH treatment (without exercise) might increase muscle anabolism and function in the elderly. Instead, it suggests that GH administration may not further enhance muscle anabolism when combined with the anabolic effects of resistance exercise training in the elderly.

SUMMARY

It is clear that the anthropometric ramifications, especially with respect to muscle mass, of the metabolic actions of GH and IGF-I treatment in intact and GH-deficient adults require further study. At present, it appears that daily GH or IGF-I treatment modestly increases nitrogen retention in most normal adults, probably by separate but permissive mechanisms, but only for a short period of time ($\approx$1 month). During prolonged GH administration, resistance to the anabolic actions of GH seems to occur, and optimizing the anabolic effects of GH or IGF-I treatment will require a better understanding of the interactions among GH, GHBP, IGF-I production, IGFBPs, the GH dose regimen, and other unidentified regulatory factors.

On the basis of the similar increases in muscle protein synthesis, muscle cross-sectional area, and muscle strength observed in placebo and GH-treated exercising young adults, it is doubtful that the nitrogen retention associated with daily GH treatment results in an increase in contractile protein, improved muscle function, strength and athletic performance. Even in catabolic or GH-deficient populations, GH treatment provides only modest increments in nitrogen retention, muscle size, strength, and exercise capacity. Further, the side effects of GH treatment (water retention, carpal tunnel compression, insulin resistance) would be a detriment, rather than an aid, to athletic performance. In addition, whether prolonged (>6 months) GH treatment alone or in combination with other agents used by athletes (e.g., anabolic steroids, ß-agonists) is associated with other adverse side effects (e.g., cancer, diabetes) has not been evaluated. Therefore, health professionals should continue to discourage the use of GH by exercise enthusiasts.

ACKNOWLEDGMENTS

The comments and suggestions of Dr. Jeffrey Zachwieja and Dr. Dennis Bier are appreciated. Jill Campbell, Barbara Wilhelm, Brigid Dodson, and Dr. Ted Angelopoulos provided technical assistance. This research was supported by Genentech, Inc. and NIH grants AG00444, AG05562, RR00954, and RR00036.

REFERENCES

1. Adamafio, N. A., and F. M. Ng. Effects of growth hormone on lipogenesis and glucose oxidation in genetically GH-deficient mice. *Mol. Cell. Endocrinol.* 37:241–244, 1984.
2. Adamson, U., and S. Efendic. Insulin-like and diabetogenic effects of growth hormone in healthy subjects, diabetics, and low insulin responders. *J. Clin. Endocrinol. Metab.* 49:456–461, 1979.
3. Ahrén, K., A. Hjalmarson, and O. Isaksson. Failure of growth hormone to exert an acute inhibitory effect on glucose uptake in the rat diaphragm. *Acta Physiol. Scand.* 78:574–576, 1970.
4. Altszuler, N., I. Rathgeb, B. Winkler, R. C. deBodo, and R. S. Steele. The effects of growth hormone on carbohydrate and lipid metabolism in the dog. *Ann. NY Acad. Sci.* 148:441–458, 1968.
5. Ammann, A. J. Growth hormone and immunity. L. E. Underwood (ed). *Human Growth Hormone Progress and Challenges.* New York: Marcel Dekker, 1988, pp. 243–253.
6. Arends, J., K. E. Yarasheski, T. Arlt, D. M. Bier, E. Kuse, et al. Effect of biosynthetic human growth hormone (hGH) on post-operative protein metabolism after orthotopic liver transplantation. *Infusionstherapie* 18:78, 1991.

7. Bartoli, A. J., C. I. Reed, and H. C. Struck. Total nitrogen content of skeletal muscle of the rat in various nutritional states. *Proc. Soc. Exp. Biol. N.Y.* 35:528–532, 1937.
8. Bak, J. F., and N. Moller, and O. Schmitz. Effects of growth hormone on fuel utilization and muscle glycogen synthase activity in normal humans. *Am. J. Physiol.* 260 (Endocrinol. Metab. 23): E736–E742, 1991.
9. Baxter, R. C. Insulin-like growth factor (IGF) binding proteins: the role of serum IGFBP's in regulating IGF availability. *Acta Paediatr. Scand.* 372:107–114, 1991.
10. Baxter, R. C. Physiological roles of IGF binding proteins. E. M. Spencer (ed). *Modern Concepts of Insulin-Like Growth Factors.* New York: Elsevier, 1991, pp. 371–379.
11. Bigland, B., and B. Jehring. Muscle performance in rats, normal and treated with growth hormone. *J. Physiol.* 116:129–136, 1952.
12. Birnbaum, R. S. and H. M. Goodman. Studies on the mechanism of the antilipolytic effects of growth hormone. *Endocrinology* 99:1336–1345, 1976.
13. Bolodia, G. and F. G. Young. Growth hormone and carbohydrate metabolism in vitro. *Nature* 215:960–961, 1967.
14. Bowers, C. Y., G. A. Reynolds, D. Durham, C. M. Barrera, S. S. Pezzoli, and M. O. Thorner. Growth hormone-releasing peptide stimulates GH release in normal men and acts synergistically with GH-releasing hormone. *J. Clin. Endocrinol. Metab.* 70:975–982, 1990.
15. Butler, P., E. Kryshak, and R. Rizza. Mechanism of growth hormone-induced postprandial carbohydrate intolerance in humans. *Am. J. Physiol.* 260 (*Endocrinol. Metab.* 23):E513–E520, 1991.
16. Canalis, E. Effect of insulin like growth factor I on DNA and protein synthesis in cultured rat calvaria. *J. Clin. Invest.* 66:709–719, 1980.
17. Canalis, E. The hormonal and local regulation of bone formation. *Endocrine Rev.* 4:62–77, 1983.
18. Chesley, A., J. D. MacDougall, M. A. Tarnopolsky, S. A. Atkinson, and K. Smith. Changes in human muscle protein synthesis after resistance exercise. *J. Appl. Physiol.* 73:1383–1388, 1992.
19. Christiansen, J. S., J. O. Jorgensen, S. A. Pedersen, J. Muller, J. Jorgensen, et al. GH-replacement therapy in adults. *Horm. Res.* 36(suppl. 1):66–72, 1991.
20. Clemmons, D. R. Role of insulin-like growth factor-1 in reversing catabolism. *J. Clin. Endocrinol. Metab.* 75:1183–1185, 1992.
21. Clemmons, D. R., C. Camacho-Hubner, J. I. Jones, R. H. McCusker, and W. H. Busby, Jr. Insulin-like growth factor binding proteins: Mechanisms of action at the cellular level. E. M. Spencer (ed). *Modern Concepts of Insulin-Like Growth Factors.* New York: Elsevier, 1991, pp. 475–486.
22. Clemmons, D. R., A. Smith-Banks, and L. E. Underwood. Reversal of diet-induced catabolism by infusion of recombinant insulin-like growth factor-I in humans. *J. Clin. Endocrinol. Metab.* 75:234–238, 1992.
23. Cowart, V. S. Human growth hormone: the latest ergogenic aid? *Phys. Sportsmed.* 16:175–185, 1988.
24. Conover, C. A. Glycosylation of insulin-like growth factor binding protein-3 (IGFBP-3) is not required for potentiation of IGF-I action: evidence for processing of cell-bound IGFBP-3. *Endocrinology* 129:3259–3268, 1991.
25. Crist, D. M., G. T. Peake, P. A. Egan, and D. L. Waters. Body composition response to exogenous GH during training in highly conditioned adults. *J. Appl. Physiol.* 65:579–584, 1988.
26. Cuneo, R. C., F. Salomon, C. M. Wiles, R. Hesp, and P. H. Sönksen. Growth hormone treatment in growth hormone-deficient adults. I. Effects on muscle mass and strength. *J. Appl. Physiol.* 70:688–694, 1991.
27. Cuneo, R. C., F. Salomon, C. M. Wiles, R. Hesp, and P. H. Sönksen. Growth hormone treatment in growth hormone-deficient adults. II. Effects on exercise performance. *J. Appl. Physiol.* 70:695–700, 1991.

28. Daughaday, W. H. The anterior pituitary. J. D. Wilson and D. W. Foster (ed). *Williams Textbook of Endocrinology*. Philadelphia: W. B. Saunders, 1985, pp. 568–613.
29. Daughaday, W. H., and D. M. Kipnis. The growth promoting and anti-insulin actions of somatotropin. *Recent Prog. Hormone Res.* 22:49–93, 1966.
30. Daughaday, W. H., and P. Rotwein. Insulin-like growth factors I and II. Peptide, messenger ribonucleic acid and gene structures, serum and tissue concentration. *Endocrine Rev.* 10:68–91, 1989.
31. Davidson, M. B. Effect of growth hormone on carbohydrate and lipid metabolism. *Endocrine Rev.* 8:115–213, 1987.
32. Dempsher, D. P., D. M. Bier, S. E. Tollefsen, P. S. Rotwein, W. H. Daughaday, et al. Whole body nitrogen kinetics and their relationship to growth in short children treated with recombinant human growth hormone. *Pediatr. Res.* 28:394–400, 1990.
33. D'Ercole, A. J., A. D. Stiles, and L. E. Underwood. Tissue concentrations of somatomedin C: further evidence for multiple sites of synthesis and paracrine or autocrine mechanisms of action. *Proc. Natl. Acad. Sci. USA* 81:935–939, 1984.
34. DeVol, D. L., P. Rotwein, J. L. Sadow, J. Novakofski, and P. J. Bechtel. Activation of insulin-like growth factor gene expression during work-induced muscle growth. *Am. J. Physiol.* 259 (*Endocrinol. Metabl.* 22):E89–E95, 1990.
35. Deyssig, R., H. Frisch, W. F. Blum, and T. Waldhör. Effect of growth hormone treatment on hormonal parameters, body composition and strength in athletes. *Acta Endocrinol.* 128:313–318, 1993.
36. Douglas, R. G., P. D. Gluckman, K. Ball, B. Breier, and J. H. F. Shaw. The effects of infusion of insulin like growth factor (IGF)I, IGF-II, and insulin on glucose and protein metabolism in fasted lambs. *J. Clin. Invest.* 88:614–622, 1991.
37. Elahi, D., M. McAloon-Dyke, N. K. Fukagawa, G. Wong, K. L. Minaker, et al. Hemodynamic and metabolic responses to human insulin-like growth factore I (IGF-I) in men. E. M. Spencer (ed). *Modern Concepts of Insulin-Like Growth Factors*. New York: Elsevier, 1991, pp. 219–224.
38. Elgin, R. G., W. H. Busby, and D. F. Clemmons. An insulin-like growth factor (IGF) binding protein enhances the biologic response to IGF-I. *Proc. Natl. Acad. Sci. USA* 84:3254–3258, 1987.
39. Evans, H. M., and J. A. Long. The effect of the anterior lobe administered intraperitoneally upon growth, maturity, and oestrous cycles of the rat. *Anat. Rec.* 21:62–63, 1921.
40. Felsing, N. E., J. A. Brasel, and D. M. Cooper. Effect of low and high intensity exercise on circulating growth hormone in men. *J. Clin. Endocrinol. Metab.* 75:157–162, 1992.
41. Fineberg, S. E., and T. J. Merimee. Acute metabolic effects of human growth hormone. *Diabetes* 23:499–504, 1974.
42. Fong, Y., M. Rosenbaum, K. J. Tracey, G. Raman, D. G. Hesse, et al. Recombinant growth hormone enhances muscle myosin heavy-chain mRNA accumulation and amino acid accrual in humans. *Proc. Natl. Acad. Sci. USA* 86:3371–3374, 1989.
43. Foster, C. M., J. A. Shafer, F. W. Rozsa, X. Y. Wang, S. D. Lewis, et al. Growth hormone promoted tyrosyl phosphorylation of growth hormone receptors in murine 3T3-F442A fibroblasts and adipocytes. *Biochemistry* 27:326–334, 1988.
44. Frohman, L. A., M. H. MacGillivray, and T. Aceto, Jr. Acute effects of human growth hormone on insulin secretion and glucose utilization in normal and growth hormone deficient subjects. *J. Clin. Endocrinol.* 27:561–567, 1967.
45. Fryburg, D. A., R. A. Gelfand, and E. J. Barrett. Growth hormone acutely stimulates forearm muscle protein synthesis in normal humans. *Am. J. Physiol.* 260 (*Endocrinol. Metab.* 23):E499–E504, 1991.
46. Fryburg, D. A., R. J. Louard, K. E. Gerow, R. A. Gelfand, and E. J. Barrett. Growth hormone stimulates skeletal muscle protein synthesis and antagonizes insulin's antiproteolytic action in humans. *Diabetes* 41:424–429, 1992.
47. Fukagawa, N. K., K. L. Minaker, W. Rowe, M. N. Goodman, D. E. Matthews, et al.

Insulin-mediated reduction of whole body protein breakdown. Dose-response effects on leucine metabolism in postabsorptive man. *J. Clin. Invest.* 76:2306–2311, 1985.

48. Gelfand, R. A., and E. J. Barrett. Effect of physiologic hyperinsulinemia on skeletal muscle protein synthesis and breakdown in man. *J. Clin. Invest.* 80:1–6, 1987.

49. Goldberg, A. L. Work-induced growth of skeletal muscle in normal and hypophysecto-mized rats. *Am. J. Physiol.* 213:1193–1198, 1967.

50. Goldberg, A. L., J. D. Etlinger, D. F. Goldspink, and C. Jablecki. Mechanism of work-induced hypertrophy of skeletal muscle. *Med. Sci. Sports* 7:248–261, 1975.

51. Goldberg, A. L., and H. M. Goodman. Relationship between growth hormone and muscular work in determining muscle size. *J. Physiol.* 200:655–666, 1969.

52. Goodman, H. M. Effects of growth hormone on glucose utilization in diaphragm muscle in the absence of increased lipolysis. *Endocrinology* 81:1099–1103, 1967.

53. Goodman, H. M. Growth hormone and the metabolism of carbohydrate and lipid in adipose tissue. *Ann. NY Acad. Sci.* 148:419–440, 1968.

54. Goodman, H. M. Multiple effects of growth hormone on lipolysis. *Endocrinology* 83:300–308, 1968.

55. Goodman, H. M. Failure of growth hormone alone to potentiate epinephrine-induced lipolysis. *Proc. Soc. Exp. Biol. Med.* 132:821–824, 1969.

56. Goodman, H. M. Antilipolytic effects of growth hormone. *Metabolism* 19:849–855, 1970.

57. Goodman, H. M., and J. Schwartz. Growth hormone and lipid metabolism. E. Knobil and W. H. Sawyer (eds). *Handbook of Physiology*, vol. 4, part 2. Washington, D.C.: American Physiological Society, 1974, pp. 211–232.

58. Gore, D. C., D. Honeycutt, F. Jahoor, T. Rutan, R. R. Wolfe, and D. N. Herndon. Effect of exogenous growth hormone on glucose utilization in burn patients. *J. Surg. Res.* 51:518–523, 1991.

59. Green, H., M. Morikawa, and T. Nixon. A dual effector theory of growth hormone action. *Differentiation* 29:195–198, 1985.

60. Grindeland, R. E., R. R. Roy, V. R. Edgerton, E. Grossman, I. Rudolph, et al. Exercise and growth hormone have synergistic effects on skeletal muscle and tibias of suspended rats. *FASEB J.* 5:A1037, 1991.

61. Guler, H. P., J. Zapf, E. Scheiwiller, and E. R. Froesch. Recombinant human insulin-like growth factor-I stimulates growth and has distinct effects on organ size in hypophysecto-mized rats. *Proc. Natl. Acad. Sci. USA* 85:4889–4893, 1988.

62. Harris, W. H., R. P. Heaney, J. Jowsey, J. Cockin, C. Atkins, et al. Growth hormone the effect on skeletal renewal in the adult dog. I. Morphometric studies. *Calcif. Tissue Res.* 10:1–13, 1972.

63. Hearings before the Subcommittee on Health and the Environment of the House of Representatives Committee on Energy and Commerce, 100th Congress, 1st session. Ser. no. 100–34. In *Medical Devices and Drug Issues*. Washington, D.C.: Government Printing Office, 1987.

64. Henneman, P. H., A. P. Forbes, M. Moldauer, E. F. Dempsey, and E. L. Carroll. Effects of human growth hormone in man. *J. Clin. Invest.* 39:1223–1238, 1960.

65. Ho, K. Y., and J. J. Kelly. Role of growth hormone and fluid homeostasis. *Horm. Res.* 36(suppl.1):44–48, 1991.

66. Hochberg, Z., T. Amit, and M. B. H. Youdim. The growth hormone binding protein as a paradigm of the erythropoietin superfamily of receptors. *Cellular Signalling* 3:85–91, 1991.

67. Horber, F. F., and M. W. Haymond. Human growth hormone prevents the protein catabolic side effects of prednisone in humans. *J. Clin. Invest.* 86:265–272, 1990.

68. Ikkos, D., R. Luft, and B. Sjögren. Body water and sodium in patients with acromegaly. *J. Clin. Invest.* 33:989–994, 1954.

69. Isaksson, O. G. P., S. Eden, and J. O. Jansson. Mode of action of pituitary growth hormone on target cells. *Annu. Rev. Physiol.* 47:483–499, 1985.

70. Jacobs, S., E. Barrett, G. Plewe, K. D. Fagin, and R. J. Sherwin. Acute effects of insulin-like

growth factor-I on glucose and amino acid metabolism in the awake fasted rat. *J. Clin. Invest.* 83:1717–1723, 1989.

71. Jiang, B., R. R. Roy, C. Navarro, and V. R. Edgerton. Absence of a growth hormone effect on rat soleus atrophy during a 4-day space flight. *J. Appl. Physiol.* 74:527–531, 1993.

72. Jorgensen, J. O. L., S. A. Pedersen, L. Thuesen, J. Jorgensen, T. Ingemann-Hansen, et al. Beneficial effects of growth hormone treatment in GH-deficient adults. *Lancet* 1:1221–1225, 1989.

73. Knauer, D. J., and G. L. Smith. Inhibition of biological activity of multiplication-stimulating activity by binding to its carrier protein. *Proc. Natl. Acad. Sci. USA* 77:7252–7256, 1980.

74. Knobil, E. Direct evidence for fatty acid mobilization in response to growth hormone in rat. *Proc. Soc. Exp. Biol. Med.* 101:288–289, 1959.

75. Kostyo, J. L. Rapid effects of growth hormone on amino acid transport and protein synthesis. *Ann. NY Acad. Sci.* 148:389–407, 1968.

76. Kostyo, J. L., and D. F. Nutting. Growth hormone and protein metabolism. E. Knobil and W. H. Sawyer (eds). *Handbook of Physiology*, vol. 4, part 2. Washington, D.C.: American Physiological Society, 1974, pp. 187–210.

77. Kupfer, S. R., L. E. Underwood, R. C. Baxter, and D. R. Clemmons. Enhancement of the anabolic effect of growth hormone and insulin-like growth factor I by use of both agents simultaneously. *J. Clin. Invest.* 91:391–396, 1993.

78. Lee, M. O., and N. K. Schaffer. Anterior pituitary growth hormone and the composition of growth. *J. Nutr.* 7:337–363, 1934.

79. Linderman, J. K., K. L. Gosselink, R. E. Grindeland, F. W. Booth, and V. R. Mukku. The synergistic effect of exercise and growth hormone on skeletal muscle atrophy during hindlimb suspension. *FASEB J.* 7:A668, 1993.

80. MacDougall, J. D. Morphological changes in human skeletal muscle following strength training and immobilization. N. L. Jones, N. McCartney, and A. J. McComas (eds). *Human Muscle Power*. Champaign, IL: Human Kinetics, 269–285, 1986.

81. Maiter, D., L. E. Underwood, M. Maes, M. L. Davenport, and J. M. Ketelslegers. Different effects of intermittent and continuous growth hormone (GH) administration on serum somatomedin-C/insulin-like growth factor I and liver GH receptors in hypophysectomized rats. *Endocrinology* 123:1053–1059, 1988.

82. Maor, G., Z. Hochberg, K. von der Mark, D. Heingard, and M. Silbermann. Human growth hormone enhances chondrogenesis and osteogenesis in a tissue culture system of chondroprogenitor cells. *Endocrinology* 125:1239–1245, 1989.

83. Marcus, R., G. Butterfield, L. Holloway, L. Gilliland, D. J. Baylink, et al. Effects of short term administration of recombinant human growth hormone to elderly people. *J. Clin. Endocrinol. Metab.* 70:519–527, 1990.

84. Mauras, N., F. F. Horber, and M. W. Haymond. Low dose recombinant human insulin-like growth factor-I fails to affect protein anabolism but inhibits islet cell secretion in humans. *J. Clin. Endocrinol. Metab.* 75:1192–1197, 1992.

85. McCusker, R. H., and D. R. Clemmons. Insulin-like growth factor binding protein secretion by muscle cells: effects of cellular differentiation and proliferation. *J. Cell. Physiol.* 137:505–512, 1988.

86. Metcalfe, P., D.G. Johnston, R. Nosadini, H. Orksov, and K. G. M. M. Alberti. Metabolic effects of acute and prolonged growth hormone excess in normal and insulin-deficient man. *Diabetologia* 20:123–128, 1981.

87. Moller, N., J. O. L. Jorgensen, O. Schmitz, J. Moller, J. S. Christiansen, et al. Effects of a growth hormone pulse on total and forearm substrate fluxes in humans. *Am. J. Physiol.* 258 (*Endocrinol. Metab.* 21):E86–E91, 1990.

88. Murphy, L.J., G. I. Bell, M. L. Duckworth, and H. G. Friesen. Identification, characterization, and regulation of a rat complementary deoxyribonucleic acid which encodes insulin-like growth factor-I. *Endocrinology* 121:684–691, 1987.

89. Murphy, L. J., G. I. Bell, and H. G. Friesen. Tissue distribution of insulin-like growth factor I and II messenger ribonucleic acid in the adult rat. *Endocrinology* 120:1279–1282, 1987.

90. Nagulesparen, M., R. Trickey, M. J. Davies, and J. S. Jenkins. Muscle changes in acromegaly. *Br. Med. J.* 2:914–915, 1976.

91. Nyberg, G., S. Boström, R. Johansson, and U. Smith. Reduced glucose incorporation to triglycerides following chronic exposure of human fat cells to growth hormone. *Acta Endocrinol. (Copenh.)* 95:129–133, 1980.

92. Pape, G. S., M. Friedman, L. E. Underwood, and D. R. Clemmons. The effect of growth hormone on weight gain and pulmonary function in patients with chronic obstructive lung disease. *Chest* 99:1495–1500, 1991.

93. Plattener, E. B., and C. I. Reed. A study of muscular efficiency in rats injected with anterior pituitary growth factor. *Endocrinology* 25:401–404, 1939.

94. Press, M. Growth hormone and metabolism. *Diabetes Metab. Rev.* 4:391–441, 1988.

95. Rechler, M. M., and S. P. Nissley. The nature and regulation of the receptors for insulin-like growth factors. *Annu. Rev. Physiol.* 47:425–442, 1989.

96. Rizza, R. A., L. J. Mandarino, and J. E. Gerich. Effects of growth hormone on insulin action in man: mechanisms of insulin resistance, impaired suppression of glucose production, and impaired stimulation of glucose utilization. *Diabetes* 31:663–669, 1982.

97. Rogol, A. D. Growth hormone: physiology, therapeutic use, and potential for abuse. K. B. Pandolf (ed). *Exercise and Sport Sciences Reviews*. Baltimore: Williams & Wilkins, 1989, pp. 353–377.

98. Rudman, D. Growth hormone, body composition and aging. *J. Am. Geriatr. Soc.* 11:800–807, 1985.

99. Rudman, D., A. G. Feller, H. S. Nagraj, G. A. Gergans, P. Y. Lalitha, et al. Effects of human growth hormone in men over 60 years old. *N. Engl. J. Med.* 323:1–6, 1990.

100. Salomon, F., R. C. Cuneo, R. Hesp, and P. H. Sönksen. The effects of treatment with recombinant human growth hormone on body composition and metabolism in adults with growth hormone deficiency. *N. Engl. J. Med.* 321:1797–1803, 1989.

101. Schwartz, J. Growth hormone directly alters glucose utilization in 3T3 adipocytes. *Biochem. Biophys. Res. Commun.* 125:237–243, 1984.

102. Schwartz, J., and H. M. Goodman. Lipolytic response to growth hormone in acutely nephrectomized rats. *J. Endocrinol.* 68:481–482, 1976.

103. Smith, P. E. Hypophysectomy and a replacement therapy in the rat. *Am. J. Anat.* 45:205–273, 1930.

104. Smith, R. G., K. Cheng, W. R. Schoen, S. Pong, G. Hickey, et al. A nonpeptidyl growth hormone secretagogue. *Science* 260:1640–1643, 1993.

105. Snyder, D. K., D. R. Clemmons, and L. E. Underwood. Treatment of obese, diet-restricted subjects with growth hormone for 11 weeks: effects on anabolism, lipolysis, and body composition. *J. Clin. Endocrinol. Metab.* 67:54–61, 1988.

106. Spencer, E. M. *Modern Concepts of Insulin-Like Growth Factors*. New York: Elsevier, 1991.

107. Sturek, M., D. R. Lamb, and A. C. Snyder. Somatomedin-like activity and muscle hypertrophy. *IRCS J. Med. Sci.* 9:760, 1981.

108. Taylor, W. N. Letter to the Editor: Will synthetic growth hormone become the peril of genetic engineering? *Ann. Sports Med.* 2:197–199, 1986.

109. Turkalj, I., U. Keller, R. Innis, S. Vosmer, and W. Stauffacher. Effect of increasing doses of recombinant human insulin-like growth factor-I on glucose, lipid, and leucine metabolism. *J. Clin. Endocrinol. Metab.* 75:1186–1191, 1992.

110. Ullman, M., H. Alameddine, A. Skottner, and A. Oldfors. Effects of growth hormone on skeletal muscle. II. Studies on regeneration and denervation in adult rats. *Acta Physiol. Scand.* 135:537–543, 1989.

111. Ullrich, A., A. Gray, and A. W. Tam. Insulin-like growth factor- I receptor primary structure: comparison with insulin receptor suggests structural determinants that define functional specificity. *EMBO J.* 5:2503–2512, 1986.

112. Underwood, L. E. *Human Growth Hormone Progress and Challenges.* New York: Marcel Dekker, 1988.
113. Underwood, L. E., and J. J. Van Wyk. Normal and aberrant growth. J. D. Wilson and D. W. Foster (eds). *Williams Textbook of Endocrinology.* Philadelphia: W. B. Saunders, 1985, pp. 155–205.
114. Wadler, G. I., and B. Hainline. Human growth hormone. A. J. Ryan (ed). *Contemporary Exercise and Sports Medicine Series: Drugs and the Athlete.* Philadelphia: F. A. Davis, 1989, pp. 70–74.
115. Ward, H. C., D. Halliday, and A. J. W. Sim. Protein and energy metabolism with biosynthetic growth hormone after gastrointestinal surgery. *Ann. Surg.* 206:56–61, 1987.
116. Wolf, R. F., D. B. Pearlstone, E. Newman, M. J. Heslin, A. Gonenne, et al. Growth hormone and insulin reverse net whole body and skeletal muscle protein catabolism in cancer patients. *Ann. Sug.* 216:280–288, 1992.
117. Yarasheski, K. E. Effect of exercise on muscle mass in the elderly. H. M. Perry, J. E. Morley, and R. M. Coe (eds). *Aging and Musculoskeletal Disorders: Concepts, Diagnosis, and Treatment.* New York: Springer, 1993, pp. 199–213.
118. Yarasheski, K. E., J. A. Campbell, K. Smith, M. J. Rennie, J. O. Holloszy, and D. M. Bier. Effect of growth hormone and resistance exercise on muscle growth in young men. *Am. J. Physiol.* 262 (*Endocrinol. Metab.* 25):E261–E267, 1992.
119. Yarasheski, K. E., K. Smith, M. J. Rennie, and D. M. Bier. Measurement of muscle protein fractional synthetic rate by capillary gas chromatography/combustion isotope ratio mass spectrometry. *Biol. Mass Spectrom.* 21:486–490, 1992.
120. Yarasheski, K. E., J. J. Zachwieja, T. J. Angelopoulos, and D. M. Bier. Short-term growth hormone treatment does not increase muscle protein synthesis in experienced weight lifters. *J. Appl. Physiol.* 74:3073–3076, 1993.
121. Yarasheski, K. E., J. J. Zachwieja, and D. M. Bier. Acute effects of resistance exercise on muscle protein synthesis rate in young and elderly adults. *Am. J. Physiol.* 265 (*Endocrinol. Metab.* 28), E210–E214, 1993.
122. Yarasheski, K. E., J. J. Zachwieja, J. A. Campbell, and D. M. Bier. Effect of resistance exercise and growth hormone therapy on fat-free mass and muscle strength in older men. *Proceedings of the Annual Meeting of the Gerontological Society of America,* 1993.
123. Zorzano, A., D. E. James, N. B. Ruderman, and P. F. Pilch. Insulin-like growth factor I binding and receptor kinase in red and white muscle. *FEBS Lett.* 234:257–262, 1988.

11
Skeletal Muscle Adaptation to Chronic Low-Frequency Motor Nerve Stimulation

WILLIAM E. KRAUS, M.D.
CAROL E. TORGAN, Ph.D.
DORIS A. TAYLOR, Ph.D.

Chronic low-frequency motor nerve stimulation (CMNS) of fast-twitch skeletal muscle induces a conversion of the stimulated muscle to a slow-twitch phenotype. This transformation, possible because of the remarkable plasticity of skeletal muscle, provides a key to unlock the cellular mechanisms that determine skeletal muscle fiber type and the trophic effects of neural activity on skeletal muscles. The mechanisms that control muscle phenotype are of long-standing interest to basic cell biologists, but determinants of skeletal muscle plasticity have also recently become of concern to clinicians, because the human body uses skeletal muscle as a major means of adapting to a number of bodily stresses. For example, skeletal muscle mediates bodily adaptation to the stresses induced by changes in physical activity and exercise, as well as to chronic disease states involving skeletal muscle (muscular dystrophies) and cardiac muscle (chronic congestive heart failure) and to a myriad of nonmuscle diseases and conditions (chronic renal failure, diabetes mellitus, and malnutrition, to name only a few). Additionally, the plasticity of skeletal muscle in adapting to increases in contractile work is being used to advantage in cardiomyoplasty procedures and in the construction of cardiac assist devices. Some applied biologists have envisioned using chronic low-frequency electrical stimulation in novel clinical settings as a means of preventing the muscular atrophy observed in chronic bedridden hospitalized patients and in astronauts on long space missions. In this review we outline what CMNS has taught us about the basic mechanisms of skeletal muscle plasticity and the cellular mechanisms of skeletal muscle signaling that mediate muscle phenotype through neural activity. This is not meant to be an exhaustive review of the subject, as several excellent reviews have been published [74, 122, 123, 128, 141]. Rather, this review focuses on current knowledge as a means of elucidating possible cellular signaling pathways that may impact upon skeletal muscle gene expression and phenotype.

Skeletal muscles are diverse in their work requirements and are highly specialized in their performance characteristics. In general, fast-twitch muscle fibers, which are activated by short high-frequency nerve impulse trains, are called upon relatively rarely for short bursts of high-intensity work and fatigue rapidly. Slow-twitch fibers, in contrast, whose nerve impulses are tonic and of relatively low frequency, are called upon almost constantly for regular, low-intensity work and are slow to fatigue. Postural muscles are composed primarily of such fibers, while the extreme example of a tonically activated, nonfatiguing muscle is the heart. Compared with the heart, skeletal muscles of all fiber types readily change their morphologic characteristics. They exhibit a remarkable ability to alter their basic protein constituents of energy metabolism, ion channel function, and the contractile apparatus in response to signals generated by neural input and by environmental and physiologic stimuli, including chronic exercise [11, 146].

The functional requirements of skeletal muscles are reflected in their constituent proteins: primarily those of energy metabolism, excitation-contraction coupling, and the contractile apparatus. Each of these classes of proteins is essential for the efficient functioning of the skeletal myocyte, and there are muscle-specific isoforms for many of these proteins. Fast-twitch muscles have low amounts of mitochondria and oxidative proteins, high concentrations of glycolytic enzymes, a relatively high density of transverse (T-) tubules and sarcoplasmic reticulum (SR) [38], and fast-twitch isoforms of the contractile proteins myosin heavy chain (HC), tropomyosin (Tm), and troponin (Tn) [146]. In contrast, slow-twitch muscles have a high density of mitochondria, are highly oxidative with low glycolytic capacity, have half the T-tubular and SR content of fast-twitch muscles, and contain slow isoforms of the contractile proteins. However, the phenotype of a muscle is not fixed. Skeletal muscle shows a remarkable ability to adapt to chronic alterations in neural stimulation or contractile frequency by changing its constituent proteins through alterations in gene expression [11, 146, 174]. For example, CMNS will gradually result, after several weeks, in conversion of a fast-twitch muscle to a slow-twitch phenotype [144, 145]. The powerful nature of neural input to muscle phenotype has been appreciated since the classic cross-innervation experiments of Buller and Eccles [22, 36]. Despite knowing a great deal about the details of protein transitions that occur during CMNS and a smattering about changes in gene expression that mediate these changes, little is known about how muscle fiber type transformation takes place: how the myocyte senses a need to alter its protein content in response to CMNS, how it transfers this information to the nuclear compartment, how that information is transduced to genetic signals that result in alterations in gene expression, and what the precise neuromuscular signals and mediators are that control muscle phenotype. On a basic level, these are questions that relate to the mechanisms mediating cellular memory in skeletal myocytes.

In the course of CMNS-induced transitions, during which the muscle phenotype is transformed from fast- to slow-twitch, many changes occur at both a tissue and a cellular level. At a tissue level, there is atrophy (decrease in wet weight of approximately 70%), significant capillary growth, and activation of satellite cells with incorporation of new nuclei into muscle fibers [68, 99, 141]. On a cellular level, there is reduction in T-tubular and SR content [38], replacement of fast-twitch contractile protein isoforms by slow-twitch isoforms [174], and reduction in glycolytic enzymatic capacity and induction of oxidative capacity due to alterations in enzyme content [58, 59]. These latter, often dramatic, alterations in protein content are primarily mediated by alterations in gene transcription [86].

Methods of CMNS
The most widely employed technique for CMNS involves pacing a skeletal muscle group through direct stimulation of its motor nerve, using implantable electrodes that are well tolerated by the animal. This was first done in rabbits by implanting bipolar platinum or stainless steel electrodes on either side of the nerve to be stimulated [145]. Positioning of the electrode is crucial, not only to prevent mechanical stimulation or damage to the nerve, but also to ensure adequate stimulation of all neural fibers. Investigators now often use fully or partially implantable devices to prevent animal interference with the electrodes. After implantation in the vicinity of the motor nerve, electrodes can be externalized and connected to a portable subcutaneously implanted stimulator. Initially, the technique developed in rabbits used motor nerve stimulation at a given frequency (often 10 Hz) for 24 hours or less per day. Several improvements have since allowed extension of the technique to smaller mammals and provide varied pacing parameters. Implantation of a miniaturized receiver-coupler has permitted telestimulation [158]. Further miniaturization of the pacemaker has allowed extension of experiments to rodents. Larger mammals such as dogs and goats have also been used as a model species. The pacemaker circuit has additionally been converted to integrated circuit technology to include an optical sensing device that will permit transcutaneous manipulation of the frequency patterns [142].

In addition to species variations, investigators have studied the effects of both high- and low-frequency stimulation patterns on muscles of different fiber types, in attempts to answer questions about the hierarchy of neural signaling pathways. Unless otherwise stated, in this review CMNS will represent data acquired in rabbits, with pacing of the fast-twitch muscles of the anterior compartment of the hind limb (tibialis anterior [TA] or extensor digitorum longus [EDL]) at 10 Hz for 8–24 hours/day. The length of time during which the muscle is stimulated is an important consideration. In particular, the rapidity of cellular changes and fiber type transformation appear to be related to the integral of the stimulation time. Thus, transformations occur approximately twice as rapidly in muscles stimulated for 24 hours/day (continuous stimulation) than in those stimulated for 12 hours/day (intermittent stimulation) [144]. There may be other differences in the biology of the cellular responses as well. For example, inflammatory infiltrates may be seen in the muscle of intermittent stimulations and not those of continuous stimulations [95].

CMNS as a Model of Exercise

Although it is not a perfect reproduction of the exercise training stimulus, CMNS is a useful model for studying many of the cellular events that occur in skeletal muscle in response to exercise [11]. The alterations in some aspects of muscle phenotype that occur in response to CMNS are similar to those that occur in response to chronic exercise conditioning, but they occur more rapidly and are of much greater magnitude. Thus CMNS provides a continuum of muscle plasticity onto which exercise can be placed.

CMNS has several advantages over voluntary muscle activity as a model for the study of the trophic effects of exercise training on skeletal muscle. With electrical stimulation for 24 hours/day, the full adaptive and plastic capacity of skeletal muscle is approachable. It is very difficult to achieve complete fiber type conversion in exercised animals, where experiments are limited by physical fatigue and psychological factors, such as motivation. With CMNS, the effects of neural activation on muscle are isolated from alterations in systemic neuroendocrine pathways that occur during physical exercise (e.g., catecholamine release, suppression of insulin release). Since the changes occur faster, experiments are less expensive and generally more reproducible. CMNS is usually performed only on a single limb of a given animal. Thus, the contralateral limb serves as an excellent control for possible interanimal variations and environmental influences (e.g., diet) on skeletal muscle phenotype. The cellular changes in phenotype occur in an ordered sequence, are reversible, increase with the duration of the stimulation, and display dose-dependent relationships. Using CMNS under standardized conditions, one can readily investigate coordinated gene expression and synthesis of various proteins characteristic of skeletal myocytes, and initiate investigations of the regulatory mechanisms involved in the control of gene expression in excitable cells.

Despite these advantages, it must be emphasized that CMNS has deficiencies as a model of skeletal muscle exercise training. CMNS induces a very different type of recruitment pattern: all motor units are activated synchronously, rather than in the graded, hierarchical fashion characteristic of voluntary movement. In most experiments, neuromuscular recruitment is performed for a much more extended period (usually from 8 to 24 hours/day) than occurs with voluntarily exercising models. Thus the exercise-to-recovery ratio in CMNS and percentage of a 24-hour period spent performing contractile work is quite different.

Several assumptions are made when using CMNS. One assumes that the presence of the stimulation device and the stimulation itself do not cause any postural or locomotor asymmetry (i.e., increased weight bearing in the contralateral limb). This assumption appears valid in that observations

TABLE 11.1
Classification Schemes of Skeletal Muscle Fiber Types

Characteristic	Fiber Type		
Electrical activity pattern	Phasic High frequency		Tonic Low frequency
Morphology	*FTb*	*FTa*	*ST*
Color	White	White/red	Red
Fiber diameter	Large	Intermediate	Small
Capillaries/mm²	Low	Intermediate	High
Mitochondrial volume	Low	Intermediate	High
Histochemistry &	*IIB*	*IIA*	*I*
biochemistry	*FG*	*FOG*	*SO*
Myosin ATPase	High	High	Low
Calcium-handling capacity	High	Medium/high	Low
Glycolytic capacity	High	High	Low
Oxidative capacity	Low	Medium/high	High
Function &	*FF*	*FR*	*S*
contractility	*FT*	*FT*	*ST*
Speed of contraction	Fast	Fast	Slow
Speed of relaxation	Fast	Fast	Slow
Fatigability	High	Moderate/high	Low
Contraction strength	High	Intermediate	Low

Abbreviations: FT, fast-twitch; ST, slow-twitch; FG, fast, glycolytic; FOG, fast, oxidative, glycolytic; SO, slow, oxidative; FF, fast-contracting, fast-fatigue; FR, fast-contracting, fatigue-resistant; S, slowly contracting.

made in the control limb do not vary due to the length of stimulation [15, 41], and measurements in the contralateral limb are similar to those made in limbs of untreated animals [126]. One also assumes that all motor units are subjected to similar patterns of activity and are equally stimulated. Although some interanimal and interfiber variability in the response to CMNS in single fiber analyses are observed, these are most likely due to initial muscle fiber-type variations between animals [41] or asymmetric environmental influences, not to the stimulation itself.

PHYSIOLOGY, BIOCHEMISTRY, AND MOLECULAR BIOLOGY OF SKELETAL MUSCLE ADAPTATIONS TO CMNS

Muscle Physiology

A rudimentary understanding of skeletal muscle structure and function is assumed and can be found in any general physiology textbook. This overview highlights the range in muscle phenotype and reviews the classification schemes. The wide variation in muscle biochemical and functional characteristics has led to a generally accepted classification of fiber types. The classifications are outlined in Table 11.1 and are described below. These classifications tend to overlap but are not interchangeable. While the classification schemes have been used to interpret data from a variety of species [6], there appear to be species-specific differences in both classification as well as response to altered activity patterns [166].

Table 11.1 provides a general catalog of the divisions of muscle fiber characteristics most often encountered. However, it is more appropriate to consider these properties as arbitrary divisions drawn along a continuum. This perspective will become more evident as the changes in phenotype in response to CMNS are detailed. That is, alterations in muscle phenotype in response to a novel electrical pattern represent a shift from one part of the spectrum to another. The range of fiber types has been categorized based on various morphological, biochemical, and functional properties (for discussion, see [129]). At one end of the continuum are the fast-twitch, glycolytic, white fibers, which are activated in a phasic manner by high-frequency electrical activity. The tonically active slow-twitch, oxidative, red fibers represent the other end of the continuum.

MORPHOLOGY. On a gross level, skeletal muscle can be categorized as red or white. The red color is due to high levels of myoglobin and capillaries. Red fibers are small, and thus diffusion distances are short. Due to a high density of mitochondria, these fibers are highly suited for oxidative metabolism. White fibers tend to be large and have a paucity of myoglobin, capillaries, and mitochondria.

HISTOCHEMISTRY AND BIOCHEMISTRY. Fiber types are most often categorized according to actomyosin ATPase (mATPase) staining. The change in muscle mATPase activity from fast to slow with continuous neural stimulation reflects underlying changes in the composition of the thick filament protein, myosin. As myosin heavy chain and light chain composition are altered, mATPase changes to reflect the thick filament composition.

In a histologic section, muscle fibers can be classified depending upon the specific myosin molecule expressed within the fiber by determining the acid or alkali stability of the myofibrillar mATPase activity. mATPase activity of type II (fast) fibers is inactivated at acid pH but remains relatively stable at alkaline pH; mATPase of type I (slow) fibers remains active at acid pH but is inactivated after alkaline preincubation [14, 51, 120]. Histologic determination of mATPase activity, and antibody binding, coupled with the ability to electrophoretically separate myosin molecules, has led to classifications of fibers as fast type II (IIB, IID/X, IIAB, IIA, IIC) or slow type I.

From a biochemical standpoint, fibers may be classified according to their oxidative and glycolytic capacity. This has been used in conjunction with contraction time, to develop the classification schemes of slow, oxidative (SO); fast, oxidative, glycolytic (FOG); and fast, glycolytic (FG) [121]. Type I fibers have an abundance of oxidative machinery and are SO; type IIA fibers are intermediate and are FOG; IIB fibers are FG due to their reliance on glycolytic metabolism [121].

CONTRACTILITY. The functional characteristics of muscle depend on the energy metabolism, the calcium-handling capacity, and the rate at which myosin splits ATP via mATPase. Type I, SO fibers have a low rate of mATPase activity, which reduces the energy demand. This, in conjunction with their lower calcium-handling capabilities, creates fibers that have a slow rate of tension development and relaxation (slow-twitch or ST) but that are very fatigue resistant (FR). On the other end of the spectrum are the fibers that have high rates of mATPase and extensive calcium-handling systems but low oxidative capacities. These fibers have a rapid rate of tension development and relaxation (fast twitch or FT) but are fast-to-fatigue (FF). It should be noted that the scheme of FR, FF, and S originated as a system for the classification of motor units [24–26]. These terms tend to be associated with the muscle fibers themselves; however it is more correct to use the nomenclature "type FF (or FR or S) unit fiber" [24].

ADAPTATIONS IN SKELETAL MUSCLE FUNCTIONAL AND BIOCHEMICAL CHARACTERISTICS (PHENOTYPE) WITH CMNS. A number of overall functional changes occur as a result of CMNS. In general, the muscle gradually converts from a fast muscle to a muscle with slow characteristics [145]. Changes in isometric twitch characteristics become significant as early as 2 weeks after stimulation, whereas changes in isotonic contraction occur later. This suggests that the calcium-sequestering system and metabolic properties are altered early, but that myofibrillar changes occur after longer periods of stimulation. The sequential nature of these alterations presumably allows the muscle to maintain a relatively normal physiologic response to a different demand. Continuously stimulated muscle displays a decrease in fatigability, an increase in the time-to-peak twitch tension and half-relaxation time, as well as a decrease in the maximum rate of tetanic tension development. Maximum rate of rise of tetanic contraction, in particular, is measured under conditions that approximate full activation of the muscle, so that the decrease presumably reflects changes in the kinetics of myosin cross-bridge interaction, which results from fast-to-slow transitions of myosin isoforms [139]. However, stimulation-induced changes in contractile properties also reflect alterations in the composition of other myofibrillar proteins, including the regulatory proteins of the thin filament, troponin (Tn), tropomyosin (Tm), and α-skeletal actin.

For the purpose of this discussion and based primarily upon the transitions in the contractile proteins, we have grouped the adaptive responses of skeletal muscle to CMNS into three phases of induction. The acute phase encompasses immediate to early responses that occur up to 2 days following the institution of CMNS. The dynamic phase includes regulatory and modulatory changes that occur during the period from 2 days to 6 weeks of continuous stimulation. The maintenance phase is primarily steady state and homeostatic and occurs from 6 weeks and beyond. The division between the dynamic and maintenance phases has been set as the point at which the slow contractile protein isoforms are expressed. In this review, each phase is considered individually, where appropriate, for the following sections: morphology and ultrastructure, proteins of excitation-contraction coupling, metabolic pathways, contractile machinery, proteins of the neuromuscular junction, and factors of putative signaling pathways. Recovery from prolonged periods of CMNS will be addressed separately (see Recovery). As already noted, CMNS refers to nerve stimulation protocols of rabbit TA and EDL, for 8–24 hours/day, at 10 Hz. Other protocols are considered individually (Section IV) and as appropriate within the discussion.

Morphology, Ultrastructure, and Performance Characteristics

MORPHOLOGY AND ULTRASTRUCTURE. After a few hours of CMNS, there is some swelling of the longitudinal SR. Within the first week, there is a decrease in the terminal cisternae of the SR. By 2 weeks of stimulation, this system approaches levels typical of slow-twitch muscle [39, 41]. Hence there is a substantial and rapid reduction in the amount of membrane that functions to transport calcium. This is subsequently followed by alterations in membrane composition [41]. Within the first week, there is also a decrease in the amount of the T-tubular system. This system continues to decrease throughout the stimulation period, such that morphometrically it also becomes indistinguishable from the T-tubular system of the slow-twitch soleus [39, 41].

During the first few weeks of CMNS, the myofibrils show evidence of disruption [41, 100]. One of the most marked alterations within the myofibrils is a widening of the Z band. This takes place during the first 2–3 weeks [39, 41, 140]. It is interesting that this alteration is complete before changes in the contractile proteins are detectable. The Z-line is thought to assist in filament alignment and to help support radial mechanical forces that are generated as the fiber shortens [38]. Therefore the question is raised as to whether this initial change represents a faster rate of protein turnover or whether it functions as a scaffold for the sequential alterations in the contractile proteins.

Visually, stimulated fast muscles are deep red, rather than pale. This is due to an increase in capillary density, combined with an increase in myoglobin content. The stimulated muscles are also smaller [15, 39, 125]. There is a decrease in fiber cross-sectional area and an increase in endomysial connective tissue [16, 41, 126]. However, there is not a gross loss of fibers. Thus the atrophy is due to a decrease in fiber area and not in fiber number [125].

A marked increase in the number of mitochondria occurs by 2 weeks, such that their content can reach levels three times that of the soleus. The increase in mitochondrial volume is not secondary to fiber atrophy, but rather represents an increase in content. Both subsarcolemmal and central mitochondrial populations increase [39, 41, 132]. Coupled with the decrease in fiber cross-sectional area, there is an increase in the inner mitochondrial membrane area per fiber [126]. However, the surface-to-volume ratio of the inner membrane of the mitochondria is maintained [132], despite a change in the proportion of some of the mitochondrial enzymes. It has recently been demonstrated that stimulation induces an increase in cardiolipin, a phospholipid of the inner mitochondrial membrane, prior to increases in mitochondrial enzymes. This finding suggests that assembly of new mitochondria starts with synthesis of the lipid bilayer, followed by insertion of the proteins [175]. Following 7 weeks of continued CMNS, there is a rapid decrease in mitochondrial volume density, although the level still remains above that of the soleus [41].

The initial increase in oxygen-consuming mitochondria is accompanied by an increase in the oxygen delivery system. Significant increases in capillary density (number of capillaries per mm^2) occur after only 4 days of stimulation [16, 64]. Following 4 weeks, the capillary density can double and reach values typical of those found in slow-twitch muscles [16]. This increase is partially due to a decrease in muscle fiber diameter. However, it is also due to an increase in capillary growth [16, 64, 114]. In particular, there is an increase in the widening of the capillaries, as well as the formation of additional sprouts and loops, which leads to an increase in capillary tortuosity [114]. It is thought that the capillary growth is stimulated by factors such as shear stress or wall tension that are related to an increase in blood flow [65]. Overall, the capillaries are more numerous, sinusoidal, and wider. The combination of the increase in capillary density and the decrease in muscle fiber diameter results in a shorter diffusion distance for oxygen. The net result is an increase in perfusion and oxygen delivery.

Many morphological alterations occur that indicate increased biosynthetic activity. Following 2–3 weeks of CMNS, there is an increase in the number of nuclei per fiber. Since fiber volume is decreased, there is an increase in the number of nuclei per unit volume. This results in a decrease in the volume of sarcoplasm managed by individual nuclei [75]. Other alterations include decondensation of heterochromatin in myonuclei, larger and more rounded nuclei, and nucleolar enlargement, which suggest increased transcriptional activity [75]. The Golgi apparati are enlarged [41], and increases in ribosomes and polyribosomes in sarcoplasm, especially in the perinuclear region, are seen [75, 165]. Thus, there is morphological evidence for increased translational activity as well. Overall, chronically stimulated fast-twitch muscle takes on the ultrastructural characteristics of slow-twitch muscle. Oftentimes, it exhibits even greater mitochondrial content and capillary density and has smaller fibers than slow-twitch muscle, which renders it highly efficient for aerobic metabolism.

FUNCTION. The functional and mechanical properties of the transformed tissue are determined by the architectural arrangement (fiber alignment, sarcomere length) and the protein composition of the metabolic and contractile machinery. In response to CMNS, fast-twitch muscles take on the functional characteristics of slow-twitch muscles. Thus there is a slowing of contractile speed, a loss in force, and a greatly increased resistance to fatigue.

Within the first 5 minutes of CMNS there is a rapid loss of force, which is followed by a more gradual decline over the next few hours [49, 104]. Following 1 day of 12 hour/day intermittent stimulation, there is a decrease in isometric twitch tension and an increase in half relaxation time ($RT_{1/2}$) [85]. These alterations indicate fatigue and may represent an impairment in calcium handling [85], as swelling of the SR is evident [41].

Continuation of stimulation leads to an increase in the time to peak tension (TPT) and $RT_{1/2}$ [125, 144, 145, 167]. These changes have been observed after only 1–4 days of stimulation [16, 85]. The increase in TPT could be due to a decrease in the velocity of shortening (Vmax), as well as to a lengthening of the "active state." These factors have been distinguished by examining the tension produced during a single contraction, relative to that produced during maximal tetani (twitch-to-tetanus ratio). Although there is an initial decrease in the isometric twitch tension, after 5–10 days of 12 hour/day stimulation, it normalizes. With the continuation of stimulation, it steadily increases through 21 days. This increase is accompanied by a decrease in maximum tetanic tension. The consequence of these alterations is an increase in the twitch-to-tetanus ratio [85, 144, 145, 167]. This indicates that the duration of the active state during a single contraction is prolonged. That is, a greater proportion of the tetanic tension is produced during a single twitch [85, 125]. Hence the increased TPT and $RT_{1/2}$ are at least partially due to a prolongation of the active state, which suggests that alterations in calcium handling are involved. In particular, there appears to be a reduced capacity for calcium uptake by the SR, as well as a decrease in cytosolic calcium buffering secondary to a decrease in parvalbumin content [41, 85, 125, 167]. The increase in TPT is due to changes in myosin isoforms as well [173].

The decrease in maximum isometric tetanic tension correlates highly with both muscle wet mass and muscle cross-sectional area [15]. At the fiber level, the force per cross-sectional area is not altered following stimulation [173]. These findings indicate that the specific tension is not altered. They suggest that the internal architecture of the transformed muscle (orientation and length of fibers, density of the tissue) is maintained. These results intimate that a constant proportion of the muscle area is involved in the generation of tension, and thus the changes in noncontractile elements such as mitochondria and nuclei do not alter specific tension [15].

Stimulated muscles exhibit an increased resistance to fatigue [15, 63, 67, 126, 144]. The change is seen within a few days following the onset of CMNS [63, 168] and is due in part to fast-to-slow contractile protein transition, which results in a slower rate of cross-bridge cycling and thus lowers the energy cost [15]. More important initial determinants, however, appear to be the increases in capillary density and in oxidative capacity [15, 129]. Of these, the increase in capillary density seems to be the most important, based on the time course of alterations. That is, changes in fatigue resistance and capillary density both occur within the first week, while there is a delay before the increase in oxidative enzymes [63, 168]. In addition, the ensuing increase in oxidative enzymes is not accompanied by a further improvement in fatigue resistance [168]. Last, there is a slowing of Vmax [2], which correlates with myosin isoform content [173].

Excitation-Contraction Coupling: Calcium-Handling Proteins
In skeletal muscle, calcium homeostasis and excitation-contraction (E-C) coupling are regulated by a complex interaction of cellular proteins that are mostly localized to the SR and the T-tubules. However, muscle adaptations to CMNS have been examined for only a few of these proteins. The calcium release channel (CRC) of the SR and the slow calcium channel, or dihydropyridine receptor (DHPR) of the T-tubule, comprise two key components of E-C coupling in skeletal and cardiac muscle [29, 45]. In fast-twitch skeletal muscle, the DHPR is thought to function as a voltage sensor that is coupled to the CRC during E-C coupling [135]. Depolarization of the T-tubule results in the release of calcium stored in the SR, by way of the CRC, thereby activating muscle contraction. The cDNAs encoding the skeletal muscle CRC [102, 176, 192] and the α_1-subunits of the skeletal muscle DHPR isoform [177] have recently been isolated and characterized, which now makes it possible to study regulation of gene expression for these products.

Reuptake of calcium into the SR is mediated by the SR Ca^{2+}-ATPase. The activity of this protein appears to be regulated, in slow-twitch skeletal and cardiac muscle only, by the phosphorylation state of phospholamban, a protein that co-localizes intracellularly with the slow/cardiac isoform of the Ca^{2+}-ATPase. Other proteins involved in calcium handling include calsequestrin and parvalbumin, which are buffers of SR and cytoplasmic Ca^{2+}, respectively, and which are primarily found in fast-twitch skeletal muscle. Overall, rabbit fast-twitch muscle has 6–7 times greater Ca^{2+}-ATPase activity, 2 times greater calsequestrin, and 200 times greater parvalbumin concentrations than does slow-twitch muscle [92].

Acute. Several investigators have noted modulations of calcium concentrations inside the SR [85, 171], as well as activity of Ca^{2+}-ATPase [85], in the earliest periods after institution of CMNS. By 2 days there is a 50% reduction in Ca^{2+}-ATPase activity induced by CMNS, despite no alteration in Ca^{2+}-ATPase protein concentration or isoform expression until much later. During the acute phase, there is a transient loss of contractile force and function (increases in TPT and $RT_{1/2}$), as numerous compartments of the cell begin to adapt to the increases in contractile work [85]. The functional losses in E-C coupling and the increases in calcium concentration in the SR have been attributed to a loss of Ca^{2+}-ATPase activity, perhaps secondary to posttranslational modifications of the Ca^{2+}-ATPase molecule itself [35]. However, Kraus et al. [88] have observed an early reduction in mRNA concentrations for the DHPR and CRC (2 times and 5 times, respectively), which are presumably reflected in similar changes at the protein level for these calcium release channels. There are early decreases in the fractional volumes of the T-tubules and SR, which begin after a few days and are complete by 2 weeks of continuous CMNS [41]. Ohlendieck et al. demonstrated a reduction of protein concentration for the calcium channels in canine latissimus dorsi muscles that were stimulated for 6 weeks, but they did not investigate any earlier time points [119]. Thus, there appears to be early modulation of calcium homeostasis in the acute phase of CMNS, which may be mediated by both transcriptional and posttranslation modifications of calcium-handling proteins.

Dynamic. Most of the described changes in calcium-handling proteins occur during the dynamic phase. By 14 days, there is a 5 times increase in SR calcium concentration, which normalizes by 21 days of continued stimulation [171]. In response to a 12-hour/day stimulation pattern, there is a reduction in parvalbumin mRNA and protein, which reaches 20% of control levels by 10 days, while Ca^{2+}-ATPase protein levels are reduced to 37% of control by 14 days [93]. Phospholamban protein levels begin to change in the dynamic phase and reach concentrations normally observed in slow-twitch muscle by 35–90 days [91]. Another membrane-bound ion channel protein involved in E-C coupling, the sodium-potassium ATPase, is also regulated by CMNS and increases to 2 times control levels after 10 days of stimulation [48].

Maintenance. A number of the changes in calcium-handling proteins occur and are completed well into the maintenance phase, after the myosin isoform switches are mostly complete. Calsequestrin levels are only mildly modulated, being reduced to 80% of control levels by 50 days; whereas a dramatic decrease is observed in parvalbumin concentration [93]. There is a switch in the Ca^{2+}-ATPase isoform composition of stimulated muscles, so that the fast-twitch isoform is replaced by the slow-twitch isoform by 72 days, as shown both at the mRNA and protein levels [91]. In canine muscle subjected to 2 Hz stimulation for 6–7 weeks, there is also a switch in Ca^{2+}-ATPase isoforms from fast to slow, which is accompanied by an increase in expression of phospholamban [12]. Presumably the same phenomenon occurs in the rabbit.

Metabolic Pathways

In general, the increased contractile activity associated with CMNS results in an increased demand for energy. This demand is met by switching from a predominantly anaerobic energy system, to an aerobic one, as evidenced by a restructuring of the major metabolic pathways. The extent of this remodeling depends on the basal levels of the enzymes, which vary among species. That is, the lower the starting levels, the greater the increase, and vice versa [166]. The degree and pattern of change also depend on the extent of the energy demand. Slightly different patterns of adaptation emerge, depending on whether the muscle is stimulated for 8–12 or 24 hours/day. The alterations are outlined by system and are illustrated in Figure 11.1.

HIGH ENERGY PHOSPHATE TRANSFER SYSTEM. *Acute.* Within the first 15 minutes of continuous CMNS, levels of the high energy phosphate, phosphocreatine (PCr), drop by 50–60%. However, within a few hours the

FIGURE 11.1

Changes in substrate and enzyme activities of major metabolic pathways during CMNS. The acute phase represents the first 48 hours after initiation of CMNS, the dynamic phase represents the period from 2 (days) to 6 weeks, and the maintenance phase represents the period beyond 6 weeks. Double bars represent discontinuity on the time scale. The direction and approximate duration of changes are represented by the bars. Hence upward deviations (shaded and hatched bars) indicate increases, while downward deviations (hatched bars) indicate decreases. The dotted lines represent basal levels. The data are presented to allow relative comparisons of the temporal relationships among the pathways. They should not be taken as an absolute time course, as this varies depending on the species and the stimulation protocol (see text for discussion). Abbreviations: AK, adenylyl kinase; CK, creatine kinase; PFK, phosphofructokinase; LDH, lactate dehydrogenase; CS, citrate synthase; MDH, malate dehydrogenase; SDH, succinate dehydrogenase; BOAC, 3-hydroxyacyl-CoA dehydrogenase; CAT, carnitine acyltransferase; KACAT, 3-oxoacid CoA-transferase.

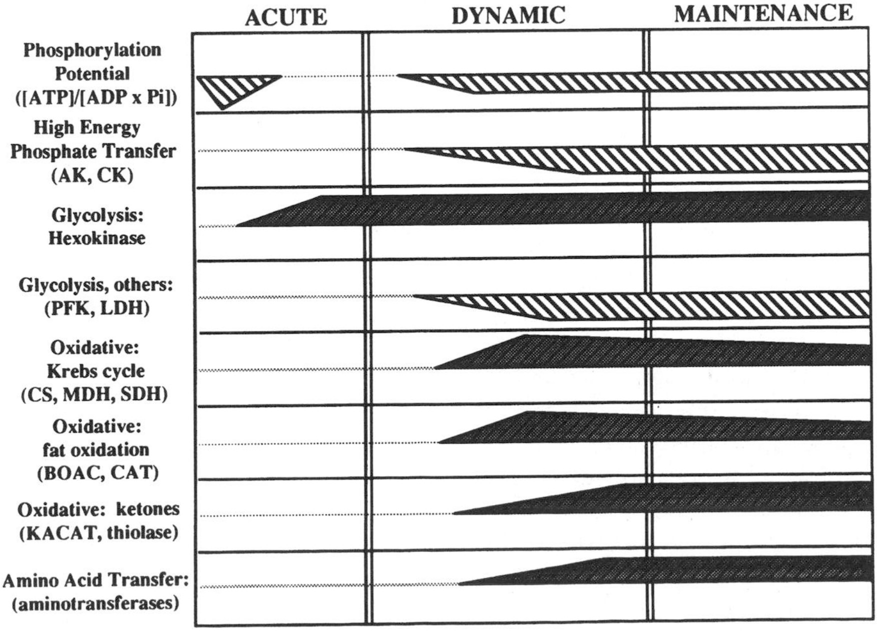

	ACUTE	DYNAMIC	MAINTENANCE
Phosphorylation Potential ([ATP]/[ADP x Pi])			
High Energy Phosphate Transfer (AK, CK)			
Glycolysis: Hexokinase			
Glycolysis, others: (PFK, LDH)			
Oxidative: Krebs cycle (CS, MDH, SDH)			
Oxidative: fat oxidation (BOAC, CAT)			
Oxidative: ketones (KACAT, thiolase)			
Amino Acid Transfer: (aminotransferases)			

concentration returns to that of unstimulated controls. As expected, creatine increases and reaches a peak at 5–15 minutes. Like PCr, the levels return to control within a few hours. By 15 minutes of stimulation there is approximately a 50% drop in ATP, which also normalizes by 24 hours [49, 104]. Changes in total AMP and ADP are negligible. Calculated free ADP and AMP (ADP_f and AMP_f) increase approximately 1.5–2 times following 60 minutes of stimulation, but they return to control levels by 12 hours. Calculated free Pi (Pi_f) increases 8 times following 15 minutes of stimulation, and by 24 hours is still 3 times greater than unstimulated levels [49]. These changes result in a drastic drop in the phosphorylation potential ($[ATP]/[ADP_f \times Pi_f]$ ratio) or ATP/ADP_f ratio during the initial 15 minutes. The ratios approach control levels by 2–3 hours [49, 104].

Dynamic/Maintenance. Although PCr levels return to normal after 12 hours of stimulation, after 2 days they again decline, so that after 10 days of stimulation they are 40–50% of control levels. Creatine levels may normalize or may become depressed [49, 60]. The ATP concentration, which after 24 hours recovers to 80% of unstimulated levels, remains slightly depressed throughout the stimulation period [49, 60]. Although ADP_f and AMP_f levels are similar to nonstimulated levels at 12 hours, they increase again and remain elevated. Pi_f similarly increases a second time and has been shown to be elevated 7–8 times above control levels. Thus the ATP phosphorylation potential declines a second time and remains depressed throughout the course of stimulation [49].

With respect to the enzymes of the high energy phosphate transfer system, after 1–2 weeks there is a gradual decline in adenylyl kinase and adenylate acid deaminase [58, 127]. There is also a gradual decline in total creatine kinase, such that by 8 weeks its level is actually lower than that found in the slow-twitch soleus [58]. The decrease in creatine kinase is due to a decrease in the large extramitochondrial fraction. In contrast, the much smaller mitochondrial fraction increases 4 times [155].

GLYCOLYSIS, GLYCOGENOLYSIS, AND GLYCOGEN SYNTHESIS. *Acute.* The immediate response to CMNS is a drastic drop in glycogen concentration. It decreases 70–90% over the first hour of CMNS and remains depressed during the initial 24 hours. There is a corresponding sharp increase in glucose, which remains elevated for 24 hours. As expected, lactate levels increase sharply and can reach values that are 10 times greater than unstimulated controls [49].

Glucose is the major fuel source in the initial stages of CMNS. As the glycogen stores become depleted, circulating glucose becomes the crucial substrate. Its delivery is enhanced by an increase in blood flow to the stimulated muscles [66]. Muscle contraction stimulates the transport of glucose across the plasma membrane [70], which most likely accounts for the increase in intracellular glucose levels. To prevent the accumulation and subsequent counter transport of glucose from the cell, it must be phosphorylated. This demand is met by a rapid increase in hexokinase levels. In particular, increased synthesis of hexokinase occurs within the first few hours following CMNS [127]. A 50% increase in hexokinase levels have been noted after the first day [54].

Dynamic/Maintenance. Although glycogen levels initially decrease, following 2 days of CMNS a 25% increase above control levels has been noted, indicating super compensation. In continuously stimulated rabbits, this phenomenon is short-lived, and levels again decline, to remain at approximately 50% of control [49, 60]. However, in rabbits stimulated intermittently, glycogen levels may continue to increase throughout a month of stimulation [16, 63]. Glucose decreases to near control levels at 2 days, and then rises to levels 3–4 times greater than control throughout the stimulation period [49, 60]. Glucose-6-phosphate falls to very low levels at 1 week and then gradually increases [60].

After approximately 1–2 weeks of continuous CMNS, there is a progressive decline in lactate dehydrogenase (LDH), phosphofructokinase (PFK), glycogen phosphorylase, and phosphoglucomutase. In continuously stimulated muscles, the levels may reach 20% of unstimulated TA levels by 10 weeks [58]. This initial lag period is not as marked in muscles stimulated for only 8, 10, or 12 hours/day, where substantial drops in LDH, PFK and phosphorylase kinase occur by 14 days of stimulation [54, 127, 133, 165]. However, in muscles stimulated for 12 hours/day, the levels of these enzymes only drop to approximately 45% of unstimulated levels [165].

As mentioned, hexokinase undergoes a rapid increase early in the stimulation period. Its levels double following 3 days of continuous stimulation and increase 4-fold by 7 days [58]. By 2 weeks, hexokinase can reach levels 2.5–5 times greater than those of the soleus [54, 58]. Substantial increases have also been noted in rat muscle after 7 days of 10 hours/day stimulation [182]. The increase in hexokinase is accompanied by an increase in the insulin-sensitive glucose transporter, GLUT-4. Levels of this protein, which functions to transport glucose across the plasma membrane, increase over 80% following 10–20 days of 8 hours/day stimulation in rats [42].

Levels of glycogen synthase, the rate-limiting enzyme in the formation of glycogen, remain fairly stable. A slight increase may occur after 2 weeks of stimulation, which is followed by a gradual decline throughout 8 weeks [54, 58]. Fructose bisphosphatase, the enzyme that regenerates glycogen from lactate, alters in parallel with the enzymes of glycogenolysis [54, 58].

OXIDATIVE METABOLISM. *Dynamic.* Most of the oxidative enzymes display a biphasic response during the first month of CMNS. In rabbits stimulated continuously, there is a 1-week latency period, after which enzymes of the Krebs cycle such as citrate synthase (CS), succinate dehydrogenase (SDH), and malate dehydrogenase (MDH) increase rapidly over the subsequent 2 weeks [58, 127]. Thus at the end of 3 weeks of stimulation, SDH has been shown to increase 8-fold, while CS and MDH increase 5-fold [58]. Rabbits stimulated for 10–12 hours/day display a slightly different biphasic response. The initial latency period is less marked. Instead, there is a slight increase in enzymes of the Krebs cycle during the first week, followed by an enhanced increase in subsequent weeks [131, 165].

Changes in enzymes involved in fatty acid oxidation, such as 3-hydroxyacyl-CoA dehydrogenase (ßOAC) and carnitine acyltransferase (CAT), parallel the pattern of alterations of the Krebs cycle enzymes in muscles stimulated for either 10 or 24 hours/day [58, 133]. 3-Oxoacid CoA-transferase (KACAT), the first enzyme in ketoacid catabolism, and thiolase, an enzyme involved in both ketone body and fatty acid metabolism, both also increase dramatically over the first few weeks, even more than the enzymes of the Krebs cycle [58, 127, 133].

Maintenance. Levels of CS, MDH, and SDH reach a peak at 3 weeks, at values that are approximately 2.5–5 times greater than control soleus. In continuously stimulated muscles, CS and SDH then gradually decline, such that by the end of 10 weeks of stimulation, levels are half of the peak value. The pattern of change for the fatty acid oxidation enzymes ßOAC and CAT is similar [58]. Despite the decreases, these enzymes still tend to be twice as high as those in the soleus [58, 59]. In muscles stimulated for 12 hours/day, peak enzyme levels are also reached around 3–4 weeks of stimulation. However, the levels appear to remain fairly stable, rather than to gradually decrease, during subsequent weeks of stimulation [165]. Unlike the Krebs cycle enzymes, KACAT continues to increase. By 8 weeks its level is 11 times greater than control unstimulated TA muscle. At the end of 10 weeks of stimulation, the level of this enzyme can be 4.5 times greater than levels noted for the soleus. This pattern has also been noted for thiolase [58].

Analysis of enzymes located within the mitochondrial matrix shows that not all enzymes in this compartment appear to be jointly regulated. That is, while enzymes of fatty acid oxidation, the Krebs cycle, and the respiratory chain increase in parallel, enzymes involved in ketone body utilization undergo greater change. Thus CMNS leads to the formation of mitochondria that have a different composition than mitochondria of unstimulated TA muscle. Alternatively, there may be distinct mitochondrial populations that differ in their enzymatic characteristics.

AMINO ACID AMINOTRANSFERASE ENZYMES. *Dynamic/Maintenance.* The enzymes aspartate aminotransferase, branched-chain-amino-acid aminotransferase, and alanine aminotransferase increase during the second to third week of CMNS. Overall, their increases tend to be lower than the enzymes of oxidative metabolism [58]. After the initial increase, the levels of these enzymes remain fairly stable. Following 10 weeks of stimulation, the levels range from approximately that of control soleus (alanine aminotransferase) to 1.9 times and 4.3 times greater than control soleus (aspartate aminotransferase and branch-chain-amino-acid aminotransferase, respectively) [58].

SUMMARY. The initial scenario is that of a fast-twitch muscle barely able to meet a sudden metabolic demand. There is a drastic collapse of both the adenylate and creatine systems, and marked glycogen depletion. Elevated intracellular glucose may represent an imbalance between glucose uptake and phosphorylation, due to the low amount of hexokinase present in fast-twitch muscle. The almost immediate increase in synthesis of hexokinase underscores the importance of glucose as a fuel source during this phase. Although the anaerobic energy systems undergo profound stress, within 24 hours, levels of many of the metabolites have normalized. Thus muscle displays a remarkable, rapid ability to recover from the initial insult to the ATP-generating systems.

During the first month of CMNS there is extensive remodeling of the enzymatic pathways, such that aerobic systems predominate, especially with respect to the utilization of fat. The increase in fatty acid oxidative machinery is accompanied by changes in substrate delivery. Fatty acid availability increases in part because of increased extracellular albumin, the major transporter of fatty acids in plasma [56], and an increase in fatty acid–binding proteins that function in intracellular lipid trafficking [76]. The increase in oxidative machinery and substrates is accompanied by increased intracellular transport of oxygen because of an increase in myoglobin [76, 127]. There is also an increase in the extracellular space. This accounts, in part, for the increase in albumin and may also function to increase metabolite exchange [56, 58]. Overall, the oxidative enzymes reach or maintain levels above those typically found in slow-twitch muscles such as the soleus. Despite this augmentation in oxidative energy production, levels of many metabolites remain altered, which raises questions about their potential roles in cellular signaling.

Contractile Machinery: Thick- and Thin-Filament Proteins
The change in myofibrillar actomyosin ATPase activity (mATPase) from fast to slow with continuous CMNS reflects underlying changes in the composition of the thick-filament protein, myosin. Myosin is a hexameric molecule comprised of 2 globular heavy chains, which contain the actin-binding site and the ATPase activity, and 2 pairs of nonidentical light chains: the alkali light chains (LC1/3) and the phosphorylatable light chains (LC2). As myosin HC and LC composition are altered, mATPase changes to reflect the thick-filament composition, which in turn is reflected in the contractile function of the muscle. Yet, stimulation-induced changes in contractile properties also reflect alterations of the composition of other myofibrillar proteins, including the regulatory proteins of the thin filament, troponin (Tn) and tropomyosin (Tm), and α-skeletal actin.

THICK-FILAMENT PROTEINS. *Acute.* No detectable changes in the mRNA encoding thick- and thin-filament proteins or in protein levels are reported within 24 hours after initiation of CMNS. Nonetheless, with continuous stimulation of rat hindlimb, changes in mRNA encoding myosin HC are detectable as early as 2 days, which suggests that a stimulation-induced signal is transmitted relatively early to the regulatory apparatus of these genes [81]. Furthermore, changes at the protein level can be seen in thick-filament gene expression within 1 week.

Dynamic. At the myofibrillar level, particular attention has been given to changes in the isoform patterns of myosin, Tn and Tm. As would be expected from changes in contractile speed and in mATPase histochemistry, CMNS leads to alterations in expression of myosin [169, 170]. Fast muscle gradually becomes "slow," as fast isoforms of myosin HC and LC are progressively replaced by slow isoforms. This is described as a sequential transition in fiber type from type IIB to type I or as a change in oxidative capacity (from FG to FOG to SO). Although the time course of this progression appears to vary with the stimulation protocol, as well as with the species, the pattern of transition appears to be similar.

The conversion from fast to slow myosin appears to result from sequential alterations in myosin mRNA expression, followed by alterations in protein synthesis. Ultimate fast to slow fiber type conversion results from a repression of fast myosin LC and HC gene expression, simultaneous with an increase in slow isoform expression. This results in transitions from fiber type IIB to IID to IIA to IIC to type I, containing myosin HC complements IIb, IId, IIa, IIa/I, and I, respectively. During this transition, hybrid fibers that contain multiple myosin isoforms can also be detected [179]. Furthermore, myosin is not replaced as a whole molecule, instead the subunits of myosin are replaced asynchronously [18, 19].

Schematically, the changes in myosin protein expression are depicted in Figure 11.2. Briefly, they can be summarized as (*a*) myosin LC conversion precedes a detectable change in HC; (*b*) replacement of the phosphorylatable light chains, LC2f, by LC2s precedes the replacement of the alkali light chains, LC1/3f, by LC1s [18]; (*c*) the decrease in fast light chains (LC1f and 3f and LC2f) and the increase in slow light chains (LC1s and LC2s) follow a symmetric time course such that the ratio between alkali and phosphorylatable LCs is maintained at approximately 1 [164]; (*d*) fast myosin HC rearrangement occurs prior to expression of slow HC; (*e*) fast HC rearrangement occurs in the order HCIIb $\Rightarrow$ HCIId $\Rightarrow$ HCIIa; (*e*) myosin HC conversion from HCIIa $\Rightarrow$ HCI represents the final step in the conversion process.

RNA Analyses. Alterations in thick-filament gene expression are detectable at the mRNA level prior to any detectable alterations in gene products, which suggests that myofibril isoform expression in response to CMNS may be transcriptionally regulated. Thus, shortly after CMNS of fast muscle begins, changes in mRNAs encoding myosin LC isoforms are detectable: in rodent, LC1/3 mRNA decreases as early as 4 days [47], whereas fast LC2f mRNA does not decrease until 7 days [83]. The decrease in LC2f message is complemented by an increase in LC2s mRNA [18].

Prior to exchange with slow LC1, the fast LC1:LC3 ratio increases, due to

FIGURE 11.2

Changes in myofibrillar protein expression during CMNS. Data cited in the text have been compiled to demonstrate schematically the temporal changes in myofibrillar protein expression in response to CMNS. The acute phase represents the first 48 hours after initiation of CMNS, the dynamic phase represents the period from 2 days to 6 weeks, and the maintenance phase represents the period beyond 6 weeks. Double bars represent discontinuity on the time scale. The direction and approximate duration of changes in protein expression are represented by the bars. In situations where conflicting data exist, an attempt has been made to synthesize the data from all available sources, including species other than rabbit. The open symbol in the HCIId panel reflects the recent reassessment of previous data which may suggest that high levels of HCIId are present prior to stimulation. The data are presented to allow relative comparisons of the temporal relationships among the myofibrillar proteins and should not be taken as an absolute time course. An exact time course of myofibrillar conversion depends upon the species, individual animal variability, and the stimulation protocol (see text for discussion). Hatched bars represent fast isoforms, shaded and hatched bars represent slow isoforms. Abbreviations: HC, myosin heavy chain; LC, myosin light chain; TnT, troponin T; f, fast; s, slow.

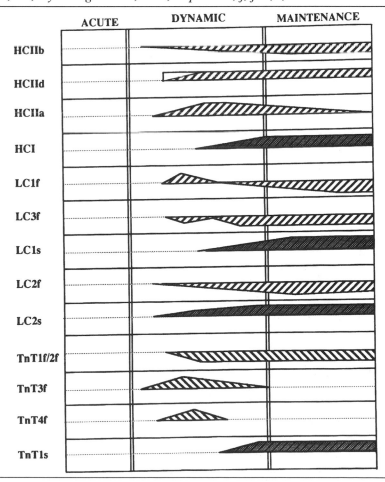

increased LC1f and decreased LC3f expression [82]. Thus, by 14 days, mRNA encoding LC1f increases significantly, and LC3f mRNA decreases [79, 82]. As stimulation continues for periods of up to 30 days, increases in mRNA encoding slow LCs are detected [79].

Alterations in myosin HC mRNA expression can also be detected during this dynamic phase. Fast myosin HC is expressed, but isoform switching gradually occurs from HCIIb, the most glycolytic, to HCIIa, the most oxidative. As early as 4 days after initiation of continuous CMNS, a repression in HCIIb mRNA is observed, which is followed by a slower increase in myosin HCIIa mRNA [20, 21, 47, 81]. By 7–21 days, the level of HCIIb mRNA is similar to that found in type I fibers [20, 129]; HCIIa mRNA increases; and slow HC mRNA is also detectable at significant levels [21]. In rabbit EDL, a 4-fold increase in slow HC mRNA is seen after 4 days of continuous stimulation [21]. This increase is delayed to longer than 20 days if stimulation only occurs 12 hours/day [79]. Examination of expression of HCIId mRNA awaits isolation of appropriate molecular probes. These shifts in mRNA precede changes in protein expression but generally reflect the transitions that occur at the protein level.

Increases in steady-state levels of mRNA can result from increased transcription and/or altered mRNA stability. The appearance, in response to CMNS, of mRNAs not normally seen in fast muscle suggests that increased transcription may play a role in the regulation of these genes. However, in response to CMNS, total RNA in rabbit TA increases to concentrations similar to that seen in adult soleus. At least 80% of this RNA is ribosomal RNA, which suggests that more translational machinery is also available within the cell after chronic stimulation (see discussion in Implications for Mechanisms of Fiber Type Conversion).

Protein Analyses. Throughout the first 6 weeks after initiation of continuous CMNS, myosin isoform switching reflects changes seen earlier in mRNA expression. Changes in myosin LC expression can first be detected prior to 3 weeks [18, 164, 170], but most of the changes in LC expression occur later than 3 weeks [17, 18, 164]. Brown et al. report that fast LC2 is rapidly replaced by slow LC2 between 2 and 7 weeks after stimulation is initiated [18]. During this replacement, a relative excess of fast LC2 is found in the cellular pool, compared with that bound to myosin HC. Exchange of slow for fast LC1/3 also occurs by 7 weeks but is delayed relative to the change in LC2 [18]. This does not appear to simply reflect the half-life of the protein or protein turnover, since the reverse process, which occurs with the removal of stimulation, does not demonstrate a lag period. These data suggest that with continuous CMNS, most changes in myosin LC expression are complete by approximately 6 weeks after CMNS is begun. The exact time course, however, is somewhat in dispute [164] and appears to reflect differences in stimulation protocols, species, and individual animal variability.

During the dynamic phase, a conversion among fast isoforms of myosin

HC also occurs. This conversion can be detected at approximately the same time as changes in LC2 become detectable: 2–3 weeks after initiation of continuous CMNS [179]. Although the final conversion is from fast to slow HC, initially a sequential rearrangement in the expression of fast HC isoforms occurs, which appears to depend upon the stimulation protocol and species. For example, in rat TA subjected to 10 Hz stimulation for 10 hours/day, myosin HCIIb decreases within 8 days. However, this decrease does not become significant for 3 weeks [179]. Schmitt and Pette report that under similar stimulation conditions at 35 days and thereafter, no HCIIb is detected in single rabbit fiber analyses [154]. Similarly, HCIIa increases as early as 8 days after initiation of stimulation, but significant differences are not detected before 18 days [179]. However, this increase in HCIIa is not maintained, so that by 90 days only minute amounts of HCIIa can be detected [154]. In rabbits, Brown et al. report that after 12 days of stimulation, the type of fast myosin HC is altered, but no slow myosin HC is expressed. By 14 days, slow myosin HC is detectable, but it only becomes significantly elevated by 21 days [17]. Although slow myosin HC is increasingly abundant, fast myosin HC protein is still detectable at 5 weeks but is undetectable by 7 weeks [17]. Little or no neonatal myosin HC is present at any time during this transition [17], which suggests that fiber regeneration is not the primary mechanism contributing to this shift. Pette and co-workers also report the expression of up to four HC isoforms in a transforming fiber: HCIIb/IId/IIa/I, [180], which suggests that a persistence of isoforms that are no longer synthesized may occur due to relatively slow degradation rates of myosin HC [103]. These data taken together suggest that at a single-fiber level, conversion from fast to slow thick-filament myosin isoforms involves an ordered, sequential replacement of the myosin molecule.

Maintenance. The mATPase activity of stimulated fast-twitch muscles progressively declines to that of slow-twitch fibers after long periods of stimulation. Although it appears that the sequence of the fiber type conversion is established (HCIIB $\Rightarrow$ HCIID $\Rightarrow$ HCIIA $\Rightarrow$ IIC $\Rightarrow$ HCI), the plasticity of the system and the differences in stimulation protocols complicate discussion of an exact time course. Depending upon the stimulation protocol and the species, this can vary widely. For example, in rabbits undergoing continuous CMNS, the isoform shifts in thick- and thin-filament proteins appear to be complete by about 6 weeks [139, 154]. However, if the stimulation is intermittent (8–12 hours/day), the conversion may take longer than 21 weeks [125, 164]. The fiber type shift from IIB to type IIC appears to occur relatively rapidly (within 3–4 weeks); however, the final shift from type IIC to type I takes longer. The expression of HCI is then maintained for the duration of the stimulation time course.

Changes in the time course of myosin conversion can also vary with species. CMNS-induced increases in the number of slow fibers, as well as the transition from fast to slow myosin LCs, have been demonstrated in rabbit

[136], cat [33, 44], dog [30, 61], sheep [28, 46], goat [101, 130], and human [98]. Interestingly, conflicting reports exist about the ability of CMNS to increase slow fiber number in rat. Several groups have reported little success in eliciting a conversion of type II fibers to type I fibers in rat [33, 90, 182, 183]. Instead, with stimulation times up to 56 days, investigators have seen a rearrangement of the fast paradigm of gene expression, as if a fiber progresses through the conversion to the point of expressing type HCIIa but then does not shift to type I [80]. However, recently Jarvis et al. reported that with 55–61 days of 10 or 20 Hz continuous stimulation, from 6 to 89% of the fibers in the rat TA are type I and express functional characteristics of slow fibers. These include a decrease in maximum tetanic tension and an increase in time to peak twitch-contraction and time-to-half-relaxation relative to the unstimulated contra-lateral control muscle [73].

This picture is even more complex if the role of hormonal influences is considered. Kirschbaum et al. have demonstrated that chronic stimulation, which can not induce HCI in euthyroid rat, enhances HCI expression in the hypothyroid state [80]. Furthermore, their data suggest that thyroid hormone and CMNS are antagonistic, mediating opposite effects on muscle. Thyroid hormone attenuates the stimulation-induced increase in HCI mRNA, whereas thyroid hormone-induced increases in HCIIb mRNA are suppressed by increased neuromuscular activity [80].

MYOSIN LIGHT CHAIN KINASE. CMNS for periods between 2 and 73 days reduces myosin light chain kinase activity in a time-dependent manner [84]. The reduction in MLCK activity occurs as early as 5 days after stimulation, and by 33–73 days of activity approaches that of slow skeletal muscle. This is interesting in light of the suggestion that phosphorylation of LC2 of myosin causes the potentiation of isometric twitch tension that accompanies low-frequency and/or tetanic stimulation [111].

THIN-FILAMENT PROTEINS. *Dynamic.* Schachat and colleagues have focused on the early stages of CMNS to determine whether the transitions in thin-filament and Z-line proteins yield information about the adaptive response to chronic stimulation and whether transitions in thin-filament and Z-line proteins are coordinately regulated in response to chronic stimulation [148]. They have defined three patterns of expression of the fast thin-filament calcium-regulatory complex, troponin-tropomyosin, and the Z-line protein, α-actinin. These programs, designated the TnT1f, TnT2f, and TnT3f programs [13, 147, 149, 150], differ in the troponin T (TnT), tropomyosin and α-actinin isoforms expressed and in the contractile properties they confer on fibers that express predominantly one or another of the programs [150].

A priori, the transition between fast and slow contractile expression can occur either by immediate change to expression of the slow thin-filament and Z-line proteins or by adaptive transitions in expression of the fast thin-filament Z-line programs prior to the change to slow-protein expression. Previous ultrastructural analysis of fibers subjected to CMNS suggests that there is an immediate change to slow thin-filament and Z-line protein expression [41]; however, this is not what occurs in the case of the thin-filament calcium-regulatory complex. The earliest response is a transition from the most calcium-responsive fast program, the TnT2f program, to the least calcium-responsive fast program, the TnT3f program. Initially fibers express primarily TnT1f and 2f, αß-Tm, and equal levels of α-actinin 1f/s and 2f. This is depicted schematically in Figure 11.2. Within the first week of stimulation, TnT1f, 2f, and α-actinin 2f decrease, and TnT3f, α-actinin 1f/s, and a combination of αß, ß2-Tm predominate [150]. This results in a decrease in fast α-tropomyosin and an increase in slow α-tropomyosin, such that the α/ß subunit ratio is not altered. Long-term stimulated muscles can contain appreciable amounts of fast α-Tm but only traces of fast TnT, which indicates that predominant slow TnT isoforms may be capable of interacting with fast Tm in these muscles. TnT isoforms disappear in the order TnT2f, 4f, 1f, 3f [154]. Because the calcium responsiveness of the TnT3f program is more like that of the slow fibers, these observations argue that the early response to chronic stimulation in thin filament proteins is characterized by adaptive transitions to patterns of expression that result in fiber physiology more like that of slow fibers.

This transition in fast thin-filament programs also leads to a reinterpretation of the increase in Z-line width, which has been interpreted as reflecting an immediate transition from fast to slow expression. The transition from the TnT2f to the TnT3f program is accompanied by a change in expression of α-actinin isoforms from α-actinin2f to α-actinin1f/s. As shown by Schachat et al., expression of the α-actinin1f/s isoform would result in the increased Z-line width observed in fibers subjected to chronic stimulation, without their moving to a slow pattern of contractile protein expression [149].

During the dynamic phase when myosin rearrangement occurs, thin-filament gene expression changes as well. When HCIIa is expressed, the predominant isoform of TnT is TnT3f, with some 1f, 2f, or 4f seen after shorter stimulation protocols. Fibers that coexpress HCIIa and HCI express TnT3f, as well as the slow isoforms TnT1s and 2s. It appears that with increasing amounts of HCI, the ratio of TnT1s + TnT2s/TnT3f also increases, which suggests that these genes may be regulated similarly in response to chronic stimulation. Thus, as the fibers switch from IIB to I, the TnT isoforms disappear in the order TnT2f, 4f, 1f, 3f. However, the decrease in TnT2f is slower than that of HCIIB, so that fibers with HCIIA and TnT2f can be found. This suggests differences in turnover rates of these proteins may exist and that different thick- and thin-filament components may associate [154].

Thus with regard to thin-filament protein expression, the earliest response to CMNS is not a shift to slow thin-filament protein expression, but a coordinated transition in fast contractile protein expression to produce a fiber that is slower in its physiological response to calcium and in its ultrastructural properties. The kinetics of the transitions in contractile protein expression indicate that the limiting factor in changing fast TnT-Tm isoforms following chronic stimulation is protein turnover.

Maintenance. As changes in myosin occur, coordinated rearrangements in thin-filament protein expression also occur. As the fibers switch from IIB to IIA to IIC to I, the fast TnT isoforms disappear in the order TnT2f, 4f, 1f, 3f. It appears that with increasing amounts of HCI, the ratio of slow TnT isoforms (TnT1s + TnT 2s) to TnT3f also increases, which suggests that these genes may be regulated similarly in response to chronic stimulation. CMNS also elicits a fast-to-slow shift of troponin I (TnI) and troponin C (TnC) [53]. However, even after long periods of stimulation, considerable amounts of fast TnI may still be expressed. Thus, fibers may contain heteromeric forms of Tn, as they have both fast and slow subunits [53].

CORRELATION OF ATPASE WITH METABOLIC ENZYME EXPRESSION. Upon examining expression of multiple glycolytic and oxidative enzymes during this phase of the transition and comparing those activities with muscle mATPase activities, Henriksson, et al. [59] report no real correlation between mATPase pattern and enzyme levels. As some enzymes shift toward slow levels, others, such as citrate synthase, greatly exceed the range expressed in slow muscle. Furthermore, some oxidative enzymes that initially show marked increases, decline toward the level in slow muscle at later times of stimulation but remain 1.7–2.8 times as high. This biphasic response occurs with a time course similar to the switch from type II to type I HC.

After 5 weeks of CMNS, metabolic enzyme activities change differently depending on the mATPase type of the fiber in which they are measured [59]. Henriksson et al. interpret the data as suggesting that (*a*) many enzymes of glycogenolysis and some of oxidation change in synchrony with the changes in mATPase fiber type, so that the concentrations of these enzymes are adjusted to the levels appropriate to the new fiber type; (*b*) many enzymes of oxidative metabolism increase beyond levels appropriate to fiber type and without synchronization to fiber type but perhaps in synchrony with each other; (*c*) other enzymes appear to change according to other rules. Thus, this group believes that although pattern of use is a major determinant of a fiber's metabolic enzyme profile, an effect is also exerted by the specific myosin isoform complement of the fiber [59].

SUMMARY. Immediately after initiation of continuous CMNS, alterations in morphology and calcium handling can been seen. However these are not obviously reflected at the myofibril level for several days. Yet, within a week of CMNS muscle enters a dynamic phase during which multiple changes at the contractile apparatus are seen. The exact time at which these changes occur depends upon the stimulation protocol, the muscle involved, and the species. However, the progression from fast to slow phenotype is reflected by an ordered conversion of the contractile apparatus, which proceeds asynchronously. Within the thick filament, a conversion of myosin LC2 from fast to slow occurs early and is followed approximately 2 weeks later by a switch in the composition of the alkali LC from LC1f/LC3f to LC1s. This asynchrony in myosin LC conversion does not appear to reflect simple differences in protein half-life because, with cessation of chronic stimulation, the reversal of this process does not demonstrate a corresponding lag. At about the same time the changes in LC2 become detectable, alterations in the composition of the myosin HC begin. In fast fibers, a rapid decrease in the glycolytic HC, HCIIb, is seen followed by an increase in HCIId. This is followed by an ordered conversion to HCIIa and finally to HCI. This conversion can be complete as early as 6 weeks after the initiation of stimulation. The enzyme responsible for phosphorylation of myosin LC2, MLCK, decreases to levels found in slow muscle during the first 35 days of stimulation. As changes in myosin occur, coordinated rearrangements in thin-filament protein expression also occur. As the fibers switch from IIB to I, the fast TnT isoforms disappear in the order TnT2f, 4f, 1f, 3f. It appears that with increasing amounts of HCI, the ratio of slow TnT isoforms (TnT1s + TnT2s) to TnT3f also increases, which suggests that these genes may be regulated similarly in response to chronic stimulation.

Once the conversion toward type I phenotype takes place, it appears to remain intact as long as the stimulation protocol is maintained. During this time, the muscle exhibits contractile patterns and mATPase staining consistent with a conversion to the slow phenotype. Furthermore, thick- and thin-filament gene expression after long-term, sustained CMNS are essentially indistinguishable from those in type I fibers.

Proteins of the Neuromuscular Junction
The neuromuscular junction (NMJ) is a specialized synaptic region that provides functional contact between the neuron and the muscle. Within this region, expression of presynaptic and postsynaptic molecules affects the neuronal influence on muscle. Within the NMJ, nicotinic acetylcholine receptors (nAChR) are expressed at high levels, whereas extrajunctional expression is low [7, 109]. Denervation induces up to a 100-fold increase in nAChR number, results in denervation supersensitivity of the muscle, and is reflected throughout the cascade of muscle responses to stimulation [7, 108, 109]. In cases of long-term denervation of muscle, there is necrosis and fiber loss. Electrical stimulation of the muscle after such periods can maintain sarcomeres and probably prevent the normal necrosis and degeneration [153]. In addition, chronic stimulation of long-term denervated muscles increases the force generation in rat EDL and soleus, although full tension generation cannot be recovered in the absence of neural input [3].

The mechanism by which this occurs is unclear, but the role of electrical stimulation on molecules induced by denervation, as well as on the nerve itself, warrants some mention. For example, electrical stimulation of denervated muscle can prevent or reverse the increase in nAChR subunits that occurs with denervation [37, 57]. Furthermore, electrical activity affects the type of receptor expressed. For example, in the denervated state, or in the absence of mature innervation during development, a distinct antigenic (fetal) isoform of nAChR is expressed throughout the fiber [57]. Other postsynaptic molecules may also be affected by electrical activity. In denervated chicken slow- or fast-twitch muscle, electrical stimulation alters both the amount and type of butyrylcholinesterase expressed [77]. However, the specific effect varies with muscle fiber type, despite the application of identical firing patterns to each. The specific cholinesterase that degrades acetylcholine, acetylcholinesterase, appears to be expressed with a pattern similar to that of nAChR. Although developmental and functional data suggest these molecules may be regulated in response to similar stimuli, the role of electrical activity on the expression of this molecule awaits elucidation.

Many of the studies that have examined the effects of motoneuron input on muscle are conducted after denervation, presumably to remove any trophic effects that may play a role in neuronal modulation of muscle gene expression. Several studies, however, have examined the role of electrical activity and/or trophic effects on molecules normally expressed either within the nerve itself or at the muscle membrane. O'Malley et al. [118] show that neither muscle activity nor innervation alone, but a combination of the two, is required for normal expression of the fetal nAChR isoform. Furthermore, Kraus et al. demonstrate an increase in muscle ß-adrenergic receptors in response to CMNS [86]. Conceivably, the effects of alterations in expression of either of these molecules could be reflected downstream within the muscle cascade in response to neuronal input. Similarly, Leighton and Arnolda show that immunoreactivity to calcitonin gene–related peptide, a potent regulator of glycogen metabolism, decreases significantly, immediately upon stimulation of soleus and EDL muscles at a low frequency [94]. This could obviously be involved in further responses of the muscle to neural stimulation.

Data that involve stimulation of a fast nerve with a low frequency, or conversely, a slow nerve with a phasic high frequency, suggest that the activity pattern itself causes muscle transformation. However, the mechanism by which this occurs remains elusive and could necessarily involve a retrograde effect on the motoneuron, which in itself could alter any trophic effects on the muscle. Recent data to suggest that chronic stimulation does in fact alter the properties of the nerve are those of Cameron et al. [27], in which intermittent low-frequency stimulation of the peroneal sciatic nerve of diabetic rats corrects a conduction deficit normally seen in unstimulated nerve. Furthermore, this group demonstrated that peroneal stimulation increases resistance to hypoxia and sciatic vascular conductance. Thus, the role of chronic stimulation on the nerve itself cannot be ignored.

Putative Signaling Pathways

MYOGENIC REGULATORY PROTEINS. A major step toward understanding skeletal myocyte determination and differentiation was made with the finding, by Davis et al. [31], that a single gene product, MyoD1, could induce nonmuscle fibroblasts to commit to the myogenic lineage and express muscle-specific genes. Since the initial description of MyoD1, a total of four DNA-binding proteins have been identified [31, 134, 191]. These comprise the myogenic regulatory protein (MRP) family and are required for terminal differentiation of muscle cells. Since MRPs are required for the proper expression of several muscle-specific genes during muscle differentiation, it is reasonable to assume that they play a regulatory role in skeletal muscle adaptations to CMNS, specifically in control of satellite cell differentiation and muscle gene expression. Several investigators have reported the regulation of gene expression for the MRPs in response to a number of physiologic stimuli. With denervation in murine soleus, MRP gene expression is induced and can be prevented with direct high-frequency electrical stimulation of the muscle [23, 37]. In very similar experiments in neonatal chicken, direct high-frequency electrical stimulation reverses the induction of MRP gene expression in denervated hind limb muscles [116]. Also in chicken, stretch-induced injury leads to an induction of MRP gene expression that is attributed to reexpression within the myonuclei of intact fibers, before induction of satellite cell proliferation [105]. Kraus et al. observed that CMNS repressed MyoD1 expression in the stimulated limb to less than 20% of control levels at 3 days (unpublished observations), just prior to the time of satellite cell activation. Perhaps repression of MRP gene expression by direct or neural electrical stimulation may permit proliferation of satellite cells and thereby contribute to adaptive mechanisms during CMNS.

SIGNALING THROUGH SECOND MESSENGERS AND GROWTH FACTORS. Little is known about the cellular signaling pathways that mediate alterations in gene expression induced by increases in contractile work of skeletal muscles. In a series of investigations designed to explore potential signaling pathways that may be mediating changes in gene expression for proteins of oxidative and glycolytic metabolism during CMNS, Kraus et al. observed that the induction of gene expression for oxidative and mitochondrial proteins correlates temporally and directionally with the induction of muscle cAMP content [86], adenylyl cyclase activity [87], ß-adrenergic receptor number [86], and tissue levels of fibroblast growth factor [113]. However, the induction of these putative signaling molecules is not inhibited by administration of a ß-adrenergic receptor blocker during CMNS, which implies that induction of adenylyl cyclase and cAMP by CMNS is not mediated through the ß-adrenergic receptor, but likely through other signaling pathways that have adenylyl cyclases as their molecular targets (e.g., stretch receptors or cross-talk with the inositol trisphosphate–protein kinase C signaling pathway). These data also imply that some genes coding for proteins of oxidative metabolism may be regulated by cellular levels of cAMP. In contrast, during CMNS, repression of gene expression for the aldolase A gene is inhibited by ß-adrenergic receptor blockade [86]. This implies that repressed expression for this gene of glycolytic metabolism is not regulated by cAMP, but through another mechanism.

RECOVERY

Once the conversion toward type I fibers occurs as a result of CMNS, it appears to remain intact as long as the stimulation protocol is maintained. However, recovery from this conversion takes place if the stimulus is removed. The time course of recovery is more prolonged than that of the original transformation, but is consistent with progressive restoration of a histochemical appearance of fast muscle by about 12 weeks [21]. Reversion seems to take place in the reverse sequence of that involved in the initial transformation and exhibits a "first in, last out" phenomenon [15]. Reversion seems to occur more rapidly in the rabbit EDL than the TA [15, 21]. Contractile characteristics and posttetanic potentiation typical of fast muscle are restored within 3–4 weeks, whereas changes in fatigue resistance, capillary density, and enzyme activity follow a more prolonged time course [15]. Typically, increases in glycolytic enzymes occur more rapidly than the corresponding decreases in oxidative enzymes, which in turn correspond closely to the changes established for mitochondrial volume density [15, 39]. Reversal of changes in the T-tubular system occurs sooner and appears to be complete by 2–4 weeks [39].

Reversal of changes in the myofibrillar apparatus is somewhat slower. However, changes in mRNA encoding myosin HC can be seen very rapidly after cessation of stimulation [20, 81]. The rapidity of these changes appears to depend upon the duration of the stimulation [21]. In 15-day-stimulated rat TA, myosin HCIIb mRNA is detectable as early as 21 hours after stimulation is interrupted [81], whereas in rabbit TA and EDL, slow HC content declines rapidly by 4 days. With longer periods of initial stimulation, similar qualitative patterns are observed, but the time course is prolonged. In rabbits stimulated for 6 weeks, slow myosin HC mRNA decreases to 54 and 42% of control in TA and EDL, respectively, within 12 days after cessation of stimulation. By 3–4 weeks, this is reflected as a decrease in the percentage of type I fibers from approximately 70% to control levels [15]. This is accompanied by a corresponding increase in fast myosin HCIIb mRNA and protein. However, as with the initial transformation, there is no apparent coordination between the switching of fast and slow myosin HC genes. Both LC1/3 and LC2 recover with similar kinetics and exhibit no differential turnover rate. Thus the 2-week delay in LC1/3 conversion during stimulation [17] presumably reflects a difference in gene regulation, rather than in turnover.

In summary, these data suggest that the plasticity associated with fast-to-slow conversion is completely reversible at the gene level and that the signals involved in reprogramming the muscle during the initial conversion do not obligate the muscle to retain the slow phenotype. Furthermore, the ability of transformed fibers to completely recover upon cessation of stimulation without the obvious recruitment of satellite cells suggests that the plasticity associated with muscle transformation from fast to slow does not necessarily involve muscle degeneration and regeneration. This ability of muscle to recover rapidly also has important clinical implications. Muscles used in cardiomyoplasty or as ventricular assist devices require pretraining and conversion to the slow phenotype to prevent failure. Ideally, pretrained muscles used in these assist devices would retain the trained phenotype upon removal of the stimulus. However, this does not appear to be the case, suggesting that further investigations into the mechanisms of conversion and maintenance of the altered phenotype are necessary.

ALTERNATIVE STIMULATION PROTOCOLS

The time course and ultimate conversion of type II to type I fibers appear to depend upon the stimulation protocol, the muscle involved, and the species. For example, in rabbit EDL and TA stimulated at 10 Hz for 8 hours/day for up to 6 weeks, no change in myosin LC pattern or in fiber population can be discerned [124, 125]. This is in obvious contrast to results obtained with 24-hours/day stimulation at 10 Hz, where conversion from type IIb to type I is essentially complete by 6 weeks. Similarly, less dramatic changes in TnT and LC patterns are seen after 60 days of intermittent stimulation than are seen at 21 days of continuous stimulation [124, 125].

Hudlicka and colleagues compared stimulation of rabbit TA at two different frequencies for 2–28 days at 8 hours/day [67]. Under both conditions, they see myosin LCs characteristic of slow muscles at 28 days. No changes in myosin LCs are seen before 28 days with either stimulation protocol. They conclude that long-term electrical stimulation of fast muscles can transform some muscle contractile properties to those of slow muscles irrespective of frequency of stimulation, provided the total number of stimuli is comparable, the duration is greater than 2 weeks, and all motor units are activated.

Two groups have demonstrated that stimulation with 30 Hz or 60 Hz intermittent stimulation is as effective as continuous 10 Hz stimulation in transforming fast into slow muscles [44, 172]. Furthermore, Mabuchi et al. examined the effect of 40 Hz stimulation (2.5 seconds on, 7.5 seconds off) for 3–5 days and determined that the pattern of conversion from type IIB to type I fibers follows the same progression seen at lower-frequency stimulation, except that changes occur sooner with 40 Hz stimulation than with 10 Hz 12-hours/day stimulation [96]. They demonstrate that after 40 Hz stimulation for 3 days, many fibers contain IIa and IIb myosin, while no evidence of type I myosin expression is seen in any mixed fiber. The type I fibers present are presumed to represent the low percentage of type I fibers in normal rabbit TA. By 6 days, mixed fibers that contain myosin HC IIb/IIa and IIa/I are observed, but no IIb/I mixed fibers are observed. By 7 weeks, fibers with HCIIa/I and I are observable, but virtually no fibers that contain HCIIb/IIa or IIa alone are seen. At no time during the conversion are embryonic, neonatal, or IId type myosin HC expressed. Thus, in this case, the stimulation protocol affects the time course of the transition of myosin expression.

A dependence upon the stimulation protocol for conversion of fiber type is even more obvious in the rat, where numerous investigators have been unable to complete the conversions to type I fibers despite long periods of stimulation [33, 90, 182, 183]. However, recently Jarvis et al. reported that with a more prolonged stimulation pattern of 55–61 days at 10 or 20 Hz continuous stimulation, from 6 to 89% of the fibers in the rat TA are type I and express functional characteristics of slow fibers. These include a decrease in maximum tetanic tension and an increase in time to peak twitch-contraction and time-to-half-relaxation, relative to unstimulated contralateral control muscle [73].

IMPLICATIONS FOR MECHANISMS OF FIBER TYPE CONVERSION

As we have just reviewed, the adaptation of skeletal muscle to CMNS involves a complex series of regulatory events that involve numerous cellular protein compartments and results in ultrastructural, physiologic, and functional consequences. A summary of these events is presented in graphic form in Figure 11.3. It is hoped that such a representation will aid in the study of temporal and quantitative relationships and will facilitate the formation of hypotheses about common signaling and regulatory pathways that may mediate these changes. Several hypotheses that are a consequence of such an analysis are presented.

Phases of Adaptations in Metabolic Pathways
The adaptation of metabolic pathways to CMNS appears to occur in several phases, which implies changing or different signals are responsible for the regulation of each phase. The primary contributors to regulation in the initial acute phase appear to be energy metabolites and changes in ion fluxes. In the second dynamic phase, classical second messengers, known growth factors, or other messengers appear to be primary candidates for regulators.

A number of patterns emerge after dissecting out the time course of the changes that occur in the various metabolic pathways during the dynamic phase. Three stages exist for enzymes and their gene activities. There is an initial latency stage that lasts 1–2 weeks, a stage of rapid change from baseline levels, and a stage of more gradual changes with a return toward, but never reaching, baseline values. The most notable exception to this pattern is hexokinase, where measurable increases are noted after only a few hours of stimulation. For hexokinase and several of the enzymes that are substrate-regulated, measurable changes in activity levels in the acute phase may be mediated by phosphorylation potential, metabolite levels, or other factors that rapidly change with the onset of CMNS.

The alterations in oxidative enzymes may at first glance be viewed as an overshoot phenomenon. Another explanation is that during the later part of the dynamic phase, the switch from fast-twitch to slow-twitch contractile proteins occurs. Thus, the contractile apparatus may be more efficient in energy utilization and may not demand the high level of oxidative capacity required at earlier stages.

The high-energy phosphate system also displays a triphasic response. Although the severe initial perturbations are normalized, usually within 24 hours, a second set of alterations results in a depressed phosphorylation potential throughout the remainder of the stimulation period. This pattern raises the possibility that phosphorylation potential may play a role in signaling the transformation of various proteins.

During the programmed switch in muscle phenotype from fast to slow-twitch during CMNS, the alteration in muscle metabolic phenotype, as reflected by alterations in enzyme activities for many metabolic proteins, appears to be primarily the result of changes in gene transcription [5, 86, 183, 184, 185]. There may be up-regulation of gene expression for some classes of genes, down-regulation for others, and differential promoter usage within the same gene for still other sets of genes. Observations of these patterns of gene regulation during CMNS suggest that distinct classes of genes are regulated by distinct signaling mechanisms. Kraus et al. explored the temporal response of steady-state mRNA levels of several muscle-specific genes to CMNS ([86], for review see [89]). Based upon the observation that the regulation patterns of these genes appear to differ markedly in latency, duration, magnitude, and direction, there appears to exist a diverse set of molecular signaling mechanisms that control muscle metabolic gene expression in response to exercise stimuli. Because of the coordinated regulation of oxidative gene activity, adenylyl cyclase activity, and cAMP levels (Fig. 11.3), it is possible that cAMP is responsible for regulation of gene transcription for oxidative proteins. It is clear from examination of Figure 11.3 that myogenic regulatory proteins, which are responsible for induction of muscle-specific gene transcription during myogenesis, are unlikely to be a major regulator for changes in muscle-specific gene expression during CMNS, since MRP gene activity is repressed by electrical stimulation of skeletal muscle [23, 37].

Reversion of Phenotype Following Cessation of CMNS

Data derived from transformation experiments, combined with data derived from reversion experiments, where CMNS is terminated and the muscles are permitted to revert to the fast phenotype (see Recovery), imply that muscle transformation mediated by CMNS may be regulated by a hierarchy of cellular signaling pathways (for discussion, see [139]). Such a hierarchy may also be active during development and maturation of mammalian skeletal muscle. For example, slow-twitch signals, when induced by prolonged CMNS, may be dominant over coexisting fast-twitch signals. When CMNS is withdrawn, the tonic, yet subordinate fast-twitch regulators once again assume their regulatory role, and the fiber reverts to its former phenotype. Such a mechanism could be invoked to explain reversion of slow-twitch muscles to fast-twitch and the appearance of embryonic phenotypes upon denervation. Such a model would explain the "first in, last out" phenomenon observed in recovery experiments [139].

FIGURE 11.3

Changes in muscle function, morphology, expression of classes of muscle genes, and potential signaling activity during CMNS. Data in this figure were synthesized from references cited in the text. They schematically depict the direction and duration of alterations but do not indicate the magnitude of the changes. The acute phase represents the first 48 hours after initiation of CMNS, the dynamic phase represents the period from 2 days to 6 weeks, and the maintenance phase represents the period beyond 6 weeks. The division between the dynamic and maintenance phases has been set as the point at which the contractile proteins have essentially completed their transition. Bars are present during the time in which changes occur; the absence of a bar indicates that no significant change is occurring or that no data are available for the time point. Termination of the bar indicates the completion of change. For example, during the acute phase, no bar is present for thick-filament protein or mRNA, as no changes have been documented at less than 48 hours after initiation of CMNS. Similarly no changes in β-adrenergic receptor density have been noted prior to 10 days, or after 21 days. Striped bars represent total RNA or mRNA, whereas solid or open bars represent protein or activity. Abbreviations: TPT, time-to-peak tension; $RT_{1/2}$, time to half-relaxation; SR/T-tubule systems, sarcoplasmic reticulum and transverse-tubules; satellite cell activity, time of active regeneration and ^3H thymidine incorporation into myotubes; myogenic proteins, MyoD, myf-5, myogenin, and MRF-4; thick filament, total fast (F) or slow (S) myosin heavy chain and F or S myosin light chain; thin filament, F or S troponin T, I, C and tropomyosin; glycolytic metabolism, enzymes of glycolysis such as lactate dehydrogenase and phosphofructo-kinase (this does not include hexokinase); oxidative metabolism, enzymes of the Krebs cycle and fatty acid oxidation such as citrate synthase and carnitine acyltransferase; calcium ATPase, F, or S/cardiac protein and mRNA isoforms; calcium channels, calcium release channel and dihydropyridine receptor; β-adrenergic receptors, membrane density; phosphorylation potential, ([ATP]/[ADPxPi]).

Total RNA and Cellular Regulation

It is apparent from observations made in several laboratories that CMNS results in increases in total cellular transcriptional activity. Heilig and Pette observed a 2–3 times increase in total RNA concentration during CMNS [55]. This finding was confirmed by Kraus et al., who found that total RNA yields per wet weight of muscle increased to 1.5 times control at 3 days, 2

FIGURE 11.3

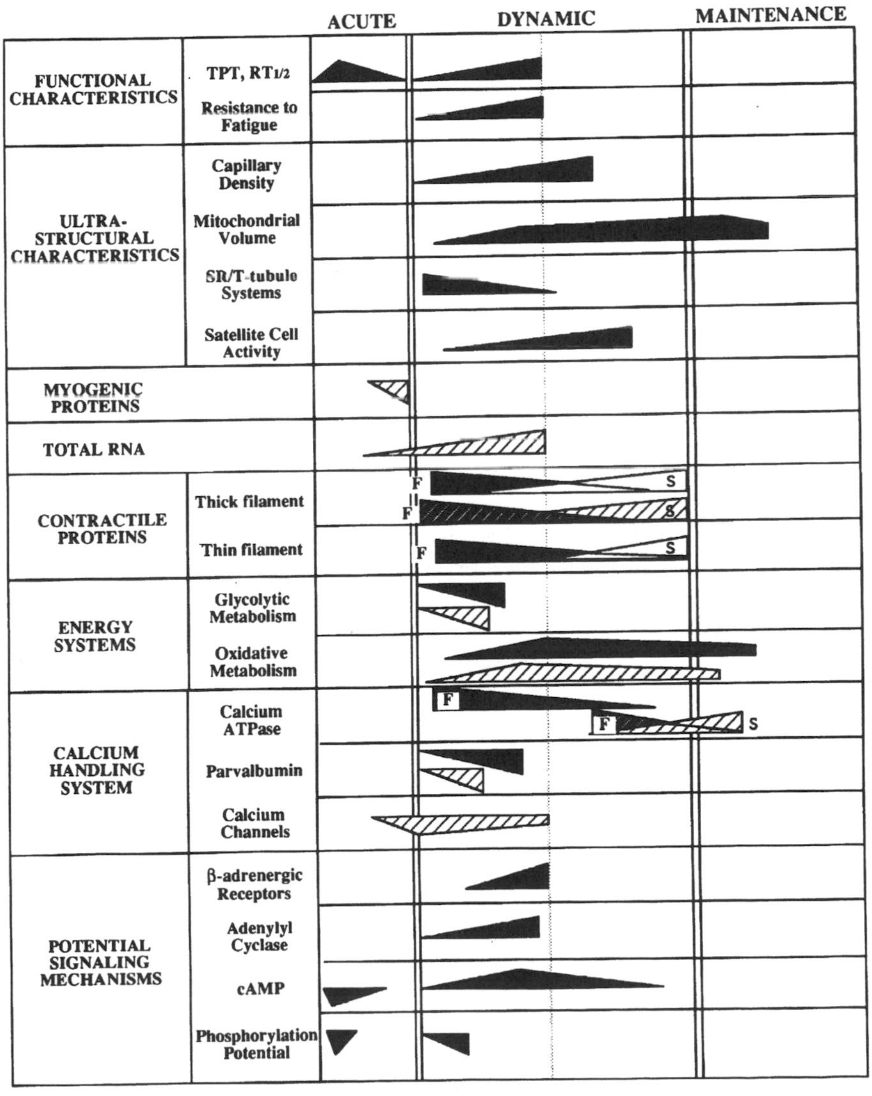

		ACUTE	DYNAMIC	MAINTENANCE
FUNCTIONAL CHARACTERISTICS	TPT, RT1/2			
	Resistance to Fatigue			
ULTRA-STRUCTURAL CHARACTERISTICS	Capillary Density			
	Mitochondrial Volume			
	SR/T-tubule Systems			
	Satellite Cell Activity			
MYOGENIC PROTEINS				
TOTAL RNA				
CONTRACTILE PROTEINS	Thick filament	F / F		S / S
	Thin filament	F		S
ENERGY SYSTEMS	Glycolytic Metabolism			
	Oxidative Metabolism			
CALCIUM HANDLING SYSTEM	Calcium ATPase	F	F	S
	Parvalbumin			
	Calcium Channels			
POTENTIAL SIGNALING MECHANISMS	β-adrenergic Receptors			
	Adenylyl Cyclase			
	cAMP			
	Phosphorylation Potential			

times control at 10 days, and 2.5 times control at 21 days of CMNS (unpublished observations). Since total muscle wet weight is decreased by approximately 30% at 21 days, with no significant changes in fiber number, these observations imply that total RNA per fiber is increased significantly by CMNS. Ninety-five to 97% of total RNA is ribosomal RNA, so these increases in total RNA represent significant increases in the translational capacity of stimulated muscle. This is reflected in a 3–5 times increase in total protein synthesis with CMNS [129]. However, these dramatic increases in total RNA and cellular protein synthesis create several difficulties regarding normalization when reporting and interpreting findings. For example, should changes in gene-specific mRNA be normalized to total RNA, to DNA content, to total protein, to fiber number, or to wet weight? Depending upon the normalization strategy that is used, one could interpret alterations in gene activity for a given protein to be an increase, a decrease, or no change. This consideration, of course, does not change conclusions regarding relative changes in gene expression in comparative analyses. Therefore, it does not alter the implication that different classes of genes are regulated by different signaling pathways, based upon the findings that they have different temporal patterns of regulation (e.g., different directions, latency, rapidity, or duration), but it does point to the need for consistency in presenting experimental results.

Tissue Degeneration and Satellite Cell Activation
Much of the plasticity associated with skeletal muscle is attributed to the ability of reserve muscle myoblasts (satellite cells) to either fuse to form new myofibers or to incorporate into existing fibers to cause regeneration after injury. Thus, in response to chronic stimulation, muscle transformation could be explained not only by alterations within an existing fiber, but also by a selective degeneration of fast fibers and regeneration of slow fibers. Recently, Maier et al. provided histologic and immunohistochemical evidence to demonstrate that stimulation at a low frequency can induce injury and subsequent regeneration in 10–20% of muscle fibers [99, 100]. This is in contrast to previously reported data that at the light- or electron-microscopic level, no damage after chronic stimulation is observed [41]. Lexell et al. more recently compared the differences in experimental design in these two studies, specifically the effects of sampling, the choice of muscle, and the stimulation protocols [95]. Their analyses demonstrate that fiber type degeneration and regeneration vary among animals and between sample areas within an animal; the EDL consistently shows more degeneration than the TA, and degeneration is less extensive with an intermittent period of stimulation that delivers half the aggregate number of electrical impulses [95]. These studies point to the importance of optimizing the stimulation protocol for the application involved, the requirement for making comparisons within a muscle rather than generalizing data for muscle transformation across muscle groups,

and the necessity of adequate sampling to assess stimulation-induced alterations.

To further complicate the issue, Eisenberg and Jacobs-El demonstrate an increase in nuclear incorporation after chronic stimulation in the absence of obvious damage, which suggests that the addition of nuclei may play a role in initiating myosin isoform switching [40]. Yet, expression of developmentally regulated isoforms of myosin in chicken muscle does not require fusion of satellite cells [105], and new myosin isoform expression can occur in the absence of satellite cell proliferation and fusion [137]. Jacobs-El et al. observed expression of multiple isoforms of myosin in the vicinity of a single nucleus in a mature muscle fiber subjected to CMNS [71], which suggests that transformation of intact muscle fibers does not require satellite cell incorporation. Yet, an increase in the number of myocyte nuclei has been demonstrated in response to changing the functional demand of muscle [106, 152, 186]. It is possible that this increased number of myocyte nuclei may be involved in maintaining a myofiber volume per nucleus appropriate for the muscle type [157]: slow oxidative fibers have a smaller cytoplasmic domain per nucleus than more glycolytic fibers [156].

Taken together, these data suggest that muscle transformation is a complex process, that it may vary with the muscle, and that it may reflect both fiber transformation and fiber regeneration. Addition to myocyte nuclei may be required, even in the absence of degeneration, to maintain an appropriate ratio of cytoplasm to nucleus. However, the ability of transformed fibers to completely recover upon cessation of stimulation without the obvious recruitment of satellite cells suggests that the plasticity associated with muscle transformation from fast to slow does not necessarily involve muscle degeneration and regeneration.

APPLICATIONS AND FUTURE DIRECTIONS

Exercise Science

A number of laboratories have demonstrated histochemically that increased contractile activity associated with exercise may induce qualitatively similar changes to chronic nerve stimulation [4, 10, 62, 122]. They further demonstrate that endurance training not only affects the metabolic properties of the fiber, but also causes fast-to-slow transitions in the calcium-handling system and the myofibrillar apparatus. These changes are reflected by a decrease in type IIB fibers, with an increase in type IIA [4, 69] and type I fibers [62], as well as by changes in parvalbumin content and the peptide pattern of SR [50]. Single-fiber analyses have provided further evidence for contractile protein changes with endurance training, including decreases in fast myosin, increases in slow myosin, and the appearance of hybrid fibers containing both fast and slow myosin [151]. In summary, it appears that endurance training in humans produces changes in fast muscle that fall along the continuum of changes seen with CMNS and that knowledge gained from studies with CMNS may aid in elucidating some of the putative regulatory steps involved in skeletal muscle conditioning.

Clinical Applications

The remarkable ability of skeletal muscle to adapt to the increased demands induced by artificial electrical stimulation raises many exciting questions about the potential for therapeutic applications. Given the dynamic range demonstrated by normal tissue, it is possible that even diseased muscle can be induced to adapt favorably to electrical nerve stimulation. The clinical applications are numerous and will briefly be summarized here.

A devastating consequence of neuromuscular diseases, as well as many other disabling diseases, is the profound atrophy and deconditioning that occurs in peripheral muscles. The myofiber atrophy can be tempered or even abated by physical therapy that relies upon a combination of passive and active muscle contraction; however, active muscle use is often severely limited by the underlying disease process. Passive muscle exercise, during which there is little or no recruitment of motor neurons, is physiologically very different from active motor function that involves neural recruitment of motor units [181]. This knowledge has led to increased interest in neuromuscular electrical stimulation for the treatment of the muscle atrophy that occurs in some neuromuscular and disabling diseases.

A major goal of using electrical stimulation in a clinical setting is to reverse weakness and/or increase strength. Stimulation has been used to treat muscle atrophy associated with immobilization and denervation (for review see [52]) and with weightlessness [34]. It also appears useful in reversing or retarding the muscle wasting associated with such diseases as multiple sclerosis [190] and muscular dystrophy [159, 162]. Following prolonged chronic low-frequency stimulation at 8–10 Hz, muscles of adults show increased resistance to fatigue, whereas low-frequency stimulation has little or no effect on the skeletal muscle of normal children [160]. However, chronic low-frequency stimulation of the quadriceps femoris of young children with Duchenne muscular dystrophy (DMD) appears to retard muscle deterioration [159] and results in a significant increase in mean maximum voluntary contraction as compared with the mean forces exerted by the unstimulated control muscles of the contralateral leg [161]. More recently, it has been shown that chronic high-frequency stimulation has a deleterious effect on children with DMD. This effect can be reversed by chronic low-frequency stimulation. Taken together, these data suggest that more investigation is necessary, but that chronic stimulation may play a therapeutic role in the treatment of some neuromuscular diseases.

Electrical stimulation has been used in a number of ways to retrain and condition muscles whose function has been lost due to injury, especially of the spinal cord. For example, it has been used for restoration of micturition [163], standing [178], arm [115] and hand [78] movement, and fecal continence [138] after trauma or stroke. Other applications include diaphragm pacing for diaphragmatic paralysis [163], correction of idiopathic scoliosis [163], management of foot drop [163], and treatment of facial paralysis [43]. It has also been used to train the gracilis to serve as an anal sphincter following abdominoperineal resection [107].

Since chronically stimulated skeletal muscle takes on some of the physiological characteristics of cardiac muscle, it is logical to consider the use of transformed skeletal muscle to augment cardiac function. Currently, the plasticity of skeletal muscle is being exploited in imaginative approaches to treat patients with limited cardiovascular reserve. For example, electrically paced skeletal muscle flaps are being transplanted into the chest to serve as ventricular assist devices and artificial ventricles (for review, see [1, 117]). The techniques offer treatments that do not require immunosuppressive or antibiotic therapy, or cumbersome wires and tubes. Procedures currently being developed offer hope for treatment of conditions that include congenital heart deformities and congestive heart failure. However, success of the procedures requires preconditioning of the skeletal muscle by CMNS and secondary transformation of the muscle phenotype to one of low glycolytic, but high oxidative, capacity.

Recently, work has intensified in this area (for review see [97]). Dynamic cardiomyoplasties have been used clinically for a number of years [112], while other techniques are currently being tested in animal models [110]. However, a number of obstacles remain. Although the use of chronic electrical stimulation for conditioning increases fatigue resistance, it also decreases force and shortening velocity, as well as muscle mass. In addition, skeletal muscle cannot completely reproduce the power required for pumping [8, 143]. These current limitations offer exciting opportunities for exploring the capabilities of transformed skeletal muscle in a functional capacity. Novel stimulation patterns may help overcome some of these obstacles [72]. This task will require a cross-disciplinary approach among physiologists, physicians, and clinicians, working together to implement, test, and evaluate future cardiac-assist models.

Basic Mechanisms of Skeletal Muscle Plasticity
Investigators interested in using CMNS to explore the dynamic state of skeletal muscle have described many of the details of the protein transitions that occur during CMNS. Elucidation of changes in gene expression is still preliminary but implies that many of the observed protein transitions are due to altered transcription. Definition of the cellular signals and specific genetic targets of the signals that result in alterations in gene expression is one of the challenges of the next stage of investigation. These studies are not trivial and will likely require genetic manipulation of the whole animal

before they can be effectively performed. Experiments designed to develop the tools necessary for these experiments are under way in a number of laboratories [9, 32, 187, 188, 189].

The adaptation of skeletal muscle to chronic low-frequency motor nerve stimulation involves remodeling of the tissue by a complex process of protein degradation, synthesis, and assembly. Many of the tissue and cellular components involved in skeletal muscle signaling and contraction have been investigated in an active and thorough fashion and summarized in this review and others. However, investigations into many areas are still very preliminary. Specifically, studies of expression and activity of tissue growth factors, extracellular matrix molecules, and other agents that modulate skeletal myocyte gene expression during muscle transformation are in their infancy. For example, during skeletal muscle remodeling, when the basic scaffolding of the tissue must be maintained, the roles of the extracellular matrix, the exo- and endo-sarcomeric cytoskeleton, and the nuclear matrix will presumably be important. Other signaling pathways such as the inositol trisphosphate system, intracellular ion fluxes, cyclic nucleotides, and novel lipid pathways also await investigation of their role in the transformation process. The results of these studies should provide insight into basic questions of cellular memory in skeletal myocytes, which presumably is involved in cellular transformation.

ACKNOWLEDGMENTS

The authors gratefully acknowledge Stanley Salmons, Brenda Russell, and Fred Schachat for their contributions, as well as Phyllis Howerton for secretarial assistance. W. E. K. is an Established Investigator of the American Heart Association, C. E. T. is supported by a National Research Service Award from the N. I. H. The authors acknowledge partial support of this research through the N. I. H. (RZ9AR1448, PS0HL17670).

REFERENCES

1. Acker, M. A., R. L. Hammond, J. D. Mannion, S. Salmons, and L. W. Stephenson. Skeletal muscle as the potential power source for a cardiovascular pump: assessment in vivo. *Science* 236:236–327, 1987.
2. Al-Amood, W. S., A. J. Buller, and R. Pope. Long-term stimulation of cat fast-twitch skeletal muscle. *Nature* 244:225–227, 1973.
3. Al-Amood, W. S., D. M. Lewis, and H. Schmalbruch. Effects of chronic electrical stimulation on contractile properties of long-term denervated rat skeletal muscle. *J. Physiol. (Lond.)* 441:243–256, 1991.
4. Anderson, P., and J. Henriksson. Training induced changes in the subgroups of human type II skeletal muscle fibres. *Acta Physiol. Scand.* 99:123–125, 1977.
5. Annex, B. H., W. E. Kraus, G. L. Dohm, and R. S. Williams. Mitochondrial biogenesis in striated muscles: rapid induction of citrate synthase mRNA by nerve stimulation. *Am. J. Physiol.* 260:C266–270, 1991.

6. Ariano, M. A., R. B. Armstrong, and V. R. Edgerton. Hindlimb muscle fiber populations of five mammals. *J. Histochem. Cytochem.* 21:51–55, 1973.

7. Axelsson, J., and T. Thesleff. A study of supersensitivity in denervated mammalian skeletal muscle. *J. Physiol. (Lond.)* 147:178–193, 1959.

8. Badylak, S. F. The potential power output for skeletal muscle to provide cardiac assistance. *Sem. Thorac. Cardiovasc. Surg.* 3:116–118, 1991.

9. Barr, E., and J. M. Leiden. Systemic delivery of recombinant proteins by genetically modified myoblasts. *Science* 254:1507–1509, 1991.

10. Baumann, H., M. Jaggi, H. Howald, and M. C. Schaub. Exercise training induces transitions of myosin isoform subunits within histochemically typed human muscle fibers. *Pflügers Arch.* 409:349–360, 1987.

11. Booth, F.W., and D. B. Thompson. Molecular and cellular adaption of muscle in response to exercise: perspective of various models. *Physiol. Rev.* 71:1–45, 1991.

12. Briggs, F. N., K. F. Lee, A. W. Wechsler, and L. R. Jones. Phospholamban expressed in slow-twitch and chronically stimulated fast-twitch muscles minimally affects calcium affinity of sarcoplasmic reticulum $Ca(2+)$-ATPase. *J. Biol. Chem.* 267:26056–26061, 1992.

13. Briggs, M. M., J. J. C. Lin, and F. H. Schachat. The extent of amino-terminal heterogeneity in rabbit fast skeletal muscle troponin T. *J. Musc. Res. Cell Motil.* 8:1–12, 1987.

14. Brooke, M. H., and K. K. Kaiser. Some comments on the histochemical characterization of muscle adenosine triphosphatase. *J. Histochem. Cytochem.* 17:431–432, 1969.

15. Brown, J. M. C., J. Henriksson, and S. Salmons. Restoration of fast muscle characteristics following cessation of chronic stimulation: Physiological, histochemical and metabolic changes during slow-to-fast transformation. *Proc. R. Soc. Lond.* 235:321–346, 1989.

16. Brown, M.D., M. A. Cotter, O. Hudlicka, and G. Vrbová. The effects of different patterns of muscle activity on capillary density, mechanical properties and structure of slow and fast rabbit muscles. *Pflügers Arch.* 361:241–250, 1976.

17. Brown, W. E., S. Salmons, and R. C. Whalen. The sequential replacement of myosin subunit isoforms during muscle type transformation induced by long term electrical stimulation. *J. Biol. Chem.* 258:14686–14692, 1983.

18. Brown, W. E., S. Salmons, and R. G. Whalen. Mechanisms underlying the asynchronous replacement of myosin light chain isoforms during stimulation-induced fibre-type transformation of skeletal muscle. *FEBS Lett.* 192:235–238, 1985.

19. Brown, W. E., R. G. Whalen, and S. Salmons 5th Int. Cong. Neuromuscul. Diseases abstr. TH60, 1982.

20. Brownson, C., H. Isenberg, W. Brown, S. Salmons, and Y. Edwards. Changes in skeletal muscle gene transcription induced by chronic stimulation. *Muscle Nerve* 11:1183–1189, 1988.

21. Brownson, C., P. Little, J. C. Jarvis, and S. Salmons. Reciprocal changes in myosin isoform mRNAs of rabbit skeletal muscle in response to the initiation and cessation of chronic electrical stimulation. *Muscle Nerve* 15:694–700, 1992.

22. Buller, A. J., J. C. Eccles and R. M. Eccles. Interactions between motoneurons and muscles in respect of the characteristic speeds of their responses. *J. Physiol.* 150:417–439, 1960.

23. Buonanno, A., L. Apone, M. I. Morasso, R. Beers, H. R. Brenner, and R. Eftimie. The MyoD family of myogenic factors is regulated by electrical activity: isolation and characterization of a mouse myf-5 cDNA. *Nucleic Acid Res.* 20:539–544, 1992.

24. Burke, R. E. The correlation of physiological properties with histochemical characteristics in single muscle units. *Ann. N.Y. Acad. Sci.* 228:145–159, 1974.

25. Burke, R. E., D. N. Levine, P. Tsairis, and F. E. Zajac III. Physiological types and histochemical profiles in motor units of the cat gastrocnemius. *J. Physiol. (Lond)* 234:723–748, 1973.

26. Burke, R. E., D. N. Levine, F. E. Zajac III, P. Tsairis, and W. K. Engel. Mammalian motor units: physiological-histochemical correlation in three types in cat gastrocnemius. *Science* 174:709–711, 1971.

27. Cameron, N. E., M. A. Cotter, S. Robertson, and E. K. Maxfield. Nerve function in

experimental diabetes in rats: effects of electrical stimulation. *Am. J. Physiol.* 264:E161–E166, 1993.

28. Carraro, U., C. Catani, L. Saggin, M. Zrunek, M. Szaboles, et al. Isomyosin changes after functional electrostimulation of denervated sheep muscle. *Muscle Nerve* 11:1016–1028, 1988.

29. Catterall, W. Excitation-contraction coupling in vertebrate skeletal muscle: a tale of two calcium channels. *Cell* 64:871–874, 1991.

30. Ciesielski, T. E., Y. Fukuda, W. W. L. Glenn, J. Gorfein, K. Jeffrey, and J. F. Hogan. Response of the diaphragm muscle to electrical stimulation of the phrenic nerve. *J. Neurosurg.* 58:92–100, 1983.

31. Davis, R. L., H. Weintraub, and A. B. Lassar. Expression of a single transfected cDNA converts fibroblasts to myoblasts. *Cell* 51:987–1000, 1987.

32. Dhawan, J., L. C. Pan, G. K. Pavlath, M. A. Travis, A. M. Lanctot, and H. M. Blau. Systemic delivery of growth hormone by injection of genetically engineered myoblasts. *Science* 254:1509–1512, 1991.

33. Donselaar, Y., O. Eerbeek, D. Kernell, and B. A. Verhey. Fibre sizes and histochemical staining characteristics in normal and chronically stimulated fast muscle of the cat. *J. Physiol. (Lond)* 382:237–254, 1987.

34. Duvoisin, M. R., V. A. Convertino, P. Buchanan, P. D. Gollnick, and G. A. Dudley. Characteristics and preliminary observations of the influence of electromyostimulation on the size and function of human skeletal muscle during 30 days of simulated microgravity. *Aviat. Space Environ. Med.* 60:671–678, 1989.

35. Dux, L., H. J. Green, and D. Pette. Chronic low-frequency stimulation of rabbit fast-twitch muscle induces partial inactivation of the sarcoplasmic reticulum Ca^{2+}-ATPase and changes in its triptic cleavage. *Eur. J. Biochem.* 192:95–100, 1990.

36. Eccles, J. C., E. Gutman, and P. Hnik (eds). *The Effects of Use and Disuse on Neuromuscular Functions.* Prague: Czech. Acad. of Sci., 1963, pp. 111–128.

37. Eftimie, R., H. R. Brenner, and A. Buonanno. Myogenin and MyoD join a family of skeletal muscle genes regulated by electrical activity. *Proc. Natl. Acad. Sci. USA* 88:1349–1353, 1991.

38. Eisenberg, B. R. Quantitative ultrastructure of mammalian skeletal muscle. L. D. Peachey, R. H. Adrian, and S. R. Geiger (eds). *Handbook of Physiology: Skeletal Muscle.* Baltimore: Williams & Wilkins, 1983, pp. 73–112.

39. Eisenberg, B. R., J. M. C. Brown, and S. Salmons. Restoration of fast muscle characteristics following cessation of chronic stimulation. The ultratructure of slow-to-fast transformation. *Cell Tissue Res.* 238:221–230, 1984.

40. Eisenberg, B. R., and J. Jacobs-El. Are satellite cells essential for isomyosin switching? D. Pette (ed). *The Dynamic State of Muscle Fibers.* Berlin, New York: Walter de Gruyter, 1990, pp. 681–691.

41. Eisenberg, B. R., and S. Salmons. The reorganization of subcellular structure in muscle undergoing fast-to-slow type transformation: a stereologic study. *Cell Tissue Res.* 220:449–471, 1981.

42. Etgen, G. E., R. P. Farrar, and J. L. Ivy. Effect of chronic electrical stimulation on GLUT-4 protein content in fast-twitch muscle. *Am. J. Physiol.* 264:R816–R819, 1993.

43. Farragher, D. J. Electrical stimulation: a method of treatment for facial paralysis. F. C. Rose, R. Jones, and G. Vrbová (eds). *Neuromuscular Stimulation: Basic Concepts and Clinical Implications.* New York: Demos Publications, 1989, pp. 303–306.

44. Ferguson, A. S., H. E. Stone, U. Roessmann, M. Burke, E. Tisdale, and J. T. Mortimer. Muscle plasticity: comparison of 30-Hz burst with 10-Hz continuous stimulation. *J. Appl. Physiol.* 66:1143–1151, 1989.

45. Fleisher, S., and M. Inui. Biochemistry and biophysics of excitation-contraction coupling. *Annu. Rev. Biophys. Biophys. Chem.* 18:333–364, 1989.

46. Frey, M., H. Thoma, H. Gruber, H. Stöhr, L. Huber, and M. Havel. The chronically stimulated psoas muscle as an energy source for artificial organs: an experimental study in

sheep. R. C.-J. Chiu (ed). *Biomechanical Cardiac Assist: Cardiomyoplasty and Muscle-powered Devices.* Mount Kisco: Futura Publishing, 1986, pp. 179–191.

47. Goldspink, G., A. Scutt, P. T. Loughna, D. J. Wells., T. Jaenicke, and G. F. Gerlach. Gene expression in skeletal muscle in response to stretch and force generation. *Am. J. Physiol.* 262:R356–R363, 1992.

48. Green, H. J., M. Ball-Burnett, E. R. Chin, L. Dux, and D. Pette. Time-dependent increases in Na$^+$, K$^+$-ATPase content of low-frequency-stimulated rabbit muscle. 310:129–131, 1992.

49. Green, H. J., S. Dusterhoft, L. Dux, and D. Pette. Metabolite patterns related to exhaustion, recovery and transformation of chronically stimulated rabbit fast-twitch muscle. *Pflügers Arch.* 420:359–366, 1992.

50. Green, H. J., G. A. Klug, H. Reichmann, U. Seedorf, W. Wiehrer, and D. Pette. Exercise-induced fibre type transitions with regard to myosin, parvalbumin, and sarcoplasmic reticulum in muscles of the rat. *Pflügers Arch.* 400:432–438, 1984.

51. Guth, L., and F. J. Samaha. Procedure for the histochemical demonstration of actomyosin ATPase. *Exp. Neurol.* 28:365–367, 1970.

52. Hainaut, K., and J. Duchateau. Neuromuscular electrical stimulation and voluntary exercise. *Sports Med.* 14:100–113, 1992.

53. Hartner, K. T., B. J. Kirschbaum, and D. Pette. The multiplicity of troponin T isoforms. *Eur. J. Biochem.* 179:31–38, 1989.

54. Heilig, A., and D. Pette. Changes induced in the enzyme activity pattern by electrical stimulation of fast-twitch muscle. D. Pette (ed). *Plasticity of Muscle.* Berlin, New York: Walter de Gruyter, 1980, pp. 409–420.

55. Heilig, A., and D. Pette. Changes in transcriptional activity of chronically stimulated fast twitch muscle. 151:211–214, 1983.

56. Heilig, A., and D. Pette. Albumin in rabbit skeletal muscle. Origin, distribution, and regulation by contractile activity. *Eur. J. Biochem.* 171:503–508, 1988.

57. Heinemann, S., G. Asouline, M. Ballivet, J. Boulter, J. Connolly, et al. Molecular biology of the neural and muscle acetylcholine receptors. S. Heinemann, and J. Patrick (eds). *Molecular Neurobiology: Recombinant DNA Approaches.* New York: Plenum Press, 1987, pp. 45–96.

58. Henriksson, J., M. M.-Y. Chi, S. Hintz, D. A. Young, K. K. Kaiser, et al. Chronic stimulation of mammalian muscle: changes in enzymes of six metabolic pathways. *Am. J. Physiol.* 251:C614–C632, 1986.

59. Henriksson, J., P. M. Nemeth, K. Borg, S. Salmons, and O. H. Lowry. Fibre type-specific enzyme activity profiles. A single fibre study of the effects of chronic stimulation on the rabbit fast-twitch tibialis anterior muscle. D. Pette (ed). *The Dynamic State of Muscle Fibers.* Berlin: Walter de Gruyter, 1990, pp. 385–398.

60. Henriksson, J., S. Salmons, M. M. Y. Chi, C. S. Hintz, and O. H. Lowry. Chronic stimulation of mammalian muscle: changes in metabolite concentrations in individual fibers. *Am. J. Physiol.* 255:C543–C551, 1988.

61. Hoffman, R. K., B. Gambke, L. W. Stephenson, and N. A. Rubenstein. Myosin transitions in chronic stimulation do not involve embryonic isozymes. *Muscle Nerve* 8:796–805, 1985.

62. Howald, H., H. Hoppeler, H. Claassen, O. Mathieu, and R. Straub. Influences of endurance training on the ultrastructural comparison of the different muscle fiber types in humans. *Pflügers Arch.* 403:369–376, 1985.

63. Hudlicka, O., M. Brown, M. Cotter, M. Smith, and G. Vrbova. The effect of long-term stimulations of fast muscles on their blood flow, metabolism and ability to withstand fatigue. *Pflügers Arch.* 369:141–149, 1977.

64. Hudlicka, O., L. Dodd, E. M. Renkin, and S. D. Gray. Early changes in fiber profile and capillary density in long-term stimulated muscles. *Am. J. Physiol.* 243:H528–H535, 1982.

65. Hudlicka, O., and S. Price. The role of blood flow and/or muscle hypoxia in capillary growth in chronically stimulated fast muscles. *Pflügers Arch.* 417:67–72, 1990.

66. Hudlicka, O., K. R. Tyler, and T. Ailman. The effect of long-term electrical stimulation on

fuel uptake and performance in fast skeletal muscles. D. Pette (ed). *Plasticity of Muscle*. New York: Walter de Gruyter, 1980, pp. 401–408.

67. Hudlicka, O., K. R. Tyler, T. Srihari, and D. Pette. The effect of different patterns of long-term stimulation on contractile properties and myosin light chains in rabbit fast muscles. *Pflügers Arch*. 393:164–170, 1982.

68. Hudlika, O. Growth of capillaries in skeletal and cardiac muscle. *Circ. Res*. 50:451–461, 1982.

69. Ingjer, F. Effects of endurance training on muscle fiber ATPase activity, capillary supply and mitochondrial content in man. *J. Physiol. (Lond.)* 294:419–432, 1979.

70. Ivy, J. L. The insulin-like effects of muscle contraction. K. B. Pandolf (ed). *Exercise and Sports Sciences Reviews*. New York: Mcmillan, 1987, pp. 29–51.

71. Jacobs-El, J., W. Ashley, and B. Russell. IIX and slow myosin expression follow mitochondrial increases in transforming muscle fibers. *Am. J. Physiol*. 265:C79–C84, 1993.

72. Jarvis. J. C., C. N. Mayne, and S. Salmons. Basic studies on skeletal muscle for cardiac assistance. *J. Cardiac Surg*. 6:204–209, 1991.

73. Jarvis, J. C., T. Mokrusch, C. N. Mayne, M. M. N. Kwende, S. Gilroy, et al. Fast-to-slow fibre type conversion does occur in continuously stimulated rat hind limb muscle. *J. Physiol*. 467:11P, 1993.

74. Jolesz, F., and F. A. Sreter. Development, innervation, and activity-pattern induced changes in skeletal muscle. *Annu. Rev. Physiol*. 43:531–552, 1981.

75. Joplin, R. E., L. L. Franchi, and S. Salmons. Changes in the size and synthetic activity of nuclear populations in chronically stimulated rabbit skeletal muscle. *J. Anat*. 155:39–50, 1987.

76. Kaufmann, M., J. A. Simoneau, J. H. Veerkamp, and D. Pette. Electrostimulation-induced increases in fatty acid-binding protein and myoglobin in rat fast-twitch muscle and comparison with tissue levels in heart. *FEBS Lett*. 245:181–184, 1989.

77. Khaskiye, A., J. P. Sine, B. Colas, and D. Renaud. Effects of electrical stimulation on molecular forms of butyrylcholinesterase in denervated fast and slow latissimus dorsi muscles of newly hatched chicken. *J. Neurochem*. 54:828–833, 1990.

78. Kidd, G. L., and J. A. Oldham. Functional rehabilitation of the hand: an application of a new electrotherapy. F. C. Rose, R. Jones, and G. Vrbova (eds). *Neuromuscular Stimulation: Basic Concepts and Clinical Implications*. New York: Demos Publications, 1989, pp. 285–294.

79. Kirschbaum, B. J., A. Heilig, K.-T. Hartner, and D. Pette. Electrostimulation-induced fast-to-slow transitions of myosin light and heavy chains in rabbit fast-twitch muscle at the mRNA level. *FEBS Lett*. 243:123–126, 1989.

80. Kirschbaum, B. J., H. B. Kucher, A. Termin, A. M. Kelly, and D. Pette. Antagonistic effects of chronic low frequency stimulation and thyroid hormone on myosin expression in rat fast-twitch muscle. *J. Biol. Chem*. 265:13974–13980, 1990.

81. Kirschbaum, B. J., S. Schneider, S. Izumo, V. Mahdavi, B. Nadal-Ginard, and D. Pette. Rapid and reversible changes in myosin heavy chain expression in response to increased neuromuscular activity of rat fast-twitch muscle. *FEBS Lett*. 268:75–78, 1990.

82. Kirschbaum, B. J., J. A. Simoneau, A. Bar, P. J. R. Barton, M. E. Buckingham, and D. Pette. Chronic stimulation-induced changes of myosin light chains at the mRNA and protein levels in rat fast-twitch muscle. *Eur. J. Biochem*. 179:23–29, 1989.

83. Kirschbaum, B. J., J. A. Simoneau, and D. Pette. Dynamics of myosin expression during the induced transformation of adult rat fast-twitch muscle. F. Stockdale, and L. Kedes (eds). *Cellular and Molecular Biology of Muscle Development*. New York: Alan R. Liss, 1989, pp. 461–469.

84. Klug, G. A., M. E. Houston, J. T. Stull, and D. Pette. Decrease in myosin light chain kinase activity of rabbit fast muscle by chronic stimulation. *FEBS Lett*. 200:352–354, 1986.

85. Klug, G. A., E. Leberer, E. Leisner, J. A. Simoneau, and D. Pette. Relationship between parvalbumin content and the speed of relaxation in chronically stimulated rabbit fast-twitch muscle. *Pflügers Arch*. 411:126–131, 1988.

86. Kraus, W. E., T. S. Bernard, and R. S. Williams. Interactions between sustained contractile

activity and ß-adrenergic receptors in the regulation of gene expression in skeletal muscles. *Am. J. Physiol.* 256:C506–C514, 1989.

87. Kraus, W. E., J. P. Longabaugh, and S. B. Liggett. Electrical pacing induces increases in adenylyl cyclase activity in rabbit skeletal muscle that are independent of the ß-adrenergic receptor. *Am. J. Physiol.* 263:E226–E230, 1992.

88. Kraus, W. E., J. W. Moore, and A. R. Marks. Sustained contractile activity negatively regulates the expression of the calcium release channel gene in skeletal muscle. *J. Cell. Biochem.* 15C:170, 1991.

89. Kraus, W. E., and R. S. Williams. Intracellular signals mediating contraction-induced changes in the oxidative capacity of skeletal muscle. D. Pette (ed). *The Dynamic State of Muscle Fibers.* Berlin: Walter de Gruyter, 1990, pp. 601–615.

90. Kwong, W. H., and G. Vrbova. Effects of low frequency stimulation on fast and slow muscles of the rat. *Pflügers Arch.* 391:200–207, 1981.

91. Leberer, E., K.-T. Härtner, C. J. Brandl, J. Fujii, M. Tada, et al. Slow/cardiac sarcoplasmic reticulum Ca^{2+}-ATPase and phospholamban mRNAs are expressed in chronically stimulated rabbit fast-twitch muscle. *Eur. J. Biochem.* 185:51–54, 1989.

92. Leberer, E., and D. Pette. Immunochemical quantification of sarcoplasmic reticulum Ca-ATPase, of calsequestrin and of parvalbumin in rabbit skeletal muscles of defined fiber composition. *Eur. J. Biochem.* 156:489–496, 1986.

93. Leberer, E., U. Seedorf, and D. Pette. Neural control of gene expression in skeletal muscle. *Biochem. J.* 239:295–300, 1986.

94. Leighton, B., and L. Arnolda. Effect of electrical stimulation of the sciatic nerve in anaesthetized rats on content of CGRP in rat skeletal muscle. *Biochem. Soc. Trans.* 19:134S, 1991.

95. Lexell, J., J. Jarvis, D. Downham, and S. Salmons. Quantitative morphology of stimulation-induced damage in rabbit fast-twitch skeletal muscles. *Cell Tissue Res.* 269:195–204, 1992.

96. Mabuchi, K., F. A. Sreter, J. Gergely, and A. O. Jorgensen. Myosin and sarcoplasmic reticulum Ca^{2+}-ATPase isoforms in electrically stimulated rabbit fast muscle. D. Pette (ed). *The Dynamic State of Muscle Fibers.* Berlin, New York: Walter de Gruyter, 1990, pp. 445–462.

97. Magovern, G. J. Introduction to the history and development of skeletal muscle plasticity and its clinical application to cardiomyoplasty and skeletal muscle ventricle. *Semi. Thorac. Cardiovasc. Surg.* 3:95–97, 1991.

98. Magovern, G. J., F. R. Heckler, S. B. Park, I. Y. Christlieb, G. A. Liebler, et al. Paced skeletal muscle for dynamic cardiomyoplasty. *Ann. Thorac. Surg.* 44:379–388, 1988.

99. Maier, A., B. Gambke, and D. Pette. Degeneration-regeneration as a mechanism contributing to the fast to slow conversion of chronically stimulated fast-twitch rabbit muscle. *Cell Tissue Res.* 244:635–643, 1986.

100. Maier, A., L. Gorza, S. Schiaffino, and D. Pette. A combined histochemical and immunohistochemical study on the dynamics of fast-to-slow fiber transformation in chronically stimulated rabbit muscle. *Cell Tissue Res.* 254:59–68, 1988.

101. Mannion, J. D., J. Shannon, W. Chen, W. E. Brown, and D. R. Gale. Skeletal muscle-powered assistance for the heart: assessment of a goat model. R. C.-J. Chiu and I. Bourgeois (eds). *Transformed Muscle for Cardiac Assist and Repair.* Mount Kisco, NY: Futura, 1990, pp. 117–127.

102. Marks, A. R., P. Tempst, K. S. Hwang, M. B. Taubman, M. Inui, et al. Molecular cloning and characterization of the ryanodine receptor/junctional channel complex cDNA from skeletal muscle sarcoplasmic reticulum. *Proc. Natl. Acad. Sci. USA* 86:8683–8687, 1989.

103. Martin, A. F., M. Rabinowitz, G. Blough, G. Prior, and R. Zak. *J. Biol. Chem.* 252:3422–3429, 1977.

104. Mayne, C. N., J. C. Jarvis, and S. Salmons. Dissociation between metabolite levels and force fatigue in the early stages of stimulation-induced transformation of mammalian skeletal muscle. *Basic Appl. Myol.* 1:63–70, 1991.

105. McCormick, K., and E. Schultz. Embryonic fibers in avian muscle following wing weighting. *J. Cell Biol.* 111:35a, 1990.

106. McCormick, K. M., and E. Schultz. Mechanisms of nascent fiber formation during avian skeletal muscle hypertrophy. *Dev. Biol.* 150:319–334, 1992.

107. Mercati, U., V. Trancanelli, P. Castagnoli, A. Mariotti, and R. Ciaccarini. Use of the gracilis muscles for sphincteric construction after abdominoperineal resection. *Dis. Colon Rectum* 34:1085–1089, 1991.

108. Merlie, J. P., K. E. Isenberg, S. D. Russell, and J. R. Sanes. Denervation supersensitivity in skeletal muscle: analysis with a cloned cDNA probe. *J. Cell Biol.* 99:332–335, 1984.

109. Miledi, R. The acetylcholine sensitivity of frog muscle fibers after complete or partial denervation. *J. Physiol (Lond.)* 151:1–23, 1960.

110. Mocek, F. W., D. R. Anderson, A. Pochettino, R. L. Hammond, A. Spanta, et al. Skeletal muscle ventricles in circulation long-term: One hundred ninety-one to eight hundred thirty-six days. *J. Heart Lung Transplant* 11:S334, 1992.

111. Moore, R. L., and J. T. Stull. Am. J. Physiol. 1984. Myosin light chain phosphorylation in fast and slow skeletal muscles in situ. Am. J. Physiol. Z47:C462–C471, 1984.

112. Moreira, L. F. P., N. A. G. Stolf, and A. D. Jatene. Benefits of cardiomyoplasty for dilated cardiomyopathy. *Semin. Thorac. Cardiovasc. Surg.* 3:140–144, 1991.

113. Morrow, N. G., W. E. Kraus, J. W. Moore, R. S. Williams, and J. L. Swain. Increased expression of fibroblast growth factors in a rabbit skeletal muscle model of exercise conditioning. *J. Clin. Invest.* 85:1816–1820, 1990.

114. Myrhage, R., and O. Hudlicka. Capillary growth in chronically stimulated adult skeletal muscle as studied by intravital microscopy and histological methods in rabbits and rats. *Microvasc. Res.* 16:73–90, 1978.

115. Nathan, R. H. Generation of functional arm movements in C4 quadriplegics by neuromuscular stimulation. F. C. Rose, R. Jones, and G. Vrbova (eds). *Neuromuscular Stimulation: Basic Concepts and Clinical Implications.* New York: Demos Publications, 1989, pp. 273–284.

116. Neville, C. M., M. Schmidt, and J. Schmidt. Response of myogenic determination factors to cessation and resumption of electrical activity in skeletal muscle: a possible role for myogenin in denervation supersensitivity. *Cell. Mol. Neurobiol.* 12:511–527, 1992.

117. Niinami, H., A. Pochettino, and L. W. Stephenson. Use of skeletal muscle grafts for cardiac assist. *Trends Cardiovasc. Med.* 1:122–126, 1991.

118. O'Malley, J. P., R. G. Mills, and J. J. Bray. Effects of electrical stimulation and tetrodotoxin paralysis on antigenic properties of acetylcholine receptors in rat skeletal muscle. *Neurosci. Lett.* 120:224–226, 1990.

119. Ohlendieck, K., F. N. Briggs, K. F. Lee, A. W. Wechsler, and K. P. Campbell. Analysis of excitation-contraction-coupling components in chronically stimulated canine skeletal muscle. *Eur. J. Biochem.* 739–747, 1991.

120. Padykula, H. A., and E. Herman. Factors affecting the activity of adenosine triphosphatase and other phosphatases as measured by histochemical techniques. *J. Histo-chem. Cytochem.* 3:161–195, 1955.

121. Peter, J. B., R. J. Barnard, V. R. Edgerton, C. A. Gillespie, and K. E. Stempel. Metabolic profiles of three fiber types of skeletal muscle in guinea pigs and rabbits. *Biochemistry* 11:2627–2632, 1972.

122. Pette, D. Activity-induced fast to slow transition in mammalian muscle. *Med. Sci. Sports Exerc.* 16:517–528, 1984.

123. Pette, D., and S. Dusterhoft. Altered gene expression in fast-twitch muscle induced by chronic low-frequency stimulation. *Am. J. Physiol.* 262:R333–R338, 1992.

124. Pette, D., and C. Heilmann. Transformation of morphological, functional and metabolic properties of fast-twitch muscle as induced by long-term electrical stimulation. *Basic Res. Cardiol.* 72:247–253, 1977.

125. Pette, D., W. Muller, E. Leisner, and G. Vrbova. Time dependent effects on contractile properties, fibre population, myosin light chains and enzymes of energy metabolism in

intermittently and continuously stimulated fast twitch muscles of the rabbit. *Pflügers Arch.* 364:103–112, 1976.

126. Pette, D., B. U. Ramirez, W. Muller, R. Simon, G. U. Exner, and R. Hildebrand. Influence of intermittent long-term stimulation on contractile, histochemical and metabolic properties of fibre populations in fast and slow rabbit muscles. *Pflügers Arch.* 361:1–7, 1975.

127. Pette, D., M. E. Smith, H. W. Staudte, and G. Vrbova. Effects of long-term electrical stimulation on some contractile and metabolic characteristics of fast rabbit muscles. *Pflügers Arch.* 338:257–272, 1973.

128. Pette, D., and G. Vrbova. Invited review: neural control of phenotypic expression in mammalian muscle fibers. *Muscle Nerve* 8:676–689, 1985.

129. Pette, D., and G. Vrbova. Adaptation of mammalian skeletal muscle fibers to chronic electrical stimulation. *Rev. Physiol. Biochem. Pharmacol.* 120:116–183, 1992.

130. Radermecker, M. A., F. E. Sluse, B. Focant, M. Reznik, J. Fourney, and R. Limet. Influence of tension reduction and peripheral dissection on histologic, biochemical and bioenergetic profiles, and kinetics of skeletal muscle fast-to-slow transformation. *J. Cardiac Surg.* 6:195–203, 1991.

131. Reichel, R., I. Kovesdi, and J. R. Nevins. Developmental control of a promotor-specific factor that is also regulated by the E1A gene product. *Cell* 48:501–506, 1987.

132. Reichmann. H., H. Hoppeler, O. Mathieu-Costello, F. von Bergen, and D. Pette. Biochemical and ultrastructural changes of skeletal muscle mitochondria after chronic electrical stimulation in rabbits. *Pflügers Arch.* 404:1–9, 1985.

133. Reichmann, H., R. Wasl, J. A. Simoneau, and D. Pette. Enzyme activities of fatty acid oxidation and the respiratory chain in chronically stimulated fast-twitch muscle of the rabbit. *Pflügers Arch.* 418:572–574, 1991.

134. Rhodes, S. J., and S. F. Konieczny. Identification of MRF4: a new member of the muscle regulatory gene family. *Genes Dev.* 3:2050–2061, 1989.

135. Rios, E., and G. Brum. Involvement of dihydropyridine receptors in excitation-contraction coupling in skeletal muscle. *Nature* 325:717–720, 1987.

136. Romanul, F. C. A., F. A. Sréter, S. Salmons, and J. Gergeley. The effect of changed pattern of activity on histochemical characteristics of muscle fibers. A. T. Milhorat (ed). *Exploratory Concepts in Muscular Dystrophy, Vol 2*. Amsterdam: Excepta Medica, 1974, pp. 309–316.

137. Rosenblatt, J. D., and D. J. Parry. Gamma irradiation prevents compensatory hypertrophy of overloaded mouse extensor digitorum longus muscle. *J. Appl. Physiol.* 73:2538–2543, 1992.

138. Sackier, J. M., and C. B. Wood. The anal sphincter. F. C. Rose, R. Jones, and G. Vrbova (eds). *Neuromuscular Stimulation: Basic Concepts and Clinical Implications*. New York: Demos Publications, 1989, pp. 331–349.

139. Salmons, S. On the reversibility of stimulation-induced muscle transformation. D. Pette (ed). *The Dynamic State of Muscle Fibers*. Berlin, New York: Walter de Gruyter, 1990, pp. 401–414.

140. Salmons, S., D. R. Gale, and F. A. Sreter. Ultrastructural aspects of the transformation of muscle fibre type by long term stimulation: changes in Z discs and mitochondria. *J. Anat.* 127:17–31, 1978.

141. Salmons, S., and J. Henriksson. The adaptive response of skeletal muscle to increased use. *Muscle Nerve* 4:94–105, 1981.

142. Salmons, S., and J. C. Jarvis. Simple optical switch for implantable devices. *Med Biol. Eng. Comput.* 29:554–556, 1991.

143. Salmons, S., and J. C. Jarvis. Cardiac assistance from skeletal muscle: a critical appraisal of the various approaches. *Br. Heart J.* 68:333–338, 1992.

144. Salmons, S., and F. A. Sreter. Significance of impulse activity in the transformation of skeletal muscle type. *Nature* 263:30–34, 1976.

145. Salmons, S., and G. Vrbová. The influence of activity on some contractile characteristics of mammalian fast and slow muscles. *J. Physiol. (Lond.)* 20:535–549, 1969.

146. Saltin, B., and P. D. Gollnick. Skeletal muscle adaptability: significance for metabolism and performance. L. D. Peachey, R. H. Adrian, and S. R. Geiger (eds). *Handbook of Physiology: Skeletal Muscle.* Bethesda, MD: American Physiological Society, 1983, pp. 555–632.

147. Schachat, F., M. Briggs, H. D. McGinnis, E. K. Williamson, M. S. Diamond, and P. W. Brandt. Expression of fast thin filament proteins: defining fiber archetypes in a multidimensional continuum. D. Pette (ed). *The Dynamic State of Muscle Fibers.* Berlin: Walter DeGruyter, 1990, pp. 279–291.

148. Schachat, F., R. S. Williams, and C. A. Schnurr. Coordinate changes in fast thin filament and Z-line protein expression in the early response to chronic stimulation. *J. Biol. Chem.* 263:13975–13978, 1988.

149. Schachat, F. H., D. D. Bronson, and O. B. McDonald. Heterogeneity of contractile proteins: a continuum of troponin-tropomyosin expression in rabbit skeletal muscle. *J. Biol. Chem.* 260:1108–1113, 1985.

150. Schachat, F. H., M. S. Diamond, and P. W. Brandt. The effect of different troponin T-tropomyosin combinations on thin filament activation. *J. Mol. Biol.* 198:551–554, 1987.

151. Schantz, P. G., and G. K. Dhoot. Coexistence of slow and fast isoforms of contractile and regulatory proteins in human skeletal muscle fibres induced by endurance training. *Acta Physiol. Scand.* 131:147–154, 1989.

152. Schiaffino, S., S. P. Bormioli, and M. Aloisi. The fate of newly formed satellite cells during compensatory muscle hypertrophy. *Virchows Arch. [B]* 21:113–118, 1976.

153. Schmalbruch, H., W. S. Al-Amood, and D. M. Lewis. Morphology of long-term denervated rat soleus muscle and the effects of chronic electrical stimulation. *J. Physiol. (Lond.)* 441:233–241, 1991.

154. Schmidt, T. L., and D. Pette. Correlations between troponin-T and myosin heavy chain isoforms in normal and transforming rabbit muscle fibers. D. Pette (ed). *The Dynamic State of Muscle Fibers.* Berlin, New York: Walter de Gruyter, 1990, pp. 293–302.

155. Schmitt, T., and D. Pette. Increased mitochondrial creatine kinase in chronically stimulated fast-twitch rabbit muscle. *FEBS Lett.* 188:341–344, 1985.

156. Schultz, E., and K. C. Darr. The role of satellite cells in adaptive or induced fiber transformation. D. Pette (ed). *The Dynamic State of Muscle Fibers.* New York: Walter de Gruyter, 1990, pp. 667–679.

157. Schultz, E., and K. M. McCormick. Skeletal muscle satellite cells. *Rev. Physiol. Biochem. Pharmacol.* (in press), 1994.

158. Schwarz, G., E. Leisner, and D. Pette. Two telestimulation systems for chronic indirect muscle stimulation in caged rabbits and mice. *Pflügers Arch.* 398:130–133, 1983.

159. Scott, O. M., S. A. Hyde, G. Vrbova, and V. Dubowitz. Therapeutic possibilities of chronic low frequency electrical stimulation in children with Duchenne muscular dystrophy. *J. Neurol. Sci.* 95:171–182, 1990.

160. Scott, O. M., G. Vrbová, S. A. Hyde, and V. Dubowitz. Effects of chronic low frequency electrical stimulation on normal human tibialis anterior muscle. *J. Neurol. Neurosurg. Psych.* 48:774–781, 1985.

161. Scott, O. M., G. Vrbová, S. A. Hyde, and V. Dubowitz. Responses of muscles of patients with Duchenne muscular dystrophy to chronic electrical stimulation. *J. Neurol. Neurosurg. Psychiatry* 49:1427–1434, 1986.

162. Scott, O. M., G. Vrbová, S. A. Hyde, and V. Dubowitz. Chronic electrical stimulation: Muscle function studies in children with neuromuscular disease. F. C. Rose., R. Jones, and G. Vrbová (eds). *Neuromuscular Stimulation: Basic Concepts and Clinical Implication.* New York: Demos Publications, 1989, pp. 307–313.

163. Sedgwick, E. M. Therapeutic uses of neuromuscular stimulation. F. C. Rose, R. Jones, and

G. Vrbová (eds). *Neuromuscular Stimulation Basic Concepts and Clinical Implications.* New York: Demos Publishers, 1989, pp. 233–243.

164. Seedorf, K., U. Seedorf, and D. Pette. Coordinate expression of alkali and DTNB myosin light chains during transformation of rabbit fast muscle by chronic stimulation. *FEBS Lett.* 158:321–324, 1983.

165. Seedorf, U., E. Leberer, B. J. Kirschbaum, and D. Pette. Neural control of gene expression in skeletal muscle. *Biochem. J.* 239:115–120, 1986.

166. Simoneau. J. A. Species-specific ranges of metabolic adaptations in skeletal muscle. D. Pette (ed). *The Dynamic State of Muscle Fibers.* Berlin, New York: Walter de Gruyter, 1990, pp. 587–599.

167. Simoneau, J. A., M. Kaufman, K. T. Hartner, and D. Pette. Relations between chronic stimulation-induced properties and the Ca^{2+}-sequestering system of rat and rabbit fast-twitch muscles. *Pflügers Arch.* 414:629–633, 1989.

168. Simoneau, J. A., M. Kaufman, and D. Pette. Asynchronous increases in oxidative capacity and resistance to fatigue of electrostimulated muscles of rat and rabbit, *J. Physiol. (Lond.)* 460:573–580, 1993.

169. Sréter, F. A., M. Elzinga, K. Mabuchi, S. Salmons, and A. R. Luff. The Nτ-methylhistidine content of myosin in stimulated and cross-reinnervated skeletal muscles of the rabbit. *FEBS Lett.* 57:107–111, 1975.

170. Sréter, F. A., J. Gergely, S. Salmons, and F. Romanul. Synthesis by fast muscle of myosin light chains characteristic of slow muscle in response to long term stimulation. *Nature New Biol.* 241:17–19, 1973.

171. Sréter, F. A., J. R. Lopez, L. Alamo, K. Mabuchi, and J. Gergely. Changes in intracellular ionized Ca concentration associated with muscle fiber type transformation. *Am. J. Physiol.* 253:C296–C300, 1987.

172. Sréter, F. A., K. Pintér, F. Jolesz, and K. Mabuchi. Fast to slow transformation of fast muscles in response to long-term stimulation. *Exp. Neurol.* 75:95–102, 1982.

173. Sweeney, H. L., M. J. Kushmerick, K. Mabuchi, J. Gergely, and F. A. Sréter. Velocity of shortening and myosin isozymes in two types of rabbit fast-twitch muscle fibers. *Am. J. Physiol.* 251:C431–C434, 1986.

174. Swynghedauw, B. Developmental and functional adaption of contractile proteins in cardiac and skeletal muscles. *Physiol. Rev.* 66:710–771, 1986.

175. Takahashi, M., and D. A. Hood. Chronic stimulation-induced changes in mitochondria and performance in rat skeletal muscle. *J. Appl. Physiol.* 74:934–941, 1993.

176. Takeshima, H., S. Nishimura, T. Matsumoto, H. Ishida, K. Kangawa, et al. Primary structure and expression from complementary DNA of skeletal muscle ryanodine receptor. *Nature* 339:439–445, 1989.

177. Tanabe, T., H. Takeshima, A. Mikami, V. Flockerzi, H. Takahashi, et al. Primary structure of the receptor for calcium channel blockers from skeletal muscle. *Nature* 328:313–318, 1987.

178. Taylor, P. N., B. A. Fox, D. J. Ewins, S. J. Biss, and I. D. Swain. Exercise regime for paraplegics prior to standing using functional electrical stimulation. F. C. Rose, R. Jones, and G. Vrbová (eds). *Neuromuscular Stimulation Basic Concepts and Clinical Implications.* New York: Demos Publishers, 1989, pp. 245–251.

179. Termin, A., R. S. Staron, and D. Pette. Changes in myosin heavy chain isoforms during chronic low-frequency stimulation of rat fast hindlimb muscles. *Eur. J. Biochem.* 186:749–754, 1989.

180. Termin, A., R. S. Staron, and D. Pette. Myosin heavy chain isoforms in single fibers of transforming rat muscle. D. Pette (ed). *The Dynamic State of Muscle Fibers.* Berlin, New York: Walter de Gruyter, 1990, pp. 463–472.

181. Trimble, M. H., and R. M. Enoka. Mechanisms underlying the training effects associated with neuromuscular electrical stimulation. *Phys. Ther.* 71:273–280, 1991.

182. Weber, F. E., and D. Pette. Contractile activity enhances the synthesis of hexokinase II in rat skeletal muscle. *FEBS Lett.* 238:71–73. 1988.

183. Williams, R. S. Mitochondrial gene expression in mammalian striated muscle: evidence that variation in gene dosage is the major regulatory event. *J. Biol. Chem.* 261:12390–12394, 1986.

184. Williams, R. S., M. Garcia-Moll, J. Mellor, S. Salmons, and W. Harlan. Adaptation of skeletal muscle to increased contractile activity. *J. Biol. Chem.* 262:2764–2767, 1987.

185. Williams, R. S., S. Salmons, E. A. Newsholme, R. E. Kaufman, and J. Mellor. Regulation of nuclear and mitochondrial gene expression by contractile activity in skeletal muscle. *J. Biol. Chem.* 261:376–380, 1986.

186. Winchester, P. K., and W. J. Gonyea. Regional injury and the terminal differentiation of satellite cells in stretched avian slow tonic muscle. *Dev. Biol.* 151:459–472, 1992.

187. Wolff, J. A., G. Acsadi, A. Jani, P. Williams, and W. Chong. Long-term stable expression of foreign genes directly transferred into mouse muscle. *J. Cell. Biochem.* 15C:90, 1991.

188. Wolff, J. A., R. W. Malone, P. Williams, W. Chong, G. Acsadi, et al. Direct gene transfer into mouse muscle in vivo. *Science* 247:1465–1468, 1990.

189. Wolff, J. A., P. Williams, G. Ascadi, S. Jiao, A. Jani, and W. Chong. Conditions affecting direct gene transfer into rodent muscle in vivo. *Biotechniques* 11:474–485, 1991.

190. Worthington, J. A., and L. H. De Souza. A pilot study investigating use of neuromuscular stimulation in multiple sclerosis patients. F. C. Rose, R. Jones, and G. Vrbová (eds). *Neuromuscular Stimulation: Basic Concepts and Clinical Implications.* New York: Demos Publications, 1989, pp. 295–302.

191. Wright, W. E., D. A. Sassoon, and V. K. Lin. Myogenin, a factor regulating myogenesis, has a domain homologous to MyoD. *Cell* 56:607–617, 1989.

192. Zorzato, F., J. Fujii, K. Otso, M. Phillips, N. M. Green, et al. Molecular cloning of cDNA encoding human and rabbit forms of the Ca^{2+} release channel (ryanodine receptor) of the skeletal muscle sarcoplasmic reticulum. *J. Biol. Chem.* 265:2244–2256, 1990.

12
Transgenic Animal Models

RICHARD W. TSIKA, Ph.D.

Morphological, biochemical, and physiological experimental approaches used during past decades have established a critical quantitative and qualitative body of information detailing adaptations that occur in response to both chronic and acute exercise regimens. This has led to new questions concerning the cellular and molecular mechanisms underlying specific exercise adaptations. Today we are faced with the task of defining the genetic basis of the interrelationship that exists between a given exercise perturbation and the observed adaptation. The integrative nature of exercise presents a considerable challenge to understanding the adaptive processes at the subcellular, cellular, and organismic levels. The coordinate synthesis of these data will then form the basis for a better understanding of complex physiological adaptations.

As a result of the development of cellular and molecular techniques, it is now feasible to begin to elucidate the molecular mechanisms that underlie these complex physiological processes. One of the most powerful techniques for genetic analysis that has been developed in the last 10 years is the generation of transgenic animals. Transgenic animals harbor a foreign gene, an exogenous piece of DNA called a transgene, which is integrated into the genome and is generally transmitted via germ line cells to subsequent generations. This permits investigation of the response of a specific gene in the intact animal to a full array of physiologically relevant regulatory signals throughout the entire life span and during various physiological states.

This review first describes the methods of generating transgenic mice, along with some practical aspects that must be considered before initiating the production of large transgenic colonies. *Pronuclear microinjection* for the generation of transgenic animals is emphasized, since this is currently the most widely used method. Second, other methods are described that are being used to study mechanisms of gene transcription and expression in vivo. These techniques include (*a*) gene targeting/homologous recombination, (*b*) retroviral-mediated gene transfer, (*c*) adenoviral gene transfer, (*d*) direct DNA injection into tissue, and (*e*) biolistic transfection. Finally, the application of transgenic models to exercise studies is discussed briefly. The topic of molecular approaches in exercise studies has recently been reviewed in depth [6, 7].

WHY USE TRANSGENIC MODELS?

The identification of DNA regulatory sequences and the corresponding *trans*-acting factors is fundamental to the understanding of gene expression. Historically, this aspect of transcriptional control has been studied using permanent cell lines or primary cell cultures where the impact of serial deletions or mutations of the promoter sequences of a gene are evaluated using transient expression assays [10, 22, 53, 55, 56, 60]. These studies have provided us with a basic understanding of the mechanisms that underlie cell-specific, developmental stage–specific, and inducible expression. Although gene regulatory mechanisms delineated in primary cell cultures appear to more closely represent regulation in the intact animal, both permanent cell lines and primary cell cultures lack many control mechanisms present in the intact tissue [50]. Given the complexity of the interactions that occur between cells and organs in vivo, the extent to which the findings in cell culture can be extrapolated to the intact animal is unknown. Importantly, studies of gene regulation in cultured cells are hampered with problems such as (*a*) representative cell lines (permanent) do not exist for all tissue types, (*b*) transfection efficiencies vary depending on transfection procedure and cell line used [3, 27, 37, 41], (*c*) the gene expression pattern of cells in culture does not always reflect that of intact tissue [5, 50], and (*d*) certain perturbations cannot be adequately simulated in culture, in particular, those of exercise. Furthermore, even when appropriate cell culture models exist for the study of transcriptional regulation, the regulatory mechanisms observed in vitro provide only a limited insight into gene regulation and may not adequately represent in vivo regulation [50].

The use of transgenic mice provides a means to study the plasticity of gene regulation in response to a normal repertoire of regulatory signals in the intact adult animal. This model system is likely to reveal a broader range of regulatory mechanisms not evident in cell cultures, allowing the identification of additional *cis*-acting regulatory elements and *trans*-acting factors. Several recent reports point out the discrepancies between comparing gene regulation studies done in vitro (cell culture) to those in vivo (intact animal). Deletion of the sequences between nucleotides -3300 and -1256 of the mouse muscle creatine kinase (MCK) gene showed no significant quantitative difference when tested by transient expression assays in cultures of differentiated skeletal muscle cells. In contrast, a 10-fold reduction in activity was observed in transgenic mice when these sequences were deleted from the MCK gene, suggesting a positive *cis*-acting regulatory element(s) in the deleted sequences [46]. Similar differences were uncovered when transgenics were used to study enhancer-promoter interactions of the elastase I [84] and prolactin genes [20]. In addition, recent in vitro promoter analysis of the MCK [2], cardiac troponin T [43], phosphoglycerate mutase [65], myosin light chain 2 [66], and α-MHC [95] genes revealed that for full promoter activity in cardiac muscle, these genes required an intact MEF-2 site. In contrast, transgenic analysis of the α-MHC gene promoter determined that the presence of a mutated MEF-2 element resulted in elevated levels of expression over wild type levels [2]. Similarly, in vitro analysis of MyoD and Myf-5 function suggests that these two genes would be indispensable for muscle development [24, 70, 90, 94]. However, two recent studies employing gene targeting to "knockout" or "inactivate" these two genes revealed that such is not the case [9, 79]. Other examples of this kind have recently been reported [21, 81]. Furthermore, Mirkovitch and Darnell [59] have found that some, but not all, of the *cis*-acting sequences of the mouse transthyretin gene, which produces a thyroxine binding protein, identified in transient expression assays were bound by proteins, using an in vivo footprinting technique. They concluded that not all binding sites demonstrable in vitro or functional elements in cultured cells are involved in ongoing transcription and that in vivo studies may reveal additional and probably more relevant sites. The incongruities between in vivo and in vitro studies probably represent the differences in the sensitivity of the two methods used to study gene regulation as well as subtle nuances in the regulatory mechanism represented in the intact animal but not in cultured cells.

WHY USE MICE?

In recent years transgenic models that use mammalian species such as rats, sheep, rabbits, goats, and pigs have been reported [35]. For example, many correlations exist between the pig and the human cardiovascular systems, and therefore the generation of pig transgenic lines would seem appropriate for the study of human cardiovascular disease. However, an investigator needs to consider that an estimated cost to generate a single transgenic pig line can be as high as $25,000 U.S. Clearly, the technology for the efficient production of these species has not yet been optimized. From a practical point of view, some of these species would also require a tremendous amount of specialized space, time, and money to use for experimentation. One transgenic pig experiment requires at least three or four participants to handle and anesthetize the animal, compared with only one person, usually the experimenter alone, to work with a mouse. This single factor can triple technical labor costs when using any large animal for experimentation.

The rat is another appealing experimental animal model extensively used for physiological and exercise physiological studies [31]. Although transgenic rats have been used successfully, [34, 35], they have not been widely used because of the following technical problems: (*a*) housing costs are higher, since more space and food are required because of their larger size; (*b*) the pronuclei are not well defined, perhaps because of the granular appearance of the rat egg cytoplasm; (c) the rat pronuclei are smaller than mouse pronuclei, therefore microinjection is difficult; and (d) hormones appear to be ineffective in producing superovulation. Consequently, more rats are required to provide enough eggs for microinjection than are necessary when using mice.

Conversely, the mouse has been extensively used, and as a result, the procedures for their production as well as for gene targeting are well documented [12, 13, 15, 28, 29, 36, 38, 40, 44, 71, 72, 82, 86, 96]. In addition, the mouse genetics and embryology have been more thoroughly studied. At this time, these factors make this model the more efficient and economical choice for most basic physiological transgenic studies. Each investigator, however, must consider the direct research application when choosing an animal model.

PRODUCTION OF TRANSGENIC MICE

Pronuclear Microinjection

Pronuclear microinjection was first successfully employed by Gordon et al [32] in 1980. Since then, its application in all disciplines of the biological sciences has grown steadily, and it is the most widely and successfully used method. With this approach, transgenic mice are generated by direct injection of recombinant DNA into the pronuclei of fertilized mouse eggs. The injected eggs are then transferred to a foster mother, where the embryo develops to birth. Offspring are checked for transgene incorporation 3 weeks after birth. Animals that are positive for transgene incorporation are bred to generate transgenic lines or in some cases analyzed for expression.

A typical transgenic experiment using pronuclear microinjection to generate transgenic mice would proceed as follows. Approximately 10–15 female donor mice are induced hormonally to superovulate by injection of pregnant mare's serum gonadotropin (PMS) and human chorionic gonadotropin (hCG) (see Fig. 12.1). This procedure increases the number of eggs from 10 to approximately 30 per superovulated mouse, which can be recovered for microinjection. After hormone treatment, females are mated with males. The following morning, the oviducts of the donor mice are removed, and the fertilized one-cell embryos are flushed from the oviduct, placed in culture, and treated with hyaluronidase to remove cumulus cells. At this time two pronuclei are visible, the larger one being the male pronucleus, which is generally the one to be injected (see Fig. 12.2A). Microinjection usually results in the delivery of 100–400 copies of purified recombinant DNA molecules into the male pronuclei of the zygotes. However, on occasion many more recombinant DNA molecules are delivered. The pronucleus will swell when injected with the DNA solution, indicating a successful penetration and injection (see Fig. 12.2C).

FIGURE 12.1

Typical breeding scheme to produce transgenic founder mice. The process from isolating eggs to transferring eggs does not necessarily need to be done in 1 day. If pseudopregnancy does not occur by evidence of a copulation plug, the eggs can be incubated overnight for transfer the next AM. For breeding these founder mice to homozygousity see Table 12.1. (Illustrated by GuoLiang Wu.)

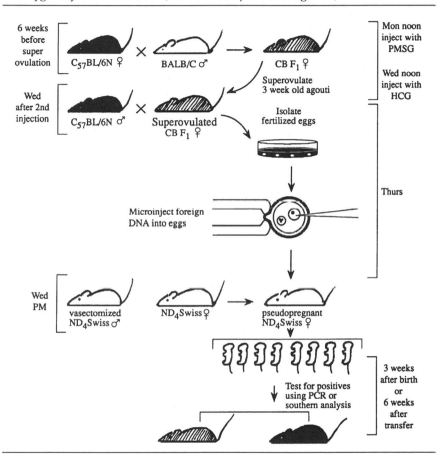

Microinjection of DNA into the pronucleus of fertilized mouse eggs can lead to the stable integration of as few as one to as many as a thousand copies of the injected DNA into the host genome [78]. In most cases, transgenes integrate randomly into the mouse genome and are arranged as tandem arrays in a head-to-tail orientation [11]. Following injection, surviving zygotes can be transferred to the oviduct of a pseudopregnant foster mother, where they will be nurtured to term. Pseudopregnant foster mothers are produced by mating vasectomized males with adult females.

Transferring the eggs on the day of injection returns the eggs to their

FIGURE 12.2

Microinjection of fertilized eggs. (Modified from ref 40; illustrated by GuoLiang Wu.)

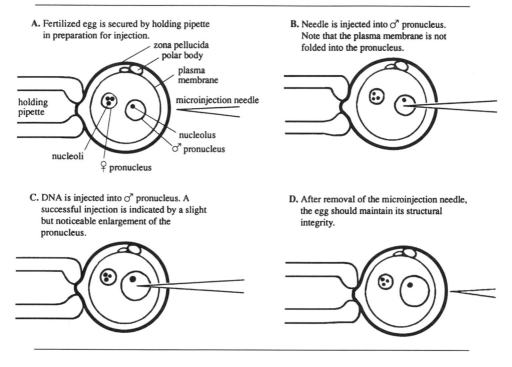

A. Fertilized egg is secured by holding pipette in preparation for injection.

zona pellucida
polar body
plasma membrane
holding pipette
microinjection needle
nucleolus
♂ pronucleus
nucleoli
♀ pronucleus

B. Needle is injected into ♂ pronucleus. Note that the plasma membrane is not folded into the pronucleus.

C. DNA is injected into ♂ pronucleus. A successful injection is indicated by a slight but noticeable enlargement of the pronucleus.

D. After removal of the microinjection needle, the egg should maintain its structural integrity.

natural environment without a prolonged delay. Alternatively, these eggs can be cultured overnight and transferred to a pseudopregnant foster mother the following morning. The advantage in this case is that the investigator can visualize the number of embryos that have progressed to the two-cell stage (see Fig. 12.3). The transferred eggs that have survived the microinjection and transfer procedures will then develop to term 3 weeks later. Two to 3 weeks after birth, the offspring are tested for transgene incorporation (see Fig. 12.1). This can be accomplished using dot blot or Southern blot hybridization or by the polymerase chain reaction (discussed in the section on identification of transgenics). Mice containing an integrated transgene are called founder mice, and they are heterozygous for the transgene. Individual transgenic lines are developed by backcross mating each positive founder mouse to its nontransgenic parental strain. The integrated transgene will be passed on to subsequent generations in a Mendelian fashion. If the transgene integrated into the genome of the fertilized egg before the first round of DNA replication, then 50% of the progeny from the backcross should test positive for the transgene. If germ line integration does not occur, the founder mouse will be mosaic for the transgene. This means that germ line cells most likely will

FIGURE 12.3

Stages of embryos at approximate times after fertilization. (Illustrated by GuoLiang Wu.)

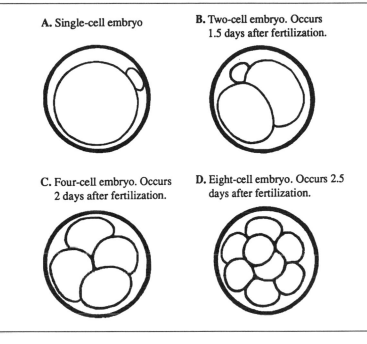

A. Single-cell embryo

B. Two-cell embryo. Occurs 1.5 days after fertilization.

C. Four-cell embryo. Occurs 2 days after fertilization.

D. Eight-cell embryo. Occurs 2.5 days after fertilization.

not contain the transgene, and therefore the transgene will not be transmitted to subsequent generations. On occasion, germ line cells can themselves be mosaic for the integrated transgene, and thus with subsequent breeding it is possible to develop the transgenic line. Backcross siblings that are transgene-positive will then undergo intercross mating for the development of homozygous lines. From this heterozygous intercross you can expect the progeny to be 25% nontransgenic, 50% heterozygous, and 25% homozygous. To test for homozygosity, a testcross to a non-transgenic parental strain is done. Mice that are homozygous will produce heterozygous progeny that all test positive for the transgene, i.e., 100% transmission [40] (see Table 12.1). The considerable time initially spent developing homozygous lines is a good investment, since all subsequent offspring will carry the transgene, thereby eliminating future screening procedures.

Factors Affecting Success

The success of this method depends in part on the dexterity of the experimenter as well as the purity, concentration, and form of the foreign DNA to be injected. The purity of DNA is a crucial factor for which specific methods have been developed and are described in detail by Constantini

TABLE 12.1
Homozygosity Breeding Scheme and Resulting Samples

Once a transgene positive mouse has been obtained, it is usually desirable to create a homozygous line. This scheme begins with only one heterozygous founder. Presumably, many more than one founder will be bred through to homozygosity. Note the significant number of samples that must be screened using Southern analysis or polymerase chain reactions (PCR) during this labor-intensive process.

Step 1.   Mate heterozygous founder back to the parental strain (backcross), which will produce an average litter size of 8.

Gestation	Weaning	No. of Samples
3 weeks	3 weeks	8 (average litter size)

Theoretically, this mating should produce a litter that is 50% positive.

Step 2.   For this example, it will be assumed that step 1 resulted in 2 male and 2 female positive mice. These mice should be mated 5 weeks after screening or 2 months after birth.

Each pair of positives should produce a litter that contains:

Nonpositive	Positive	Positive
Nontransgenic	Heterozygous	Homozygous
25%	50%	25%

Therefore, from a heterozygous intercross, 75% should screen positive.

Gestation	Weaning	No. of Samples
3 weeks	3 weeks	16 × 75% = 12 positives

Step 3.   To identify the homozygous lines of the 75% that screen positive in step 2, all positively screened progeny must be bred (backcross) to the parental strain. Those that produce litters that are 100% positive are homozygous. This final step will require Southern or PCR screening of 8 × 12 or approximately 96 mice. At times, breeding to homozygosity will be lethal.

and Lacy [19]. The DNA concentration must be strictly monitored, since high concentrations can be toxic to the fertilized egg. In general, the DNA concentration ranges from 1 to 5 μg/ml dissolved in TE buffer (10 mM Tris-HCl, pH 7.4, 0.1 mM EDTA) [12, 13]. Linear fragments with cohesive ends appear to integrate with a greater efficiency than other DNA forms [12, 13, 71, 72]. It is also important to eliminate prokaryotic sequences, as these can inhibit the expression of some transgenes [12, 13, 87]. Success will also depend on other less defined factors that for example, result in more efficient incorporation of some constructs.

Not all of the eggs from the superovulating female will have been fertilized, and not all the injected eggs will survive. In general, the number of eggs surviving injection will range from 50 to 90%. Of these, 10–25% give rise to offspring, and 10–30% of these pups are transgenic. Efficiencies can range from 1% to perhaps as high as 40% [19]. These normally small percentages of transgenic pups represent a precious commodity and should be carefully monitored. Not all mothers will take care of their offspring, and when this is observed, the pups should be placed with a foster mother. This is best accomplished by transferring pups dotted with the new mother's urine to disguise the scent of the old mother, thereby encouraging adoption.

Identification of Transgenics
The identification of transgene-positive animals begins with the isolation and purification of high molecular weight genomic DNA from a 1–2 cm piece of tail that is obtained from each pup at the age of 3 weeks. Once isolated, tail DNA can be analyzed for transgene incorporation by Southern [83] or slot blotting [48] or by polymerase chain reaction (PCR) [4, 25, 62]. Southern or slot blotting involves hybridization to a sequence-specific DNA probe. PCR and slot blot analyses allow large numbers of animals to be screened efficiently in a short period of time (PCR, 1 day; DNA slot blot, ≈ 2 days). In contrast, a minimum of 5 days is required if Southern blotting is used. It should be noted that DNA slot blot analysis should only be used when the transgene does not contain sequence homology to an endogenous gene, since in this situation, every sample would test positive. It is appropriate to use slot blotting when the transgene contains reporter sequences such as the chloramphenicol acetyltransferase (CAT) gene. Since the CAT gene is not present in mammals, only those samples which hybridize specifically to a DNA probe containing complementary sequences to the CAT gene will appear as transgene positive. If homologous sequences are contained within the transgene, then Southern blotting should be used, which can distinguish the transgene by size. Time spent screening for transgenic animals becomes an important planning consideration when developing a transgenic colony. For each individual transgene to be studied, a minimum of three independent lines should be generated (see section on transgene expression).

When mice test positive for transgene integration by PCR or slot blotting, further confirmation should be ascertained by Southern blot analysis. Increased sensitivity is gained by using Southern analysis because impurities not eliminated during the isolation of genomic DNA are fractionated during gel electrophoresis. As a result, the fractionated genomic DNA is cleaner and the potential problems associated with slot blotting such as high background, false positives, variable hybridization, and missing low copy number transgene-positive samples due to impurities and unfractionated DNA are substantially reduced. Because transgenes integrate into a chromosomal site as tandemly repeated DNA, digestion of genomic DNA with a restriction endonuclease that cuts the transgene only once gives rise to multiple copies of a restriction fragment whose length is the same as that of the transgene. The band corresponding to the transgene can now be easily identified by running purified transgene on each Southern blot. Because the transgene is randomly integrated into a chromosomal site (as tandemly repeated DNA), additional bands corresponding to the ends of the inserted sequence will appear. These bands will vary in size, depending on the sequence of the mouse genomic DNA flanking the junction sites where the transgene has integrated into the genome of the mouse (see Fig. 12.4). Conversely, the integration of a single copy of the transgene is characterized by the conspicuous absence of a band corresponding in size to the transgene and the appearance of two additional bands of different size (described above). Transgene copy number is determined by rehybridizing the Southern blot with a single-copy endogenous gene such as the mouse *c-myc* gene. The density of the *c-myc* band on an autoradiograph is quantified using a scanning densitometer (or Phosphor Imager), and this value is set equal to one. Densities of the test sample bands (transgene) are also quantified by densitometry, and those values are then divided by the value obtained for *c-myc* to determine transgene copy number. Alternatively, copy number determination can be accomplished by comparing the level of Southern blot hybridization (density) of the test samples to the

FIGURE 12.4

Southern blot analysis of β-MHC/CAT constructs in transgenic mice. Mouse DNA was digested with EcoRI, fractionated on a 0.8% agarose gel, transferred onto a nylon membrane and hybridized with a CAT probe. The banding pattern of two transgenic lines (line 6 and 41) are shown. Note that in lanes marked 6-21 and 6-27 there are 3 bands, indicating that multiple copies of the β-MHC/CAT transgene have integrated into a chromosomal site as a tandem head-to-tail array. The major band in the middle corresponds to the transgene and is easily identified because it migrated adjacent to the β-MCH/CAT transgene standard (lane PC). The bands that appear above and below the transgene band correspond to junctional fragments. In line 41 only a single transgene copy has integrated and therefore only two bands are visible and correspond to the junctional fragments.

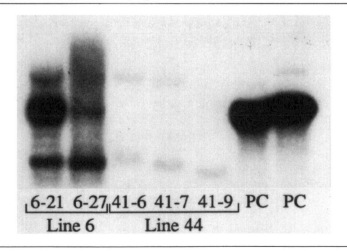

FIGURE 12.5

Southern blot analysis to determine β-MCH/CAT transgene copy number. β-MHC/ CAT transgene standards of known copy number were run adjacent to a sample of unknown copy number (line 44, animals 8 and 9). PC = β-MCH/CAT transgene. The appearance of three bands indicates that multiple copies of the transgene must have integrated into a chromosomal site. Densitometric analysis indicates that line 44, animal 9, contains approximately 100 copies of the β-MCH/CAT transgene.

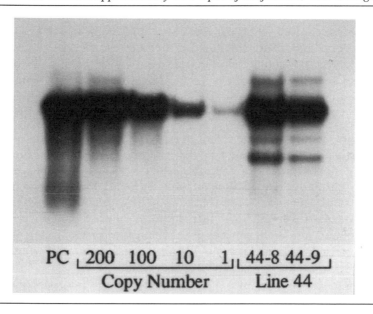

density value of transgene standards of known copy number (Fig. 12.5). Standards are prepared by diluting purified transgene stock solutions of a known concentration.

Transgene Expression

Once transgene-positive founder mice have been identified, they are generally bred and the litters checked for transgene inheritance before testing for expression. Because the transgenes integrate into a chromosomal location which is purely random, there is no way of knowing what influence the adjacent endogenous sequences will have on the transgene. The transgene may integrate into a chromosomal site that is inactive or into a site that leads to inappropriate expression in tissues or during a developmental stage when the endogenous gene is not normally expressed. The integration site can also affect levels of expression. The integration of the transgene may disrupt an endogenous gene that results in a lethal mutation or a loss of function mutant. In addition, the inappropriate aforementioned expression patterns can be due to the lack of important DNA regulatory sequences contained within the transgene rather than the fact that it did not integrate into its normal chromosomal position. To distinguish "positional effects" from missing regulatory sequences, it is important to generate multiple (three or more) independent lines of each transgene. Positional effects can be alleviated by using gene-targeting methods.

An additional factor that must be considered concerning transgene expression is that prokaryotic plasmid DNA (vector) sequences can severely interfere with transgene expression [12, 87]. When possible, transgenes should be prepared by choosing restriction endonucleases that will excise the transgene and eliminate most, if not all, of the vector sequence. Preparation of transgenes in this matter results in a linear piece of DNA, which has been shown to integrate 5-fold more efficiently than closed, circular, supercoiled DNA.

Functional Analysis of Transgenes
For studies aimed at identifying transcriptional regulatory elements contained within the promoter and upstream region of a specific gene, reporter gene assays are generally used. Reporter genes are constructed by fusing the promoter sequences of a specific gene to the coding region of a reporter gene such as CAT [33, 67], which is not endogenous to mammalian tissues. This allows differentiation between the expression of transgene and the endogenous gene. Other reporter genes that are commonly used are ß-galactosidase [16] and luciferase [8, 68] genes. The degree of transcriptional activation is determined by using a sensitive enzyme assay. Other methods of determining transgene expression include northern blotting, in situ hybridization, immunohistochemical, and histochemical; when minigenes are used as a transgene, S1 nuclease protection is used.

The following is a list of advantages and disadvantages of this method for analysis of regulatory elements in genes.

Advantages
1. The transgene is present in every cell type, including germ line cells, thus successive generations can be produced and maintained for study.
2. The transgene can be studied in a broad range of cell types. This allows one to study gene expression in tissues that are difficult to culture or transfect.
3. A transgene can be studied at every stage of development.
4. The transgene integrates into a chromosomal site. Although integration occurs at a random site, the transgene will be in an environment that more closely represents that of the endogenous gene.
5. There are no limits to the size of the DNA to be injected into the mouse egg. In fact, a recent report by Schedl et al. [80] demonstrated that large yeast artificial chromosomes (YAC) could be microinjected into the pronuclei of a fertilized mouse egg. This YAC spanned 250,000 base

pairs, which is 33–35 times greater than inserts carried by either retroviral or adenoviral vectors.

6. There are no extraneous sequences (plasmid or viral promoter/enhancer) to interfere with the expression of the integrated transgene.
7. There are no additional isolation or cloning steps necessary to produce the transgene to be injected.

Disadvantages

1. The success of this method requires considerable training time to acquire good technical skills, which are critical in the isolation and microinjection of fertilized eggs.
2. As with retroviral vectors, insertional mutagenesis or chromosomal position effects (variable expression levels between transgenic lines for the same transgene) can occur due to the random nature of integration into the host genome. Also, integration can be lethal.
3. In addition, unlike most of the other gene transfer methods, this procedure requires the use of expensive equipment ($40,000–$60,000).
4. Cost (see next section).

COST OF PRODUCING TRANSGENIC MICE

The costs incurred in generating transgenic mice are considerable. The following is an outline that *estimates* the initial investment required as well as the recurring expenses generally associated with the production, analysis, and maintenance of transgenic colonies.

Before committing to the substantial initial investment, the experimenter should thoroughly investigate the possibility of procuring transgenic mice made by a transgenic facility. A number of sources that can be contracted to make mice include local on-campus facilities and private companies. Prices for this specialized service will range from $3,000 to $10,000 per transgenic mouse, with an equal variation of associated guarantees. In most cases, when you contract a transgenic facility to generate transgenic mice, the guarantee that they will produce tail blot–positive mice does not guarantee that these founder mice will have germ-line-integrated transgenes or will express your transgene.

Equipment Investment

Microinjection of pronuclei requires specialized equipment for the proper visualization and manipulation of embryos.

The 1990 quotation on Table 12.2 is for a Narishige (Nikon) Diaphot inverted microscope, equipped for Nomarski D. I. C. transmitted light brightfield optics. It should be noted that all of the following estimates of costs will vary from institution to institution, depending on applicable discounts.

TABLE 12.2
Representative List of Necessary Transgenic Equipment

No. Needed	Description	Estimated Cost
1	Nikon Diaphot inverted microscope	$ 6,922
1	Halogen Illuminator 50W for Diaphot	142
2	12V/50W tungsten halogen bulbs	42
1	Power cord	8
2	CFDW 10× widefield, high eyepoint eyepiece	626
1	Rectangular mech stage w/coaxial XY motion	1,463
1	CF DIC 10× Plan Achromat, N.a. .25 (7.1 mm)	528
1	CF DIC 20× Achr w/correction collar (.45 mm)	632
1	CF DIC 40× Achr w/correction collar (.18 mm)	1,232
1	Nomarski DIC II attachment	7,814
1	Narishige IM5A and IM5B microinjectors	1,344
1	Narishige No202 micromanipulator	5,245
1	Narishige No204 micromanipulator	6,925
2	NM-2 manipulator (3D) condenser mount	3,990
1	NS-B mounting adapters	260
1	Vibration platform: The microscope micromanipulators and microinjectors rest on this vibration table, which provides an antivibration base. This table significantly reduces external vibrations, which is essential for the reduction of vibrations through the microscope itself, thereby reducing hazards during micromanipulating and microinjecting embryos.	3,785
1	Micropipet puller: This is for single injection needles or holding needles. The puller provides calibrated heating and pulling tension necessary for proper construction of these needles.	2,415
1	Pipet grinder: This is used to grind and smooth pipette tips at an angle for easier injection.	1,678
1	Microforge: This is used for making fine glass tubes necessary to make round edge pipettes for holding pipettes.	5,495
1	Biological safety cabinet	4,630
1	CO_2 incubator (forma scientific)	2,990
500	Microisolator cages with bottle, rubber stopper, water tube, and card holder	18,000
	Total estimated initial investment	$76,166

Breeding Colonies and Recurring Housing Costs

The generation and maintenance of a transgenic colony requires a large number of mice and time. Proper maintenance of an animal colony is absolutely critical, to assure that animals are healthy and suitable for long-term transgenic analysis. Therefore, before beginning transgenic work, the investigator should have secured space in a animal facility that can provide temperature-controlled rooms, equipment for washing, and sterilizing cages and water bottles, and access to proper veterinary care. In addition, these animals need to be monitored daily to supply food and water, and at least once a week, the bedding must be changed. This daily monitoring will also allow checking for the birth of new litters. This should be a part of your daily routine, even if the animal facility personnel generally provide these services. Since changing the bedding in the cages requires that the animals be temporarily relocated, your own staff or a well-trained and motivated general animal care worker should do this, to prevent inadvertent mixing of animals.

A transgenic colony is composed of different categories of mice, each serving a specific function. The categories of mice and their function are listed below. The strains of mice used in this example are those that have given good results. However, it should be noted that the specific strains of mice used vary from laboratory to laboratory. In general, outbred stains are used when there is no specific genetic background required. For more information on specific strains, a good reference is *Manipulating the Mouse Embryo: A Laboratory Manual* [40].

F1 BREEDING COLONY. Microinjection requires the generation of F2 hybrid fertilized one-cell eggs. For this purpose, a breeding colony is maintained for the production of F1 hybrid females. To produce F1 hybrid females, approximately 30 breeding cages are set up, each containing 1 male (Balb/c) and 1 or 2 females (C57B1/6J). At 3 weeks postbirth, the progeny (C57B1/6J X Balb/c) are weaned and separated by sex. Most of the males are sacrificed at this time. It will require an additional 6–8 weeks before the F1 hybrid female progeny can be used to produce F2 fertilized eggs. A good breeding pair can produce a litter every 3 weeks if the male is left in the cage after birth. An accurate accounting of litter size and date of birth should be maintained on a cage card. This provides a mechanism to monitor the efficiency of the breeding pairs and to identify those F1 hybrid progeny that have reached sexual maturity and can be used for the production of F2 eggs.

BREEDING COLONY FOR F2 EGG PRODUCTION. This colony consists of F1 hybrid female and stud male mice. The mating between the F1 hybrid male (C57B1/6J X Balb/c) and superovulated F1 hybrid female (C57B1/6J X Balb/c) produces the F2 fertilized eggs for microinjection. Approximately 40 cages will be required for this purpose. Of these, 20 cages will be used to house F1 stud males (1/cage) and 20 cages to house F1 females (5/cage) for superovulation. The male's performance is monitored by checking for a copulation plug the morning after the female has been placed in the male's cage. This record should be kept on cage cards, and if the male fails to mate more than 70% of the time, he should be replaced.

STERILE STUD MALES. These males (ND4/Swiss) are used to produce pseudopregnant foster mothers. Generally, males are made sterile by vasectomy at the age of 8–10 weeks. These males are housed individually (30 cages). Thirty vasectomized males are sufficient to produce 3–6 psuedopregnant females twice a week. The breeding record of these males should be recorded on cage cards. Males that fail to mate, as indicated by the absence of a copulation plug, when presented with different females more than twice should be replaced. The effectiveness of the vasectomy procedure should be checked prior to mating with foster mothers. This is done by placing each vasectomized male with 3 test females. If no litters are born after 6–8 weeks, the vasectomy can be considered successful.

FOSTER MOTHERS. F1 female mice that have been superovulated and mated are sacrificed the next morning, and the fertilized F2 eggs are collected. Once the F2 eggs have been collected and microinjected with foreign DNA, they are transferred to the uterus of a recipient pseudopregnant female (ND4/Swiss), where they will be nurtured until birth. Different coat colors should be used between the egg donor F1 hybrid female and the pseudopregnant ND4/Swiss foster mother. This provides visual assurance that the progeny are derived from the donor eggs. If the progeny are a different color than the egg donor, you know that the male (ND4/Swiss) was not properly vasectomized. Thirty cages are used to house the vasectomized stud males (1/cage), and 20 cages are used to house foster mothers (5/cage). A large number of foster mothers are necessary, because the females will be in estrus on different days. Two females should be put in with each male, to assure that at least 3–6 of the females will have been mated, as judged by the appearance of a copulation plug.

FOUNDER LINES. A total of 70 cages are ncessary for founder lines. Approximately 10 cages must be used to establish each line for each founder. Most investigators will find it necessary to establish a number of lines; however, once a line is established, 3–4 cages are sufficient to maintain these lines. It cannot be stressed enough that meticulous records need to be kept on cage cards as soon as each line is established, to prevent erroneous mixing and subsequent loss of lines. Poor record keeping is particularly hazardous when large numbers of animals are required, as is generally the case for exercise studies.

Estimated Summary of Per Diem Charges and Animal Costs
Animal cost and per diem charges will represent a large recurring expense when generating and maintaining a transgenic colony (Table 12.3). For simplicity, housing costs are calculated on a cage per day basis (this example reflects a rate of $0.55/cage/day). Some institutional vivarium rates are in fact based on this, while others are based on an animal/day basis. I have found that overall, the cage/day basis is more economical where an average of 4–5 animals can be housed per cage.

Recurring Technical Costs
It will be necessary to maintain a full-time technician dedicated to the production and maintenance of transgenic lines. Regional cost-of-living differences and the overall qualifications an individual possess will determine the actual expense. The investigator should plan to hire an individual with at least an M.S. in biology or animals sciences and place him or her into a "senior" classification.

TABLE 12.3
Transgenic Animal Colony Cost

Category	Initial Acquisition Costs*	Annual Housing Costs
Foster mothers and stud males: ND4/SWISS mice (30 males + 100 females) @ $2.00 ea.:	$260	30 cages $ 6,023
F1 Breeding colony (males): Balb/C mice (30 males) @ $8.00 ea.:	$240	50 cages $10,038
F1 Breeding colony (females): C57BL/6J mice (30 females) @ $8.00 ea.:	$240	
Founder line cages: In this example 70 cages are estimated.		70 cages $14,052
Total costs	$740	$30,113

*Initial acquisition costs refer only to the number of mice needed to initialize the colonies. The number of cages that will be necessary to maintain will be higher once breeding has begun.

HOMOLOGOUS RECOMBINATION AND GENE TARGETING

Recently, a method has been developed that allows foreign DNA to be targeted to a specific site within the mouse genome, termed "gene targeting" [15, 29]. This method is currently being used to modify specific genes in an effort to more clearly define the function of their protein products. Directed gene targeting is accomplished by utilizing a naturally occurring molecular event called "homologous recombination." Homologous recombination is facilitated by the degree of sequence homology that exists between two pieces of DNA. For efficient insertion or replacement of a targeted gene, the degree of sequence homology between the transgene (vector carrying transgene) and the host chromosomal DNA is vital [38, 86].

Direct pronuclei microinjection of foreign DNA into a fertilized one-cell stage embryo can lead to integration by homologous recombination (HR) but with a disappointingly low frequency [96]. However, the use of embryonic stem (ES) cells has resulted in substantial improvements in HR frequencies. ES cells are derived from the inner cell mass of blastocysts, are pluripotent, and have the ability to give rise to germ line cells, thereby promoting the stable inheritance of the transgene [26, 76]. Importantly, ES cells are amenable to maintenance in culture in an undifferentiated state as well as manipulation and characterization prior to microinjection into blastocyst-stage embryos.

Gene targeting used to knockout (disable) a specific gene generally starts by inserting in vitro a bacterial neomycin gene expression cassette, which acts as a positive selection marker, into the sequence of the cloned target gene. Insertion of the neomycin gene sequence interrupts the cloned target gene, rendering it incapable of generating a functional protein product. A second gene, usually the herpes simplex virus thymidine kinase (HSV-tk) gene, is also included within the vector, and it serves as a negative selection marker [54]. This gene flanks the homologous sequences and is lost if homologous recombination occurs but is retained and expressed if random integration occurs. The altered gene is then transferred into mouse ES cells by electroporation, where homologous recombination takes place between the exogenously altered cloned gene and the chromosomal target gene. The inactivated cloned gene can be delivered into ES cells in either a linearized insertion vector or in a linearized replacement vector that has been designed for positive/negative selection (PNS). If a replacement vector is used, the disrupted cloned gene recombines with the chromosomal target gene locus and replaces it. When an insertion vector is used, the disrupted cloned gene is inserted into the chromosomal target gene locus. Both homologous recombination methods are quite effective in knocking out the functional chromosomal target gene.

Once the disrupted cloned gene has been transferred into ES cells, these cells must be screened to determine which cells have stable incorporation of the altered cloned gene in their genome. Those cells in which this has occurred will be resistant to the antibiotic G418 (neo^r) and the drug gangcyclovir (HSV-tk$^-$). The product of the neomycin gene will prevent G418 from inhibiting translation, and the absence of the viral enzyme, thymidine kinase, will prevent the utilization of gangcyclovir, a toxic thymidine analog. Selection-positive ES cells are amplified and then introduced into the blastocoel cavity of blastocyst-stage embryos, which are subsequently transferred to a pseudopregnant foster mother. The modified ES cells, which have been transferred into the blastocysts, will develop along with the endogenous ES cells to produce a mouse containing cells contributed from two different mice. These mice are called chimeras and are identified by the appearance of two different coat colors. The modified ES cells originated from a mouse embryo with a black coat and are transferred to a blastocyst-stage mouse embryo with a white or agouti coat. At this point, the chimeric mice are heterozygous for the mutated (knockout) gene. The chimeric mouse is mated with a normal mouse, and the offspring are screened for transmission of the knockout gene. Positive progeny indicate that the disrupted gene was transmitted through germ line cells, and they are intercrossed to develop homozygous lines.

Gene targeting is a powerful method with which well-defined genetic alterations can be systematically employed to study the function of any gene. A complete discussion of gene targeting is beyond the scope of this review. For a more detailed description see recent reviews [15, 82, 96].

Advantages
1. Problems encountered by position effects and insertional mutagenesis are eliminated.

2. Precise mutations of a gene can be accomplished with pinpoint accuracy.
3. The effects of a gene deletion or mutation can be examined with the gene in its natural chromosomal location.
4. Many trangenics can be produced with the construct in the same location for comparative analysis of mutated or variant genes.
5. ES cells can be grown for many generations in vitro.
6. ES cells can be screened in vitro before producing animal lines.

Disadvantages
1. The development of knockout mice entails a major investment of time. Even those laboratories well endowed with highly trained labor should plan approximately 9 months to produce knockout mice if every step goes well. During a 1992 interview with Tak Mak, the *Journal of NIH Research* quotes him as saying, "It does not require the brains of an Einstein to make these mice, but it does require God smiling at you every day for nine months. . . ."[42].
2. Estimates from those performing this method predict animal costs will total between $50,000 and $100,000 annually [88].

GENE TRANSFER TECHNIQUES

The number of gene transfer methods being developed with possible applications to gene therapy and gene regulation are increasing rapidly. However, most of these techniques do not result in the stable integration of the transgene into the genome of germ line cells, thereby preventing the development of stable lines of transgenic animals.

Transgenesis by Retroviral Transfer of Foreign DNA
Retroviral-based gene transfer has been used extensively to transfer genes into various cell types and into embryos at different developmental stages [44, 45, 61, 64]. The genome of a retrovirus is composed of RNA. After infection of a target cell (new host), the RNA genome of the retrovirus is converted into DNA by the activity of the enzymes reverse transcriptase, RNase H, and DNA polymerase, resulting in a linear double-stranded piece of DNA. The linear viral DNA integrates into the host cell's genome randomly as a single copy, at which point it is referred to as a provirus. The wild-type retrovirus is not used for gene transfer, but a modified version that is replication-defective is.

A recombinant retrovirus vector is an infectious virus that has been modified in such a way that the viral proteins encoded by the virus genome are not expressed. This strategy eliminates possible autonomous replication and spread from the host cell. However, the engineered retroviral vectors still retain all the *cis*-acting regulatory elements necessary for packaging and integration into the host genome. By removing the structural genes for viral replication, a space is provided into which the foreign gene can be subcloned [17, 23, 57]. The replication-deficient retroviral vector carrying the foreign gene is first introduced into packaging cells. The packaging cells have been previously programmed to express all the necessary viral proteins so that infectious virus particles can be produced which carry the foreign gene. The resulting recombinant retrovirus can infect a replicating host cell and integrate into the host genome, which is followed by expression of the subcloned foreign gene [58]. It is important to note that the packaging cells, but not the host cells, can serve as production factories for the recombinant retrovirus because they provide the necessary proteins for virus production. The advantages and disadvantages of this technique are listed below.

Advantages
1. Retroviral gene transfer does not require the use of expensive equipment.
2. The retroviral vector carrying the gene of interest integrates into the genome randomly as a single copy.
3. There is a high efficiency of infection of susceptible cells.
4. These vectors carry strong enhancer sequences that result in high-level expression in most cell types, which can be advantageous in directing expression of a protein from a cDNA.
5. Recombinant retroviruses can be introduced into tissues at different development stages.

Disadvantages
1. There is a limitation on the size of the DNA insert that can be studied ($\approx$8–10 Kb).
2. The gene of interest must be recloned into the retroviral vector and then transferred into packaging cells where infectious recombinant viruses are produced. In addition, care must be taken to develop packaging cell lines that will produce high titers of the recombinant virus. This process can take months.
3. Low titers of the retrovirus could prevent infection of sufficient cells. If a subcloned gene contains introns, splice sites, or termination signals, this can interfere with expression and lead to even lower viral titers. Whether a newly engineered retrovirus will produce sufficient titer cannot be predicted in advance.
4. Retroviruses will only integrate into replicating cells, which precludes those cells that are postmitotic such as striated (skeletal and cardiac) muscle and neurons.
5. These vectors carry strong promoter and enhancer sequences that can

interfere with the expression (induction, tissue-specific, developmental stage) of the gene under study.

6. Retroviral infection of embryos (4–8-cell stage) can result in multiple integrations, each occurring at a different chromosomal site, within one cell or in multiple cells.

7. This method results in animals that are mosaic for the transferred gene (not all cells carry this gene), and rarely is this vector integrated into germ line cells, thus, the gene is not passed on to subsequent generations. This feature necessitates extensive breeding schemes in order to establish a homozygous line.

8. Because integration of the recombinant retrovirus into the host genome occurs at random sites, the potential for insertion mutagenesis by disrupting a host gene exist. In addition, the strong viral enhancer sequences [located in viral long terminal repeat (LTR)] may alter the expression of an adjacent host gene.

ADENOVIRUSES AS GENE TRANSFER VEHICLES

In contrast to retroviruses, adenoviruses have a DNA genome. As with retroviruses, adenoviruses can be modified to render them replication deficient and to accept foreign DNA inserts. Also, specialized cell lines (packaging) are used for the production of high titers of infectious replication-deficient recombinant viral particles [5, 30, 39, 61, 77].

Advantages
1. Recombinant replication-deficient adenoviruses have a broad host range and a high efficiency of infection. They can also be produced in high titers.

2. Most importantly, adenoviruses can infect cells that are not undergoing replication. There is no requirement for replication.

3. Recombinant replication-deficient adenovirus vectors express transgenes at high levels even though they do not integrate into a chromosomal site.

4. Adenovirus particles are stable, allowing concentration and purification.

5. Same as advantages 1, 4, and 5 for recombinant replication-deficient retroviral vectors.

Disadvantages
1. Same as disadvantages 1, 2, and 5 for recombinant retroviral vectors.

2. Adenoviruses do not integrate into the host genome, precluding the generation of stable transgenic lines for long-term study.

IN SITU DELIVERY OF FOREIGN DNA

Direct DNA Injection

Direct DNA injection is quite simple and does not require specialized equipment, only a syringe. It involves the direct injection of either recombinant DNA or RNA expression plasmids or reporter genes into muscle tissue of living animals [92, 93]. The mechanism by which striated muscle takes up the recombinant plasmids is not known. Although the foreign DNA does not integrate into a chromosomal position, its expression can be detected for several months [14]. Its application to skeletal muscle gene expression was first demonstrated by Wolff et al [92, 93] and since then has been extended to include expression in the heart [1, 49, 52, 69] but no other tissue types [1]. More recently, this method was successfully employed in the screening for tissue specific regulatory elements [73, 89], hormone responsive elements [49, 69], and elements that direct inducible gene expression [37].

Advantages
1. This procedure is technically uncomplicated and does not require any specialized equipment (very low cost).
2. The recombinant plasmids are subjected to a relevant in vivo environment. It is therefore possible to quickly screen a series of promoter constructs carrying successive 5′ deletions to determine sequences necessary for constitutive and tissue specific expression in vivo, even though the plasmid DNA remains episomal.
3. This procedure represents a simple approach to somatic cell gene therapy. A recent report demonstrated that the direct intramuscular injection of some cytokine genes (interleukin-2 (IL-2)), IL-4, and transforming growth factor ß (TGF-ß1)) resulted in the immunological effects expected from these cytokine proteins [74].

Disadvantages
1. The expression of a gene can only be studied in the injected muscle.
2. The DNA enters only those cells in close proximity to the injection site.
3. Since the plasmid DNA remains episomal, it is not passed on to subsequent generations of animals, and thus problems of reproducibility may be encountered. This results in the need for large numbers of animals to demonstrate statistically significant trends. In addition, plasmid expression is not permanent, and the magnitude of expression diminishes with time. Furthermore, chromatin structural influences cannot be studied with episomal DNA.
4. This method can produce cell injury and inflammation [93].
5. Because both control and test plasmids are injected, large amounts of plasmid DNA (100–200 µg) are needed. In addition, coinjection of

control plasmids with strong promoters may compete for transcription factors.

6. Expression of injected DNA appears to be limited to striated muscle.

Gene Transfer by DNA Biolistic Process

The use of the "biolistic process" of DNA delivery [51] provides an alternate method in which gene transfer can be accomplished in situ. This procedure involves coating microprojectiles (gold or tungsten particles) with plasmid DNA. In turn, the DNA-coated microprojectiles are spread onto microcarrier discs that are subsequently placed in the apparatus and accelerated. The accelerated microcarrier discs are prevented from leaving the apparatus, however, the DNA-coated microprojectiles exit the apparatus at high velocity and do not come to rest until they contact and penetrate the cells in the target tissue. This method has been used successfully to produce antibodies [85], to transform yeast mitochondria [47], and to test gene expression in different mammalian tissue types [18, 91].

Advantages

1. Other than the cost ($9,000–$10,000) of the apparatus, the advantages are the same as those for direct DNA injection using a syringe.
2. This method is not restricted to animal studies and is frequently used for plant investigations.

Disadvantages

1. The cost of the apparatus (see above).
2. Variability in expression levels can occur because of differences in the amount of DNA coating the microparticles and in operating the apparatus.
3. Same as issues 1 through 4 for the direct DNA injection method.

Both of these approaches, which deliver the foreign DNA directly in situ, provide an alternative to the traditional methods of gene transfer, which involve isolation, culture, transformation, and reintroduction of the target tissue into the recipient.

SUMMARY

Exercise adaptations induce the differential expression of genes that encode components of the contractile apparatus, metabolic pathways, organelle systems, and membrane components. These changes in gene expression are presumably brought about by the activation of intracellular signaling pathways. The use of transgenic technology is particularly well suited for exercise studies because it uniquely allows investigators to evaluate gene regulatory mechanisms in the intact animal at all stages of the life cycle. Transgenic mice can be generated that harbor any of the varied genes involved in exercise adaptation, for the purpose of determining what sequences within this gene regulate the response to any exercise regimen. Once the corresponding transcriptional factor(s) have been identified and the gene(s) cloned, a series of similar studies (gene networking) could be undertaken to determine the signal transduction pathway. Alternatively, transgenics can be produced that overexpress a particular protein or express an isoform of a protein in a tissue where it is not normally expressed. The goal of these studies would be to determine if function is improved and if exercise adaptation is enhanced or facilitated. Ultimately, gene targeting can be used to either mutate or knock out a gene to determine whether its gene product is indispensable for function, exercise performance, and/or adaptation.

Note: This review contains current information as of the time of submission, *15 June 1993.*

ACKNOWLEDGEMENTS

The author wishes to thank the following individuals for their critical reading of this review: Drs. Matthew Wheeler, Byron Kemper, Matilde Holzwarth, Philip Best. Special thanks to Dr. Frank Booth for encouragement and for his critical reading of this review.

REFERENCES

1. Acsadi, G., S. Jiao, A. Jani, D. Duke, P. Williams, W. Chong, and J. A. Wolff. Direct gene transfer and expression into rat heart *in vivo. The New Biol.* 3(1):71–81, 1991.
2. Adolph, E. A., A. Subramaniam, P. Cserjesi, E. N. Olson, and J. Robbins. Role of myocyte-specific enhancer-binding factor (MEF-2) in transcriptional regulation of the α-cardiac myosin heavy chain gene. *J. Biol. Chem.* 268(8):5349–5352, 1993.
3. Andreason, G. L., and G. A. Evans. Introduction and expression of DNA molecules in eukaryotic cells by electroporation. *BioTechniques* 6(7):650–660, 1988.
4. Arnheim, N., and H. Erlich. Polymerase chain reaction strategy. *Annu. Rev. Biochem.* 61:131–156, 1992.
5. Berkner, K. L. Development of adenovirus vectors for the expression of heterologous genes. *BioTechniques* 6(7):616–629, 1988.
6. Booth, F. W. Perspectives on molecular and cellular exercise physiology. *J. Appl. Physiol.* 65(4):1461–1471, 1988.
7. Booth, F. W. Application of molecular biology in exercise physiology. *Exer. Sports Sci. Rev.* 17:1–27, 1989.
8. Brasier, A. R., J. E. Tate, and J. F. Habener. Optimized use of the firefly luciferase assay as a reporter gene in mammalian cell lines. *BioTechniques* 7:1116–1122, 1989.
9. Braun, T., M. A. Rudnick, H-H. Arnold, and R. Jaenisch. Targeted inactivation of the muscle regulatory gene Myf-5 results in abnormal rib development and perinatal death. *Cell* 71:369–382, 1992.

10. Breathnach, R., and P. Chambron. Organization and expression of eukaryotic split genes coding for proteins. *Annu. Rev. Biochem.* 50:349–383, 1981.
11. Brinster, R. L., H. Y. Chen, M. E. Trumbauer, A. W. Senear, R. Warren, and R. D. Palmiter. Somatic expression of herpes thymidine kinase in mice following injection of a fusion gene into eggs. *Cell* 27:223–231, 1981.
12. Brinster, R. L., H. Y. Chen, M. E. Trumbauer, M. K. Yagle, and R. D. Palmiter. Factors affecting the efficiency of introducing foreign DNA into mice by microinjecting eggs. *Proc. Natl. Acad. Sci. USA* 82:4438–4442, 1985.
13. Brinster, R. L., and R. D. Palmiter. Introduction of genes into the germ line of animals. *The Harvey Lectures Series 80.* New York: Alan R. Liss, 1986, pp. 1–38.
14. Buttrick, P. M., A. Kass, R. N. Kitsis, M. L. Kaplan, and L. A. Leinwand. Behavior of genes directly injected into the rat heart in vivo. *Circ. Res.* 70:193–198, 1992.
15. Capecchi, M. R. The new mouse genetics: altering the genome by gene targeting. *T. I. G.* 5(3):70–76, 1989.
16. Carroll, S. L., D. J. Bergsma, and R. J. Schwartz. A 29-nucleotide DNA segment containing an evolutionarily conserved motif is required in *cis* for cell-type-restrictioned depression of the chicken α-smooth and muscle gene core promoter. *Mol. Cell. Biol.* 8:241–250, 1980.
17. Cepko, C. L., B. E. Roberts, and R. C. Mulligan. Construction and applications of a highly transmissible murine retrovirus shuttle vector. *Cell* 37:1053–1062, 1984.
18. Cheng, L., P. R. Ziegelhoffer, and N-S. Yang. In vivo promoter activity and transgene expression in mammalian somatic tissues evaluated by using particle bombardment. *Proc. Natl. Acad. Sci. USA* 90:4455–4459, 1993.
19. Constantini, F., and E. Lacy. Introduction of a rabbit ß-globin gene into the mouse germ line. *Nature* 294:92–94, 1981.
20. Crenshaw, E. B., K. Kalla, D. M. Simmons, L. W. Swanson, and M. G. Resenfeld. Cell-specific expression of the prolactin gene in transgenic mice is controlled by synergistic interactions between promoter and enhancer elements. *Genes Dev.* 3:959–972, 1989.
21. Donchower, L. A., M. Harvey, B. L. Slagle, et al. Mice deficient for p53 are deveopmentally normal but susceptible to spontaneous tumours. *Nature* 356:215–221, 1992.
22. Dynan, W. S., and R. Tjian. Control of eukaryotic messenger RNA synthesis by sequence-specific DNA-binding proteins. *Nature* 316:774–778, 1985.
23. Eglitis, M. A., and W. F. Anderson. Retroviral vectors for introduction of genes into mammalian cells. *Bio Techniques* 6:608–614, 1988.
24. Emerson, C. P. Myogenesis and myogenic control genes. *Curr. Opin. Cell Biol.* 2:1065–1075, 1990.
25. Erlich, H. A. *PCR technology.* Principles and applications for DNA amplification. Stockton Press, 1989, pp. 1–242.
26. Evans, M. J., and M. Hikaukman. Establishment in culture of pluripotential cells from mouse embryos. *Nature* 292:154–156, 1981.
27. Felgner, P. L., T. R. Gadek, M. Holm, R. Roman, H. W. Chan, et al. Lipofection: a highly efficient, lipid-mediated DNA-transfer procedure. *Proc Natl. Acad. Sci. USA.* 84:7413–7417, 1987.
28. Field, L. J. Transgenic mice in cardiovascular research. *Annu. Rev. Physiol.* 55:97–114, 1993.
29. Frohman, M. A., and G. R. Martin. Cut, paste, and save: new approaches to altering specific genes in mice. *Cell* 56:145–147, 1989.
30. Ghosh-Choudhury, G., Y. Haj-Ahmad, P. Brinkley, J. Rudy, and F. L. Graham. Human adenovirus cloning vectors based on infectious bacterial plasmids. *Gene* 50:161–171, 1986.
31. Gill, T. J., G. J. Smith, and R. W. Wissler. The rate as an experimental animal. *Science* 245:269–276, 1989.
32. Gordon, J. W., G. A. Scangos, D. J. Plotkin, J. A. Barbosa, and R. H. Ruddle. Genetic transformation of mouse embryos by microinjection of purified DNA. *Proc. Natl. Acad. Sci. USA* 77:7380–7384, 1980.

33. Gorman, C. M., L. F. Moffat, and B. M. Howard. Recombinant genomes which express chloramphenicol acetyltransferase in mammalian cells. *Mol. Cell. Biol.* 2:1044–1051, 1982.

34. Hammer, R. E., S. D. Maika, J. A. Richardson, J.-P. Tang, and J. D. Taurog. Spontaneous inflammatory disease in transgenic rats expressing HLA-B27 and human ß₂m: an animal model of HLA-B27 associated human disorders. *Cell* 63:1099–1112, 1990.

35. Hammer, R. E., A. G. Pursel, C. E. Rexroad, et al. Production of transgenic rabbits, sheep and pigs by miroinjection. *Nature* 315:680–683, 1985.

36. Hanahan, D. Transgenic mice as probes into complex systems. *Science* 246:1265–1275, 1989.

37. Harsdorf, R., R. J. Schott, Y.-T. Shen, S. F. Vatner, V. Mahdavi, and B. Nadal-Ginard. Gene injection into canine myocardium as a useful model for studying gene expression in the heart of large mammals. *Circ. Res.* 72:688–695, 1993.

38. Hasty, P. J. Rivera-Perez, and A. Bradley. The length of homology required for gene targeting in embryonic stem cells. *Mol. Cell Biol.* 11(11):5586–5591, 1991.

39. Hoffman, M. New vector delivers genes to lung cells. *Science* 252:374, 1991.

40. Hogan, B., F. Constantini, and E. Lacy. *Manipulating the Mouse Embryo: A Laboratory Manual.* New York: Cold Spring Harbor Laboratory, 1986, pp. 1–332.

41. Hollen, T., F. K. Yoshimura. Variation in enzymatic transient gene expression assays. *Anal. Biochem.* 182:411–418, 1989.

42. Hooper, C. Genetic knockouts: surprises, lessons and dreams. *J. NIH Res.* 4:34–35, 1992.

43. Iannello, R. C., J. H. Mar, and C. P. Ordahl. Characterization of a promoter element required for transcription in myocardial cells. *J. Biol. Chem.* 266:3309–3316, 1991.

44. Jaenisch, R. Transgenic animals. *Science* 240:1468–1474, 1988.

45. Jaenisch, R. D., Jahner, P. Nobis, et al. Chromosomal position and activation of retroviral genomes inserted into the germ line of mice. *Cell* 24:519–529, 1981.

46. Johnson, J. E., B. J. Wold, and S. D. Hauschka. Muscle creatine kinase sequence elements regulating skeletal muscle and cardiac muscle expression in transgenic mince. *Mol. Cell. Biol.* 9(8):3393–3399, 1989.

47. Johnston, S. A., P. W. Anziano, K. Shark, J. C. Sanford, and R. A. Butow. Mitochondrial transformation in yeast by bombardment with microprojectiles. *Science* 240:1538–1541, 1988.

48. Kafatos, F. C., C. W. Jones, and A. Efstratiadis. Determination of nucleic acid sequence homologies and relative concentrations by a dot hybridization procedure. *Nucl. Acid Res.* 7:1541–1552, 1979.

49. Kitsis, R. N., P. M. Buttrick, E. M. McNally, M. L. Kaplan, and L. A. Leinwand. Hormonal modulation of a gene injected into rat heart in vivo. *Proc. Natl. Acad. Sci. USA* 88: 4138–4142, 1991.

50. Kitsis, R. N., and L. Leinwand. Discordance between gene regulation in vitro and in vivo. *Gene Expression* 2(4):313–318, 1992.

51. Klein, T. M., R. Arentzen, P. A. Lewis, and S. Fitzpatrick-McElligott. Transformation of microbes, plants, and animals by particle bombardment. *Bio. Technol.* 10:286–291, 1992.

52. Lin, H., M. S. Parmacek, G. Morle, S. Bolling, and J. M. Leiden. Expression of recombinant genes in myocardium *in vivo* after direct injection of DNA. *Circulation* 82:2217–2221, 1990.

53. Maniatis, T., S. Goodbourn, and J. A. Fischer. Regulation of inducible and tissue-specific gene expression. *Science* 236:1237–1245, 1987.

54. Mansour, S. L., K. R. Thomas, and M. R. Capecchi. Disruption of the proto-oncogene int-w in mouse embryo-derived stem cells: a general strategy for targeting mutations to non-selectable genes. *Nature* 336:348–352, 1988.

55. McKnight, S. L., and R. C. Kingsbury. Transcriptional control signals of a eukaryotic protein-coding gene. *Science* 217:316–324, 1982.

56. McKnight, S. L., and R. Tijian. Transcriptional selectively of viral genes in mammalian cells. *Cell* 46:795–805, 1986.

57. Miller, A. D., and G. J. Rosman. Improved retroviral vectors for gene transfer and expression. *BioTechniques* 7(9):980–990, 1989.
58. Miller, D. G., M. A. Adam, and A. D. Miller. Gene transfer by retrovirus vectors occurs only in cells that are actively replicating at the time of infection. *Mol. Cell. Biol.* 10(8):4239–4242, 1990.
59. Mirkovitch, J., and J. E. Darnell, Jr. Rapid *in vivo* footprinting technique identifies proteins bound to the TTR gene in the mouse liver. *Genes Dev.* 5:83–93, 1991.
60. Mitchell, P. J., and R. Tijan. Transcriptional regulation in mammalian cells by sequence-specific DNA binding proteins. *Science* 245:371–378, 1989.
61. Mulligan, R. C. The basic science of gene therapy. *Science* 260:926–932, 1993.
62. Mullis, K. B., and I. Falcona. Specific synthesis of DNA *in vitro* via a polymerase-catalyzed chain reaction. *Methods Enzymol.* 155:335–350, 1987.
63. Mullins, J. J., J. Peters, and D. Ganten. Fulminant hypertension in transgenic rats harbouring the mouse ren-2 gene. *Nature* 344:541–548, 1990.
64. Nabel, E. G., G. Plautz, and G. J. Nabel. Site-specific gene expression in vivo by direct gene transfer into the arterial wall. *Science* 249:1285–1288, 1990.
65. Nakatsuji, Y. K., K. Hidaka, S. Tsuijino, Y. Yamamoto, T. Mukai, et al. A single MEF-2 site is a major positive regulatory element required for transcription of the muscle-specific subunit of the human phosphoglycerate mutase gene in skeletal and cardiac muscle cells. *Mol. Cell Biol.* 12:4384–4390, 1992.
66. Navankasattusas, S., H. Zhu, A. V. Garcia, S. M. Evans, and K. R. Chein. A ubiquitous factor (HF-1a) a muscle factor (HF-1b/MEF-2) form an E-box-independent pathway for cardiac muscle gene expression. *Mol. Cell Biol.* 12:1160–1170, 1992.
67. Neumann, J. R., C. A. Morency, and K. O. Russian. A novel rapid assay for chloramphenicol acetyltransferase gene expression. *BioTechniques* 5(5):444–447, 1987.
68. Nguyen, V. T., M. Morange, and O. Bensuade. Firefly luciferase luminescence assays using scintillation counters for quantitation in transfected mammalian cells. *Anal. Biochem.* 171:404–408, 1988.
69. Ojamaa, K., and I. Klein. Thyroid hormone regulation of alpha-myosin heavy chain promoter activity assessed by *in vivo* DNA transfer in rat heart. *Biochem. Biophys. Res. Commun.* 179(3):1269–1275, 1991.
70. Olson, E. P. MyoD family: a paradigm for development? *Genes Dev.* 4:1454–1461, 1990.
71. Palmiter, R. D., and R. L. Brinster. Transgenic mice. *Cell* 41:343–345, 1985.
72. Palmiter, R. D., and R. L. Brinster. Germ-line transformation of mice. Allan Campbell, editor. Ann. Reviews Inc., 1986, vol. 20, pp. 465–499.
73. Parmacek, M. S., A. J. Vora, T. Shen, E. Barr, F. Jung, and J. M. Leiden. Identification and characterization of a cardiac-specific transcriptional regulatory element in the slow/cardiac troponin C gene. *Mol. Cell. Biol.* 12(5):1967–1976, 1992.
74. Raz, E., A. Watanabe, S. M. Baird, R. A. Eisenberg, T. B. Parr, et al. Systemic immunological effects of cytokine genes injected into skeletal muscle. *Proc. Natl. Acad. Sci. USA.* 90:4523–4527, 1993.
75. Rennie, J. Essential but expendable: when do master genes regulate cell growth? *Sci. Am.* 267(6):25–26, 1992.
76. Robertson, E. J. Pluripotential stem cell lines as a route into the mouse germ line. *T. I. G.* 2:9–13, 1986.
77. Rosenfeld, M. A., W. Siegfried, K. Yoshimura, et al. Adenovirus-mediated transfer of a recombinant αl-antitrypsin gene to the lung epithelium *in vivo*. *Science* 252:431–434, 1991.
78. Rosenthal, N., J. M. Kornhauser, M. Donoghue, K. M. Rosen, and J. P. Merlie. Myosin light chain enhancer activates muscle-specific, developmentally regulated gene expression in transgenic mice. *Proc. Natl. Acad. Sci. USA* 86:7780–7784, 1989.
79. Rudnicki, M. A., T. Braun, S. Hinuma, and R. Jaenisch. Inactivation of MyoD in mice leads to up-regulation of the myogenic HLH gene Myf-5 and results in apparently normal muscle development. *Cell* 71:383–390, 1992.

80. Schedl, A., L. Montoliu, G. Kelsey, and G. Schutz. A yeast artificial chromosome covering the tyrosinase gene convers copy number-dependent expression in transgenic mice. *Nature* 362:258–261, 1993.

81. Shull, M. M., I Ormsby, A. B. Kier et al. Targeted disruption of the mouse transforming growth factor-ß1 gene results in multifocal inflammatory disease. *Nature* 359:693–699, 1992.

82. Smithies, O. Animal models of human genetic diseases. *T. I. G.* 9(4):112–116, 1993.

83. Southern, E. M. Detection of specific sequences among DNA fragments separated by gel electrophoresis. *J. Mol. Biol.* 98:503–517, 1975.

84. Swift, G. H., F. Kruse, R. J. MacDonald, and R. E. Hammer. Differntial requirements for cell-specific elastase I enhancer domains in transfected cells and transgenic mice. *Genes Dev.* 3:687–696, 1989.

85. Tang, D-c., M. DeVit, and S. A. Johnston. Genetic immunization is a simple method for eliciting and immune response. *Nature* 356:152–154, 1992.

86. Thomas, K. R., C. Deng, and M. R. Capecchi. High-fidelity gene targeting in embryonic stem cells by using sequence replacement vectors. *Mol. Cell. Biol.* 12(7):2919–2923, 1992.

87. Townes, T. M., J. B. Lingrel, H. Y. Chen, R. L. Brinster, and R. D. Palmiter. Erythroid-specific expression of human ß-globin genes in transgenic mice. *EMBO J.* 4:1715–1723, 1986.

88. Travis, J. Scoring a technical knockout in mice. *Science* 256:1392–1394, 1992.

89. Vincent, C. K., A. Gualberto, C. V. Patel, and K. Walsh. Different regulatory sequences control creatine kinase-M gene expression in directly injected skeletal and cardiac muscle. *Mol. Cell. Biol.* 13(2):1264–1272, 1993.

90. Weintraub, H., R. Davis, S. Tapscott et al. The myoD gene family: nodal point during specification of the muscle cell lineage. *Science* 251:761–766, 1991.

91. Williams, R. S., S. A. Johnston, M. Riedy, M. J. DeVit, S. G. McElligott, and J. C. Sanford. Introduction of foreign genes into tissues of living mice by DNA-coated microprojectiles. *Proc. Natl. Acad. Sci. USA* 88:2726–2730, 1991.

92. Wolff, J. A., R. W. Malone, P. Williams, W. Chong, G. Acsadi, et al. Direct gene transfer into mouse muscle *in vivo*. *Science* 247:1465–1468, 1990.

93. Wolff, J. A., P. Williams, G. Acsadi, S. Jiao, A. Jani, and W. Chong. Conditions affecting direct gene transfer into rodent muscle *in vivo*. *BioTechniques* 11(4)474–485, 1991.

94. Wright, W. E. Muscle basic helix-loop helix proteins and the regulation of myogenesis. *Curr. Opin. Gen. Dev.* 2:243–248, 1992.

95. Zhu, H., V. T. B. Nguyen, A. B. Brown, A. Pourhosseini, A. V. Garcia, et al. A novel, tissue-restricted zinc finger protein (HF-1b) binds to the cardiac regulatory element (HF-1b/MEF-2) in the rat myosin light chain 2 gene. *Mol. Cell. Biol.* 13:4432–4444, 1993.

96. Zimmer, A. Manipulating the genome by homologous recombination in embryonic stem cells. *Annu. Rev. Neurosci.* Annual Reviews Inc. 1992, pp. 115–137.

13
Physical Growth and Biological Maturation of Young Athletes

ROBERT M. MALINA, Ph.D., F.A.C.S.M.

The number of youth competing in a variety of sports at national and international levels is increasing, e.g., diving, gymnastics, swimming, and figure skating. Females appear among the elite at young ages more often than males. Significant numbers of children and youth of both sexes also begin to specialize in a sport at relatively young ages, and the process of identifying and selecting talented individuals for a given sport often begins in childhood.

The success of youth in some sports and the selection of talented individuals at young ages are not without problems. There is concern about potential negative influences of intensive training and the demands of high-performance sports on the growth and maturation of young athletes. Indeed, the treatment and some of the techniques of training young athletes for high-performance sports may fall within the bounds of child abuse. Microscopic analysis and evaluation of sport in the media contributes additional stresses. In a related matter, changes in the political systems of Eastern Europe and reevaluation of the role of sports in national agenda have placed these elaborate sport systems in jeopardy. Many of these systems had talent identification programs for young athletes, and the practices developed in some Eastern European countries, especially the former German Democratic Republic and Soviet Union, have influenced those currently used in many parts of the world. Indeed, a significant amount of data on the growth and maturation of young athletes comes from Eastern Europe.

The purpose of this review is to evaluate the growth and maturation status of young athletes. Available data are collated by sport in an attempt to describe the growth and maturity status of youngsters actively engaged in specific sports. Studies that combine athletes participating in different sports are not included. The closing section briefly addresses the effects of intensive training for sport on growth and maturation in the context of the data presented. Previous reviews have focused more on maturation [16, 111, 112] and to a lesser extent on growth [124], although both are related.

METHODOLOGICAL NOTES AND LIMITATIONS

ATHLETES. The definition of a sample as athletes was accepted as reported. Most studies include youngsters who can be classified as select, elite, junior national, or national caliber.

389

GROWTH. Growth refers to increase in the size of the body or its parts. It includes changes in size, body composition, physique, and specific body systems. This review is limited to two indicators of size, stature and body weight. When sufficient data are available, the size attained (growth status) by athletes from Europe and the Americas is plotted by sport relative to reference data for a nationally representative sample of U.S. youth [75]. Smoothed 10th (*P 10*), 25th (*P 25*), 50th (*P 50*, median), 75th (*P 75*), and 90th (*P 90*) percentiles are used for comparison, although only P 10, P 50, and P 90 are shown in the figures. When data are not extensive across the age span, the size of the athletes is simply described relative to the reference data. Limited data for young athletes from Japan and China are described relative to Japanese reference means [138].

The physique and body composition of young athletes is not considered. Physique is a selective factor in some sports, and young athletes in a given sport tend to have physiques similar to those of adult athletes in the sport [32, 34, 153]. Body composition is most often viewed in the context of the two-compartment model, fat-free mass and fat mass, and relative fatness is often the focus in many studies of athletes. Males, athletes and nonathletes, show a decline in relative fatness during adolescence, but athletes have less fatness. Relative fatness does not increase as much with age during adolescence in female athletes as it does in nonathletes. Thus, difference between female athletes and nonathletes is greater than the corresponding trend in males [119].

MATURATION. Biological maturation refers to the tempo and timing of progress toward the mature state. Skeletal (skeletal age), sexual (secondary sex characteristics), and somatic (age at peak height velocity) maturation are often used.

The hand-wrist is used to assess skeletal maturation, and the two more commonly used procedures are the Greulich-Pyle (GP, [73]) and Tanner-Whitehouse (TW, [185]) methods. The methods differ in criteria and scoring and in the reference samples upon which they are based [117, 119]. The upper limit (i.e., skeletal maturity) of the GP method is 18 years in both sexes; limits of the TW method are 16 years for girls and 18 years for boys. A youngster who reaches the upper limit is simply labeled as mature or adult, and should not be included in the calculation of mean skeletal age (SA) for a group. Both methods yield an SA that corresponds to the level of skeletal maturity attained by a child relative to the reference sample; SAs derived from each method are not equivalent.

SA is expressed relative to the child's chronological age (CA), and children are often classified as having an SA that is *advanced, average,* or *delayed*. The criteria that define the categories in this review are (*a*) *advanced*—SA is one year or more ahead of CA (early maturer); (*b*) *average*—SA is within plus or minus one year of CA (average maturer); (*c*) *delayed*—SA is one year or more behind CA (late maturer). The terms are descriptive labels and indicate nothing about factors underlying earliness or lateness.

Secondary sex characteristics include the breasts, pubic hair, and menarche in girls and the genitals and pubic hair in boys. Breast, genital, and pubic hair development are most often assessed relative to five stages or grades for each character [119]. The ratings are often used to characterize the maturity status of a sample and to group athletes by maturity status independent of CA. This presents problems because chronologically older children tend to be taller and heavier than younger children of the same stage of pubertal development [117].

Age at menarche, the first menstrual period, occurs, on average, about 13.0 years of age in samples of American and European girls [119]. Most data for athletes are based on the retrospective method, which requires that the individual recalls the age at which she experienced her first menstrual period. The retrospective method is severely limited when used with young athletes. Estimated mean ages are biased, since all subjects have not attained menarche. Allowing for error of recall, the retrospective method is useful with athletes after 17 years of age, when almost all girls have attained menarche.

In studies of young athletes, the prospective method is ideal; it requires longitudinal study in which athletes are examined at close intervals during puberty. The status quo method is a useful cross-sectional alternative with young athletes. It yields an estimate of the median age at menarche for the sample and can also be used with other secondary sex characteristics [117, 119]. Prospective and status quo data for menarche in young athletes are very limited, and only these are included in the main section of the review. A brief discussion of retrospective estimates is offered later in the review.

Peak height velocity (PHV) refers to the maximum rate of growth in stature during the adolescent spurt, and the age when PHV occurs is an indicator of somatic maturity. Longitudinal data are necessary to estimate PHV, but methods of estimation vary. PHV occurs, on average, at about 12 years in girls and 14 years in boys [17, 116, 119].

CHRONOLOGICAL AGE. Growth and maturation data are expressed relative to CA, the child's age as determined by the calendar. CA is usually reported to the nearest 0.1 year. Some reports simply refer to a whole year (e.g., 11 years of age). It is assumed that the authors refer to age at last birthday (i.e., the child is not yet 12 years). In plotting such data, 0.5 year was added to the reported age (i.e., 11.5 years). Some studies group children across several years (e.g., 11–13 years) and do not indicate the mean CA of the group. It is assumed that these ages refer to age at last birthday, and the midpoint of the range was used in plotting data. The upper age limit in this review is 18 years; the lower limit varies with available data for each sport.

COUNTRY NAMES. Given political change, several new nations have emerged. For convenience, the original names of several Eastern European countries are used: the Soviet Union, East Germany or German Democratic Republic (now a part of Germany), Czechoslovakia (now the Czech

Republic and Slovakia), and Yugoslavia. Considerable data on the growth and maturation of young athletes are from these countries.

TEAM SPORTS

Baseball

There is relatively little information on the growth and maturation of young players. Most participants in the 1955 Little League World Series were pubescent (17.0%) or postpubescent (45.5%) in pubic hair status [74], while among players in the 1957 World Series, equal numbers of boys had SAs that were classified as average (45.5%) or advanced (45.5%) relative to their CAs [102]. Maturity was also related to position and batting order; all except one starting pitcher and all boys who batted in the fourth position were postpubescent [74]. In contrast, successful interscholastic baseball players at the fifth and sixth grades (about 10–12 years) did not differ from nonparticipants in maturation [45]. Among older boys in the Medford Boys' Growth Study [45], there were no maturity differences between senior high school baseball players and nonplayers (about 15–18 years of age). The catch-up of later-maturing boys during the high school years reduces the size, strength, and skill differences so apparent in early adolescence. Also, at more competitive levels, skill is of more importance than the advantage afforded by greater size and strength at younger ages.

American Football

American football is a sport in which a large body size is an advantage and in which many boys are selected for a position by their body size. Data for 58 participants, 10.2–14.2 years of age, in a local league from two small communities indicate statures that approximate the reference median, but body weights just below P 75 [119, 124]. Pubic hair stages 1–4 were represented in the sample, and the distribution was similar to that seen in the general population. In contrast, interscholastic football players in the Medford Boys' Growth Study were advanced in SA at all ages between 10 and 15 years compared with nonparticipants, and the outstanding players were more advanced than other players [45]. At the senior high school level, SA did not differ consistently between players and nonplayers, probably reflecting the catch-up of late maturers and attainment of skeletal maturity by many boys. However, high school football "all stars" approximated the 90th percentile of the reference data for stature and weight [96].

Basketball

MALES. Mean statures and weights of basketball players often approximate or exceed P 90 from early through late adolescence (Fig. 13.1, *left*). Data from samples in Czechoslovakia indicate secular increases in stature and weight of players from the 1960s [107, 155] to the mid-1980s [97].

FIGURE 13.1

Statures and weights of male basketball and volleyball players (left) and female basketball, volleyball and handball players (right). In all figures, points connected by a solid line are mixed-longitudinal or longitudinal, and those by a dashed line are cross-sectional. Individual points: basketball (males [42, 154, 187]; females [175, 187]); volleyball (males, [97, 141, 156]; females, [93, 126, 141, 202]).

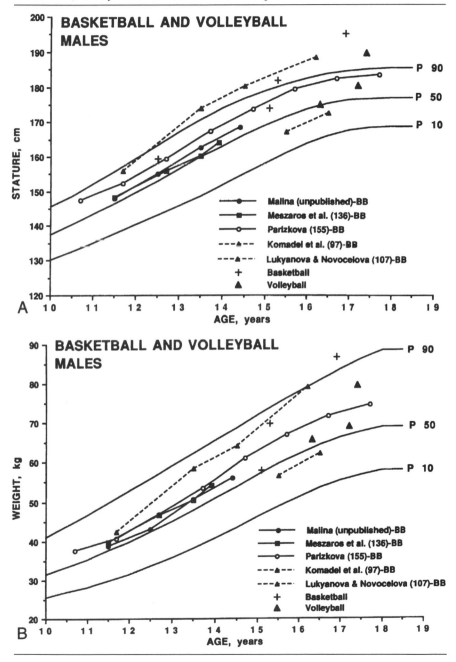

FIGURE 13.1 *(continued)*

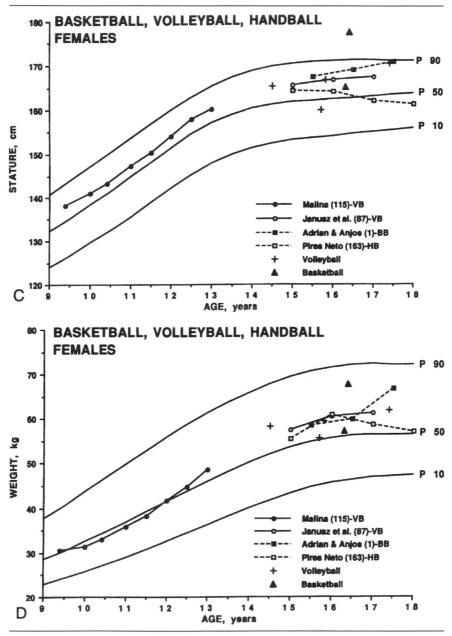

Belgian data indicate a size difference between national and regional selections of 14- to 15-year-old players [42].

Interscholastic basketball players and nonplayers 9–12 years of age did not differ in skeletal maturity [45], while select Finnish basketball players had SAs and CAs that did not differ, 12.5 ± 1.2 and 12.5 ± 0.5 years, respectively [154]. However, between 13 and 15 years of age, successful basketball players were advanced in SA [42, 45]. Among 16 Belgian nationally select players, 10 and 6, respectively, had SAs classified as advanced and average, and there were no late maturers, while among 14 regionally select players, 11 had SAs classified as average [42]. Data for older ages in the Medford Boys' Growth Study showed no differences in SA between high school basketball players and nonplayers [45].

FEMALES. Data for female basketball players are limited to late adolescence (Fig. 13.1, *right*). Mean statures for two U.S. samples [1, 175] are between P 50 and P 75, while that for an Australian selection [187] exceeds P 90. Body weights vary between P 50 and P 90. Skeletal maturation and secondary sex characteristic development of 10 Czechoslovak basketball players (mean age, 16 years) were classified as average, and none of the athletes was advanced [151].

Volleyball

MALES. Data for male volleyball players are also limited to late adolescence (Fig. 13.1, *left*). Regionally select Chilean junior players [141] have a mean stature and weight that are at the reference medians, while two select Czechoslovak samples [97, 156] show a secular increase from the late 1960s [156] to the mid-1980s [97]. The recent sample [97] has a mean stature that exceeds P 90 and a mean weight between P 75 and P 90.

FEMALES. Two samples of volleyball players, a mixed-longitudinal sample of U.S. girls 9–13 years from a well-developed parochial school program [115] and a longitudinal sample of select players 15–17 years from Poland [87], have statures close to P 75 (Fig. 13.1, *right*). Mean weights of the younger girls are at the median, while those of the adolescent players are just below P 75. Mean statures and weights for three of four samples of adolescent players from Brazil [93], the U.S. [126], and Czechoslovakia [202] are well above the median; the mean stature of the Czechoslovak tournament participants is at P 90. Stature of the Chilean juniors [141] is just below the median, and weight is at the median.

Estimated six-monthly growth rates for stature and weight in the mixed-longitudinal sample of volleyball players 10–13 years of age were similar to medians for nonathletes [115]. Hence, their larger body size is not a function of accelerated growth rates. SAs and CAs of Czechoslovak volleyball players (n=12) were virtually identical at about 14 and 17 years [150], while secondary sex characteristic development (n=10) was classified as average [151].

European Handball
Statures of a sample of junior female handball players from Brazil [163] fluctuate about P 50, while weights tend to be slightly above P 50 (Fig. 13.1, *right*).

Soccer (European Football)
Given the popularity of soccer throughout the world, there is surprisingly little information on the growth and maturation of young male soccer players. Data from Europe [10, 50, 62, 98, 107, 128, 219], the Americas [53, 92], Japan [7, 172] and China [37] indicate statures that approximate the median/mean of the respective reference data from childhood through about 15 years of age. Subsequently, statures tend to be at or below the median in late adolescent players from Europe and the Americas, with the exception of the sample from the early 1960s [107] and Chilean junior players [52]. In contrast, Chinese players tend to be slightly above the Japanese reference mean (this is also true in the Chinese population in general). Mean weights of players from Europe and the Americas tend fluctuate about median from childhood through adolescence, while those for Japanese and Chinese players are, with one exception, consistently below the reference mean for Japan.

Several studies of the skeletal maturation of young soccer players in Europe [29, 128, 211] and Japan [7, 172] indicate SAs that approximated, on average, CAs, while estimated ages at PHV in 18 Welsh (n=32) and Danish (n=8) adolescent soccer players were 14.2 ± 0.9 and 14.2 years, respectively [11, 67]. This would suggest "average" maturity status from childhood through the adolescent spurt. Data for pubertal Italian soccer players suggest a tendency for adolescent players 14–16 years of age to be advanced in SA, pubic hair development, and testicular volume, and taller and heavier than nonplayers; in contrast, pubertal players and nonplayers 10–11 and 12–13 years of age did not differ in SA, sexual maturation, and body size [29, 128]. These results may suggest a trend for boys advanced in maturity status to be more successful in soccer in later adolescence. Although numbers are small (n=18), data for 12-year-old soccer players suggest maturity-associated variation by position [10]. Strikers (n=5) and midfielders (n=4) tended to attain PHV earlier than defenders (n=7).

Ice Hockey
Data on the growth and maturation of boys participating in ice hockey, with one exception, are derived from Canada, Finland, and Czechoslovakia (Fig. 13.2). Statures tend to be variable during childhood and early adolescence, especially those from Canada. This may reflect ethnic variation; players of primarily French Canadian ancestry [21, 53] tend to be shorter. From about 15 years and older, all mean statures are at or below the median. In contrast, mean body weights from diverse samples of hockey players 8–15 years of age approximate P 50, while those of older players

FIGURE 13.2

Statures and weights of male ice hockey players. Individual points: [20, 49, 77, 104, 148, 154, 156, 158, 165].

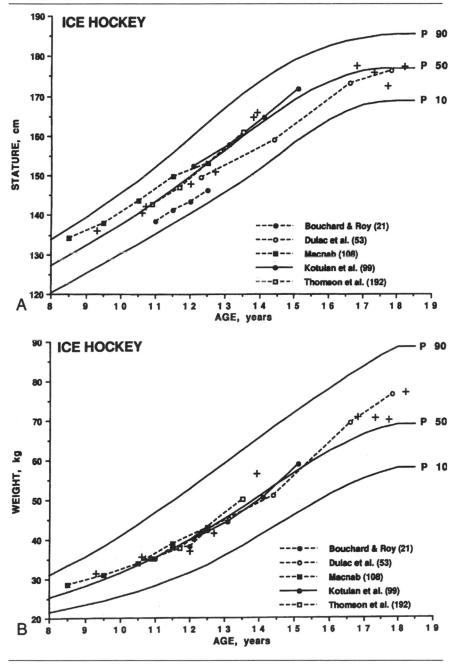

tend to be above P 50. The trend for late adolescent hockey players suggests a population that has greater weight for stature.

The maturity status of ice hockey players is consistent with the data for body size (Fig. 13.3). Cross-sectional data at 9 and 13 years of age from Finland indicate SAs and CAs that were, on average, the same [154, 165]. Longitudinal data for 16 select hockey players from Czechoslovakia indicate SAs that were behind corresponding CAs by about 0.5 years from 12 to 15 years of age [99]. This sample had an estimated age of PHV ("the point of inflection of the height growth curve") of 14.5 ± 1.0 years, which was consistent with the lag in skeletal maturation. Cross-sectional samples from Canada span 10–16 years of age. Younger groups, 10–12 years, had SAs that were behind corresponding CAs by 0.3–0.6 years [21, 49, 158]. However, among elite hockey players 13–16 years of age, SA was significantly advanced relative to CA by an average of 1.7 and 1.3 years [103]. The trend for boys advanced in maturity status to predominate among elite hockey players is illustrated in the distribution of players classified as advanced, average, or delayed in SA relative to CA. Among 12-year-old international tournament participants [124], boys classified as

FIGURE 13.3

Skeletal age versus chronological age in ice hockey players. Individual points: [21, 49, 103, 154, 158, 165].

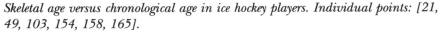

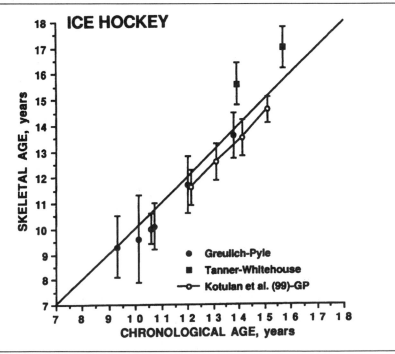

average (43%) and delayed (37%) were about equally represented, while those classified as advanced represented a small percentage (14%). However, among 13–14- and 15–16-year-old elite players [103], no boys were delayed in SA; most were advanced, 82% and 62%, respectively.

Ice hockey also shows variation in skeletal maturity (and correspondingly body size) by position among 12-year-old boys. Among tournament participants (n=205), most defensemen were average and advanced in SA, while most forwards and goalkeepers were average and delayed in SA [119]. Only 11% of the forwards and 8% of the goalkeepers were advanced, while only 15% of the defensemen were delayed in SA relative to CA. The evidence from baseball, ice hockey, and soccer among boys 12 years of age thus suggests that in addition to maturity-associated variation in body size, there is variation in maturity status by position within a given sport.

INDIVIDUAL SPORTS

Track and Field

For convenience, events comprising track and field were grouped into distance runs (one mile or further, cross-country), sprints, jumps (long, high), and throws (shot, discus). Some studies simply describe samples as track athletes or training in light athletics, or group athletes across events. These data were not considered in the comparisons.

MALES. Young distance runners 10–18 years tend to have statures that fluctuate about P 50 and body weights that tend to be below P 50 [19, 51, 55, 109, 135, 188, 193, 195, 196, 205]. Mean statures and weights of sprinters tend to be at or above P 50 [2, 19, 130, 135, 188, 195, 196]. Results are similar for Chinese and Japanese distance runners and sprinters 13–17 years [152]. U.S. Junior Olympians [196] and Belgian national selections [19] in jumping and throwing events have similar statures. Throwers are slightly taller within each sample, approximating P 90. Weights of throwers are at P 90, while those of jumpers are at P 50. Chinese and Japanese jumpers 15–17 years show similar trends [152].

Elite male (n=18) distance runners 9–15 years of age from the state of Michigan were slightly shorter and lighter than active youth not involved in distance running, but longitudinal observations over one year indicated growth rates (cm/yr) that did not differ from those of nonrunners. The smaller size may reflect the slightly delayed SA of the runners [173]. In contrast, longitudinal observations on six junior champion distance runners in Japan indicated greater statures and weights than active and control boys, and an earlier age at PHV, 12.6 years [95].

Track athletes did not differ in skeletal maturity from nonathletes in elementary school [45]. Similar observations were reported for small samples of distance runners and sprinters 10–12 years of age [135]. At older ages, track athletes in the Medford study were advanced in SA in junior high school (12–15 years), but did not differ in SA from nonathletes in senior high school (15–18 years) [45]. At more advanced competitive levels, mean SAs of male participants 12–18 years of age (n=103) in an instructional camp for track and field athletes (events not specified) were in advance of mean CA (14.9 ± 1.3 years), slightly by the GP (15.2 ± 1.7 years) and significantly by the TW (16.8 ± 1.3 years) methods [47]. Examination of the scatter plot of SA versus CA indicated that only two boys had TW SAs less than their CAs, and the greatest advancement of SA over CA was apparent between 13 and 15 years of age. Similar trends were apparent in nationally select Belgian [118] athletes 15–18 years, and Chinese and Japanese [152] junior athletes 13–17 years. The data show a pattern of advanced SA initially. At older ages, many athletes have attained skeletal maturity, but a number of later-maturing boys are also successful performers. This indicates the reduced significance of maturity-associated variation in body size on track and field performance in late adolescence.

FEMALES. Mean statures of distance runners [1, 19, 27, 84, 137, 166, 188, 193, 194, 196, 204, 216, 217] and sprinters [19, 84, 123, 166, 188, 194, 196, 217] 10–18 years tend to be at or above P 50. However, mean weights of distance runners are consistently below P 50, while those of sprinters are, with one exception, quite close to P 50. Identical trends are apparent in Chinese and Japanese junior distance runners and sprinters 13–17 years [152]. Adolescent distance runners of both sexes tend to have less weight for stature, but the tendency is more apparent in females than in males. Data for U.S. Junior Olympians [196], Olympic Development Camp participants [84], and Olympians <18 years from the Mexico City, Munich, and Montreal Olympic Games [123] indicate greater statures in jumpers than throwers, and greater weights in throwers than jumpers. The statures of jumpers and throwers generally exceed P 90; in contrast, mean weights of the throwers are close to or above P 90, while those of the jumpers are at or above P 50. Chinese and Japanese jumpers and throwers 15–17 years do not differ in stature, but the latter are heavier, and both groups of athletes are considerably larger than the reference mean [152].

Elite female (n=14) distance runners 9–15 years of age from the state of Michigan were slightly shorter and lighter than active girls not involved in distance running. Longitudinal observations over one year indicated stature growth rates (cm/yr) that were slightly greater in the runners, most likely reflecting their slightly delayed SAs [173].

Mean SA of 168 female participants 12–18 years at an instructional track and field camp was the same as mean CA (15.0 ± 1.2 years) by the TW (14.9 ± 1.3 years) method, but slightly in delay by the GP method (14.6 ± 1.3 years) [47]. The scatter plot of TW SAs versus CAs indicated reasonably equal numbers above and below the line of unity across CA, with the exception of the older ages, suggesting generally average skeletal maturity status. Similar results were reported for 10 Czechoslovak runners, 15.5 years of age [151]. Among 29 nationally select Belgian track and field athletes

15–18 years, about one-half attained skeletal maturity (n=15), which is 16.0 years in the TW method [118]. The skeletally mature and immature were equally distributed among events. Among Chinese and Japanese athletes 13–17 years, sprinters tended to be slightly advanced in SA, while distance runners were generally average in SA. The vast majority of jumpers and throwers 15–17 years had already attained skeletal maturity [152].

Information on the sexual maturation of young female track and field athletes is not extensive. The estimated median age at menarche (probit) for a status quo sample of Hungarian track athletes 10–17 years of age was 12.6 years, a value similar to nonathlete populations in Hungary [61].

Swimming
Studies of young swimmers generally treat the athletes as a group, without attention to stroke and distance. Given the wealth of information on young swimmers, the available data were grouped geographically for convenience: the Americas (largely the U.S.), Western Europe, Eastern Europe, and Japan.

MALES. With few exceptions, statures of age-group swimmers in the Americas are above the reference median. Those from the U.S. Swimming select camp program, 14–17 years [200, 201], have statures that approximate P 90 (Fig. 13.4, *left*). Mean weights of swimmers from the Americas are at, but generally above, P 50. The U.S. select swimmers are also the heaviest.

Young Western European swimmers, mostly from France [14, 36, 63, 132], have statures and weights that approximate the respective reference medians, while Belgian [207], Swedish [56, 57], and Norwegian [110] swimmers are generally taller and heavier than the medians (Fig. 13.4, *center*). Data for Eastern European swimmers are more variable (Fig. 13.4, *right*). Mean statures and weights are above and below the reference medians, and swimmers from the Soviet Union [26] are generally taller and heavier than those from the German Democratic Republic [198]. There appears to be a secular increase in size; the most recent samples from Hungary [59] and Czechoslovakia [97, 146] are taller and heavier than earlier samples. The best freestyle swimmers from East Germany in the 1960s had statures at P 50 and weights above P 50 [198].

Data for young Japanese swimmers indicate statures at the Japanese reference mean and weights above the mean [127, 145].

Male age group swimmers tend to have SAs concentrated in the average and advanced categories, with relatively few late-maturing youngsters [25, 143, 162, 183]. This trend is especially apparent in late childhood and early adolescence. At these ages, better performers also tend to be advanced in skeletal maturation [191] and secondary sex characteristic development [89, 129]. The preceding thus suggests that successful young male swimmers are advanced in maturation compared with swimming peers. This trend seems to continue at more elite levels. After about 14–15 years of age, swimmers in the U.S. Swimming select camp program [200, 201],

FIGURE 13.4

Statures and weights of male swimmers from the Americas (left), Western Europe (center), and Eastern Europe (right). Individual points: Americas [52, 131, 147, 197, 203]; Western Europe [36, 56, 110, 123]; Eastern Europe [146, 174].

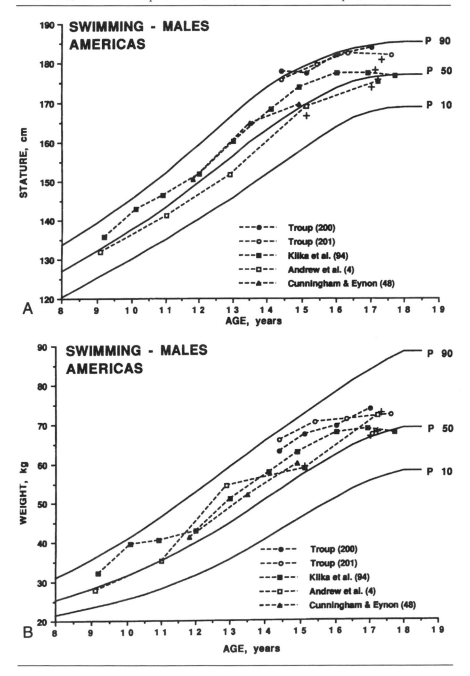

FIGURE 13.4 *(continued)*

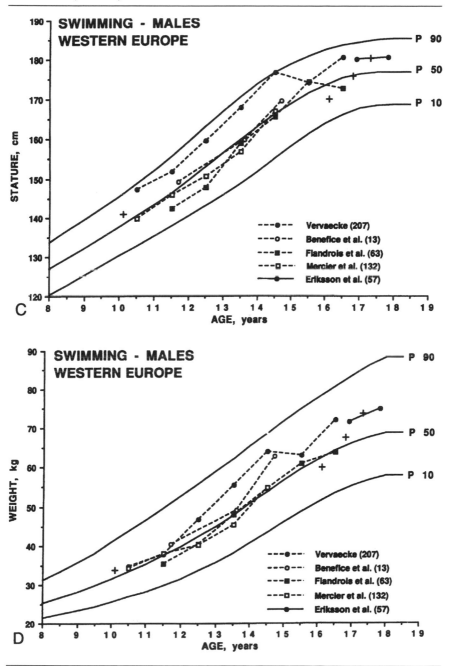

FIGURE 13.4 *(continued)*

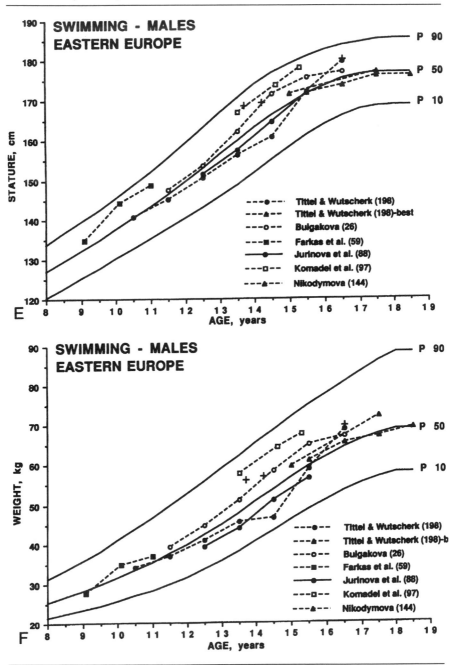

elite Belgian swimmers [207], and a small sample of Olympic swimmers under 18 years of age [120] were advanced in skeletal maturation.

FEMALES. Mean statures of female swimmers from the Americas are at and generally above P 50, while nationally select U.S. swimmers [200, 201] have statures at or just below P 90 (Fig. 13.5, *left*). In contrast, body weights are somewhat less variable and cluster at and above P 50. The nationally select U.S. swimmers do not have weights that clearly distinguish them from other samples.

Statures and weights of Western European age-group swimmers show a pattern similar to that observed in the Americas (Fig. 13.5, *center*). Data for Olympic swimmers from the Mexico City, Munich, and Montreal Olympic Games are included because most subjects were from Western European countries. From 14 to 18 years, Olympic [123] and elite Swedish [57, 208] swimmers tend to be taller and heavier than the other samples.

Statures of Eastern European swimmers are above and below P 50 during childhood and early adolescence and at or above P 50 after 14 years of age (Fig. 13.5, *right*). More recent samples of swimmers from Hungary [59] and Czechoslovakia [97, 146] are taller and heavier than earlier samples from these countries [60, 157] during childhood and early adolescence. A Czechoslovak sample 15–18 years of age from the early 1950s [144] had statures at P 50 and weights above P 50. This early sample is shorter than more recent ones, but has a similar body weight. Age-group swimmers from the Soviet Union [26] are taller and heavier than those from East Germany [198].

Several samples of Japanese female swimmers [127, 139, 145] present statures that are at or above the Japanese reference mean and weights that are generally above the mean.

In early adolescence, about 10–13 years, female swimmers tend to have SAs appropriate for their CAs, and most are classified in the average category [142, 143, 189, 190]. Studies that treat swimmers of a wider age range as a single group show similar results [25, 151, 183]. Elite Belgian swimmers with mean CAs between 13.9 and 15.3 years had SAs that were delayed by about 0.5 year, though within the average range [207]. On the other hand, 12 swimmers under 16 years of age at the Montreal Olympic Games (1976) were advanced in SA by about 0.5–0.7 years [120]. Participants in the U.S. select camp program, 13–17 years, showed variable results. Swimmers surveyed in 1989 had SAs that were, on average, in advance of CAs by about 0.7 years [200], while those surveyed in 1990 had SAs that were, on average, about equivalent to CAs, except for the 13-year-old group, in whom SA was advanced [201]. In contrast, maturity assessments for female participants in the XII Central American Swimming Championships (1981) indicated advanced SA from about 9–14 years and then delayed SA from about 14–17 years [162].

The skeletal maturity data, though somewhat variable, suggest that most female age-group swimmers are average or advanced in SA relative to CA.

FIGURE 13.5

Statures and weights of female swimmers from the Americas (left), *Western Europe* (center), *and Eastern Europe* (right). *Individual points: Americas [131, 197]; Western Europe [15, 36, 149, 160, 208]; Eastern Europe [97, 146].*

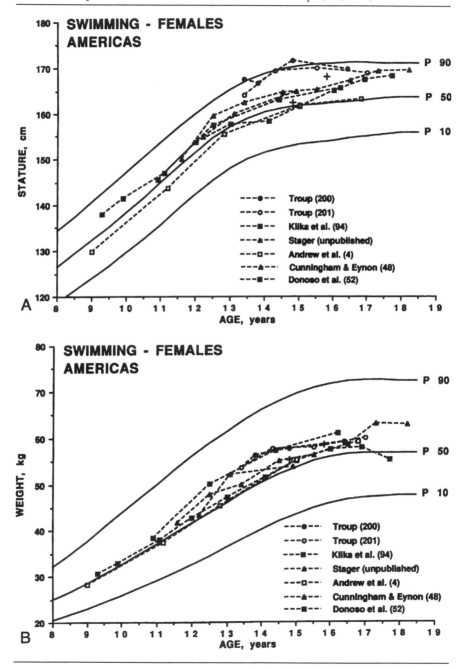

FIGURE 13.5 *(continued)*

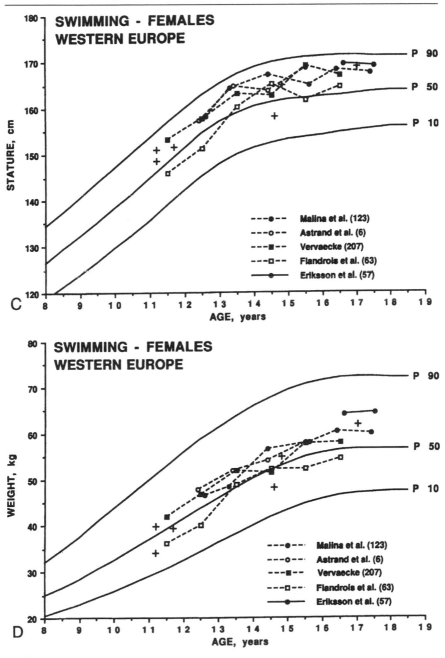

FIGURE 13.5 *(continued)*

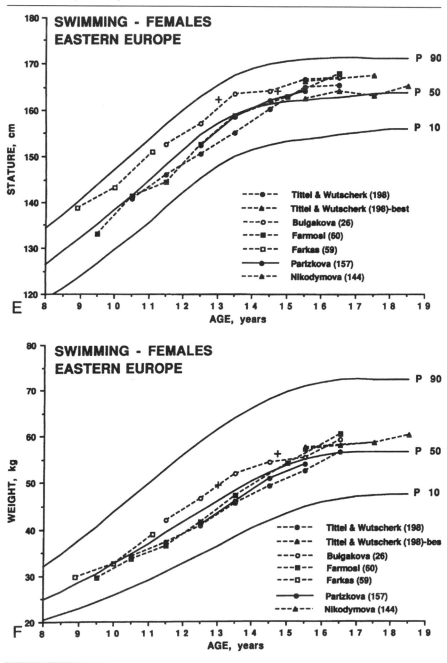

Less extensive data for secondary sex characteristics indicate similar breast and pubic hair development in age-group swimmers 8–15 years and nonswimmers [15, 129]. Estimated median ages at menarche (probit) for status quo samples of age-group swimmers from several elite programs in California, Indiana, and Texas and for an independent sample in Austin, Texas, were 13.1 ± 1.1 years and 12.7 ± 1.1 years, respectively (Malina, unpublished), which are similar to the median age for the general U.S. population. In an early study of 30 elite Swedish swimmers 11.9–16.4 years, all but one girl (12.3 years) attained menarche; the age at menarche for the remaining 29 was 12.9 ± 1.1 years [6]. On the other hand, more recent retrospective estimates of age at menarche in elite university swimmers are considerably later, 14.3 and 14.4 years [113, 181]. This issue is discussed later in the review.

Among age-group swimmers under 12 years, the more successful tended to be advanced in SA [191] and more mature in breast and pubic hair development [9]. On the other hand, in small samples (n=7 per group) of national and junior national qualifiers 15–18 years of age, the former had slightly lower breast and pubic hair ratings than the latter, even though the national qualifiers were older by 0.4 years [129].

Diving

Mean statures of male U.S. Junior Olympic divers are consistently below P 50 from 11–18 years, while weights are below P 50 from 11–15 years and at P 50 from 16–18 years [122]. A combined sample of U.S., Canadian, and Mexican junior national team members [179] has similar statures and weights, except in the oldest age group, when they are shorter and lighter. Among females, mean statures of U.S. Junior Olympic divers are slightly but consistently below P 50 [122]. Weights are also slightly below P 50 from 10–14 years, but are at P 50 from 15–18 years. The combined sample of U.S., Canadian, and Mexican junior national team members [129] are shorter than U.S. divers but have similar body weights. Single-year growth velocities for statures of both male and female Junior Olympic divers were within the range of reference data, and the estimated median age at menarche (probit) was 13.6 years ± 1.1 years [122].

Gymnastics

MALES. Statures of male gymnasts tend to cluster around P 10 of the reference data, while weights, with one exception, vary between P 50 and P 10 (Fig. 13.6, *left*). SAs are plotted relative to CAs for several samples of gymnasts in Figure 13.7 (*top*). The trend indicates no clear pattern in childhood, 6–8 years [70], but a delay of 1–2 years during adolescence [69, 91, 154]. The SA-CA difference also appears to be rather constant during this time. Data on secondary sex characteristics are consistent with those for skeletal maturation [24, 219].

FIGURE 13.6

Statures and weights of male gymnasts (left) and female gymnasts from Europe (center) and the Americas (right). Individual points: males [5, 22, 69, 86, 131, 154, 156, 174]; females, Europe [15, 58, 149, 180, 190, 206, 220]; females, Americas [5, 22, 33, 80, 106, 131, 140, 215].

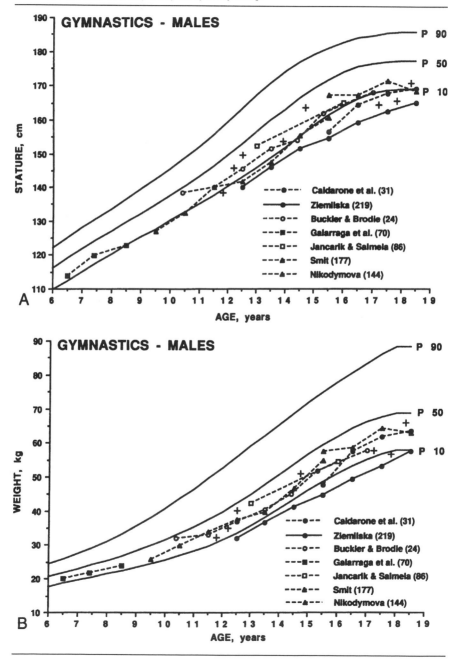

FIGURE 13.6 *(continued)*

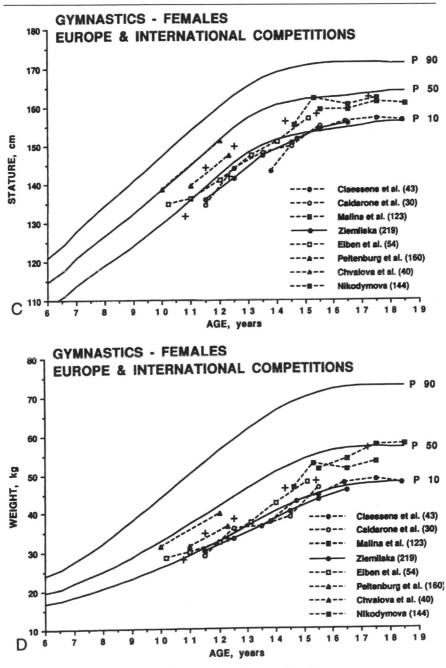

FIGURE 13.6 *(continued)*

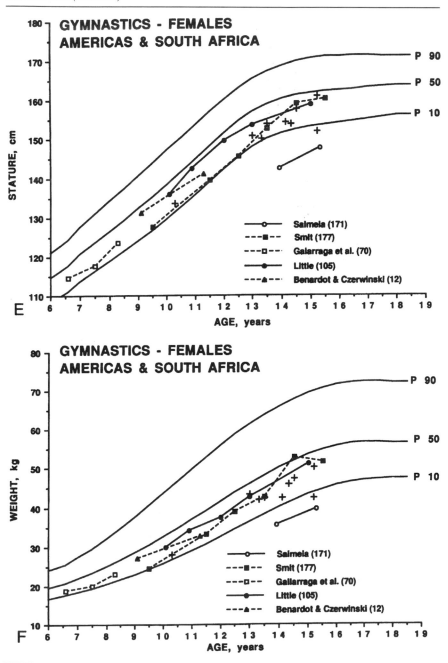

FIGURE 13.7
Skeletal age versus chronological age in male (top) and female (bottom) gymnasts.

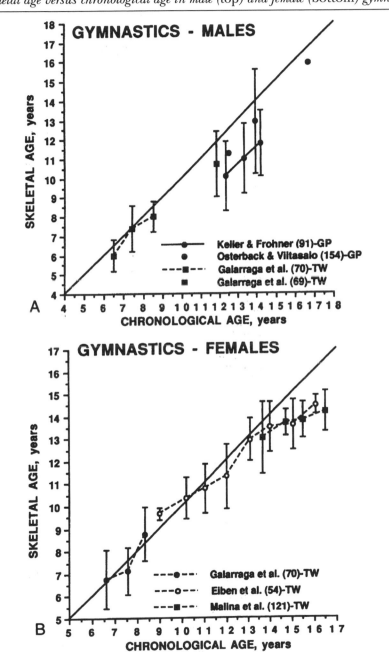

FEMALES. Data for female gymnasts are more extensive; the data are grouped for convenience: Europeans and samples from international competitions, and the Americas and South Africa. Statures and weights of gymnasts in international competitions and from Europe vary between P 50 and P 10, but most are nearer P 10 (Fig. 13.6, *center*). The earliest data are from the 1950s [144] and participants in the Mexico City, Munich, and Montreal Olympic Games, 1968–1976 [123]. More recent samples of gymnasts of the same age, 14–18 years, are shorter and lighter. This is especially apparent in participants in the 1987 world championships [43], who have statures and weights that fall on P 10. A secular trend toward smaller statures and lighter weights has thus occurred in samples of world class female gymnasts.

Statures and weights of gymnasts from the Americas and South Africa also vary between P 50 and P 10, with the exception of a small sample of elite Canadian gymnasts [171] who are well below P 10 (Fig. 13.6, *right*). In contrast to European gymnasts, statures and weights of gymnasts from the Americas do not cluster at P 10.

The skeletal maturation of female gymnasts shows a pattern similar to that for males (Fig. 13.7, *bottom*). Cross-sectional data indicate no clear pattern of SA-CA differences during childhood, 6–10 years [54, 70]. Subsequently, SA tends to lag relative to CA through about 16 years [54, 121, 189, 190]. Note that skeletal maturity of females is attained at 16.0 years in the TW method. Athletes who have already attained skeletal maturity are not included in the calculations; they are simply classified as adult. SAs of gymnasts older than 16–18 years also tend to be delayed, but group statistics are biased by the exclusion of those who already are skeletally mature [121]. In contrast, a sample of 24 Czechoslovak gymnasts observed at 12.4 and 16.5 years had SAs (local adaptation of the GP method) that were equivalent to CAs on each occasion [150].

Data on breast and pubic hair development of gymnasts are consistent with those for skeletal maturation [15, 160, 219], and more talented gymnasts are more delayed in sexual maturation than those at the local club level [160]. Age at menarche is also quite late. Prospective studies of highly trained Polish (n=9) and Swiss (n=11) gymnasts gave mean ages at menarche of 15.1 ± 0.9 [219] and 14.5 ± 1.2 [190] years, respectively. Status quo estimates for Hungarian gymnasts [54] and participants at the 1987 world championships [43] were 15.0 ± 0.6 and 15.6 ± 2.1 years, respectively. The latter sample did not include girls under 13 years of age, so the estimate is likely biased toward an older age.

Tennis

Statures of young male Italian [50], Finnish [134], and U.S. [28] tennis players tend to be below P 50, while weights are at P 50. However, two samples of Czechoslovak players 12–13 years [40, 101] are considerably taller and also heavier. The late adolescent Chilean national players [52] are shorter than P 50, but just as heavy. In nine Finnish tennis players, SAs and CAs did not differ [134].

Data for young female tennis players are quite limited, given the popularity of the sport. Statures are generally above P 50, especially in adolescence, while weights are near P 50 [28, 40, 52, 101, 187]. A sample of Czechoslovak tennis players (n=14) observed at 14.3 and 17.1 years had SAs that did not differ from their CAs on each occasion [150].

Figure Skating
Young figure skaters of both sexes tend to have statures and weights that are well below the respective reference medians, males [97, 167, 214] more than females [52, 68, 97, 100, 167, 169, 176, 214]. Four of the five samples of males have statures at or below P 10. Evidence from gonadal hormone assays in both sexes [214], and skeletal and sexual maturation in girls [150, 151] indicates later maturation in figure skaters.

Skiing
Statures and weights of male skiers vary about the respective reference medians [38, 52, 97, 159, 168, 178, 182]. In contrast, statures of female skiers are generally above the median, while weights are at the median [97, 159, 182], with the exception of the 10- and 17-year-old samples of Canadian skiers [168, 216], who are consistently shorter and lighter. Growth rates for stature (cm/yr) and weight (kg/yr) of Finnish skiers 10–14 years of age followed over two years were similar to local control subjects [159].

Cycling
Statures of male cyclists are variable, especially in late adolescence (Fig. 13.8). However, longitudinal samples from Czechoslovakia [99, 164] and Denmark [66] are above P 50 and taller than cross-sectional samples from Belgium [209, 212], who are at or below P 50. Body weights are less variable, and most cluster about P 50, although the three longitudinal samples are slightly heavier throughout. Cyclists of the Chilean national team [52] are the shortest, especially in late adolescence, but they have similar weights.

Six select Czechoslovak cyclists followed longitudinally from 12 to 15 years had SAs that were consistently advanced relative to CAs, and an earlier estimated age at PHV, 12.9 ± 0.4 years [99]. In contrast, cross-sectional samples of Belgian cyclists had equivalent SAs and CAs [210].

Rowing/Canoeing
Limited data for males indicate statures and weights greater than the respective reference medians [52, 97, 99, 216, 218]. Eleven select Czechoslovak rowers followed longitudinally from 12 to 15 years had SAs in advance of CAs, and the degree of advancement increased with age [99]. Their estimated age at PHV, 13.5 ± 0.5 years, was earlier than in control subjects by about one year. Mixed-longitudinal data for Polish female

FIGURE 13.8
Statures and weights of male cyclists.

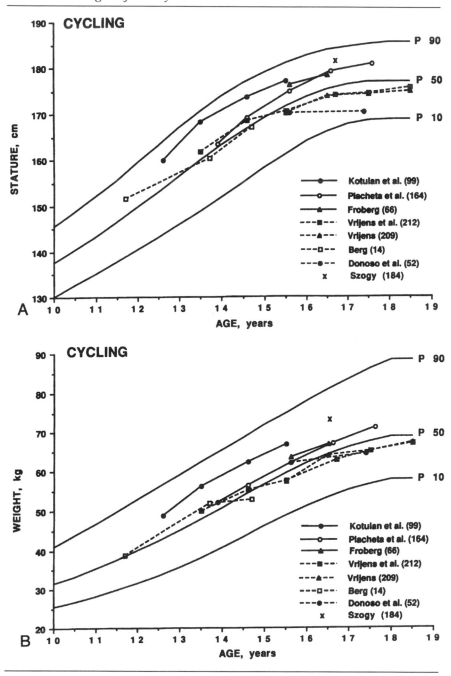

rowers 11–14 years enrolled in a sports school are similar to those for males, i.e., taller and heavier than the respective reference medians (Malina, unpublished).

Wrestling

The limited data for prepubescent wrestlers are variable [44, 170]. Mixed-longitudinal data for Polish boys 11–14 years, in a sports school, indicate statures and weights greater than the respective reference medians (Malina, unpublished). In contrast, cross-sectional data for U.S. wrestlers 14–18 years indicate statures that are generally less than P 50 and weights that are at or below P 50 [46, 83, 90, 186, 196]. Finnish wrestlers were delayed in SA, and the delay was greater in younger (CA 12.1 years, SA-CA = –0.9 years) than in older (15.7 years, SA-CA = –0.3 years) wrestlers [154].

Weight Lifting

Statures of weight lifters 13–18 years are slightly below P 50 in early adolescence, but move toward P 10 in late adolescence [39, 64, 133, 135, 199]. In contrast, body weights, with few exceptions, are generally above the reference median. SAs of four 12-year-old Finnish weight lifters were delayed by about 0.5 years [135].

Ballet

FEMALES. Data for children and youth training in ballet are available primarily for females (Fig. 13.9). Statures of Yugoslav and U.S. dancers are near P 50, while those of younger Belgian dancers are below P 50, and that of older dancers is at P 50. In contrast, weights are below P 50, approximating P 10 at some ages. Late adolescent U.S. dancers have weights at P 10. The data of Warren [213] for select dancers (which are reported only graphically) indicate a similar pattern.

Maturation data for female ballet dancers are variable. Among a select group of Belgian ballerinas 11.8–13.6 years of age, 19 of 22 dancers had TW SAs that were within ± 1 year of CAs [41]. In contrast, 15 dancers, 12–15 years of age, training to become professional dancers in New York had SAs (method not specified) classified as delayed [213]. Only one of the 22 Belgian dancers had attained menarche [41]. Prospective data for the New York dancers indicated a mean age at menarche of 15.4 ± 1.9 years [213]. The New York sample was also quite delayed in breast and pubic hair development. Status quo estimates for two samples attending ballet schools in Novi Sad, Yugoslovia, gave median menarcheal ages of 13.6 and 14.1 years, which were later than local reference data by about one year [71, 72].

MALES. Small samples of Belgian (n=8) and U.S. (n=7) male ballet dancers 12–15 years of age had mean statures and weights below the reference medians [Claessens and Beunen, unpublished; 81, 82]. Four Belgian dancers (18.1 years) had a mean stature at P 50 but a mean weight at P 10, while U.S. dancers 16.7 (n=10) and 18.8 (n=11) years had statures

FIGURE 13.9
Statures and weights of female ballet dancers.

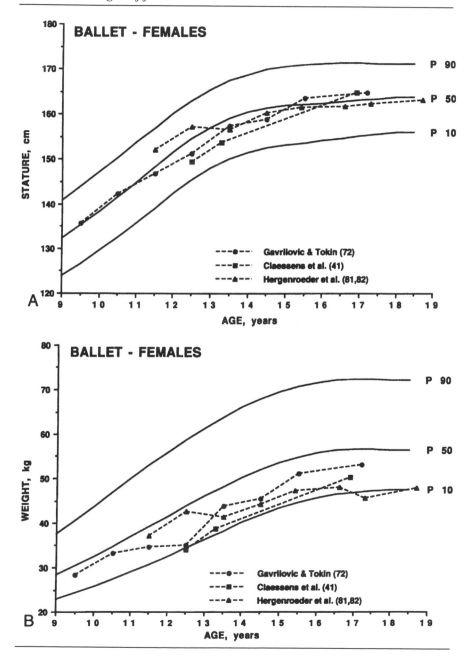

and weights at and above the respective medians. Six of the eight Belgian dancers had SAs (TW) within ± 1 year of CAs.

DOES TRAINING FOR SPORT INFLUENCE GROWTH AND MATURATION?

It is often assumed that regular physical activity, including training for sport, is important to support normal growth and maturation. Some have suggested that sport training may have a stimulatory or accelerating influence on growth and sexual maturation; more often, however, concern is expressed about potential negative influences of intensive training on growth and maturation, moreso in females than in males [114]. Others have suggested that regular training in swimming, track, ballet, and speed skating before menarche causes the late sexual maturation in these athletes [35, 65, 76, 213]. Concern about the potential influence of training for sport on the sexual maturation of girls was highlighted in a recent report of the American Medical Association and the American Dietetic Association [3, p. 4] which cautions:

> Some fitness programs may be detrimental to adolescents if they mandate prolonged, strenuous exercise and/or very low body fat to maximize their competitive edge . . . These regimes may delay sexual maturation, decrease bone growth and ultimate height. . .

In light of these views, how can the available data for young athletes in a variety of sports be interpreted?

GROWTH IN STATURE. Gymnastics is the only sport that presents a profile of short stature in both sexes. Figures skaters of both sexes and male divers and weight lifters also present, on average, short statures, though data are not extensive. Some samples of female ballet dancers indicate shorter stature during early adolescence, but late adolescent statures do not differ from the reference median. On the other hand, athletes of both sexes in other sports have, on average, statures that equal or exceed the reference median. And, in many of these sports, training is as intense as, or more intense than, training in gymnastics, figure skating, and ballet.

The data for gymnasts must be considered in the context of extremely selective criteria applied to this sport, including selection at an early age for small body size and physique characteristics associated with later maturation [8, 79]. The short stature of gymnasts is also familial. Their parents are significantly shorter than those of swimmers and nonathletes [161, 189]. Retrospective growth data also indicate that select gymnasts had statures that were about one standard deviation score below average by 2 years of age, long before they were nationally selected; recreational and locally select gymnasts were also smaller, about one-half of a standard deviation score, by 2 years of age [161]. The short stature is also related to later skeletal and sexual maturation; data on the age at PHV for gymnasts are not available. Longitudinal observations on elite East German male gymnasts from 12 to 14 years indicate similar gains in SA, CA, and stature, leading the authors to conclude that the delayed growth and maturation are "more a sequelae of selecting than caused by the influence of sports activities" [91, p. 18]. It is thus difficult to implicate the stress of training as the causative factor in the slower growth and smaller size of gymnasts.

Diet is a potentially confounding factor. For example, young East German female gymnasts were on a dietary regime "intended to maintain the optimal body weight, i.e., a slightly negative energy balance, and thus (had) a limited energy depot over a long period" [85, p. 98]. This may be chronic mild undernutrition. Other factors that may interact with marginal caloric status and perhaps altered eating habits merit closer attention. These may include the psychological and emotional stress associated with maintaining body weight when the natural course of growth is to gain, year-long training (often before school in the morning and after school in the late afternoon), frequent competitions, altered social relationships with peers, and perhaps overbearing and demanding coaches.

Gymnasts of both sexes are often described as having relatively short legs for their stature [24] or as having been selected for short limbs [85]. It is also suggested that growth rate of leg length is stunted in highly trained gymnasts [8, 190], leading to disproportionately short legs and short stature. However, cross-sectional data for several samples of male and female gymnasts, including three from international competitions, indicate sitting height/stature ratios that are quite similar to reference data for European and American white youth [30, 31, 43, 123, 219]. Although gymnasts are absolutely shorter, the results suggest similar proportional relationships of the legs and trunk relative to nonathletes. Longitudinal data that span late childhood through late adolescence are necessary to satisfactorily address this issue.

The size attained by athletes of both sexes in other sports does not appear to be affected by intensive training. Available longitudinal studies indicate mean statures that maintain their position relative to the reference values over time, and several short-term studies indicate growth rates in stature that are within the range of rates observed in the nonathlete population [115, 122, 159, 173].

MATURATION. Short-term longitudinal studies of boys and girls in several sports [91, 99, 150, 172] indicate similar gains in both SA and CA, which would imply no effect of training on skeletal maturation. Although methods for estimating PHV vary, the available data indicate no effect of training on the age at PHV in boys in several sports [11, 67, 95, 99, 114]. There are presently no corresponding estimates of age at PHV of young female athletes.

Sexual maturation data are more available for young female than male athletes. The data, however, are largely cross-sectional, so inferences about the effects of training are hazardous. Prospective studies of female gymnasts [190, 219] and ballet dancers [213] indicate later ages at menarche. Status quo estimate for Hungarian [54] and world class [43] gymnasts give a similar late age at menarche, while those for girls in Yugoslav ballet schools [71, 72] are earlier. The late menarche and late attainment of adult stature in select ballet dancers [213] is similar to the pattern of growth characteristic of late-maturing children [119]. Like gymnastics, ballet has rigid selection criteria that place an emphasis on thinness and linearity [78], and significant numbers of young ballerinas have eating problems [76].

Later mean ages at menarche are commonly reported for late adolescent and adult athletes [16, 18, 111, 113, 119]. Standard deviations are about one year or more; hence, it is important to note that not all athletes experience menarche late. These data are retrospective and are thus limited to some extent by error of recall. Status quo data for Hungarian [54] and world class [43] gymnasts and Junior Olympic divers [122] are generally consistent with the retrospective data, but status quo estimates for track athletes [61] and age-group swimmers (Malina, unpublished) are earlier than retrospective estimates. It is especially evident in swimmers. Data for young swimmers, Olympic swimmers, and national level swimmers from several countries, collected in the 1950s–1970s, indicate mean ages at menarche that approximate the mean of the general population [111]; however, university level swimmers from elite programs in the U.S. in the mid-1980s had mean ages at menarche of 14.3 and 14.4 years [113, 181]. This trend probably reflects enhanced opportunities for girls in swimming. In the 1950s–1970s, it was common for female swimmers to retire by 16–17 years of age. With the advent of Title IX legislation in the U.S., many universities added and/or improved their swim programs so that more opportunities were available. Also, later-maturing age-group swimmers, catching-up to their peers in size and strength in late adolescence, probably experienced more success in swimming and persisted in the sport. Another factor may be change in the size and physique of female swimmers. A comparison of university level female swimmers in the late-1980s with those in the mid-1970s indicated that the former were taller and more linear (Malina, unpublished), a physique characteristic of later maturers.

The later recalled mean ages at menarche of athletes in a variety of sports and correlations with years of training before menarche are often used to infer that training prior to menarche "delays" this physiological event. Association does not imply a cause-effect sequence between training and sexual maturation. Further, athletes who take up regular training in a sport after menarche are excluded. Other factors known to influence menarche also need to be considered. For example, there is a familial tendency for later maturation in athletes. Mothers of ballet dancers [23] and university level athletes in several sports [125] attain menarche later than mothers of nonathletes, and sisters of elite swimmers [181] and university athletes [125] attain menarche later than average. Ages at menarche of the mothers and sisters are not as late as those of the athletes. Mother-daughter and sister-sister correlations in families of athletes are similar to those for the general population [125]. Another factor is number of siblings in the family. Girls from larger families tend to attain menarche later than those from smaller families, and the estimated magnitude of the sibling number effect is similar in athletes and nonathletes [113].

In adequately nourished individuals, sexual maturation is a genotypically mediated process. Linearity of physique is associated with later maturation in both sexes, and some sports select for this characteristic of body build. Dietary practices associated with an emphasis on thinness or an optimal weight for performance may possibly influence growth and maturation, especially if they involve energy deficiency for prolonged periods. The demands of training compete with those of growth and maturational processes for available energy. Psychological and emotional stresses associated with training and competition are additional concerns. Nevertheless, if training for sport is related to later menarche, it most likely interacts with or is confounded by other factors, so that the specific effect of training per se may be impossible to extract. In the vast majority of athletes, intensive training for sport has no effect on growth and maturational processes.

ACKNOWLEDGMENTS

I would like to thank the following colleagues for providing raw data and/or unpublished data for use in this review: Gaston Beunen and Albrecht Claessens of the Catholic University of Leuven, Claude Bouchard of Laval University, Albert Hergenroeder and William Klish of the Baylor College of Medicine, Georges Lariviere of the University of Montreal, Michael Little of the State University of New York at Binghamton, and Joel Stager of Indiana University.

REFERENCES

1. Adrian, M. J., and L. A. dos Anjos. Comparison of physical characteristics between young female basketball players and cross-country runners. In M. J. Adrian (ed). *Sports Women.* Basel: Karger, 1987, pp. 30–39.
2. Alabin, V., and T. Yushkevitch. Talent selection in the sprint. *Legkaya Atletika* 5:15, 1978 (reprinted in *Sov. Sports Rev.* 16:34–35, 1981).
3. American Medical Association/American Dietetic Association. *Targets for Adolescent Health: Nutrition and Physical Fitness.* Chicago: American Medical Association, 1991.
4. Andrew, G. M., M. R. Becklake, J. S. Guleria, and D. V. Bates. Heart and lung functions in swimmers and nonathletes during growth. *J. Appl. Physiol.* 32:245–251, 1972.

5. Araujo, C. G. S., and Moutinho, M. F. C. S. Somatotipo e composicao corporal de ginastas olimpicos adolescentes. *Caderno Artus de Medicina Desportiva* (Rio de Janiero) 1:39–42, 1978.

6. Astrand, P. -O., L. Engstrom, B. O. Eriksson, P. Karlberg, I. Nylander, et al. Girls swimmers, with special reference to respiratory and circulatory adaptation and gynaecological and psychiatric aspects. *Acta Paediatr.* Suppl. 147:1–75, 1963.

7. Atomi, Y., Y. Kuroda, T. Asami, and T. Kawahara. HDL_2-cholesterol of children (10 to 12 years of age) related to VO_2 max, body fat, and sex. J. Rutenfranz, R. Mocellin, and F. Klimt (eds). *Children and Exercise XII.* Champaign, IL: Human Kinetics, 1986, pp. 167–172.

8. Bajin, B. Talent identification program for Canadian female gymnasts. B. Petiot, J. H. Salmela, and T. B. Hoshizaki (eds). *World Identification for Gymnastic Talent.* Montreal: Sports Psyche Editions, 1987, pp. 34–44.

9. Bar-Or, O. Predicting athletic performance. *Physician Sportsmed.* 3:81–85, 1975.

10. Bell, W. Physiological characteristics of 12-year-old soccer players. T. Reilly, A. Lees, K. Davids, and W. J. Murphy (eds). *Science and Football.* London: Spon, 1988, pp. 175–180.

11. Bell, W. Body size and shape: a longitudinal investigation of active and sedentary boys during adolescence. *J. Sports Sci.* 11:127–138, 1993.

12. Benardot, D., and C. Czerwinski. Selected body composition and growth measures of junior elite gymnasts. *J. Am. Diet. Assoc.* 91:29–33, 1991.

13. Benefice, E., J. Mercier, M. J. Guerin, and C. Prefaut. Differences in aerobic and anthropometric characteristics between peripubertal swimmers and non-swimmers. *Int. J. Sports Med.* 11:456–460, 1990.

14. Berg, K. Body composition and nutrition of adolescent boys training for bicycle racing. *Nutr. Metab.* 14:172–180, 1972.

15. Bernink, M. J. E., W. B. M. Erich, A. L. Peltenburg, M. L. Zonderland, and I. A. Huisveld. Height, body composition, biological maturation and training in relation to socioeconomic status in girl gymnasts, swimmers, and controls. *Growth* 47:1–12, 1983.

16. Beunen, G. Biological age in pediatric exercise research. O. Bar-Or (ed). *Advances in Pediatric Sport Sciences. Vol. 3. Biological Issues.* Champaign, IL: Human Kinetics, 1989, pp. 1–19.

17. Beunen, G., and R. M. Malina. Growth and physical performance relative to the timing of the adolescent spurt. *Exerc. Sport Sci. Rev.* 16:503–540, 1988.

18. Beunen, G., and R. M. Malina. Growth and biological maturation: Relevance to athletic performance. O. Bar-Or (ed). *The Encyclopedia of Sports Medicine: The Child and Adolescent Athlete.* Oxford: Blackwell Scientific Publications (in press).

19. Beunen, G., R. M. Malina, A. Claessens, and R. Wellens. Skeletale maturiteit en lichaamsafmetingen bij jonge Belgische atletiekbeoefenaars. *Hermes (Leuven)* 20:157–169, 1989.

20. Bouchard, C., F. Landry, C. Leblanc, and J. -C. Mondor. Quelques-unes des caracteristiques physiques et physiologiques des joueurs de hockey et leurs relations avec la performance. *Mouvement* 9:95–110, 1974.

21. Bouchard, C., and B. Roy. L'age osseux des jeunes participants du Tournoi International de Hockey Pee-Wee de Quebec. *Mouvement* 4:225–232, 1969.

22. Broekhoff, J., A. Nadgir, and W. Pieter. Morphological differences between young gymnasts and non-athletes matched for age and gender. T. Reilly, J. Watkins, and J. Borms (eds). *Kinanthropometry III.* London: Spon, 1986, pp. 204–210.

23. Brooks-Gunn, J., and M. P. Warren. Mother-daughter differences in menarcheal age in adolescent girls attending national dance company schools and non-dancers. *Ann. Hum. Biol.* 15:35–43, 1988.

24. Buckler, J. M. H., and D. A. Brodie. Growth and maturity characteristics of schoolboy gymnasts. *Ann. Hum. Biol.* 4:455–463, 1977.

25. Bugyi, B., and I. Kausz. Radiographic determination of the skeletal age of the young swimmers. *J. Sports Med. Phys. Fitness* 10:269–270, 1970.

26. Bulgakova, N. Z. *Selection and Training of Young Swimmers.* Moscow: Physical Culture and Sports, 1978.

27. Burke, E. J., and F. Brush. Physiological and anthropometric assessment of successful teenage female distance runners. *Res. Q.* 50:180–187, 1979.

28. Buti, T., B. Elliot, and A. Morton. Physiological and anthropometric profiles of elite prepubescent tennis players. *Physician Sportsmed.* 12:111–116, 1984.

29. Cacciari, E., L. Mazzanti, D. Tassinari, R. Bergamaschi, C. Magnani, et al. Effects of sport (football) on growth: auxological, anthropometric and hormonal aspects. *Eur. J. Appl. Physiol.* 61:149–158, 1990.

30. Caldarone, G., M. Leglise, M. Giampietro, and G. Berlutti. Anthropometric measurements, body composition, biological maturation and growth predictions in young female gymnasts of high agonistic level. *J. Sports Med.* 26:263–273, 1986.

31. Caldarone, G., M. Leglise, M. Giampietro, and G. Berlutti. Anthropometric measurements, body composition, biological maturation and growth predictions in young male gymnasts of high agonistic level. *J. Sports Med.* 26:406–415, 1986.

32. Carter, J. E. L. Somatotypes of children in sports. R. M. Malina (ed). *Young Athletes: Biological, Psychological, and Educational Perspectives.* Champaign, IL: Human Kinetics, 1988, pp. 153–165.

33. Carter, J. E. L., and R. M. Brallier. Physiques of specially selected young female gymnasts. R. M. Malina (ed). *Young Athletes: Biological, Psychological, and Educational Perspectives.* Champaign, IL: Human Kinetics, 1988, pp. 167–175.

34. Carter, J. E. L., and B. H. Heath. *Somatotyping: Development and Applications.* Cambridge: Cambridge University Press, 1990.

35. Casey, M. J., E. C. Jones, C. Foster, and M. L. Pollock. Effect of the onset and intensity of training on menarchal age and menstrual irregularity among elite speedskaters. D. M. Landers (ed). *Sport and Elite Performers.* Champaign, IL: Human Kinetics, 1986, pp. 33–44.

36. Chatard, J. C., J. M. Lavoie, B. Bourgoin, and J. R. Lacour. The contribution of passive drag as a determinant of swimming performance. *Int. J. Sports Med.* 11:367–372, 1990.

37. Chen, J. D. Growth, exercise, nutrition and fitness in China. R. J. Shephard and J. Parizkova (eds). *Human Growth, Physical Fitness and Nutrition.* Basel: Karger, 1991, pp. 19–32.

38. Chovanova, E. Problematika vyberu talentovanych lyziarov-zjazdarov zo somatickeho hladiska. *Teor. Praxe Tel. Vych.* 29:212–218, 1981.

39. Chovanova, E., L. Pataki, and D. Vavrovic. Somatotypologicka charakteristika mladych vzpieracov. *Teor. Praxe Tel. Vych.* 31:32–35, 1983.

40. Chvalova, O., J. Chytrackova, and V. Kasalicka. Vysledky mereni somatotypy u mladych tenistu. *Teor. Praxe Tel. Vych.* 36:211–215, 1988.

41. Claessens, A. L., G. P. Beunen, M. M. Nuyts, J. A. Lefevre, and R. E. Wellens. Body structure, somatotype, maturation and motor performance of girls in ballet schooling. *J. Sports Med.* 27:310–317, 1987.

42. Claessens, A., J. Boutmans, and G. Beunen. Body structure, somatotype, and motor fitness of young Belgian basketball players of different competitive levels. *Anthrop. Kozl.* 30:227–231, 1986.

43. Claessens, A. L., R. M. Malina, J. Lefevre, G. Beunen, V. Stijnen, et al. Growth and menarcheal status of elite female gymnasts. *Med. Sci. Sports Exerc.* 24:755–763, 1992.

44. Clarke, D. H., P. Vaccaro, and N. M. Andresen. Physiological alterations in 7- to 9-year-old boys following a season of competitive wrestling. *Res. Q. Exerc. Sport* 55:318–322, 1984.

45. Clarke, H. H. *Physical and Motor Tests in the Medford Boys' Growth Study.* Englewood Cliffs, NJ: Prentice-Hall, 1971.

46. Clarke, K. C. Predicting certified weight of young wrestlers: A field study of the Tcheng-Tipton method. *Med. Sci. Sports* 6:52–57, 1974.

47. Cumming, G. R. Correlation of athletic performance and aerobic power in 12 to 17 year old children with bone age, calf muscle, total body potassium, heart volume and two

indices of anaerobic power. O. Bar-Or (ed). *Pediatric Work Physiology.* Nantaya, Israel: Wingate Institute for Physical Education and Sport, 1973, pp. 109–134.

48. Cunningham, D. A., and R. B. Eynon. The working capacity of young competitive swimmers, 10–16 years of age. *Med. Sci. Sports* 5:227–231, 1973.
49. Cunningham, D. A., P. Telford, and G. T. Swart. The cardiopulmonary capacities of young hockey players: age 10. *Med. Sci. Sports* 8:23–25, 1976.
50. Dal Monte, A., L. M. Leonardi, F. Sardella, M. Faina, and P. Gallippi. Evaluation test of the alternate aerobic-anaerobic potential in subjects at development age. L. Vecchiet (ed). *1st International Congress on Sports Medicine Applied to Football, Proceedings Vol. II.* Rome: D. Guanella, 1980, pp. 788–794.
51. Daniels, J., and N. Oldridge. Changes in oxygen consumption of young boys during growth and running training. *Med. Sci. Sports* 3:161–165, 1971.
52. Donoso, H., G. Quintana, A. Rodriguez, J. Huberman, M. Holz, and G. Godoy. Algunas caracteristicas antropometricas y maximo consumo de oxigeno en 368 deportistas seleccionados Chilenos. *Arch. Soc. Chilena Med.* 25:7–17, 1980.
53. Dulac, S., G. Lariviere, and M. Boulay. Relations entre diverses mesures physiologiques et la performance a des tests de patinage. F. Landry and W. A. R. Orban (eds). *Ice Hockey.* Miami: Symposia Specialists, 1978, pp. 55–63.
54. Eiben, O. G., E. Panto, G. Gyenis, and J. Frohlich. Physique of young female gymnasts. *Anthrop. Kozl.* 30:209–220, 1986.
55. Elovainio, R., and S. Sundberg. A five year follow-up study on cardiorespiratory function in adolescent elite endurance runners. *Acta Paediatr. Scand.* 72:351–356, 1983.
56. Eriksson, B. O., K. Berg, and J. Taranger. Physiological analysis of young boys starting intensive training in swimming. B. Eriksson and B. Furberg (eds). *Swimming Medicine IV.* Baltimore: University Park Press, 1978, pp. 147–160.
57. Eriksson, B. O., I. Holmer, and A. Lundin. Physiological effects of training in elite swimmers. B. Eriksson and B. Furberg (eds). *Swimming Medicine IV.* Baltimore: University Park Press, 1978, pp. 177–187.
58. Eston, R. G., and M. Maridaki. Body composition of trained and untrained premenarcheal girls. T. Reilly, J. Watkins, and J. Borms (eds). *Kinanthropometry III.* London: Spon, 1986, pp. 197–203.
59. Farkas, A., J. Mohacsi, and J. Meszaros. Four styles of swimming performance and anthropometry of child swimmers. S. Oseid and K. -H. Carlsen (eds). *Children and Exercise XIII.* Champaign, IL: Human Kinetics, 1989, pp. 129–134.
60. Farmosi, I. Az uszonok testalkatanak es teljesitmenyenek osszefuggese. L. Nadori (ed). *A Sport Es Testneveles Idoszeru Kerdesei, No. 23.* Budapest: Sport, 1980, pp. 77–121.
61. Farmosi, I. Data concerning the menarche age of Hungarian female athletes. *J. Sports Med.* 23:89–94, 1983.
62. Farmosi, I., and L. Nadori. If jusagi labdarugok alkati es motorikus vizsgalatanak nehany eredmenye. *Testnevelesi Foiskola Kozlemenyei* 1:173–179, 1981.
63. Flandrois, R., M. Grandmontagne, M. H. Mayet, R. Favier, and J. Frutoso. La consommation maximale d'oxygene chez le jeune francais, sa variation avec l'age, le sexe et l'entrainement. *J. Physiol. Paris* 78:186–194, 1982.
64. Fleck, S. J., P. M. Pattany, M. H. Stone, W. J. Kraemer, J. Thrush, and K. Wong. Magnetic resonance imaging determination of left ventricular mass: Junior Olympic weightlifters. *Med. Sci. Sports Exerc.* 25:522–527, 1993.
65. Frisch, R. E., A. B. Gotz-Welbergen, J. W. McArthur, T. Albright, J. Witschi, et al. Delayed menarche and amenorrhea of college athletes in relation to age of onset of training. *JAMA* 246:1559–1563, 1981.
66. Froberg, K. Prediction of performance in young competitive bicyclists. S. Oseid and K. -H. Carlsen (eds). *Children and Exercise XIII.* Champaign, IL: Human Kinetics, 1989, pp. 57–66.
67. Froberg, K., B. Andersen, and O. Lammert. Maximal oxygen uptake and respiratory functions during puberty in boy groups of different physical activity. R. Frenkl and I.

Szmodis (eds). *Children and Exercise. Pediatric Work Physiology XV.* Budapest: National Institute for Health Promotion, 1991, pp. 265–280.

68. Gaisl, G., and G. Wiesspeiner. Training prescriptions for 9- to 17-year old figure skaters based on lactate assessment in the laboratory and on the ice. J. Rutenfranz, R. Mocellin, and F. Klimt (eds). *Children and Exercise XII.* Champaign, IL: Human Kinetics, 1986, pp. 59–65.

69. Galarraga, A. L., C. R. Alonso, J. Jordan, E. G. More, and O. G. Guerra. Relacion de la edad biologica con indicadores morfologicos y funcionales en ninos de 11–12 anos. *Rev. Cub. Pediatr.* 54:49–64, 1982.

70. Galarraga, A. L., I. P. Segredo, E. G. More, and O. G. Guerra. El uso de indicadores antropometricos como criterio de madurez biologica en ninos gimnastas de 6 a 8 anos de edad. *Rev. Cub. Pediatr.* 54:64–76, 1982.

71. Gavrilovic, Z. Uticaj telesne aktivnosti na vreme pojave menarhe. M. Milojevic and B. Beric (eds). *Zena i Sport.* Novi Sad, Yugoslavia: Fakultet Fizicke Kulture, OOUR Institut, Fizicke Kulture Univerziteta, 1983, pp. 53–59.

72. Gavrilovic, Z., and S. Tokin. Neke antropometrijske mere i menarha ucenica baletske skole u Novom Sad. *Zena u Fizicko Kulturi: Zbornik Radova.* Novi Sad, Yugoslavia; Fakultet Fizicke Kulture, OOUR Institut, Fizicke Kulture Univerziteta, 1983, pp. 199–206.

73. Greulich, W. W., and S. I. Pyle. *Radiographic Atlas of Skeletal Development of the Hand and Wrist, 2nd ed.* Stanford, CA: Stanford University Press, 1959.

74. Hale, C. J. Physiologic maturity of Little League baseball players. *Res. Q.* 27:276–284, 1956.

75. Hamill, P. V. V., R. A. Drizd, C. L. Johnson, R. D. Reed, and A. F. Roche. NCHS growth charts for children, birth–18 years, United States. *Vital Health Stat. Series 11,* No. 165, 1977.

76. Hamilton, L. H., J. Brooks-Gunn, M. P. Warren, and W. G. Hamilton. The role of selectivity in the pathogenesis of eating problems in ballet dancers. *Med. Sci. Sports Exerc.* 20:560–565, 1988.

77. Hamilton, P., and G. M. Andrew. Influence of growth and athletic training on heart and lung functions. *Eur. J. Appl. Physiol.* 36:27–38, 1976.

78. Hamilton, W. G. Physical prerequisites for ballet dancers: Selectivity that can enhance (or nullify) a career. *J. Musculoskel. Med.* 3:61–66, 1986.

79. Hartley, G. A comparative view of talent selection for sport in two socialist states—the USSR and the GDR—with particular reference to gymnastics. *The Growing Child in Competitive Sport.* Leeds: The National Coaching Foundation, 1988, pp. 50–56.

80. Haywood, K. M. Strength and flexibility in gymnasts before and after menarche. *Br. J. Sports Med.* 14:189–192, 1980.

81. Hergenroeder, A. C., B. Brown, and W. J. Klish. Anthropometric measurements and estimating body composition in ballet dancers. *Med. Sci. Sports Exerc.* 25:145–150, 1993.

82. Hergenroeder, A. C., M. L. Fiorotto, and W. J. Klish. Body composition in ballet dancers measured by total body electrical conductivity. *Med. Sci. Sports Exerc.* 23:528–533, 1991.

83. Housz, T. J., G. O. Johnson, R. A. Hughes, D. J. Housz, R. J. Hughes, et al. Isokinetic strength and body composition of high school wrestlers across age. *Med. Sci. Sports Exerc.* 21:105–109, 1989.

84. Housz, T. J., W. G. Thorland, G. D. Tharp, G. O. Johnson, and C. J. Cisar. Isokinetic leg flexion and extension strength of elite adolescent female track and field athletes. *Res. Q. Exerc. Sport* 55:347–350, 1984.

85. Jahreis, G., E. Kauf, G. Frohner, and H. E. Schmidt. Influence of intensive exercise on insulin-like growth factor I, thyroid and steroid hormones in female gymnasts. *Growth Regul.* 1:95–99, 1991.

86. Jancarik, A., and J. H. Salmela. Longitudinal changes in physical, organic and perceptual factors in Canadian male gymnasts. B. Petiot, J. H. Salmela, and T. B. Hoshizaki (eds). *World Identification Systems for Gymnastic Talent.* Montreal: Sport Psyche Editions, 1987, pp. 151–159.

87. Janusz, A., A. Jarosinska, and J. Steslicki. Wplyw treningu siatkarskiego na budowe ciala dziewczat. *Przegl. Antropol.* 51:139–144, 1985.

88. Jurinova, I., S. Sprynarova, and J. Cermak. Vztah mezi svalovou silou, maximalni sportrebou kysliku a velikosti srdecni u 12–15 letych plavcu. *Teor. Praxe Tel. Vych.* 23:470–474, 1975.

89. Kanitz, M., and O. Bar-Or. Relationship between anthropometric, developmental and physiological parameters and achievement in swimming in 10- to 12-year-old boys. (Abstract). *Isr. J. Med. Sci.* 10:289, 1974.

90. Katch, F. I., and Michael, E. D. Body composition of high school wrestlers according to age and wrestling weight category. *Med. Sci. Sports* 3:190–194, 1971.

91. Keller, E., and G. Frohner. Growth and development of boys with intensive training in gymnastics during puberty. Z. Laron and A. D. Rogol (eds). *Hormones and Sport.* New York: Raven Press, 1989, pp. 11–20.

92. Kirkendall, D. T. The applied sport science of soccer. *Physician Sportsmed.* 13:53–59, 1985.

93. Kiss, M. A., M. B. Rocha Ferreira, C. P. Souza, M. R. Vasconcelos, F. B. Santos, et al. Potencia maxima aerobica em atletas de selecoes Paulistas e Brasileiras. *Med. Esporte* (Porto Alegre) 1:23–30, 1973.

94. Klika, R., B. W. Meleski, and R. M. Malina. Growth and body composition of age group swimmers (in preparation).

95. Kobayashi, K., K. Kitamura, M. Miura, H. Sodeyama, Y. Murase, et al. Aerobic power as related to body growth and training in Japanese boys: a longitudinal study. *J. Appl. Physiol.* 44:666–672, 1978.

96. Kollias, J., E. R. Buskirk, E. T. Howley, and J. L. Loomis. Cardiorespiratory and body composition measurements of a select group of high school football players. *Res. Q.* 43:472–478, 1972.

97. Komadel, L., D. Hamar, and J. Kadlecik. Somaticke a funkcne charakteristiky mladeze vzhladom na vek a treningove zatazenie vo vybranych druhoch sportu. *Acta Facultatis Educationis Physicae Universitatis Comenianae,* Publicatio XXVII. Bratislava: Slovenske Pedagogicke Nakladatel'stvo, 1989, pp. 63–72.

98. Kosava, A., S. Hlatky, W. Lilge, and H. Holdhaus. Physical structure and performance of young soccer players. *Anthropol. Kozl.* 33:267–272, 1991.

99. Kotulan, J., M. Reznickova, and Z. Placheta. Exercise and growth. Z. Placheta (ed). *Youth and Physical Activity.* Brno: J. E. Purkyne University Medical Faculty, 1980, pp. 61–117.

100. Kovalcikova, J., A. Zrubak, and E. Mikulova. Antropometricka a somatotypologicka charakteristika vrcholovych sportovkyn. *Teor. Praxe Tel. Vych.* 29:152–161, 1981.

101. Kovalcikova, J., A. Zrubak, E. Mikulova, and F. Zak. Somatotypologicka charakteristikas tenistov a tenistiek TSM CSSR. *Teor. Praxe Tel. Vych.* 37:408–418, 1989.

102. Krogman, W. M. Maturation age of 55 boys in the Little League World Series, 1957. *Res. Q.* 30:54–56, 1959.

103. Lariviere, G., and A. Lafond. Physical maturity in young elite ice hockey players. *Can. J. Appl. Sport Sci.* 11:24P, 1986.

104. Lariviere, G., H. Lavallee, and R. J. Shephard. A simple skating test for ice hockey players. (Abstract). *Can. J. Appl. Sport Sci.* 1:223–228, 1976.

105. Little, M. A. Growth of girl gymnasts aged 7–17 years. Unpublished manuscript, 1986.

106. Lopez, A., and J. Rojas. Somatotype et composition du corps chez les gymnastes de haut niveau. *Cinesiologie* 18:5–18, 1979.

107. Lukyanova, R. P., and N. I. Novocelova. Physical development and physical preparation of young athletes in track and field, soccer and basketball. *Theory and Practice of Physical Culture* 6:38–41, 1964 (reprinted in *Yessis Translation Review* 2:18–22, 1967).

108. Macnab, R. B. J. A longitudinal study of ice hockey in boys aged 8–12. *Can. J. Appl. Sport Sci.* 4:11–17, 1979.

109. Maffulli, N., V. Testa, A. Lancia, G. Capasso, and S. Lombardi. Indices of sustained aerobic power in young middle distance runners. *Med. Sci. Sports Exerc.* 23:1090–1096, 1991.

110. Magel, J. R., and K. Lange Andersen. Pulmonary diffusing capacity and cardiac output in

young trained Norwegian swimmers and untrained subjects. *Med. Sci. Sports* 1:131–139, 1969.

111. Malina, R. M. Menarche in athletes: a synthesis and hypothesis. *Ann. Hum. Biol.* 10:1–24, 1983.

112. Malina, R. M. Biological maturity status of young athletes. R. M. Malina (ed). *Young Athletes: Biological, Psychological, and Educational Perspectives.* Champaign, IL: Human Kinetics, 1988, pp. 121–140.

113. Malina, R. M. Darwinian fitness, physical fitness and physical activity. C. G. N. Mascie-Taylor and G. W. Lasker (eds). *Applications of Biological Anthropology to Human Affairs.* Cambridge: Cambridge University Press, 1991, pp. 143–184.

114. Malina, R. M. Effects of habitual physical activity and training for sport on growth in stature and the adolescent growth spurt. *Med. Sci. Sports Exerc.* (accepted for publication).

115. Malina, R. M. Attained size and growth rate of female volleyball players 9–13 years of age. *Pediatr. Exerc. Sci.* (Accepted for publication).

116. Malina, R. M., and G. Beunen. Growth and maturation: Methods of monitoring. O. Bar-Or (ed). *The Encyclopedia of Sports Medicine: The Child and Adolescent Athlete.* Oxford: Blackwell Scientific Publications (in press).

117. Malina, R. M., and G. Beunen. Matching of opponents in youth sports. O. Bar-Or (ed). *The Encyclopedia of Sports Medicine: The Child and Adolescent Athlete.* Oxford: Blackwell Scientific Publications (in press).

118. Malina, R. M., G. Beunen, R. Wellens, and A. Claessens. Skeletal maturity and body size of teenage Belgian track and field athletes. *Ann. Hum. Biol.* 13:331–339, 1986.

119. Malina, R. M., and C. Bouchard. *Growth, Maturation, and Physical Activity.* Champaign, IL: Human Kinetics, 1991.

120. Malina, R. M., C. Bouchard, R. F. Shoup, A. Demirjian, and G. Lariviere. Growth and maturity status of Montreal Olympic athletes less than 18 years of age. J. E. L. Carter (ed). *Physical Structure of Olympic Athletes. Part I. The Montreal Olympic Games Anthropological Project.* Basel: Karger, 1982, pp. 117–127.

121. Malina, R. M., A. L. Claessens, J. Lefevre, G. Beunen, V. Stijnen, et al. Maturity-associated variation in the growth of elite female gymnasts. (in progress)

122. Malina, R. M., and C. A. Geithner. Background in sport, growth status, and growth rate of Junior Olympic Divers. R. M. Malina and J. L. Gabriel (eds). *United States Diving Sports Science Seminar.* 1993 Proceedings. Indianapolis, IN: U. S. Diving, 1993, pp. 26–35.

123. Malina, R. M., B. B. Little, C. Bouchard, J. E. L. Carter, P. C. R. Hughes, et al. Growth status of Olympic athletes less than 18 years of age: young athletes at the Mexico City, Munich, and Montreal Olympic Games. J. E. L. Carter (ed). *Physical Structure of Olympic Athletes. Part II. Kinanthropometry of Olympic Athletes.* Basel: Karger, 1984, pp. 183–201.

124. Malina, R. M., B. W. Meleski, and R. F. Shoup. Anthropometric, body composition, and maturity characteristics of selected school-age athletes. *Pediatr. Clin. North Am.* 29:1305–1323, 1982.

125. Malina, R. M., R. C. Ryan, and C. M. Bonci. Age at menarche in athletes and their mothers and sisters. *Ann. Hum. Biol.* (Accepted for publication).

126. Malina, R. M., and R. F. Shoup. Anthropometric and physique characteristics of female volleyball players at three competitive levels. *Humanbiol. Budapest.* 16:105–112, 1985.

127. Matsui, H., Miyashita, M., Miura, M., Kobayashi, K., Hoshikawa, T., and Kamei, S. Maximum oxygen uptake and its relationship to body weight of Japanese adolescents. *Med. Sci. Sports* 4:27–32, 1972.

128. Mazzanti, L., D. Tassinari, R. Bergamaschi, G. Nanni, C. Magnani, et al. Hormonal, auxological and anthropometric aspects in young football players. In J. R. Bierich, E. Cacciari, and S. Raiti (eds). *Growth Abnormalities.* New York: Raven Press, 1989, pp. 363–369.

129. Meleski, B. W. Growth, maturity, body composition, and selected familial characteristics of competitive swimmers 8 to 18 years of age. Doctoral dissertation. Austin: University of Texas, 1980.

130. Melichna, J., L. Havlickova, J. Vranova, Z. Bartunek, V. Seliger, et al. Muscle fibre composition and physical performance of sprinters and long distance runners. *Acta Univ. Carol. Gymnica* 18:95–123, 1982.

131. Mendez de Perez, B. *Los Atletas Venezolanos: Su Tipo Fisico.* Caracas: Universidad Central de Venezuela, 1981.

132. Mercier, J., P. Vago, M. Ramonatxo, C. Bauer, and C. Prefaut. Effect of aerobic training quantity on the VO_2 max of circumpubertal swimmers. *Int. J. Sports Med.* 8:26–30, 1987.

133. Mero, A., K. Hakkinen, and H. Kauhanen. Hormonal profile and strength development in young weight lifters. *J. Hum. Mov. Stud.* 16:255–266, 1989.

134. Mero, A., L. Jaakkola, and P. V. Komi. Neuromuscular, metabolic and hormonal profiles of young tennis players and untrained boys. *J. Sports Med.* 7:95–100, 1989.

135. Mero, A., H. Kauhanen, E. Peltola, and T. Vuorimaa. Changes in endurance, strength and speed capacity of different prepubescent athletic groups during one year of training. *J. Hum. Mov. Stud.* 14:219–239, 1988.

136. Meszaros, J., J. Mohacsi, and I. Szmodis. A four-year study of physique in young basketball players. *Anthrop. Kozl.* 24:153–157, 1980.

137. Michael, E., J. Evert, and K. Jeffers. Physiological changes of teenage girls during five months of detraining. *Med. Sci. Sports* 4:214–218, 1972.

138. Ministry of Health and Welfare. *The 1988 National Nutrition Survey of Japan.* Tokyo: Dai-ichi Shuppan Co., 1990.

139. Miyashita, M., Y. Hayashi,, and H. Furuhashi. Maximum oxygen uptake of Japanese top swimmers. *J. Sports Med. Phys. Fitness* 10:211–216, 1970.

140. Moffatt, R. J., B. Surina, B. Golden, and N. Ayres. Body composition and physiological characteristics of female high school gymnasts. *Res. Q. Exerc. Sport* 55:80–84, 1984.

141. Montecinos, R. M., J. E. Guajardo, L. Lara, F. Jara, and P. Gatica. Evaluation of physical capacity in Chilean volleyball players. P. V. Komi (ed). *Exercise and Sport Biology.* Champaign, IL: Human Kinetics, 1982, pp. 213–221.

142. Ness, G. W., D. A. Cunningham, R. B. Eynon, and D. B. Shaw. Cardiopulmonary function in prospective competitive swimmers and their parents. *J. Appl. Physiol.* 37:27–31, 1974.

143. Newble, D. I., and S. D. R. Homan. The development of a scientific testing programme for age group swimmers. *Aust. J. Sports Med.* 10:77–81, 1978.

144. Nikodymova, L. Contribution a l'etude de l'influence du sport pratique systematique-ment sur le developpement physique des adolescents. *Teorie a Praxe Telesne Vychovy a Sportu.* Prague: Comite d'Etat pour l'Education Physique et le Sport, 1956, pp.60–75.

145. Nomura, T. The influence of training and age on VO_2 max during swimming in Japanese elite age group and Olympic swimmers. A. P. Hollander, P. A. Huijing, and G. de Groot (eds). *Biomechanics and Medicine in Swimming.* Champaign, IL: Human Kinetics, 1983, pp. 251–257.

146. Novak, J., T. Jurimae, V. Bunc, E. V. Mackova, M. Cermak, and T. Paul. Response to maximal ergometric load of different types and relation to cardiorespiratory parameters to specific performance in young swimmers. H. Lollgen and H. Mellerowicz (eds). *Progress in Ergometry: Quality Control and Test Criteria.* Berlin: Springer-Verlag, 1984, pp. 251–259.

147. Novak, L. P. Effect of competitive swimming on body composition of adolescent boys. *Youth and Sports.* Magglingen: Research Institute of the Swiss School for Physical Education and Sports, 1983, pp. 43–54.

148. Novak, L. P. Maximal aerobic capacity, pulmonary functions, body composition, and anthropometry of adolescent hockey players. *Youth and Sports.* Magglingen: Research Institute of the Swiss School for Physical Education and Sports, 1983, pp. 55–68.

149. Novak, L. P., M. Bierbaum, and H. Mellerowicz. Maximal oxygen consumption, pulmonary function, body composition, and anthropometry of adolescent female athletes. *Int. Z. Angew. Physiol.* 31:103–119, 1973.

150. Novotny, V. V. Veranderungen des Knochenalters im Verlauf einer mehrjahrigen sportlichen Belastung. *Med. Sport* 21:44–47, 1981.

151. Novotny, V. V., and D. Kucerova. Rapports entre le developpement morphologique et l'aptitude fonctionnelle chez la jeunesse adolescente. *Anthropologie* 6:9–14, 1968.
152. Ohtsuki, F., I. Kita, T. Uetake, K. Tsukagoshi, T. Asami, and H. Matsui. Skeletal ages with regard to the physical performance for track and field junior athletes. H. Matsui (ed), *Chino-Japanese Cooperative Study on Physical Fitness of Junior Track and Field Athletes, I.* Tokyo: Hokuetsu Publ. Co., 1988, pp. 18–26.
153. Orvanova, E. Physical structure of winter sports athletes. *J. Sports Sci.* 5:197–248, 1987.
154. Osterback, L. L., and J. Viitasalo. Growth selection of young boys participating in different sports. J. Rutenfranz, R. Mocellin, and F. Klimt (eds). *Children and Exercise XII.* Champaign, IL: Human Kinetics, 1986, pp. 373–380.
155. Parizkova, J. Longitudinal study of the relationship between body composition and anthropometric characteristics in boys during growth and development. *Glas. Antropol. Drustva Jugoslav.* 7:33–38, 1970.
156. Parizkova, J. La masse active, la graisse deposee et la constitution corporelle chez les sportifs de haut niveau. *Kinanthropologie* 4:95–106, 1972.
157. Parizkova, J. *Body Fat and Physical Fitness.* The Hague: Martinus Nijhoff, 1977.
158. Paterson, D. H., D. A. Cunningham, D. S. Penny, M. Lefcoe, and S. Sangal. Heart rate telemetry and estimated energy metabolism in minor league ice hockey. *Can. J. Appl. Sport Sci.* 2:71–75, 1977.
159. Pekkarinen, H. A., and S. Mahlamaki. Anthropometric measures of young Finnish cross-country skiers and control children. J. Rutenfranz, R. Mocellin, and F. Klimt (eds). *Children and Exercise XII.* Champaign, IL: Human Kinetics, 1986, pp. 363–372.
160. Peltenburg, A. L., W. B. M. Erich, J. J. H. Thijssen, W. Veeman, M. Jansen, et al. Sex hormone profiles of premenarcheal athletes. *Eur. J. Appl. Physiol.* 52:385–392, 1984.
161. Peltenburg, A. L., W. B. M. Erich, M. L. Zonderland, M. J. E. Bernink, J. L. van den Brande, and I. A. Huisveld. A retrospective growth study of female gymnasts and girl swimmers. *Int. J. Sports Med.* 5:262–267, 1984.
162. Pena, M. E., E. Cardenas, and J. L. del Olmo. Crecimiento y maduracion osea en deportistas preadolescentes y adolescentes. R. Ramos Galvan and R. M. Ramos Rodriguez (eds). *Estudios de Antropologia Biologica. II Coloquio de Antropologia Fisica Juan Comas, 1982.* Mexico City: Instituto de Investigaciones Antropologicas, 1974, pp. 453–466.
163. Pires Neto, C. S. Determinacao do percentual de gordura corporal em handebolistas femininas. *Kinesia* 1:69–81, 1985.
164. Placheta, Z., T. Havlat, and O. Necasova. Development of some factors limiting physical performance during 4-year endurance training of boys aged 14–18. *Scr. Med. (Brno)* 48:621–645, 1975.
165. Rahkila, P., T. Lintunen, M. Silvennoinen, and L. Osterback. Physical fitness of novice ice hockey players in relation to skeletal age. R. M. Malina (ed). *Young Athletes: Biological, Psychological, and Educational Perspectives.* Champaign, IL: Human Kinetics, 1988, pp. 193–202.
166. Raven, R. B., B. L. Drinkwater, and S. M. Horvath. Cardiovascular responses of young female track athletes during exercise. *Med. Sci. Sports* 4:205–209, 1972.
167. Ross, W. D., S. R. Brown, J. W. Yu, and R. A. Faulkner. Somatotype of Canadian figure skaters. *J. Sports Med.* 17:195–205, 1977.
168. Ross, W. D., and J. A. P. Day. Physique and performance of young skiers. *J. Sports Med. Phys. Fitness* 12:30–37, 1972.
169. Ross, W. D., D. T. Drinkwater, N. O. Whittingham, and R. A. Faulkner. Anthropometric prototypes: Ages six to eighteen years. K. Berg and B. O. Eriksson (eds). *Children and Exercise IX.* Baltimore: University Park Press, 1980, pp. 3–12.
170. Sady, S. P., W. H. Thomson, K. Berg, and M. Savage. Physiological characteristics of high-ability prepubescent wrestlers. *Med. Sci. Sports Exerc.* 16:72–76, 1984.
171. Salmela, J. H. Growth patterns of elite French-Canadian female gymnasts. *Can. J. Appl. Sport Sci.* 4:219–222, 1979.

172. Satake, T., Y. Okajima, Y. Atomi, T. Asami, and Y. Kuroda. Effect of physical exercise on physical growth and maturation. *J. Phys. Fitness Japan* 35:104–110, 1986.
173. Seefeldt, V., J. Haubenstricker, C. F. Branta, and S. Evans. Physical characteristics of elite distance runners. E. W. Brown and C. F. Branta (eds). *Competitive Sports for Children and Youth.* Champaign, IL: Human Kinetics, 1988, pp. 247–258.
174. Seliger, V. The influence of sports training on the efficiency of juniors. *Int. Z. Angew. Physiol. Einschl. Arbeitsphysiol.* 26:309–322, 1968.
175. Shoup, R. F., and R. M. Malina. Anthropometric and physique characteristics of female high school varsity athletes in three sports. *Humanbiol. Budapest.* 16:169–177, 1985.
176. Slemenda, C. W., and C. C. Johnston. High intensity activities in young women: site specific bone mass effects among female figure skaters. *Bone Miner* 20:125–132, 1993.
177. Smit, P. J. Anthropometric observations on South African gymnasts. *Afr. Med. J.* 47:480–485, 1973.
178. Song, T. M. K. Relationship of physiological characteristics to skiing performance. *Physician Sportsmed.* 10:97–102, 1982.
179. Sovak, D., M. R. Hawes, and K. Plant. Morphological proportionality in elite age group North American divers. *J. Sports Sci.* 10:451–465, 1992.
180. Sprynarova, S., and J. Parizkova. Comparison of the functional, circulatory and respiratory capacity in girl gymnasts and swimmers. *J. Sports Med. Phys. Fitness* 9:165–171, 1969.
181. Stager, J. M., and L. K. Hatler. Menarche in athletes: the influence of genetics and prepubertal training. *Med. Sci. Sports Exerc.* 20:369–373, 1988.
182. Stepnicka, J., and T. Broda. Somatotype mladych sjezdaru. *Teor. Praxe Tel. Vych.* 25:166–169, 1977.
183. Szabo, S., J. Doka, P. Apor, and K. Somogyvari. Die Beziehung zwischen Knochenlebensalter, funktionellen anthropometrischen Daten und der aeroben Kapazitat. *Schweiz. Z. Sportmed.* 20:109–115, 1972.
184. Szogy, A. The influence of speed and strength characteristics on the anaerobic capacity of adolescent cyclists. S. Oseid and K. -H. Carlsen (eds). *Children and Exercise XIII.* Champaign, IL: Human Kinetics, 1989, pp. 67–73.
185. Tanner, J. M., R. H. Whitehouse, N. Cameron, W. A. Marshall, M. J. R. Healy, and H. Goldstein. *Assessment of Skeletal Maturity and Prediction of Adult Height, 2nd ed.* New York: Academic Press, 1983.
186. Tcheng, T-K., and C. M. Tipton. Iowa Wrestling Study: anthropometric measurements and the prediction of a "minimal" body weight for high school wrestlers. *Med. Sci. Sports* 5:1–10, 1973.
187. Telford, R. D., R. B. Cunningham, V. Deakin, and D. A. Kerr. Iron status and diet in athletes. *Med. Sci. Sports Exerc.* 25:796–800, 1993.
188. Tharp, G. G., G. O. Johnson, and W. G. Thorland. Measurement of anaerobic power and capacity in elite young track athletes using the Wingate test. *J. Sports Med.* 24:100–106, 1984.
189. Theintz, G. E., H. Howald, Y. Allemann, and P. C. Sizonenko. Growth and pubertal development of young female gymnasts and swimmers: a correlation with parental data. *Int. J. Sports Med.* 10:87–91, 1989.
190. Theintz, G. E., H. Howald, U. Weiss, and P. C. Sizonenko. Evidence for a reduction of growth potential in adolescent female gymnasts. *J. Pediatr.* 122:306–313, 1993.
191. Thompson, G. G., B. A. Blanksby, and G. Doran. Maturity and performance in age group competitive swimmers. *Aust. J. Phys. Educ.* 64:21–25, 1974.
192. Thomson, M. J., D. A. Cunningham, and G. A. Wearring. Eating habits and caloric intake of physically active young boys, ages 10 to 14 years. *Can. J. Appl. Sport Sci.* 5:9–14, 1980.
193. Thoren, C. A. R., and K. Asano. Functional capacity and cardiac function in 10-year-old boys and girls with high and low running performance. J. Ilmarinen and I. Valimaki (eds). *Children and Sport.* Berlin: Springer-Verlag, 1984, pp. 182–188.

194. Thorland, W. G., G. O. Johnson, C. J. Cisar, T. J. Housh, and G. D. Tharp. Strength and anaerobic responses of elite young female sprint and distance runners. *Med. Sci. Sports Exerc.* 19:56–61, 1987.

195. Thorland, W. G., G. O. Johnson, C. J. Cisar, T. J. Housh, and G. D. Tharp. Muscular strength and power in elite young male runners. *Pediatr. Exerc. Sci.* 2:73–82, 1990.

196. Thorland, W. G., G. O. Johnson, T. G. Fagot, G. D. Tharp, and R. W. Hammer. Body composition and somatotype characteristics of Junior Olympic athletes. *Med. Sci. Sports Exerc.* 13:332–338, 1981.

197. Thorland, W. G., G. O. Johnson, T. J. Housh, and M. J. Refsell. Anthropometric characteristics of elite adolescent competitive swimmers. *Hum. Biol.* 55:735–748, 1983.

198. Tittel, K., and H. Wutscherk. *Sportanthropometrie.* Leipzig: Johan Ambrosius Barth, 1972.

199. Toteva, M. Somatotype characteristics of young Bulgarian athletes in age aspect. Paper presented at the IV European Congress on Sports Medicine, Prague, 1985 (as cited by Orvanova, E. Somatotypes of weight lifters. *J. Sports Sci.* 8:119–137, 1990).

200. Troup J. P. *International Center for Aquatic Research Annual: Studies by the International Center for Aquatic Research 1989–1990.* Colorado Springs: United States Swimming Press, 1990.

201. Troup J. P. *International Center for Aquatic Research Annual: Studies by the International Center for Aquatic Research 1990–91.* Colorado Springs: United States Swimming Press, 1991.

202. Ulbrichova, M., and E. Packova. Somaticky stav dorostenek v odbijene. *Teor. Praxe Tel. Vych.* 27:332–337, 1979.

203. Vaccaro, P., D. H. Clarke, and A. F. Morris. Physiological characteristics of young well-trained swimmers. *Eur. J. Appl. Physiol.* 44:61–66, 1980.

204. Vaccaro, P., and A. Poffenbarger. Resting and exercise respiratory function in young female child runners. *J. Sports Med.* 22:102–107, 1982.

205. Vandewalle, H., G. Peres, J. Heller, J. Panel, and H. Monod. Force-velocity relationship and maximal aerobic power on a cycle ergometer. *Eur. J. Appl. Physiol.* 56:650–656, 1987.

206. van Erp-Baart, M. -A., L. W. H. M. Fredrix, R. A. Binkhorst, T. C. L. Lavaleye, P. C. J. Vergouwen, and W. H. M. Saris. Energy intake and energy expenditure in top female gymnasts. R. A. Binkhorst, H. C. G. Kemper, and W. H. M. Saris (eds). *Children and Exercise XI.* Champaign, IL: Human Kinetics, 1985, pp. 218–223.

207. Vervaecke, H. Somatische en Motorische Determinanten van de Sprintsnelheid en van de Bewegingsuitvoering bij Elitezwemmers. Doctoral dissertation. Institute of Physical Education, Catholic University of Leuven, Belgium, 1983.

208. von Dobeln, W., and I. Holmer. Body composition, sinking force, and oxygen uptake of man treading water. *J. Appl. Physiol.* 37:55–59, 1974.

209. Vrijens J. Morfo-fysiologische aspecten van de wielersport bij de jongeren. *Werken van de Belgische Geneeskundige Vereniging voor Lichamelijke Opvoeding en Sport* 23:105–115, 1972–1973.

210. Vrijens, J. Studie van de morfologische en functionele prestatiefactoren in de wielersport. *Werken van de Belgische Geneeskundige Vereniging voor Lichamelijke Opvoeding en Sport* 28:15–26, 1979–1980.

211. Vrijens, J., and C. Van Cauter. Physical performance capacity and specific skills in young soccer players. R. A. Binkhorst, H. C. G. Kemper, and W. H. M. Saris (eds). *Children and Exercise XI.* Champaign, IL: Human Kinetics, 1985, pp. 285–292.

212. Vrijens, J., J. L. Pannier, and J. Bouckaert. Physiological profile of competitive road cyclists. *J. Sports Med. Phys. Fitness* 22:207–216, 1982.

213. Warren, M. P. The effects of exercise on pubertal progression and reproductive function in girls. *J. Clin. Endocrinol. Metab.* 51:1150–1157, 1980.

214. Weaver, W. G., and J. M. Thomson. Changes in somatotypic and cardiopulmonary factors over puberty in elite age-group figure skaters. F. J. Nagle and H. J. Montoye (eds). *Exercise in Health and Disease.* Springfield, IL: Charles C Thomas, 1981, pp. 43–59.

215. Webster, B. L., and S. Barr. Body composition analysis of female adolescent athletes: Comparing six regression equations. *Med. Sci. Sports Exerc.* 25:648–653, 1993.

216. Wells, C. L., E. W. Scrutton, L. D. Archibald, W. P. Cooke, and J. W. De La Mothe. Physical working capacity and maximal oxygen uptake of teenaged athletes. *Med. Sci. Sports* 5:232–238, 1973.

217. Wilmore, J. H., C. H. Brown, and J. A. Davis. Body physique and composition of the female distance runner. *Ann. N. Y. Acad. Sci.* 301:764–776, 1977.

218. Wright, G. R., J. Nicoletti, and R. J. Shephard. Selection, training and development of youth oarsmen. H. Lavalle and R. J. Shephard (eds). *Frontiers of Activity and Child Health.* Quebec: Editions du Pelican, 1977, pp. 293–305.

219. Ziemilska, A. *Wplyw intensywnego treningu gimnastycznego na rozwooj somatyczny i dojrzewanie dzieci.* Warsaw: Akademia Wychowania Fizycznego, 1981.

220. Zonderland, M. L., W. B. M. Erich, A. L. Peltenburg, M. J. E. Bernink, L. Havekes, A. M. J. van Erp-Baart, and W. H. M. Saris. Lipoprotein profiles and nutrition of prepubertal female athletes. R. M. Malina (ed). *Young Athletes: Biological, Psychological, and Educational Perspectives.* Champaign, IL: Human Kinetics, 1988, pp. 177–191.

14
Assessment and Interpretation of Aerobic Fitness in Children and Adolescents

NEIL ARMSTRONG, Ph.D.
JOANNE R. WELSMAN, Ph.D.

Aerobic fitness depends upon pulmonary, cardiovascular, and hematological components of oxygen delivery and the oxidative mechanisms of the exercising muscle. Maximal oxygen uptake ($\dot{V}O_2$max), the highest rate at which an individual can consume oxygen during exercise, limits the capacity to perform aerobic exercise and therefore serves as the most popular index of adults' aerobic fitness. Aerobic exercise training in adult subjects typically induces improvements in submaximal blood lactate indices that are greater than improvements in $\dot{V}O_2$max [46, 66]. This occurs because there is much greater scope for increasing the oxidative profile of skeletal muscle than there is for enhancing the central mechanisms that appear to limit $\dot{V}O_2$max [73]. Consequently, various submaximal measures of blood lactate have been accepted as valid and sensitive indices of aerobic fitness.

Protocols for the determination of adult athletes' $\dot{V}O_2$max and blood lactate responses to exercise are well-established and used routinely in sport science laboratories [74, 197]. The data are analyzed, interpreted, and used to advise the athlete and coach on how to improve subsequent performance. Methodologies for the determination of untrained children and adolescents' $\dot{V}O_2$max and blood lactate responses to exercise are less secure than those for adult athletes, and they are limited by ethical considerations. The appropriate analysis and interpretation of experimental data collected from young subjects are problematic and must be considered in relation to the growth and maturation of the child.

This chapter focuses on $\dot{V}O_2$max and blood lactate data collected from normal (i.e., healthy but untrained) children and adolescents with reference to sex, chronological age, growth, and maturation. It examines the methodological problems involved in determining $\dot{V}O_2$max and appropriate submaximal blood lactate indices in children and adolescents and explores means of interpreting aerobic fitness in relation to growth and functional development.

ETHICAL CONSIDERATIONS

There are clear ethical issues concerning the consent of children to participate in research in the exercise sciences. The legality and ethics of involving children as subjects in research have been debated at length [136, 221, 222]. It is generally agreed that research that involves a child and is of no direct benefit to that child (nontherapeutic research) is not necessarily either unethical or illegal. However, children should take part in research only if the relevant knowledge could not be gained by research in adults [221, 222]. It is advisable to seek the informed consent of both child and parents, and researchers should consider carefully the maturity and independence of the children to be approached and the likely expectations of their parents. When a child lacks sufficient understanding to consent, willing co-operation should always be sought. Research procedures should involve "negligible risk" to the child (i.e., not greater than risks of harm ordinarily encountered in daily life). The Medical Research Council Working Party on Research in Children [222] cites procedures involving negligible risk as including observation of behavior, noninvasive physiological monitoring, developmental assessments and physical examinations, changes in diet, and obtaining blood and urine specimens.

A child's participation in research in the exercise sciences should not be through coercion, and it can only be ethical if it places that child at no more than negligible risk of harm and is therefore not against his or her interests.

MAXIMAL AND PEAK OXYGEN UPTAKE

Measurement of Maximal and Peak Oxygen Uptake
ESTIMATION OF MAXIMAL OXYGEN UPTAKE FROM SUBMAXIMAL RESPONSES AND PERFORMANCE TESTS. The measurement of $\dot{V}O_2$max requires the subject to exercise almost to exhaustion. Several investigators have been reluctant to carry out this type of test with children and have therefore attempted to estimate $\dot{V}O_2$max from submaximal data. The most common procedure is to use a single submaximal heart rate measurement and the corresponding oxygen consumption (or power output) to predict $\dot{V}O_2$max using the Astrand nomogram [14]. The nomogram was, however, derived from data on an adult population, and several incorrect assumptions are made when it is applied to children. The cardiopulmonary responses of children during submaximal exercise do not always parallel those of adults, and the maximal heart rates of children are often higher than those of adults and have a greater range. The Astrands have never seriously tested their nomogram with individuals below the age of 20 years, but others persist in doing so. The available data confirm that the prediction of $\dot{V}O_2$max from submaximal data is subject to large errors [27,30], and Woynarowska's, [223] report that the Astrand nomogram underestimates

the directly determined $\dot{V}O_2$max in boys by an average of 26% and in girls by an average of 23% is typical.

Some experimenters have used maximal performance tests such as the 12-minute run [99, 170] and the 20m progressive shuttle run [10, 20] to estimate $\dot{V}O_2$max, but this type of test is more a reflection of the environment, the child's pace judgment, and the potency of the motivational conditions under which the test takes place than the $\dot{V}O_2$max. Cumming [37] stated that in normal children the prediction of $\dot{V}O_2$max from an endurance run is little better than can be obtained from height, weight, and skinfold measurements. Shephard [171] commented that performance tests are a complicated way of identifying tall or fat children. It appears that with children and adolescents there is no valid substitute for a direct determination of $\dot{V}O_2$max.

MAXIMAL OXYGEN UPTAKE OR PEAK OXYGEN UPTAKE? Following a series of classical experiments, Hill and his colleagues [82, 83] reported that oxygen consumption increases with running speed up to a critical velocity beyond which no further increase in oxygen consumption takes place, even though the subject is still able to increase speed. It was assumed that running at speeds beyond the point of leveling of oxygen consumption was supported by anaerobic energy sources, resulting in an intracellular accumulation of lactate, acidosis, and inevitably exhaustion. Although both theoretical [137] and methodological [132] bases of the $\dot{V}O_2$ plateau phenomenon have been challenged, it is traditionally used as the criterion for establishing $\dot{V}O_2$max during a laboratory test [14, 131, 172]. Since an absolute leveling of oxygen consumption with increasing exercise intensity is uncommon, several less stringent criteria of a $\dot{V}O_2$ plateau have been proposed. These include a rise in $\dot{V}O_2$ during the final exercise period of less than 150 ml or 2.1 ml/min · kg for a 2.5% increase in treadmill speed [195], a rise in $\dot{V}O_2$ of less than 2 standard deviations below that of the mean of changes between previous exercise intensities [128], and a rise in $\dot{V}O_2$ of not more than 2 ml/min · kg for a 5–10% increase in exercise intensity [169].

Regardless of the criterion used, only a minority of children and adolescents demonstrate a plateau in $\dot{V}O_2$ during treadmill exercise [42, 154]. During cycle ergometer exercise, even fewer children and adolescents exhibit a $\dot{V}O_2$max plateau [8, 18, 35]. Nevertheless, it is well documented that children can exercise to exhaustion without demonstrating a $\dot{V}O_2$ plateau [35, 147, 154]. Several studies have demonstrated that children who exhibit a $\dot{V}O_2$ plateau are indistinguishable from those that do not [35, 44, 147]. The requirement of a plateau does not therefore appear to be a useful criterion for defining $\dot{V}O_2$max in children and adolescents.

Maximal tests with children and adolescents are usually terminated by voluntary exhaustion, i.e., when the child, despite strong verbal encouragement from the experimenters is unwilling or unable to continue. The appropriate term is therefore peak oxygen uptake (peak $\dot{V}O_2$), which represents the highest oxygen consumption elicited during an exercise test to exhaustion, rather than $\dot{V}O_2max$, which conventionally implies the existence of a $\dot{V}O_2$ plateau. If the subject has been habituated to the test procedures and environment and shows signs of intense effort (hyperpnea, facial flushing and grimacing, unsteady gait, sweating), peak heart rate has leveled off prior to the final exercise intensity at a value at least 95% of maximal heart rate as predicted by age, and respiratory exchange ratio is at least unity, peak $\dot{V}O_2$ can be confidently accepted as a maximal index [8, 152]. Some laboratories recommend high postexercise blood lactate levels (e.g., 6–7 mM) as a subsidiary criterion of maximal exercise [40, 108, 147], but in the light of methodological influences upon blood lactate measures (discussed later in this chapter) and the considerable variability in postexercise blood lactate levels observed in children, this recommendation appears to be problematic. In addition, as it is advisable to encourage children to cool down with exercise of gradually reducing intensity following maximal exertion, if postexercise blood samples are taken, they should be taken immediately exercise terminates rather than after a delay to allow blood lactate peaking.

Reliability coefficients using treadmill peak $\dot{V}O_2$ protocols with children and adolescents range from 0.53 to 0.99 [28, 64]. Cumming and his associates [38] found a mean variation of 4.5% for children exercising to exhaustion during 12 cycle ergometer experiments. Boileau et al. [28] reported a 5.3% variation in peak $\dot{V}O_2$ on successive cycle ergometer tests. Paterson et al. [142] examined the reliability of walking, jogging, and running protocols by repeating each test three times in eight boys aged 10–12 years. They reported reliability coefficients of r = 0.56 for the walking protocol, r = 0.91 for the jogging protocol, and r = 0.90 for the running protocol. Paterson [142] concluded that peak $\dot{V}O_2$ measured using a jogging or running protocol is as consistent (reliable and reproducible) in children as $\dot{V}O_2max$ in adult groups. Although it has been suggested that better reliability is achieved when a $\dot{V}O_2$ plateau criterion is used [64], it appears that acceptable reliability can be obtained even if the traditional criterion is not always satisfied [108]. Habituation to the laboratory environment is, however, vital before testing young subjects.

EXERCISE ERGOMETERS AND PROTOCOLS. The choice of laboratory ergometer for the measurement of peak $\dot{V}O_2$ lies between step bench, cycle ergometer, and treadmill. It is difficult to persuade young children to climb a step with a consistent rhythm, and problems may arise from differences in leg length, but the major drawback is the young subject's lack of mass. In our experience, stepping exercise with children is seldom terminated by cardiopulmonary insufficiency, and peak $\dot{V}O_2$ is between 25 and 30% less than that elicited during treadmill exercise. As a result, the step bench is seldom the ergometer of choice in the laboratory, although studies have been reported from remote areas [31].

The treadmill engages a larger muscle mass in the exercise than the cycle ergometer, and the peak $\dot{V}O_2$ obtained is therefore more likely to be limited by central rather than peripheral factors [169, 172]. In cycle ergometry, a higher proportion of the total power output is developed by the quadriceps muscle [98], and the effort required is large in relation to muscle strength [84]. Blood flow through the quadriceps is therefore limited [69, 96], resulting in increased anaerobic metabolism [28, 183] and consequent termination of exercise by peripheral muscle pain [220]. Cycle ergometers need to be modified for young children [86] who often find difficulty in maintaining the required pedal rhythm [11]. It has also been reported that children may improve their cycle ergometer peak $\dot{V}O_2$ merely by becoming accustomed to the test [167].

Boileau et al. [28] compared peak $\dot{V}O_2$ values of 21 11- to 14-year-old boys on a treadmill and a cycle ergometer. They reported a correlation of 0.95 between the two scores, but the treadmill values were 7.4–7.9% higher than the cycle values. Macek and his co-workers [120] reported similar results with younger children. Armstrong and Davies [6] found the mean treadmill peak $\dot{V}O_2$ of 14-year-old boys to be 9% higher than the mean value elicited during cycle ergometry. The correlation between cycle and treadmill scores was 0.89, but these authors pointed out that although on average treadmill scores were higher than cycle ergometer values, some children do achieve a higher peak $\dot{V}O_2$ on a cycle ergometer. This observation questions the validity of Krahenbuhl et al.'s [108] technique of raising cycle ergometer values by a fixed constant and pooling cycle and treadmill data to provide normal values of children's peak $\dot{V}O_2$.

Both treadmill and cycle ergometer have been shown to be suitable for use with children of 10 years of age or older, and the choice of ergometer often depends upon the ancillary variables being assessed [28, 172]. In a well-equipped laboratory, the treadmill is usually the machine of choice, but studies of children may involve mobile laboratories [99] or temporary laboratories established in schools [9]. Under these circumstances, the use of a treadmill is often not appropriate due to its bulk, noise, and general lack of mobility.

It appears that during treadmill exercise, running protocols elicit higher peak $\dot{V}O_2$ than walking protocols [142, 168], but no differences are apparent between continuous and discontinuous tests [168]. Skinner et al. [182] compared continuous and intermittent treadmill tests for determining peak $\dot{V}O_2$ with 144 children. They concluded that if one is interested in obtaining only maximal values of children, then it makes little difference whether a continuous or discontinuous protocol is used. The advantage of a continuous protocol is that it is less time consuming, but many children find a discontinuous test more acceptable, and this kind of protocol facilitates submaximal ancillary measures such as blood sampling.

DIURNAL AND SEASONAL VARIATION IN PEAK OXYGEN UPTAKE. Diurnal and seasonal variations in children's peak $\dot{V}O_2$ are not well documented.

Cumming and his co-workers [36] tested 12 13- to 16-year-olds, six times in the morning and six times in the afternoon, and detected no differences in peak $\dot{V}O_2$. Similarly, Cumming [37] was unable to detect any significant seasonal changes in the peak $\dot{V}O_2$ of Canadian children. Astrand [12] noted an improvement in the "working capacity" of Swedish children during the school year with deterioration during the summer vacation. Cunningham et al. [44] recorded a springtime in boys' peak $\dot{V}O_2$ but related it to training and competitive seasons. Shephard [169] considered seasonal variation and concluded that

> the intensity of activity in and out of school and the relative restrictions on physical activity imposed by climatic conditions are so variable from one region of the world to another that it would indeed be surprising if any useful generalizations could be made.[p. 326]

In a later study, however, Shephard et al. [175] reported cyclic variations in peak $\dot{V}O_2$, with the highest score being recorded in the period November to December, but in subsequent work [173] he found that "fitness scores were uninfluenced by the season of sampling." Kemper [99], in his longitudinal analysis of teenagers, indicated that there were no time or measurement effects on peak $\dot{V}O_2$. In general, children and adolescents' peak $\dot{V}O_2$ values are recorded without regard for any seasonal or diurnal variations that may exist.

Peak Oxygen Uptake and Age
Malina and Bouchard [123] claim that reliable determinations of peak $\dot{V}O_2$ in children under 8 years of age are almost impossible to make. Young children typically have short attention spans and often poor motivation, thereby decreasing the likelihood of achieving maximal data [21, 177]. Equipment and protocols designed for adults make testing with young children more difficult. Children have a relatively low tidal volume, and therefore pediatric gas analysis equipment should have a small dead space. The influence of children using respiratory valves, mouthpieces, tubing, and mixing chambers designed for use with adults requires further evaluation [33, 150], but the smaller the child the greater the potential problem.

Despite methodological problems, data have been reported from children aged 4 through 7 years. Whether the children exhibited maximal values is unclear in some studies that did not report the incidence of recognized criteria [36, 148, 230]. Small sample sizes are common [45, 163], and recent, well-controlled studies have reported combined male and female data [107, 177]. This review therefore examines the more secure data base of males and females aged 8–16 years.

The world literature contains a substantial amount of cross-sectional data on the peak $\dot{V}O_2$ of untrained children, and several longitudinal studies

FIGURE 14.1

Relationship in children and adolescents between peak VO₂ (liters/min) determined on a treadmill and chronological age. Data points are mean values drawn from the literature and represent 3703 male and 1234 female peak VO₂ determinations.

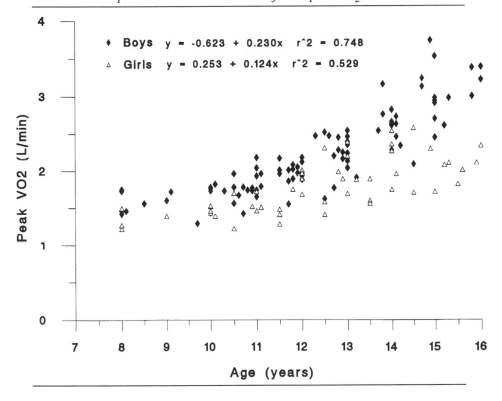

have been reported. Studies from which relevant data can be extracted are summarized in Figures 14.1 and 14.2. Krahenbuhl et al. [108] summarized data representing 5793 males and 3508 females aged 6 to 16 years, but they appear to have included both trained and untrained children in the analysis, and they combined data collected during various forms of ergometry. For reasons expressed earlier, we have graphed cycle ergometer and treadmill data separately. Care has been taken to exclude trained children where studies include both trained and untrained subjects and to avoid duplication of studies that involve dual publication of the same data base in a different format. The figures represent 10,154 peak V̇O₂ data points from subjects aged 8–16 years, but they must be interpreted cautiously, as the data points represent reported means from longitudinal and cross-sectional studies with varying sample sizes. No information appears to be available on randomly selected groups of youngsters, and since volunteers are generally used as subjects, selection bias cannot be

FIGURE 14.2

Relationship in children and adolescents between peak VO₂ (liters/min) determined on a cycle ergometer and chronological age. Data points are mean values drawn from the literature and represent 3050 male and 2167 female peak VO₂ determinations.

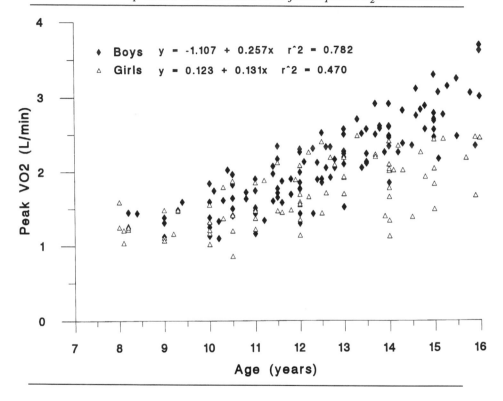

ruled out, as relatively few subjects are likely to be drawn from the markedly sedentary or overweight sections of the population.

The gradual increase of boys' peak $\dot{V}O_2$ in relation to chronological age is clearly illustrated in Figures 14.1 and 14.2. Ten longitudinal studies [2, 19, 104, 127, 156, 185] from Europe, Japan, and North America have provided a consistent picture of a progressive rise in boys' peak $\dot{V}O_2$ from 8 to 16 years. A Canadian study [127] assessed 75 boys annually throughout the period covered by this review and reported an average yearly increase in peak $\dot{V}O_2$ of 11.1%. The largest absolute increases occurred between 12 and 13 years (0.31 liter/min) and 13 and 14 years (0.32 liter/min).

With girls, Figures 14.1 and 14.2 illustrate a similar but less consistent trend. From age 8 to 13 years, girls' peak $\dot{V}O_2$ appears to increase with chronological age. Mirwald and Bailey's [127] longitudinal study of 22 8- to 13-year-old girls demonstrated an average annual increase of 11.6% in peak $\dot{V}O_2$, with the highest absolute rises of 0.25 liter/min and 0.23 liter/min occurring between 11 and 12 years and 12 and 13 years, respectively. Several cross-sectional studies, however, have indicated a leveling-off or even a fall in peak $\dot{V}O_2$ from 13 to 15 years (e.g., [32, 133, 228]). Yoshizawa's [228] data are the most striking, with a 0.61 liter/min fall off in peak $\dot{V}O_2$ demonstrated between 14 and 15 years in urban Japanese girls, although interestingly, this was not reflected in the same author's study of rural Japanese girls [228]. Andersen and his associates [2, 156], in their longitudinal studies of Norwegian girls (aged 10.3–15.2 years) and German girls (aged 12.7–15.7 years), found peak $\dot{V}O_2$ to reach its highest value at 13.3 years in Norway and at 14.7 in Germany.

Krahenbuhl et al. [108] reported that using the quadratic and cubic regression lines they generated as a guide, boys and girls had similar peak $\dot{V}O_2$ until age 12 years. At age 14 years the difference in peak $\dot{V}O_2$ was 25%, and by age 16 years the difference exceeded 50%. However, substituting age into their published regression equations results in female peak $\dot{V}O_2$ being predicted as higher than male peak $\dot{V}O_2$ at each age studied. Our analysis (Figs. 14.1 and 14.2) suggests that from age 10 years, male peak $\dot{V}O_2$ values are greater than those of similarly aged females. We found linear regression to be the method of choice, and using the regressions as a guide, treadmill determined peak $\dot{V}O_2$ is about 12% higher in males than females at age 10 years, increasing to 23% higher at age 12, 31% higher at age 14, and 37% higher at 16 years of age. Cycle ergometer–determined peak $\dot{V}O_2$ differences illustrate the same trend, with male scores higher than female scores by 2% at 10 years, 17% at 12 years, 27% at 14 years, and 37% at 16 years of age. The longitudinal studies that have assessed gender differences [2, 127, 156] support the cross-sectional findings, although the percentage differences between the sexes are less pronounced.

Boys appear to have higher levels of habitual physical activity than girls [3, 188], and this has been suggested as contributing to boys' higher peak $\dot{V}O_2$ values [108]. The evidence relating habitual physical activity to peak $\dot{V}O_2$ is, however, conflicting [4, 17, 99], and the problem is confounded by the difficulties involved in accurately assessing children's habitual physical activity [164]. Children and adolescents' current physical activity patterns [3, 5] indicate that they rarely experience the levels of physical activity associated with increases in peak $\dot{V}O_2$ [158, 200], and habitual physical activity is therefore unlikely to make a major contribution to peak $\dot{V}O_2$ values.

The sex difference between older children and adolescents' peak $\dot{V}O_2$ values has been attributed to differences in hemoglobin concentration [8, 100]. Hemoglobin concentration is positively related to peak $\dot{V}O_2$ in both sexes, even when the effect of age on both variables is partialled out [8]. The differences in hemoglobin concentration between the sexes generally reflect the differences in peak $\dot{V}O_2$ and indicate that sex differences in hemoglobin may well contribute to sex differences in peak $\dot{V}O_2$. However, Armstrong and his associates [7] have demonstrated that with young children this does not appear to be the case, as boys' peak $\dot{V}O_2$ may be significantly higher than that of girls, despite no difference in hemoglobin concentration. The sex differences in peak $\dot{V}O_2$ among young children may be related to variations in body composition, since boys possess a greater percentage of lean body mass, even in the prepubertal years [150]. Davies et al. [45] suggested that the lower peak $\dot{V}O_2$ of girls during cycle ergometry is due mainly to their smaller leg volume. Kemper et al. [101] reported that in their longitudinal study, although the differences were reduced when peak $\dot{V}O_2$ was related to fat free mass, the value for boys remained higher than those for girls at all years of measurement. The issue is confounded, however, by the fact that growth and development evoke changes in body composition that affect the conceptual basis for estimating fatness and leanness in children [112].

Peak Oxygen Uptake and Maturity
The development of peak $\dot{V}O_2$ appears to be influenced by a body size–maturation interaction [43], but although the relationship between peak $\dot{V}O_2$ and body size is well documented and often misrepresented (see following sections), relatively few studies have investigated the relationship between peak $\dot{V}O_2$ and maturation [8, 57]. No single means of maturity assessment provides a complete description of maturity during adolescence. Nevertheless, Malina [122] has argued that although there is a variation in the development of secondary sex characteristics, skeletal maturity, and peak height velocity within each sex during adolescence, these maturity indicators are sufficiently interrelated to indicate a general maturity factor during adolescence.

The use of the secondary sex characteristic rating of puberty developed by Tanner [192] is particularly applicable to cross-sectional studies. There is some lack of precision in the use of Tanner's indices of maturity, since an individual in, say, the early phase of stage 3 pubic hair development is rated the same as an individual in the late phase of this stage. Similarly, there is no consistent relationship between the age at which secondary sex characteristics develop and the rate of progress through the stages. As Malina (personal communication) has pointed out, ideally chronological age should also be incorporated into the analysis. Nevertheless, these indices have been shown to provide a valid classification of children in cross-sectional studies, and Tanner [194] has reported a high concordance of sexual maturity rating with, for example, skeletal age.

Several studies have used Tanner's methodology to classify subjects as pre-pubertal or pubertal (e.g., [7, 159, 161]), but only one substantial study [8] appears to have considered peak $\dot{V}O_2$ at each maturational stage, probably because of the large number of subjects required for a worthwhile analysis.

Armstrong and his associates [8] classified 184 boys and 136 girls into the appropriate maturity stage according to Tanner [192]. They reported that the more mature boys had a higher peak $\dot{V}O_2$ than less mature boys, probably due to greater muscle mass (indicated by a higher body mass but no difference in skinfold thickness) and higher hemoglobin concentration. With girls, they found peak $\dot{V}O_2$ in relation to maturity stage to be ergometer specific. On the treadmill, the only significant difference between group means was between Tanner stage 4 (2.09 liter/min) and stage 2 (1.69 liter/min); whereas, on the cycle ergometer the more mature girls (stages 4 and 5) had significantly higher mean peak $\dot{V}O_2$ than the less mature girls (stages 1, 2, and 3). Armstrong speculated that this may have been an artifact of the methodology, with less mature girls terminating the exercise with peripheral fatigue due to an inability to maintain the pedal rate against a relatively heavy resistance. On both ergometers the differences between the peak $\dot{V}O_2$ of the boys and girls were more pronounced in the mature children, probably reflecting the boys' greater muscle mass and hemoglobin concentration.

Kemper and Verschuur [100] assessed peak $\dot{V}O_2$ in relation to skeletal age in 375 children aged 13 and 14 years. The skeletal age of the sample ranged from 9 to 16 years, and a multiple regression analysis revealed that the increase in peak $\dot{V}O_2$ with increasing skeletal age was almost completely due to the increase in body size. Shephard et al. [175] studied 770 children and concluded that skeletal age adds little to the description of physiological variables yielded by chronological age, height, and mass. The value of skeletal age analysis in this context appears to be limited. The determination of skeletal age is expensive [196], and the ethics of exposing children to x-rays must be considered very carefully [23, and our section on Ethical Considerations].

Some longitudinal studies of peak $\dot{V}O_2$ in children and adolescents have used peak height velocity (PHV) to standardize maturation [99, 104, 127], but with the exception of the Saskatchewan Growth Study [127], a limited number of annual observations render the mathematical models currently available for fitting individual curves unsuitable. The results of these studies must therefore be interpreted with caution. Mirwald and Bailey [127] reported that the maximal increase in peak $\dot{V}O_2$ occurred in the year of PHV in both boys and girls, although it is important to note that the attainment of PHV occurs early in adolescence in girls and late in boys [194].

Beunen and Malina [26], in their excellent review of the literature concerned with growth, physical performance, and the adolescent spurt, concluded that the evidence suggests an adolescent growth spurt in peak $\dot{V}O_2$ in boys, with the spurt reaching a maximum gain near the time of PHV, but secure data are insufficient to offer any generalization for girls.

Peak Oxygen Uptake and Body Size
Numerous investigations have found high correlations (approx. r = 0.7/0.8) between children and adolescents' peak $\dot{V}O_2$ and either body mass or height (e.g., [8, 45]). As most physical activity involves moving body mass

from one place to another, to compare the peak $\dot{V}O_2$ of individuals who differ in body mass, peak $\dot{V}O_2$ is conventionally expressed in relation to mass as ml/min · kg.

When peak $\dot{V}O_2$ is expressed relative to body mass, a different picture emerges from that apparent when absolute values are used. Longitudinal studies show boys' mass-related peak $\dot{V}O_2$ to be fairly consistent over the age range 8 to 16 years [2, 127], although there are reports of both an increase [185] and a fall [156] in mass-related peak $\dot{V}O_2$ between 12 and 14 years of age. Girls' longitudinal data demonstrate unequivocally a decrease in mass-related peak $\dot{V}O_2$ with age [2, 19, 127]. Cross-sectional data are more difficult to interpret because of the variation in samples studied, but boys' values are higher than girls' values of peak $\dot{V}O_2$ throughout the age range reviewed. The trend is clearly illustrated in Figures 14.3 and

FIGURE 14.3

Relationship in children and adolescents between treadmill-determined peak VO₂ expressed relative to body mass (ml/min · kg) and chronological age. Data points are mean values drawn from the literature and represent 4355 male and 1375 female peak VO₂ determinations.

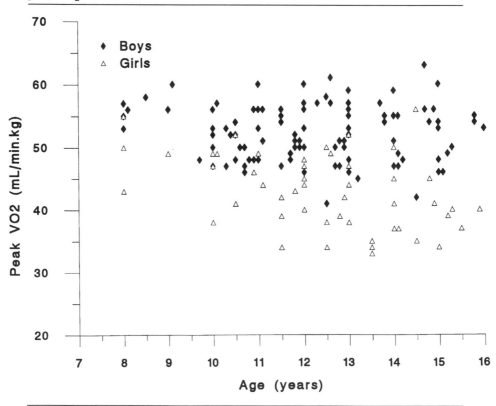

FIGURE 14.4

Relationship in children and adolescents between cycle ergometer–determined peak
VO₂ expressed relative to body mass (ml/min · kg) and chronological age. Data points
are mean values drawn from the literature and represent 3538 male and 2392 female
peak VO₂ determinations.

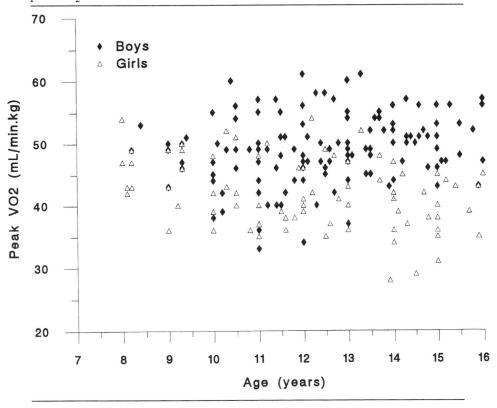

14.4, which represent 11,660 peak $\dot{V}O_2$ data points from subjects aged
8–16 years. In addition to the factors discussed earlier, the most popular
explanation for boys' superior mass-related peak $\dot{V}O_2$ concerns the girls'
greater accumulation of subcutaneous body fat during the
circumpubertal years [2, 13, 36].

Mass-related peak $\dot{V}O_2$ remains the most popular method of expressing
peak $\dot{V}O_2$, and earlier reviews have focused on the effects of growth and
maturation on mass-related peak $\dot{V}O_2$ (e.g., [21, 108]). Bar-Or [21] has
suggested that for practical purposes there is no advantage to be gained by
using other than body mass or height for growth-related comparisons.
However, we believe that this type of analysis may cloud our understanding
of growth and maturational changes in peak $\dot{V}O_2$, and in the following
section we explore some alternative approaches.

Interpreting Growth-related Changes in Peak Oxygen Uptake by Scaling for Differences in Body Size

RATIO STANDARDS. The interpretation of developmental changes in peak $\dot{V}O_2$, such as the identification and comparison of mean values for particular age and sex groups, is confounded by the need to somehow account for differences in body size. As described in the previous section, it is conventional to express peak $\dot{V}O_2$ in ratio with body-mass. Simply by dividing the absolute value of $\dot{V}O_2$ (liters/min) by body mass, ratio standards can be constructed to provide values that are then used for statistical comparison and correlation with other physiological measures. This division of peak $\dot{V}O_2$ by body mass is assumed to adequately partition out the influence of body size.

In 1949 Tanner [191] published a paper that clearly demonstrated the theoretical and statistical limitations of this procedure: The ratio standard assumes that the relationship between peak $\dot{V}O_2$ and body mass takes the form:

$$Y = a \cdot x \qquad (\text{peak } \dot{V}O_2 = a \cdot \text{body mass}),$$

where a is the constant derived from the mean values of peak $\dot{V}O_2$ and body mass for the series of data it describes (i.e., the line of the equation passes through the point of the two means and the origin). The ratio standard should only be applied in those cases where the coefficient of variation (V) for body mass divided by the coefficient of variation for peak $\dot{V}O_2$ equals the Pearson product moment correlation coefficient (r) obtained between the two variables, i.e. $Vx/Vy = r\,x,y$ [95, 191]. Where this equation is not satisfied, the use of the ratio standard will distort the data, with the size of the distortion increasing as the discrepancy between Vx/Vy and $r\,x,y$ increases. Specifically, inappropriate application of the ratio standard to peak $\dot{V}O_2$ data will overestimate values for individuals of low body mass and underestimate values for those of high body mass.

REGRESSION STANDARDS. Mathematically, the relationship between peak $\dot{V}O_2$ and body mass is better described by the regression equation:

$$Y = a + b \cdot x \qquad (\text{peak } \dot{V}O_2 = a + b \cdot \text{mass}),$$

where a is the intercept of the regression line on the y axis and b is the slope of the line. This analysis permits the construction of regression standards against which an individual's peak $\dot{V}O_2$ may be compared with that predicted from the regression equation [191]. Subsequently Tanner used this technique to illustrate differences in physique among Olympic athletes from various disciplines [193].

Where intergroup comparisons are required, such as peak $\dot{V}O_2$ differences in children of different age, maturity, or sex groups, analysis of covariance [184] should be the statistical technique of choice. Where a strong linear relationship between the two variables under consideration can be demonstrated (e.g., between peak $\dot{V}O_2$ and age) and both variables share a linear relationship with a third variable—a covariate (e.g., peak $\dot{V}O_2$ and age are both highly correlated with body mass), analysis of covariance successfully partitions out the influence of the covariate through the calculation and statistical comparison of adjusted means.

Despite his clear demonstration of the inadequacies of ratio standards to describe many physiological performance variables, Tanner's recommendations failed to excite much interest within the exercise sciences, even when the issues he raised were endorsed and developed by Katch and associates [95, 97]. These authors developed the concept of "spurious correlation," which results when ratio standards are inappropriately used in correlations with other physiological performance variables. They demonstrated that calculation of "weight-regressed" or "weight-adjusted" oxygen uptake scores would produce correlations between endurance performance and peak $\dot{V}O_2$ that were independent of body mass.

Recently, however, there has been a renewal of interest in the issue of partitioning out the influence of body size (scaling) during the interpretation of physiological performance variables in both children and adults [134, 150, 219]. Several studies have produced findings that illustrate how inappropriate scaling using ratio standards can lead to misplaced interpretation of physiological mechanisms. In adults, Winter et al. [219] used analysis of covariance to demonstrate significant sex differences in maximal exercise performance. These results suggested the existence of qualitative differences in muscle between males and females rather than simple quantitative differences that were indicated by the results based on ratio comparisons. Similarly, child-adult differences in submaximal oxygen uptake (running economy), which have been frequently documented [153, 155], have been shown to disappear when regression standards form the basis of the comparison and body mass is appropriately controlled for [56]. In recent studies we have specifically addressed the interpretation of growth-related peak $\dot{V}O_2$. Williams et al. [217] compared peak $\dot{V}O_2$ in 10- and 15-year-old boys, using both conventional comparison of per body mass ratios and analysis of covariance. As expected, no significant difference was noted between peak $\dot{V}O_2$ expressed in ratio with body mass. However the regression lines for the relationship between peak $\dot{V}O_2$ and body mass, illustrated in Figure 14.5, describe quite clearly two different populations. The analysis of covariance produced adjusted means of 2.21 and 2.30 liters/min for the 10- and 15-year-old boys, respectively. These values were significantly different, leading to the conclusion that for a given body mass, older boys have a significantly higher peak $\dot{V}O_2$ than younger ones. Similar results were obtained when the data were examined in relation to biological age. Subsequently, we extended this type of analysis to compare

FIGURE 14.5

The relationship between peak oxygen uptake and body mass in 10- and 15-year-old boys.

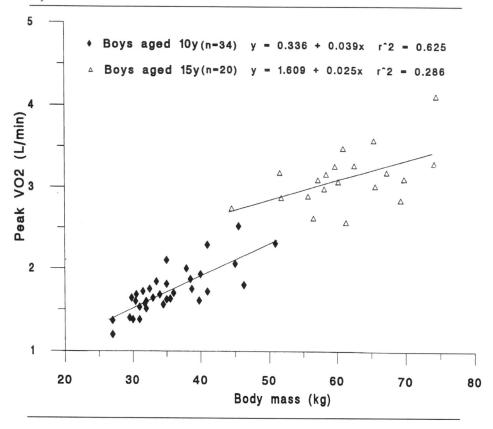

peak $\dot{V}O_2$ in prepubertal males and females with pubertal and adult groups (Welsman, Armstrong, Winter, and Kirby, unpublished observations). Once again, traditional ratio standard comparisons replicated accepted findings. In contrast, analysis of covariance on logarithmic plots of body mass and peak $\dot{V}O_2$ produced adjusted means for peak $\dot{V}O_2$ of 1.99, 2.19, and 2.14 liters/min for prepubertal, pubertal, and adult females, respectively. Values for corresponding male groups were 2.25, 2.51, and 2.80 liters/min. These findings confirmed that the increase in peak $\dot{V}O_2$ suggested by Williams et al. [217] extended from prepuberty to adulthood in males and demonstrated that peak $\dot{V}O_2$ actually increases in females from prepuberty to puberty and, importantly, that values appear to be maintained into adulthood rather than declining, as so frequently reported [21, 108].

POWER FUNCTIONS. Although scaling methods based upon linear regression may statistically provide a better fit for data in terms of reduction in residual error [134], some degree of caution must accompany their use [218]. Positive intercepts are common, which suggest that for zero body mass there still exists a physiological response, and therefore investigators must avoid extrapolation beyond actual data points. Furthermore, many relationships between physiological and anthropometric variables are not linear [166], and more sensitive models must be applied.

Allometric analyses have a long history of use in the biological sciences for describing and interpreting changes in physiological function with changes in size [71, 81, 166], but apart from a few notable exceptions (e.g., [34, 125, 151]), their application in developmental exercise physiology has not become established.

Allometric relationships are most frequently described by the power function:

$$y = a \cdot x^b$$

The values for a and b are derived from the regression equation obtained from the logarithmic transformation of the variables involved, thus:

$$\ln y = \ln a + b \cdot \ln x$$

This expression of the power function as a linear model opens up two further possibilities for statistical comparison. Firstly, analysis of covariance may be applied to the log-transformed data, although as Winter [218] emphasizes, the normal distribution of the transformed variables should be verified [176]. Secondly, the identification of the b exponent permits the construction of power function ratios, Y/x^b, which partition out body size differences correctly and facilitate intergroup comparisons.

The application of power function models has several advantages over the linear method of scaling described above, although the improvement in statistical fit in terms of reduction in residual error may be minimal [71, 134]. Firstly, the statistical procedures involved in the generation and comparison of power function ratios is less daunting than the calculation and interpretation involved in analysis of covariance. Power function ratios may be compared using simple t-test or analysis of variance techniques according to the number of groups under scrutiny. Secondly, and importantly, scaling models based upon linear regression assume an additive error term, whereas the power function model assumes a multiplicative error term. For example, the data presented in Figure 14.6 indicate a tendency toward greater spread in peak $\dot{V}O_2$ scores with increasing body size, which suggests a multiplicative rather than an additive error term, thus confirming that the power function analysis may be preferable. Analyses based upon power function modeling may be further

FIGURE 14.6

The power function relationship between peak oxygen uptake and body mass in males and females.

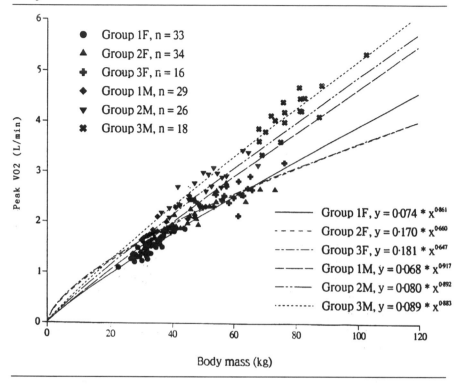

refined if the natural logarithms of the power function ratios are computed and compared [134].

Few studies have applied allometric principles to the investigation of peak $\dot{V}O_2$ development in children, and the results have been mixed. If peak $\dot{V}O_2$ increases linearly with body mass during growth, a b exponent of 1.0 would be expected—in other words, the simple ratio standard would apply. In adults, exponents of 0.5 and 0.47 have been reported for trained and untrained males, respectively, and 0.74 for female athletes [25]. The mean exponent for all male and female groups examined within this study was 0.74. This approximates the value 0.67 (2/3) predicted from the theory of geometric similarity [166]. Similar results were reported by Nevill et al. [134], with exponents of 0.63 and 0.72 observed in untrained males and females, respectively. These exponents were not significantly different, and the common exponent 0.67 corresponds to the theoretically predicted value.

However, growth in children is not a regular process, and differential or nonisometric changes occur in the proportions of body segments [166].

Therefore this theoretical exponent may not be appropriate for all age groups. In children, Cooper et al. [35] reported an exponent of 1.01 for boys and girls aged 11–18 years, which suggests that peak $\dot{V}O_2$ increases in proportion to body size, and thus the simple ratio standard is appropriate for use with children. We applied power function models to the peak $\dot{V}O_2$ data mentioned above, and the results are illustrated in Figure 14.6 (Welsman, Armstrong, Winter, and Kirby, unpublished observations). Both linear regression and power function models were shown to provide a better fit for the data in terms of the reduction in the residual error, compared with that associated with the ratio standard.

Power function exponents for prepubertal, pubertal, and adult females suggested a downward trend (.861, .660 and .647 respectively) but were not significantly different. Exponents for males of the same biological age were .917, .892, and .883 and were not significantly different. As exponents for males and females were not significantly different, a common exponent of .798 could be identified. These findings suggest, therefore, that in prepubertal children to adults, peak $\dot{V}O_2$ changes with increases in body size in the same fashion, but the increase is less than proportional to the change in body size.

It is notable that the studies reporting exponents greater than the theoretical value of .67 have included children who are still growing and developing. An explanation for these elevated values has recently been proposed by Nevill (personal communication), based upon work by Alexander et al. [1]. These authors demonstrated that in mammals, leg muscle mass represents a greater proportion of overall body mass in the larger mammals, i.e., leg muscle mass is proportional to mass, $m^{1.1}$. Therefore, Nevill suggests that when modeling a physiological variable such as peak $\dot{V}O_2$, height, as well as body mass must be incorporated into the allometric equation. This allows the influence of body mass to be separated from the additional effect of the disproportionate increase in muscle mass with increasing body size and produces mass exponents close to .67.

Comparisons based upon allometric relationships must include consideration of differences in the second numerical term in the equation (a) as well as those in the b exponents, i.e., the constant multipliers [134] or proportionality coefficients [166]. Using this technique, we identified significant differences in the constant multipliers between prepubertal girls (a=.091) and both groups of older females (pubertal a=.100, adult a=.097) and between all three groups of males (a=.103, .115, and .128 for prepubertal, pubertal, and adult males). These observations confirmed those indicated by the above-mentioned comparison of regression standards [217]; namely that there are functional improvements in peak $\dot{V}O_2$ between prepuberty and puberty in girls, with no decline between puberty and young adulthood, and in boys significant increases across all three age groups.

These findings obtained from the linear regression and power function scaling techniques, which have been demonstrated to be theoretically and statistically the best fit for examining peak $\dot{V}O_2$ in relation to body size [134, 191], are clearly at odds with traditional interpretation of growth-related peak $\dot{V}O_2$ based on conventional analyses and recommendations that peak $\dot{V}O_2$ expressed as a simple ratio standard be used for growth-related comparisons [21, 171]. Moreover, they support Rowland's conclusion [150], based on examination of growth-related changes in metabolic scope, that "the capacity to deliver oxygen to the working muscles improves during the childhood years independent of gains in body size."

Can this interpretation be explained in terms of current understanding of the growth of physiological processes that have a bearing upon the delivery and utilization of oxygen? The increase in oxygen-consuming muscle mass as a percentage of total body mass in males during maturation [121] is consistent with the observed increases in peak $\dot{V}O_2$ [217]. The earlier maturation of girls [192] with increases in fat mass but no significant gains in muscle mass following puberty [121] also conforms to the female pattern of peak $\dot{V}O_2$ described. Increases in other components of the oxygen transport chain such as hemoglobin concentration are documented [150], but further research is indicated to examine how the components of peak $\dot{V}O_2$ such as arteriovenous oxygen difference and stroke volume develop during growth and maturation.

MULTILEVEL MODELING. Multilevel modeling [70] may prove an invaluable technique for future longitudinal analyses of developmental changes in aerobic function where the influence of factors such as body size and composition need to be controlled for. This type of modeling will also, for example, distinguish the influence of training on peak $\dot{V}O_2$ from the normal increments expected with growth and development. Using multilevel modeling to examine changes in peak $\dot{V}O_2$ in children undergoing intensive training, Jones [91] identified an increase in peak $\dot{V}O_2$ toward the end of puberty in boys, but no similar change in girls. Despite the complexity of the statistics involved, further development of this type of analysis may provide clarification of our understanding of the development of aerobic function in children and adolescents.

BLOOD LACTATE RESPONSES TO EXERCISE

Methodological Influences upon Blood Lactate Measures during Exercise
Before proceeding with the discussion of patterns of blood lactate change with exercise in children, it is important to highlight the numerous methodological factors that may influence actual levels measured during an exercise test. These factors must always be considered during comparisons of results from different studies and include the mode of exercise (e.g., cycling vs running [90]) and the test protocol used [61]. Differences

in measured blood lactate concentrations may also be attributed to the site of blood sampling and the specific lactate assay methodology used. Reports and interpretations of children's blood lactate responses have tended to overlook these factors, although the differences may be considerable. Direct interstudy of comparisons of blood lactate responses and derived measures such as exercise intensities at fixed blood lactate reference values are, therefore, only appropriate where identical techniques have been used [63, 216].

Arterial arm blood is the preferred indicator of muscle lactate production, as lactate levels here closely approximate those in the femoral venous blood draining the muscle groups active during leg exercise [135, 162]. Because arterial sampling is not feasible for routine laboratory assessment, many investigators have sampled venous blood. However, femoral lactate levels are not well reflected by venous arm blood [68]. Furthermore, during cycle ergometry, lactate concentrations are significantly lower in venous blood than in simultaneously sampled arterial or capillary blood [63, 224, 227]. During treadmill exercise, lower venous (compared with capillary) blood lactates have been reported during treadmill running [49]. In contrast, Williams et al. [216] failed to find significant differences in lactate levels measured simultaneously in arterial, venous, and capillary blood, although a trend toward lower venous values was noted. Therefore, as long as a good blood flow is maintained [72], capillary sampling is preferred, as not only will the lactate levels reflect arterial levels but it is not technically difficult and is a less traumatic prospect for children and adolescents. The application of topical anesthetic creams may reduce anxiety in young subjects.

The lactate concentration measured will also depend upon the lactate analysis technique used and more specifically the blood preparation that is assayed. Many sports science laboratories and coaches in the field use the modern semiportable and portable lactate analyzers that are based upon an enzymatic electrochemical assay. These analyzers are popular because they can provide rapid results (generally within 30–60 seconds) and require very small (25µl) blood samples that can be easily drawn from the fingertip or earlobe. Furthermore, blood is assayed "whole" (i.e., without further preparation), although these analyzers can also assay blood that has been hemolyzed [65, 144, 216] or plasma [216]. However, because of the small sample volume, care must be taken to guard against sweat contamination [197].

Chemical assays such as the enzymatic-spectrophotometric [85] and enzymatic-fluorimetric [113, 124] methods are restricted to laboratory use, as the techniques are more cumbersome and require additional blood preparation (e.g., to obtain plasma, serum, or a protein-precipitated sample).

The differences in the results obtained from the use of different blood preparations can be considerable. They reflect the presence or absence of cellular material in the assay sample [208] and whether or not the lactate from the erythrocytes is included following chemical lysis. Therefore, lactate levels in lysed blood tend to exceed those in nonlysed blood [65], and levels in plasma and protein-free samples will exceed those in lysed blood [217] and whole blood [65, 207, 216]. To illustrate the extent of the differences: using the regression equations generated by Williams et al. [216], a whole blood lactate of 4.0 mM corresponds to a lysed blood value of 4.4 mM and a plasma value of 5.5 mM.

Postpeak Oxygen Uptake Blood Lactate Levels
Increases with age in the level of blood lactate measured following incremental treadmill or cycle ergometer exercise to exhaustion have been documented frequently since the earliest laboratory-based studies of exercise physiology in children. For example, Astrand [11] reported postpeak $\dot{V}O_2$ lactates of 8.5 mM in 7- to 9-year-old boys, rising to 10.9 mM at 16–20 years. In girls of the same age, values were 8.0 and 11.5 mM, respectively. Several more recent studies have supported these trends [39, 165, 190]. However, there are a few notable exceptions: Two longitudinal studies have indicated an absence of change in postpeak $\dot{V}O_2$ lactates in children between the ages of 12 and 19 [105, 181]. Similarly, a recent cross-sectional study of 210 11- to 16-year-old children demonstrated no change in postpeak $\dot{V}O_2$ blood lactate levels across this range whether examined by chronological or maturational age [213], although children's values remained significantly lower than values obtained from adults tested under identical conditions. What is apparent, however, is that within any age group, interindividual variation is considerable. For example, in the youngest children studied by Cumming et al. [40], the mean ± 2 standard deviations covered the range 4.9–14.1 mM.

Immediately following an incremental exercise test to peak $\dot{V}O_2$, blood lactate levels continue to rise as lactate diffuses from the active muscles into the blood. In adults, peak levels are reached approximately five minutes postexercise [146, 187]. In children, peak blood lactate levels are seen one to two minutes postexercise [60, 174]. This earlier peaking may reflect children's smaller body size and reduced diffusion distance between capillaries [40]. Different lengths of delay between exercise and sampling must, therefore, be considered when interpreting interstudy differences in postexercise lactate concentrations. Such factors may contribute to the discrepancies in age-related findings described above.

Sex differences in postpeak $\dot{V}O_2$ blood lactate levels have proved difficult to identify consistently. While there is evidence to suggest that similar values are obtained in young boys and girls [11, 115, 116], it appears that up to the age of 14–15 years, girls elicit higher values [39, 165, 213], although there is evidence to the contrary [41, 44]. The higher postexercise lactates in girls (compared with boys) have been suggested to reflect differences in muscle metabolism linked to the advanced maturational status of girls compared with boys of similar chronological age [189]. However, substantive evidence of maturity-linked changes in blood lactate responses is lacking [213], an aspect that is discussed in more detail later.

Blood Lactate as a Criterion for the Attainment of Peak Oxygen Uptake
It has been recommended that in the absence of a plateau in $\dot{V}O_2$, the attainment of peak $\dot{V}O_2$ is confirmed by a postexercise plasma lactate level of 10.0 mM in adults [198]. The application of a similar subsidiary criterion to the assessment of peak $\dot{V}O_2$ in children is particularly attractive, considering that most children do not demonstrate $\dot{V}O_2$max plateaux (see earlier discussion). In the light of the methodological influences described above and the considerable variability in postexercise blood lactate levels observed in children, the recommendation that children should attain a certain level of blood lactate for a peak $\dot{V}O_2$ to be accepted as a maximal effort [39, 40] seems untenable. That high levels of blood lactate are not a prerequisite for the attainment of peak $\dot{V}O_2$ is evident from those studies that have shown no significant differences in peak cardiopulmonary responses between children who elicit high levels of lactate at peak $\dot{V}O_2$ and those who do not [40]. To illustrate the extent to which simple differences in blood lactate assay influence the results obtained, Cumming's [40] recommendation for a 6.0 mM criterion was based upon a plasma assay. This would approximate a whole blood lactate value of 4.0 mM [216].

Lactate Thresholds and Fixed Blood Lactate Reference Values
Although peak $\dot{V}O_2$ limits the performance of maximal aerobic exercise, submaximal blood lactate measures have been shown to be better predictors of an individual's potential for submaximal aerobic exercise [210, 226]. Therefore, monitoring blood lactate levels has become a recommended adjunct to the measurement of peak $\dot{V}O_2$ during routine laboratory evaluation of aerobic fitness [74, 197].

Exercise at the same relative submaximal intensity elicits a lower blood lactate response in children than in adults [55, 111], and an age-related increase toward adult values during development has been described [50, 120, 220]. However, the true pattern of change in blood lactate responses to exercise with age and the mechanisms underlying the differences between children and adults are difficult to tease out from the available literature, largely due to theoretical and methodological differences between studies. Various terms have been applied to submaximal measures of blood lactate during incremental exercise, and most exercise physiologists are familiar with the "anaerobic threshold," which has tended to become their generic term.

Originally, anaerobic threshold was described quite specifically as "the level of work or O_2 consumption just below that at which metabolic acidosis and the associated changes in gas exchange occur" [206]. The theoretical bases of the anaerobic threshold relating to an imbalance between oxygen supply and demand were also clearly specified [205]. The onset of anaerobic metabolism during incremental exercise was, therefore, determined invasively from the point at which blood lactate first increased above resting levels during incremental exercise [206]. Central to the theory was the postulated casual link between the first increase in blood lactate and certain predictable changes in gas exchange parameters. This led to the inference that the anaerobic (lactate) threshold could be accurately determined from noninvasive ventilatory measures such as the breakaway in ventilation or specific changes in the relationship between the ventilatory equivalents for oxygen and carbon dioxide [206]. The true nature and significance of an "anaerobic threshold" has been widely debated and reviewed (e.g., [201, 206, 225]), but the majority view now appears to be that the level of lactate measured in the blood reflects the balance between lactate production and elimination [29]. The first increase in lactate levels observed during incremental exercise therefore reflects the intensity at which processes of production and diffusion from muscle to blood exceed those of elimination and metabolism, rather than indicating the onset of anaerobiosis in the muscle cell.

Several authors have referred to a relatively higher anaerobic threshold in children than adults [17, 202, 204], but many of the studies cited to support this assumption have determined the anaerobic threshold from noninvasive, ventilatory measures [92, 139, 145, 211]. However, results from studies that have demonstrated a lack of coincidence between the lactate and ventilatory anaerobic thresholds [59, 87, 179] suggest that it is unsound to infer developmental changes in blood lactate levels from these indirect measures of gas exchange during exercise.

Other investigators have preferred to measure cardiopulmonary variables at a fixed blood lactate reference level of 4.0 mM. This has been variously termed anaerobic threshold [103] or the onset of blood lactate accumulation (OBLA) [180]. The specific theoretical underpinning of the use of the 4.0 mM level is quite different from that of the classical anaerobic threshold described by Wasserman. Careful scrutiny of exactly which "threshold" has been measured must therefore accompany interpretation of children's blood lactate responses. Such methodological differences make it difficult to identify changing patterns in lactate responses during development, as rarely have two studies employed similar methodology. For example, Rotstein et al. [149] measured the running velocity at which the inflection point of the lactate curve occurred during a discontinuous treadmill exercise protocol with stages of 5 minutes. The inflection point was determined from calculating two regression lines for points clearly above and below the inflection and recording their meeting point. Tanaka and Shindo [190] defined their lactate threshold as the running velocity at a blood lactate level slightly below 2.0 mM, derived from a series of incremental track runs of 4 minutes each. Other authors have used the 4.0

mM level to represent the anaerobic threshold measured during incremental treadmill exercise [67].

The use of fixed blood lactate reference levels to evaluate aerobic fitness may be preferable, as many of the problems associated with the accurate detection of some threshold point are avoided and the influence of varying baseline lactate levels may be minimized [94]. Furthermore, during treadmill exercise with untrained children, it is often difficult to obtain enough data points from a sufficiently low intensity to identify thresholds with precision.

Determination of lactate measures during laboratory testing with adults usually requires each incremental stage to last 4 minutes. This duration is necessary to ensure adequate diffusion of lactate from muscle to blood so that the blood lactate measure reflects the exercise intensity at which it was drawn [93]. With children and adolescents, the duration of exercise stage may be reduced to 3 minutes [74].

Because of children's generally low blood lactate levels during exercise, concern has been expressed that the 4.0 mM fixed level is not an appropriate criterion measure of submaximal aerobic fitness [203, 215]. Williams [215] demonstrated in 12-year-old children exercised to peak $\dot{V}O_2$ that 30% of the boys and 12% of the girls tested did not reach a whole blood lactate level of 4.0 mM. Similarly, Yoshizawa et al. [229] noted that the 4.0 mM level occurred close to maximum effort in 5- to 6-year-old children. Consequently a fixed reference level of 2.5 mM has been recommended for use with children and adolescents [214].

Part of the original justification of the 4.0 mM level was the suggestion that it corresponded to the highest exercise intensity that could be sustained without a progressive increase in blood lactate levels, i.e., a maximal lactate steady state (MLaSS). At this intensity an equilibrium between processes of lactate accumulation and elimination is reached [80]. Mean levels of blood lactate at the MLaSS of 4.0 mM in adults have been reported [80], although a considerable interindividual range has been identified [79, 186].

In a similar investigation with children, Williams and Armstrong [214] used a series of 10-minute treadmill running bouts to examine the relationships between the MLaSS and fixed reference levels in 13-year-old untrained children. Using a whole blood assay, the MLaSS occurred at lactate levels of 2.1mM and 2.3mM in boys and girls, respectively. When cardiopulmonary responses at the MLaSS were compared with those corresponding to the 2.5 and 4.0 mM levels, no significant differences existed between $\dot{V}O_2$ and heart rate values at the 2.5 mM level and the MLaSS, but values at the 4.0 mM level were significantly higher. These findings supported the use of the 2.5 mM level in children.

In contrast to these results, steady states of 4.6 mM [130] and 5.0 mM [129] have been reported in 11- to 12-year-old boys. Although some of the discrepancy in results compared with the previous study may be explained by differences in the lactate assay used, these values appear higher than might be expected considering the general pattern of blood lactate responses in children and the values reported for adults. One explanation might be that the protocol used by Mocellin et al. [129, 130] resulted in an overestimation of the true MLaSS. Although subjects ran for a total of 16 minutes at each intensity, this was made up of 3.5-minute bouts of running interspersed with 30-second rest periods for blood sampling. This may have altered patterns of lactate production and elimination, compared with a continuous exercise bout in these "active" boys, such that the MLaSS was overestimated.

Table 14.1 summarizes the findings of studies that have assessed cardiopulmonary variables at various submaximal blood lactate measures in untrained children. Differences in methodology preclude the combining of data from several studies to form a composite picture of children's submaximal blood lactate responses during development. Furthermore, the predominance of adolescent boys in the subject population restricts extrapolation to other groups, particularly girls, for whom information is notably sparse.

To what extent are age-related changes evident from these findings? Tanaka and Shindo [190] reported a decline in the heart rate at the lactate threshold with increasing age in boys. When expressed as a percentage of peak heart rate, an inverse relationship with chronological age was observed (r=−0.57, P<0.01). Simon et al. [178] reported a higher heart rate at the intensity eliciting a blood lactate of 4.0 mM in 13- to 15-year-olds, compared with adults, although differences were virtually removed when expressed in relative terms. Greater child-adult differences were reported by Izumi and Ishiko [89] during cycle ergometer assessment of lactate threshold. Whether expressed in terms of heart rate or $\dot{V}O_2$, they found that children were able to exercise considerably closer to peak exercise levels than adults (73% vs. 63% peak $\dot{V}O_2$) before the lactate threshold was reached.

In a comprehensive survey of performance at fixed blood lactate reference values of 4.0 and 2.5 mM in relation to chronological age, Williams and Armstrong [213] found no significant correlation between age and % peak $\dot{V}O_2$ at the 4.0 mM level in 11- to 16-year-old boys and girls. However, a significant correlation was observed at the 2.5 mM level, although coefficients were low (−0.226 for boys and −0.272 for girls). When child-adult differences in % peak $\dot{V}O_2$ at the two reference levels were examined (Williams, unpublished observations), a sex difference was noted; although in both males and females the 4.0 mM occurred at a significantly higher % peak $\dot{V}O_2$ in the children (boys 91% vs. men 86%; girls 90% vs. women 85%), the 2.5 mM level corresponded to a significantly higher % peak $\dot{V}O_2$ in the boys, compared with the men (83% vs. 75%), but

TABLE 14.1
Submaximal Blood Lactate Variables in Children: Lactate Thresholds and Fixed Blood Lactate Reference Values

Study*	Sex	n	Age (yr)	Lactate Variable	VO_2 (ml/min·kg)	% Peak VO_2	Heart Rate (b/min)	% Peak VO_2	Lactate (mM)	Velocity (km/hr)
89.	M	11	13.3	LT†	35.8	72.7	164	85	3.84	
190.	M	15	8.8	LT			185	93		11.3
	M	11	10.9	LT			185	92		11.4
	M	11	12.7	LT			173	90		11.0
	M	19	14.6	LT			173	87		10.9
17.	M	11	10.4	LT	36.7	71	169	84		
15, 16.	M	13	11.8	LT	33.2	63.7			1.6	
15.	M	11	19.6	LT	35.9	70.9			1.9	
149.	M	28	10.8	LT		82.24				
	M	28	10.8	LT		85.07				
213.	M	84	11–16	2.5 mM	41	83	186	93		
	F	65	11–16	2.5 mM	32	77	184	92		
199.	M	26	11	2.5 mM		85				
	M	26	14	2.5 mM		85				
	M	26	11	4.0 mM		94				
	M	26	14	4.0 mM		92				
102.	M		10–14	4.0 mM			190			
213.	M	81	11–16	4.0 mM	45	91	195	97		10.04
	F	81	11–16	4.0 mM	37	90	193	96		10.36

*All studies reflect treadmill testing except the first study, which used cycle ergometry.
†Lactate threshold, i.e., point of onset of rapid increase in blood lactate concentration.

no difference was evident between the younger and older female subjects (77% vs. 76%).

Sex differences are difficult to determine from the available literature. Some authors have identified a higher "anaerobic threshold" in boys than in girls, indicating an earlier onset of aerobic metabolism in girls (see [203]). However, Williams and Armstrong [213] identified no significant differences in performance at the two reference levels examined, although a trend toward a lower percentage of peak $\dot{V}O_2$ in the girls was evident.

CHILD-ADULT DIFFERENCES IN BLOOD LACTATE RESPONSES TO EXERCISE. The lower glycogen utilization rates and lower maximal muscle lactate concentrations observed by Eriksson in 11- to 15-year-old boys [53, 55] suggest that glycogenolysis and consequent ability to produce lactate is limited in children and adolescents, compared with adults. The similarly reduced activity of phosphofructokinase (PFK) measured in five 11-year-old boys was offered in explanation [51]. Eriksson himself urged caution in drawing general conclusions from such a limited sample [52], although support for these findings was provided by Fournier et al. [62].

The tendency to cite Eriksson's findings of lower PFK levels in children as the major cause of children's lower blood lactate responses overlooks the more recent evidence that has failed to identify any significant differences in the maximal activities of a variety of glycolytic enzymes in children aged 11–14 years [76–78]. However, the elevated levels of oxidative enzymes such as succinic dehydrogenase (SDH) and isocitric dehydrogenase (ICDH) in children and adolescents [51, 62, 77] compared with adults are evidence that children have an enhanced ability to provide energy via oxidative pathways. Furthermore, the difference in the ratios of PFK to ICDH observed between adults (1.633) and children (0.844) suggests that the Krebs cycle functions at a higher rate in children and reflects an enhanced ability to oxidize pyruvate [77].

The increased availability of fat as a fuel during exercise may alter the lactate response pattern during incremental exercise by shifting the lactate curve to the right [88]. Greater intramuscular lipid stores may also indicate a greater availability of fatty acids and contribute to lower glycogen utilization during exercise [190]. Higher lipid storage [24] and muscle blood flow [106] have been noted in children, compared with adults. The combination of these two factors might be suggested to contribute to lower levels of lactate accumulation in children. However, small subject numbers in these studies limit extrapolation, and evidence that fat mobilization and utilization in children differ little from those in adults is available. Levels of free glycerol in blood reflect the extent of adipose tissue lipolysis [120]. In children during prolonged exercise, no significant differences in glycerol levels compared with adults have been identified [54, 120]. Similarly, the mean pattern of increase in the fat-mobilizing human growth hormone (HGH) was the same in prepubertal boys during prolonged exercise at 70% peak $\dot{V}O_2$ as in adults [138]. Neither were relationships between the

HGH response and blood lactate levels identified; a finding supported by Wirth et al. [220], who also failed to identify differences in free fatty acid levels during exercise in prepubertal, pubertal, and postpubertal children.

The speed at which oxygen uptake reaches a steady-state value following the onset of exercise reflects the ability of the circulatory systems to deliver and the working muscles to utilize oxygen [212]. A faster adjustment of the $\dot{V}O_2$ response in children has frequently been suggested to contribute to their lower lactate response to exercise [114, 118]. Documentation of children's transient $\dot{V}O_2$ is scarce, and methodological discrepancies between the studies preclude direct comparison and interpretation. At exercise intensities close to or exceeding peak $\dot{V}O_2$, children achieve a higher percentage of peak $\dot{V}O_2$ after 30-seconds exercise than adults [117, 118, 148]. Support for a faster oxygen on-transient in children has come from more recent studies of the $t^1/2\dot{V}O_2$ (the time taken for the $\dot{V}O_2$ to reach 50% of its asymptotic value) [143, 157]. Macek et al. [119] reported $t^1/2\dot{V}O_2$ values of 11.7 and 29.1 seconds in boys and adults, respectively, with correspondingly lower blood lactate concentrations in the boys. Sady [157] reported similarly large child-adult differences during cycling exercise at an intensity set to theoretically elicit 110% peak $\dot{V}O_2$. However, results from a carefully designed study of the $t^1/2\dot{V}O_2$ during submaximal exercise failed to identify child-adult differences. Sady et al. [160] reported $t^1/2\dot{V}O_2$ values of 18.5 and 17.4 seconds in children and adults, respectively, during exercise at 40% peak $\dot{V}O_2$. Thus, the contention that lower muscle and blood lactate during submaximal exercise result from faster oxygen on-transients [50] remains to be confirmed. Further studies using breath-by-breath $\dot{V}O_2$ measurement are required to elucidate this matter further.

Several authors have implied that children have a natural propensity for high levels of physical activity [22, 43]. These assumed high levels of activity have been used to explain the low trainability of childrens' aerobic capacity reported by some investigators [22, 23, 75]. If this is the case, then might the differences between adults' and children's blood lactate responses reflect a training effect in children due to a higher levels of habitual activity? Such an effect is improbable in the light of recent evidence that has shown not only that few 10- to 16-year-old children demonstrate the frequency, duration, and intensity of exercise likely to improve cardiopulmonary fitness [3–5], but specifically, that there are no relationships between levels of habitual physical activity assessed from 3-day minute-by-minute heart rate recordings and % peak $\dot{V}O_2$ at submaximal blood lactate measures in prepubertal [7] or 13-year-old [209] children.

Blood Lactate and Maturation
Eriksson et al. [53] observed an "almost significant" correlation between testicular volume and muscle lactate concentration during exercise in a small sample of 13- to 15-year-old boys and postulated that lactate production is influenced by sexual maturation. These findings have often

been cited as evidence that the ability to derive energy from glycolysis depends upon maturation [60, 141].

The results from studies on animals, which have identified relationships between testosterone levels and the maturation of skeletal muscle glycolytic capacity [47, 48, 109], and human studies, which have identified moderate correlations between various blood lactate responses to exercise and salivary testosterone levels in boys [55, 58, 126], have supported this contention. Others have reached a similar conclusion [190] based upon the relationship between skeletal age (which reflects androgen levels) and performance at the lactate threshold. However, these studies have not examined the full maturational range, and there has been a notable failure to address the issue of maturation and lactate production in girls. Testosterone levels in girls during puberty are minimal, but clearly their ability to produce lactate is not compromised.

Several studies have failed to identify links between blood lactate responses to exercise and sexual maturation. Paterson and Cunningham [140] found no significant differences in postexercise blood lactates between early and late maturers of the same chronological age, despite a 2-year differential in biological (skeletal) age. A recent examination of submaximal blood lactate responses between groups of boys and girls rated according to the development of the secondary sexual characteristics [192] failed to identify significant alterations in the percentage peak $\dot{V}O_2$ at 2.5 and 4.0 mM reference levels, although there was a trend toward a reduction in values at the lower reference level [213].

In 38 of the boys from the above study, aged 11–16 years, serum testosterone levels were examined in relation to blood lactate variables. No significant correlations were obtained between testosterone level and percentage peak $\dot{V}O_2$ at blood lactate levels of 2.5 or 4.0 mM (Welsman and Armstrong, unpublished observations). Bar-Or [21] suggested that it was premature to assume that differences in glycolytic capacity between boys and men are explained by differences in male hormone activity. These data support that view and suggest that testosterone plays a minimal role in the development of glycolytic capacity. Future studies using longitudinal measures to follow hormonal markers of maturity, including dehydroepi-androsterone (DHA) in girls [110], in relation to exercise blood lactate responses are required to elucidate this issue further.

SUMMARY

Our understanding of the development of children and adolescents' aerobic fitness is limited by ethical considerations and methodological constraints. Protocols, apparatus, and criteria of maximal effort used with adults are often unsuitable for use with children. In normal children and adolescents, peak $\dot{V}O_2$ increases with growth and maturation, although there are indications that girls' peak $\dot{V}O_2$ may level off around 14 years of age. Males exhibit higher values of peak $\dot{V}O_2$ than females, and the sex difference increases as they progress through adolescence. The difference between males and females has been attributed to the boys' greater muscle mass and hemoglobin concentration. It appears that boys experience an adolescent growth spurt in peak $\dot{V}O_2$, which reaches a maximum gain near the time of PHV, but data are insufficient to offer any generalization for girls. Peak $\dot{V}O_2$ has usually been expressed in relation to body mass, and with this convention it appears that boys' values are consistent throughout the developmental period, whereas girls' values decrease as they get older. This type of analysis may, however, have clouded our understanding of growth and maturational changes in peak $\dot{V}O_2$, and scaling for differences in body size may provide further clarification. If differences are shown where none were previously thought to exist, then physiological explanations must be sought.

Methodological issues have also hindered the understanding of how children's blood lactate responses to exercise develop. The actual lactate level recorded during an exercise test is influenced by the site of sampling and the blood handling and assay techniques. Valid interstudy comparisons can only be made where similar procedures have been employed. In general, children demonstrate lower blood lactate levels at peak $\dot{V}O_2$ than adults, although individual variation is wide. Therefore the use of blood lactate measures to confirm the attainment of peak $\dot{V}O_2$ cannot be supported. Exercise at the same relative submaximal intensity elicits a lower blood lactate in children than in adults, but interpretation and identification of developmental and maturational patterns of response are limited by the use of different testing conditions and reference points (e.g., lactate threshold and fixed level reference points). There is growing evidence that the 2.5 mM reference level should be used in preference to the 4.0 mM level, as the adult criterion occurs close to maximal exercise in many children and adolescents. Explanations for child-adult differences in blood lactate responses to exercise are difficult to elucidate. Conclusive evidence is lacking for the conventional explanations that differences are caused by insufficient testosterone and glycolytic enzymes, faster oxygen on-transients, a greater reliance on fat as a fuel, or high levels of physical activity.

(*Note:* Source references for Figures 14.1–14.4 are available from the authors on request.)

REFERENCES

1. Alexander, R. McN., A. S. Jayes, G. M. O. Maloiy, and E. M. Wathuta. Allometry of the leg muscles of mammals. *J. Zool. Lond.* 194:539–552, 1981.
2. Andersen, K. L., V. Seliger, J. Rutenfranz, and J. Skrobak-Kaczynski. Physical performance capacity of children in Norway. Part IV—The rate of growth in maximal aerobic power

and the influence of improved physical education of children in a rural community. *Eur. J. Appl. Physiol.* 35:49–58, 1976.

3. Armstrong, N., J. Balding, P. Gentle, and B. Kirby. Patterns of physical activity among 11 to 16 year old British children. *Br. Med. J.* 301:203–205, 1990.

4. Armstrong, N., J. Balding, P. Gentle, J. Williams, and B. Kirby. Peak oxygen uptake and habitual physical activity in 11 to 16 years old. *Pediatr. Exerc. Sci.* 2:349–358, 1990.

5. Armstrong, N., and S. Bray. Physical activity patterns defined by heart rate monitoring. *Arch. Dis. Child.* 66:245–247, 1991.

6. Armstrong, N., and B. Davies. An ergometric analysis of age group swimmers. *Br. J. Sports Med.* 15:20–26, 1981.

7. Armstrong, N., J. Welsman, and B. Kirby. Daily physical activity estimated from continuous heart rate monitoring and laboratory indices of aerobic fitness in pre-adolescent children. *Res. Q. Exerc. Sport.* 64:(Suppl)A24, 1993.

8. Armstrong, N., J. Williams, J. Balding, P. Gentle, and B. Kirby. The peak oxygen uptake of British children with reference to age, sex and sexual maturity. *Eur. J. Appl. Physiol.* 62:369–375, 1991.

9. Armstrong, N., J. Williams, J. Balding, P. Gentle, and B. Kirby. Cardiopulmonary fitness, physical activity patterns, and selected coronary risk factor variables in 11- to 16-year-olds. *Pediatr. Exerc. Sci.* 3:219–228, 1991.

10. Armstrong, N., J. Williams, and D. Ringham. Peak oxygen uptake and progressive shuttle run performance in boys aged 11–14 years. *Br. J. Phys. Ed. Res. Suppl.* 4:10–11, 1988.

11. Astrand, P. O. *Experimental Studies of Physical Working Capacity in Relation to Sex and Age.* Copenhagen: Munksgaard, 1952.

12. Astrand, P. O. Personal communication cited by R. J. Shephard (ed). *Frontiers of Fitness.* Springfield, IL: Charles C. Thomas, 1971, p 336.

13. Astrand, P. O. The child in sport and physical activity—physiology. J. G. Albinson and G. M. Andrew (ed). *Child in Sport and Physical Activity.* Baltimore: University Park Press, 1976, pp. 19–33.

14. Astrand, P. O., and K. Rodahl. *Textbook of Work Physiology.* New York: McGraw-Hill, 1986.

15. Atomi, Y., T. Fukunaga, H. Hatta, and Y. Yamamoto. Relationship between lactate threshold during running and relative gastrocnemius area. *J. Appl. Physiol.* 63:2343–2347, 1987.

16. Atomi, Y., T. Fukunaga, Y. Yamamoto, and H. Hatta. Lactate threshold and VO_2max of trained and untrained boys relative to muscle mass and composition. J. Rutenfranz, R. Mocellin and F. Klimt (eds). *Children and Exercise XII*, Champaign, IL: Human Kinetics, 1986, pp. 53–58.

17. Atomi, Y., K. Iwaoka, H. Hatta, M. Miyashita, and Y. Yamamoto. Daily physical activity levels in preadolescent boys related to VO_2max and lactate threshold. *Eur. J. Appl. Physiol.* 55:156–161, 1986.

18. Bale, P. The physiological performance of pre-adolescent school children. *Phys. Ed. Rev.* 1:89–95, 1978.

19. Bale, P. Pre- and post-adolescents' physiological response to exercise. *Br. J. Sports Med.* 15:246–249, 1981.

20. Barnett, A., L. Y. S. Chan, and I. C. Bruce. A preliminary study of the 20-m multistage shuttle run as a predictor of peak VO_2 in Hong Kong Chinese students. *Pediatr. Exerc. Sci.* 5:42–50, 1993.

21. Bar-Or, O. *Pediatric Sports Medicine for the Practitioner.* New York: Springer-Verlag, 1983.

22. Bar-Or, O. The growth and development of children's physiologic and perceptional responses to exercise. J. Ilmarinen, I. Valimaki (eds). *Children and Sport.* Berlin: Springer-Verlag, 1984, pp. 13–17.

23. Bar-Or, O. Trainability of the prepubescent child. *Phys. Sports Med.* 17:65–82, 1989.

24. Bell, R. D., J. D. MacDougall, R. Billeter, and H. Howald. Muscle fibre types and morphometric analysis of skeletal muscle in six-year-old children. *Med. Sci. Sports* 12:28–31, 1980.

25. Bergh, U., B. Sjodin, A. Forsberg, and J. Svedenhag. The relationship between body mass and oxygen uptake during running in humans. *Med. Sci. Sports Exerc.* 23:205–211, 1991.

26. Beunen, G., and R. M. Malina. Growth and physical performance relative to the timing of the adolescent spurt. *Exerc. Sports Sci. Rev.* 16:503–540, 1988.

27. Binkhorst, R. A., W. H. M. Saris, A. M. Noordeloos, M. A. Van't Hof, and A. F. J. de Haan. Maximal oxygen consumption of children (6 to 18 years) predicted from maximal and submaximal values in treadmill and bicycle tests. J. Rutenfranz, R. Mocellin, and I. Klimt (eds). *Children and Exercise XII.* Champaign, IL: Human Kinetics, 1986, pp. 227–232.

28. Boileau, R. A., A. Bonen, V. H. Heyward, and B. H. Massey. Maximal aerobic capacity on the treadmill and bicycle ergometer of boys 11–14 years of age. *J. Sports Med. Phys. Fitness* 17:153–162, 1977.

29. Brooks, G. A. Anaerobic threshold: review of the concept and directions for future research. *Med Sci. Sports Exerc.* 17:22–31, 1985.

30. Buono, M. J., J. J. Roby, F. G. Micale, and J. F. Sallis. Predicting maximal oxygen uptake in children: modification of the Astrand-Ryhming test. *Pediatr. Exerc. Sci.* 1:278–283, 1989.

31. Chan, O. L., M. T. Duncan, J. W. Sundsten, T. Thinakaran, M. N. B. C. Noh, and V. Klissouras. The maximum aerobic power of the Temiars. *Med. Sci. Sports Exerc.* 8:235–238, 1976.

32. Chatterjee, S., P. K. Banerjee, P. Chatterjee, and S. R. Maitra. Aerobic capacity of young girls. *Indian J. Med Res.* 69:327–333, 1979.

33. Clarke, D. H. Children and the research process. G. A. Stull and H. M. Eckert (eds). *Effects of Physical Activity on Children.* Champaign, IL: Human Kinetics, 1986, pp. 9–13.

34. Cooper, D. M. Development of the oxygen transport system in normal children. O. Bar-Or (ed). *Advances in Pediatric Sports Sciences Vol 3.* Champaign, IL: Human Kinetics, 1989, pp.67–100.

35. Cooper, D. M., D. Weiler-Ravell, B. J. Whipp, and K. Wasserman. Aerobic parameters of exercise as a function of body size during growth in children. *J. Appl. Physiol.* 56:628–634, 1984.

36. Cumming, G. R. Current levels of fitness. *Can. Med. Assoc. J.* 96:868–877, 1967.

37. Cumming, G. R. Personal communication cited by R. J. Shephard (ed). *Frontiers of Fitness.* Springfield, IL: Charles C. Thomas, 1971, p. 336.

38. Cumming, G. R., A. Goodwin, G. Baggley, and J. Antel. Repeated measurement of aerobic capacity during a week of intensive training at a youth's track camp. *Can. J. Physiol. Pharmacol.* 45:805–811, 1967.

39. Cumming, G. R., L. Hastman, and J. McCort. Treadmill endurance times, blood lactate, and exercise blood pressures in normal children. R. A. Binkhorst, H. C. G. Kemper and W. H. M. Saris (eds). *Children and Exercise XI.* Champaign, IL: Human Kinetics, 1985, pp. 140–150.

40. Cumming, G. R., L. Hastman, J. McCort, and S. McCullough. High serum lactates do occur in children after maximal work. *Int. J. Sports Med.* 1:66–69, 1980.

41. Cunningham, D. A., and R. B. Eynon. The working capacity of young competitive swimmers 10–16 years of age. *Med. Sci. Sports Exerc.* 5:227–231, 1973.

42. Cunningham, D. A., B. MacFarlane, V. Waterschoot, D. H. Paterson, M. Lefcoe, and S. P. Sangal. Reliability and reproducibility of maximal oxygen uptake measurement in children. *Med. Sci. Sports Exerc.* 9:104–108, 1977.

43. Cunningham, D. A., D. H. Paterson, and C. J. R. Blimkie. The development of the cardiorespiratory system with growth and physical activity. R. A. Boileau (ed). *Advances in Pediatric Sport Sciences Vol 1.* Champaign, IL: Human Kinetics, 1984, pp. 85–116.

44. Cunningham, D. A., B. Van Waterschoot, D. H. Paterson, M. Lefcoe, and S. P. Sangal. Reliability and reproducibility of maximum oxygen uptake measurements in children. *Med. Sci. Sports* 9:104–108, 1977.

45. Davies, C. T. M., C. Barnes, and S. Godfrey. Body composition and maximal exercise performance in children. *Hum. Biol.* 44:195–214, 1972.

46. Denis, C., D. Dormois, and J. R. Lacour. Endurance training, V̇O₂max and OBLA: a longitudinal study of two different age groups. *Int. J. Sports Med.* 5:167–173, 1984.

47. Dux, L., E. Dux, and F. Guba. Further data on the androgenic dependency of the skeletal musculature: the effect of prepubertal castration of the structural development of the skeletal muscles. *Horm. Metab. Res.* 14:191–194, 1982.

48. Dux, L., E. Dux, H. Mazareau, and F. Guba. A non-neural regulatory effect on the metabolic differentiation of the skeletal muscle. Effect of castration and testosterone administration on the skeletal muscles of the rat. *Comp. Biochem. Physiol.* 64A:177–183, 1979.

49. El-Sayed, M. S., K. P. George, D. Wilkinson, N. Mullen, R. Fenoglio, and J. Flannigan. Fingertip and venous blood lactate concentration in response to graded treadmill exercise. *J. Sports Sci.* 11:139–143, 1993.

50. Eriksson, B. O. Physical training, oxygen supply and muscle metabolism in 11–13 year old boys. *Acta Physiol. Scand.* 384(Suppl.), 1972.

51. Eriksson, B. O., P. D. Gollnick, and B. Saltin. Muscle metabolism and enzyme activities after training in boys 11–13 years old. *Acta Physiol. Scand.* 87:485–497, 1973.

52. Eriksson, B. O., P. D. Gollnick, and B. Saltin. The effect of physical training on muscle enzyme activities and fibre composition in 11 year old boys. *Acta Paediatr. Belg.* 28(Suppl.) 245–252, 1974.

53. Eriksson, B. O., J. Karlsson, and B. Saltin. Muscle metabolites during exercise in pubertal boys. *Acta Paediatr. Scand.* 217(Suppl.):154–157, 1971.

54. Eriksson, B. O., B. Persson, and J. I. Thorell. The effects of repeated prolonged exercise on plasma growth hormone, insulin, glucose, free-fatty acids, glycerol, lactate and beta-hydroxybutyric acid in 13 year old boys and in adults. *Acta Paediatr. Scand.* 217(Suppl.):142–146, 1971.

55. Eriksson, B. O. and B. Saltin. Muscle metabolism during exercise in boys aged 11–16 years compared to adults. *Acta. Paediatr. Belg.* 28(Suppl.):257–265, 1974.

56. Eston, R. G., S. Robson, and E. Winter. A comparison of oxygen uptake during running in children and adults. J. Borms (ed). *Kinanthropometry IV*. London: E & F Spon, 1993, pp. 236–241.

57. Fahey, T. D., A. Del Valle-Zuris, G. Dehlsen, M. Trieb, and J. Seymour, Pubertal stage differences in hormonal and haematological responses to maximal exercise in males. *J. Appl Physiol.* 46:823–827, 1979.

58. Falgairette, G., M. Bedu, N. Fellmann, E. Van Praagh, J. F. Jarrige, and J. Coudert. Modifications of aerobic and anaerobic metabolisms in active boys during puberty. G. Beunen, J. Ghesquiere, T. Reybrouck and A. L. Claessens (eds). *Children and Exercise*. Suttgart: Ferdinand Enke, 1990, pp. 42–49.

59. Farrell, S. W., and J. L. Ivy. Lactate acidosis and the increase in VE/V̇O₂ during incremental exercise. *J. Appl. Physiol.* 62:1551–1555, 1987.

60. Fellmann, N., M. Bedu, H. Spielvogel, G. Falgairette, E. Van Praagh, et al. Anaerobic metabolism during pubertal development at high altitude. *J. Appl. Physiol.* 64:1382–1386, 1988.

61. Ferry, A., A. Duvallet, and M. Rieu. The effect of experimental protocol on the relationship between blood lactate and workload. *J. Sports Med. Phys. Fitness* 28:341–347, 1988.

62. Fournier, M. J., J. Ricci, A. W. Taylor, R. J. Ferguson, R. R. Montpetit, and B. R. Chaitman. Skeletal muscle adaptation in adolescent boys: sprint and endurance training and detraining. *Med. Sci. Sports Exerc.* 14:453–456, 1982.

63. Foxdal, P. B. Sjodin, H. Rudstan, C. Ostman, B. Ostman, and G. C. Hedenstierna. Lactate concentration differences in plasma, whole blood, capillary finger blood and erythrocytes during submaximal graded exercise in humans. *Eur. J. Appl. Physiol.* 61:218–222, 1990.

64. Freedson, P. S., and T. L. Goodman. Measurement of oxygen consumption. T. W. Rowland (ed). *Pediatric Laboratory Exercise Testing*. Champaign, IL: Human Kinetics. 1993, pp. 91–113.

65. Friedheim, L. C., and G. P. Town. Blood lactate methodologies compared. *Med. Sci Sports Exerc.* 21(Suppl.):S21, 1989.
66. Gaessar, G. A., and D. C. Poole. Lactate and ventilatory thresholds: disparity in time course of adaptations to training. *J. Appl. Physiol.* 61:999–1004, 1986.
67. Gaisl, G., and G. Weisspeiner. Training prescriptions for 9- to 17-year-old figure skaters based on lactate assessment in the laboratory and on the ice. J. Rutenfranz, R. Mocellin, and F. Klimt (eds). *Children and Exercise XII.* Champaign, IL:Human Kinetics, 1986, pp. 59–66.
68. Gisolfi, C., and S. Robinson. Venous blood distribution in the legs during intermittent treadmill work. *J. Appl. Physiol.* 29:368–373, 1970.
69. Glassford, R. C., G H. Y. Bayford, A. W. Sedgwick, and R. B. J. McNab. Comparison of maximal oxygen uptake values determined by predicted and actual methods. *J. Appl. Physiol.* 20:509–513, 1965.
70. Goldstein, H. Efficient statistical modeling of longitudinal data. *Ann. Hum. Biol.* 13:129–141, 1986.
71. Gould, S. J. Allometry and size in ontogeny and phylogeny. *Biol. Rev.* 41:587–640, 1966.
72. Graham, T. E. The measurement and interpretation of lactate. H. Lollgen, and H. Mellerowicz (eds). *Progress in Ergometry: Quality Control and Test Criteria.* Berlin: Springer-Verlag, 1984, pp. 51–65.
73. Hagberg, J. M. Physiological implications of lactate threshold. *Int. J. Sports Med.* 5(Suppl):106–109, 1984.
74. Hale, T., N. Armstrong, A. Hardman, P. Jakeman, C. Sharp, and E. Winter. *Position Statement on the Physiological Assessment of the Elite Competitor.* Leeds, UK: British Association of Sports Sciences, 1988.
75. Hamilton, P., and G. M. Andrew. Influence of growth and athletic training on heart and lung functions. *Eur. J. Appl. Physiol.* 36:27–38, 1976.
76. Haralambie, G. Skeletal muscle enzyme activities in female subjects of various ages. *Bull. Eur. Physiopathol. Respir.* 15:259–267, 1979.
77. Haralambie, G. Enzyme activities in skeletal muscle of 13–15 years old adolescents. *Bull. Eur. Physiol. Res.* 18:65–74, 1982.
78. Haralambie, G., and H. Reinartz. Human skeletal muscle enolase and factors influencing its activity. *Enzyme.* 23:404–409, 1978.
79. Haverty, M., W. L. Kenny, and J. L. Hodgson. Lactate and gas exchange responses to incremental and steady state running. *Br. J. Sports Med.* 2:51–54, 1988.
80. Heck, H., A. Mader, G. Hess, S. Mucke, R. Muller, and W. Hollman. Justification of the 4 mmol.1^{-1} lactate threshold. *Int. J. Sports Med.* 6:117–130, 1985.
81. Heusner, A. A. Mathematical expression of the effects of changes in body size on pulmonary function and structure. *Am. Rev. Respir. Dis.* 128:S72–S74, 1983.
82. Hill, A. V. *Muscular Activity.* London: Balliere, Tindall and Cox, 1925.
83. Hill, A. V., C. N. H. Long, and H. Lupton. Muscular exercise, lactic acid and the supply and utilization of oxygen. Parts IV–VIII. *Proc. R. Soc. Lond.* B 97:84–138, 155–176, 1924.
84. Hoes, M., R. A. Binkhorst, A. Smeekes-Kuyl, and A. C. Vissurs. Measurement of forces exerted on a pedal crank during work on the bicycle ergometer at different loads. *Int. Z. Angew. Physiol.* 26:33–42, 1968.
85. Hohorst, H. J. L-(+) Lactate determination with lactic dehydrogenase and DPN. H. V. Bergmeyer (ed). *Methods of Enzymatic Analysis.* (2nd edition), New York: Academic Press, 1965, pp. 226–270.
86. Howell, M. L., and R. B. J. MacNab. *The Physical Work Capacity of Canadian Children Aged 7 to 17.* Toronto, Ont.: Canadian Association for Health, Physical Education, and Recreation. 1968, pp. 125–135.
87. Hughes, E. F., S. C. Turner, and G. A. Brooks. Effects of glycogen depletion and pedalling speed on "anaerobic threshold." *J. Appl. Physiol.* 52:1598–1607, 1982.
88. Ivy, J. L., R. T. Withers, P. J. Van Handel, D. H. Elger, and D. L. Costill. Muscle respiratory

capacity and fibre type as determinants of the lactate threshold. *J. Appl. Physiol.* 48:523–527, 1980.

89. Izumi, I., and T. Ishiko. Lactate threshold in pubescent boys. *Jpn. J. Phys. Ed.* 28:309–314. (In Japanese), 1984.

90. Jacobs, I., and B. Sjodin. Relationship of ergometer-specific V̇O₂ max and muscle enzymes to blood lactate during submaximal exercise. *Br. J. Sports Med.* 19:77–80, 1985.

91. Jones A. Peak aerobic power in intensively trained young athletes related to puberty. *J. Sports Sci.* (Abstract) 9:418–419, 1991.

92. Kanaley, J. A., and R. A. Boileau. The onset of the anaerobic threshold at three stages of physical maturity. *J. Sports Med. Phys. Fitness* 28:367–374, 1988.

93. Karlsson, J., and I. Jacobs. Onset of blood lactate accumulation during muscular exercise as threshold concept. I. Theoretical considerations. *Int. J. Sports Med.* 3:190–201, 1982.

94. Karlsson, J., A. Holmgren, D. Linnarson, and H. Astrom. OBLA exercise stress testing in health and disease. H. Lollgen and H. Mellerowicz (eds). *Progress in Ergometry: Quality Control and Test Criteria.* Berlin: Springer-Verlag, 1984, pp. 66–91.

95. Katch, V. L. Use of the oxygen/body weight ratio in correlational analyses: spurious correlations and statistical considerations. *Med. Sci. Sports.* 5:252–257, 1973.

96. Katch, F. I., F. N. Girandola, and V. L. Katch. The relationship of body weight to maximum oxygen uptake and heavy work endurance capacity on the bicycle ergometer. *Med. Sci. Sports* 3:101–106, 1971.

97. Katch, V. L., and F. I. Katch. Use of weight-adjusted oxygen uptake scores that avoid spurious correlation. *Res. Q.* 45:447–451, 1974.

98. Kay, C., and R. J. Shephard. On muscle strength and the threshold of anaerobic work. *Int. Z. Angew. Physiol.* 27:311–328, 1969.

99. Kemper, H. C. G. (ed). Growth, health and fitness of teenagers. *Med. Sport Sci.* 20:1–202, 1985.

100. Kemper, H. C. G., and R. Verschuur. Maximal aerobic power in 13 and 14 year old teenagers in relation to biologic age. *Int. J. Sports Med.* 2:97–100, 1981.

101. Kemper, H. C. G., R. Verschuur, and L. deMey. Longitudinal changes of aerobic fitness in youth ages 12 to 23. *Pediatr. Exerc. Sci.* 1:257–270, 1989.

102. Keul, J., W. Kindermann, and G. Simon. Die aerobe und anaerobe Kapazitat als Grundlage fur die Leistungsdiagnostik. *Leistungssport.* 8:22–32, 1978.

103. Kindermann, W., G. Simon, and J. Keul. The significance of the aerobic-anaerobic transition for the determination of work load intensities during endurance training. *Eur. J. Appl. Physiol.* 42:25–34, 1979.

104. Kobayashi, K., K. Kitamura, M. Miura, H. Sodeyama, Y. Murase, et al. Aerobic power as related to body growth and training in Japanese boys: a longitudinal study. *J. Appl. Physiol.* 44:666–672, 1978.

105. Koch, G. Muscle blood flow in prepubertal boys. J. Borms and M. Hebbelinck (eds). *Medicine and Sport, Pediatric Work Physiology.* Basel: Karger, 1978, pp. 39–46.

106. Koch, G., and L. Fransson. Essential cardiovascular and respiratory determinants of physical performance at age 12–17 years during intensive physical training. J. Rutenfranz, R. Mocellin and F. Klimt (eds). *Children and Exercise XII.* Champaign, IL: Human Kinetics, 1986, pp. 275–292.

107. Krahenbuhl, G. S., R. P. Pangrazi, W. J. Stone, D. W. Morgan, and T. Williams. Fractional utilization of maximal aerobic capacity in children 6 to 8 years of age. *Pediatr. Exerc. Sci.* 1:271–277, 1989.

108. Krahenbuhl, G. S., J. S. Skinner, and W. M. Kohrt. Developmental aspects of maximal aerobic power in children. *Exerc. Sports Sci. Rev.* 13:503–538, 1985.

109. Krotkiewski, M., J. G. Kral, and J. Karlsson. Effects of castration and testosterone substitution on body composition and muscle metabolism in rats. *Acta Physiol. Scand.* 109:233–237, 1980.

110. Lac, G., P. Duché, G. Falgairette, and A. Robert. Adrenal androgen profiles in saliva

throughout puberty in both sexes. J. Coudert and E. Van Praagh (eds). *Pediatric Work Physiology*. Paris: Masson, 1992, pp. 221–223.

111. Lehmann, M., J. Keul, and U. Korsten-Reck. Einfluss einer stufenweisen Laufbandergom-etrie bei Kindern und Erwachsenen auf die Plasmacatecholamine die aerobe und anaerobe Kapazitat. *Eur. J. Appl. Physiol.* 47:301–311, 1981.

112. Lohman, T. G. Assessment of body composition in children. *Pediatr. Exerc. Sci.* 1:19–30, 1989.

113. Lowry, O. H., and J. V. Passonneau. *A Flexible System of Enzymatic Analysis*. New York: Academic Press, 1972.

114. Macek, M. Aerobic and anaerobic energy output in children. J. Rutenfranz, R. Mocellin and F. Klimt (eds). *Children and Exercise XII*. Champaign, IL: Human Kinetics, 1986, pp. 3–9.

115. Macek, M., and J. Vavra. Aerobic and anaerobic metabolism during exercise in childhood. *Malatti Cardiovasculari.* 10:409–420, 1969.

116. Macek, M., and J. Vavra. Cardiopulmonary and metabolic changes during exercise in children 6–14 years old. *J. Appl. Physiol.* 30:200–204, 1971.

117. Macek, M., and J. Vavra. Relation between aerobic and anaerobic energy supply during maximal exercise in boys. H. Lavallee and R. J. Shephard (eds). *Frontiers of Activity and Child Health*. Quebec: Editions du Pelican, 1977, pp. 157–159.

118. Macek, M., and J. Vavra. The adjustment of oxygen uptake at the onset of exercise: a comparison between prepubertal boys and young adults. *Int. J. Sports Med.* 1:75–77, 1980.

119. Macek, M., J. Vavra, H. Benesova, and J. Radvansky. The adjustment of oxygen uptake at the onset of exercise: relation to age and to workload. J. Ilmarinen and I. Valimaki (eds). *Children and Sport*. Berlin: Springer-Verlag, 1984, pp. 129–134.

120. Macek, M., J. Vavra, and J. Novosadova. Prolonged exercise in prepubertal boys. I—Cardiovascular and metabolic adjustment. *Eur. J. Appl. Physiol.* 35:291–298, 1976.

121. Malina, R. M. Quantification of fat, muscle and bone in man. *Clin. Orthop.* 65:9–20, 1969.

122. Malina, R. M. Competitive youth sports and biological maturation. E. W. Brown and C. F. Branta (eds). *Competitive Sports for Children and Youth*. Champaign, IL: Human Kinetics, 1988, pp. 227–246.

123. Malina, R. M., and C. Bouchard. *Growth, Maturation and Physical Activity*, Champaign, IL: Human Kinetics, 1991.

124. Maughan, R. J. A simple rapid method for the determination of glucose, lactate, pyruvate, alanine, 3-hydroxybutyrate and acetoacetate on a single 20 μl blood sample. *Clin. Chim. Acta* 122:231–240, 1982.

125. Mercier, J., A. Varray, M. Ramonatxo, B. Mercier, and C. Prefaut. Influence of anthropometric characteristics on changes in maximal exercise ventilation and breathing pattern during growth in boys. *Eur. J. Appl. Physiol.* 63:235–241, 1991.

126. Mero, A. Blood lactate production and recovery from anaerobic exercise in trained and untrained boys. *Eur. J. Appl. Physiol.* 57:660–666, 1988.

127. Mirwald, R. L., and D. A. Bailey. *Maximal Aerobic Power*. London, Ont.: Sports Dynamics, 1986.

128. Mitchell, J. H., B. J. Sproule, and C. B. Chapman. The physiological meaning of the maximum oxygen intake test. *J. Clin. Invest.* 37:538–547, 1958.

129. Mocellin, R., M. Heusgen, and H. P. Gildein. Anaerobic threshold and maximal steady-state blood lactate in prepubertal boys. *Eur. J. Appl. Physiol.* 62:56–60, 1991.

130. Mocellin, R., M. Heusgen, and U. Korsten-Reck. Maximal steady state blood lactate levels in 11-year-old boys. *Eur. J. Pediatr.* 149:771–773, 1990.

131. Moffatt, R. J., B. Surina, B. Golden, and N. Ayres. Body composition and physiological characteristics of female high school gymnasts. *Res. Q.* 55:80–84, 1984.

132. Myers, J., D. Walsh, M. Sullivan, and V. Froelicher. Effect of sampling on variability and plateau in oxygen uptake. *J. Appl. Physiol.* 68:404–410, 1990.

133. Nakagawa, A., and T. Ishiko. Assessment of aerobic capacity with special reference to sex and age of junior and senior high school students in Japan. *Jap. J. Physiol.* 20:118–129, 1970.

134. Nevill, A. M., R. Ramsbottom, and C. Williams. Scaling physiological measurements for individuals of different size. *Eur. J. Appl. Physiol.* 65:110–117, 1992.

135. Newton, J. L., and S. Robinson. The distribution of blood lactate and pyruvate during work and recovery. *Fed. Proc.* 24:590, 1965.

136. Nicholson, R. H. *Medical Research with Children.* Oxford: Oxford University Press, 1986.

137. Noakes, T. D. Implications of exercise testing for prediction of athletic performance: a contemporary perspective. *Med. Sci. Sports Exerc.* 20:319–330, 1988.

138. Oseid, S., and L. Hermansen. Hormonal and metabolic changes during and after prolonged work in pre-pubertal boys. *Acta Paediatr. Scand.* 217(Suppl.):147–153, 1971.

139. Palgi, Y., B. Gutin, J. Young, and D. Alejandro. Physiologic and anthropometric factors underlying endurance performance in children. *Int. J. Sports Med.* 5:67–73, 1984.

140. Paterson, D. H., and D. A. Cunningham. Development of anaerobic capacity in early and late maturing boys. R. A. Binkhorst, H. C. G. Kemper and W. H. M. Saris (eds). *Children and Exercise XI.* Champaign, IL: Human Kinetics, 1985, pp. 119–128.

141. Paterson, D. H., D. A. Cunningham, and L. A. Bumstead. Recovery O_2 and blood lactic acid: longitudinal analysis in boys aged 11–15 years. *Eur. J. Appl. Physiol.* 55:93–99, 1986.

142. Paterson, D. H., D. A. Cunningham, and A. Donner. The effect of different treadmill speeds on the variability of $\dot{V}O_2$max in children. *Eur. J. Appl. Physiol.* 47:113–122, 1981.

143. Pendergast, D. R., D. Shindell, P. Cerretelli, and D. W. Rennie. Role of central and peripheral circulatory adjustments in oxygen transport at the onset of exercise. *Int. J. Sports Med.* 1:160–170, 1980.

144. Pyne, D. B., and R. Telford. Classification of swimming training sessions by blood lactate and heart rate responses. *Excel* 5:9–12, 1988.

145. Reybrouck, T., M. Weymans, J. Ghesquiere, D. Van Gervan, and H. Stijns. Ventilatory threshold in kindergarten children during treadmill exercise. *Eur. J. Appl. Physiol.* 50:79–86, 1982.

146. Rieu, M., A. Duvallet, L. Scharapan, L. Thievlart, and A. Ferry. Blood lactate accumulation in intermittent supramaximal exercise. *Eur. J. Appl. Physiol.* 57:235–242, 1988.

147. Rivera-Brown, A. M., M. A. Rivera, and W. R. Frontera. Applicability of criteria for $\dot{V}O_2$max in active adolescents. *Pediatr. Exerc. Sci.* 4:331–339, 1992.

148. Robinson, S. Experimental studies of physical fitness in relation to age. *Arbeitsphysiologie* 10:251–323, 1938.

149. Rotstein, A., R. Dotan, O. Bar-Or, and G. Tenenbaum. Effect of training on anaerobic threshold and anaerobic performance of preadolescent boys. *Int. J. Sports Med.* 7:281–286, 1986.

150. Rowland, T. W. Developmental aspects of physiological function relating to aerobic exercise in children. *Sports Med.* 10:255–266, 1990.

151. Rowland, T. W. On body size and running economy. *Pediatr. Exerc. Sci.* 4:1–4, 1992.

152. Rowland, T. W. Aerobic exercise testing protocols. T. W. Rowland (ed). *Pediatric Laboratory Exercise Testing.* Champaign, IL: Human Kinetics. 1993, pp. 19–41.

153. Rowland, T. W., J. A. Auchinachie, T. J. Keenan, and G. M. Green. Physiologic responses to treadmill running in adult and prepubertal males. *Int. J. Sports Med.* 8:292–297, 1987.

154. Rowland, T. W., and L. N. Cunningham. Oxygen uptake plateau during maximal treadmill exercise in children. *Chest* 101:485–489, 1992.

155. Rowland, T. W., and G. M. Green. Physiological responses to treadmill exercise in females: adult-child differences. *Med. Sci. Sports Exerc.* 20:474–488, 1988.

156. Rutenfranz, J., K. L. Andersen, V. Seliger, J. Ilmarinen, F. Klimmer, et al. Maximal aerobic power affected by maturation and body growth during childhood and adolescence. *Eur. J. Pediatr.* 139:106–112, 1982.

157. Sady, S. P. Transient oxygen uptake and heart rate response at the onset of relative endurance exercise in pre-pubertal boys and adult men. *Int. J. Sports Med.* 2:240–244, 1981.

158. Sady, S. P. Cardiorespiratory exercise training in children. *Clin. Sports Med.* 5:493–514, 1986.

159. Sady, S. P., and V. L. Katch. Relative endurance and physiological responses: a study of individual differences in prepubertal boys and adult men. *Res. Q.* 52:246–255, 1981.

160. Sady, S. P., V. L. Katch, J. F. Villanacci, and T. B. Gilliam. Children-adult comparisons of oxygen uptake and heart rate kinetics during submaximum exercise. *Res. Q.* 54:55–59, 1983.

161. Sady, S. P., M. P. Savage, W. H. Thomson, and M. M. Petratis. The reliability of the VO_2-HR relation during graded treadmill exercise in prepubertal boys and adult men. *Res. Q.* 54:302–304, 1983.

162. Saltin, B., G. Blomqvist, J. H. Mitchell, R. L. Johnson, Jr., K. Wildenthal, and C. Chapman. Response to exercise after bedrest and after training. *Circulation* 38:(Suppl. 5), 1968.

163. Saris, W. H. M. *Aerobic Power and Daily Physical Activity in Children.* Meppel, Netherlands: Kripps Repro., 1982.

164. Saris, W. H. M. Habitual physical activity in children: methodology and findings in health and disease. *Med. Sci. Sports Exerc.* 18:253–263, 1986.

165. Saris, W. H. M., A. M. Noordeloos, B. E. M. Ringnalda, M. A. Van't Hof, and R. A. Binkhorst. Reference values for aerobic power of healthy 4 to 18 year old Dutch children: preliminary results. R. A. Binkhorst, H. C. G. Kemper, and W. H. M. Saris (eds). *Children and Exercise XI,* Champaign, IL: Human Kinetics, 1985, pp. 151–160.

166. Schmidt-Neilsen, K. *Scaling: Why is Animal Size So Important?* Cambridge: Cambridge University Press, 1984.

167. Schmucker, B., and W. Hollman. The aerobic capacity of trained athletes from 6 to 7 years of age. *Acta Pediatr. Belg.* 28:92–101, 1974.

168. Sheehan, J. M., T. W. Rowland, and E. J. Burke. A comparison of four treadmill protocols for determination of maximal oxygen uptake in 10 to 12 year old boys *Int. J. Sports Med.* 8:31–34, 1987.

169. Shephard, R. J. The working capacity of schoolchildren. R. J. Shephard (ed). *Frontiers of Fitness,* Springfield, IL: Charles C. Thomas, 1971, pp. 319–345.

170. Shephard, R. J. The prediction of athletic performance by laboratory and field tests—an overview. R. J. Shephard and H. Lavallee (eds). *Physical Fitness Assessment—Principles, Practice and Application,* Springfield, IL: Charles C. Thomas, 1978, pp. 113–141.

171. Shephard, R. J. *Physical Activity and Growth.* London: Year Book Medical Publishers, 1982.

172. Shephard, R. J. Tests of maximum oxygen intake. A critical review. *Sports Med.* 1:99–124, 1984.

173. Shephard, R. J. The Canada Fitness Survey, some international comparisons. *J. Sports Med. Phys. Fitness* 26:292–300, 1986.

174. Shephard, R. J., C. Allen, O. Bar-Or, C. T. M. Davies, S. Degre, et al. The working capacity of Toronto school children. *Can Med. Assoc. J.* 100:560–566, 705–714, 1969.

175. Shephard, R. J., H. Lavallée, J. C. Jéquier, R. LaBarre, M. Rajic, and C. Beaucage. Seasonal differences in aerobic power. R. J. Shephard and H. Lavellee (eds). *Physical Fitness Assessment—Principles, Practice and Application,* Springfield IL: Charles C. Thomas, 1978, pp. 194–210.

176. Sholl, D. The quantitative investigation of the vertebrate brain and the applicability of allometric formulae to its study. *Proc. R. Soc. Lond Series B.* 35:243–257, 1948.

177. Shuleva, K. M., G. R. Hunter, D. J. Hester, and D. L. Dunaway. Exercise oxygen uptake in 3 through 6 year old children. *Pediatr. Exerc. Sci.* 2:130–139, 1990.

178. Simon, G., A. Berg, H. H. Dickhuth, A. Simon-Alt, and J. Keul. Bestimmung der anaeroben Schwelle in Abhangigkeit von Alter und von der Leistungsfahigkeit. *Dtsch. Z. Sportsmed.* 32:7–14, 1981.

179. Simon, J., J. L. Young, D. K. Blood, K. R. Segal, R. B. Case, and B. Gutin. Plasma lactate and ventilation thresholds in trained and untrained cyclists. *J. Appl. Physiol.* 60:777–781, 1986.

180. Sjodin, B., and I. Jacobs. Onset of blood lactate accumulation and marathon running performance. *Int J. Sports Med.* 2:23–26, 1981.

181. Sjodin, B., and J. Svedenhag, J. Oxygen uptake during running as related to body mass in circumpubertal boys: a longitudinal study. *Eur. J. Appl. Physiol.* 65:150–157, 1992.

182. Skinner, J. S., O. Bar-Or, V. Bergsteinova, C. W. Bell, D. Royer, and E. R. Buskirk. Comparison of continuous and intermittent tests for determining maximal oxygen intake in children. *Acta Paediatr. Scand.* 217:24–28, 1971.

183. Skinner, J. S., and T. H. McLellan. The transition from aerobic to anaerobic metabolism. *Res. Q.* 51:234–248, 1980.

184. Snedecor, G. W., and W. G. Cochran. *Statistical Methods.* (7th edition). Ames: Iowa Press, 1980.

185. Sprynarova, S., J. Parizkova, and V. Bunc. Relationships between body dimensions and resting and working oxygen consumption in boys aged 11 to 18 years. *Eur. J. Appl. Physiol.* 56:725–736, 1987.

186. Stegmann, H., and W. Kindermann. Comparison of prolonged exercise tests at the individual anaerobic threshold and the fixed anaerobic threshold of 4 mmol.1^{-1}. *Int. J. Sports Med.* 3:105–110, 1982.

187. Stegmann, H., W. Kindermann, and A. Schnabel. Lactate kinetics and individual anaerobic threshold. *Int. J. Sports Med.* 2:160–165, 1981.

188. Sunnegardh, J., and L. E. Bratteby. Maximal oxygen uptake, anthropometry and physical activity in a randomly selected sample of 8 and 13 year old children in Sweden. *Eur. J. Appl. Physiol.* 56:266–272, 1987.

189. Suurnakki, T., J. Ilmarinen, C. Nygard, P. V. Komi, and J. Karlsson. Anaerobic strain in children during a cross-country skiing competition. J. Rutenfranz, R. Mocellin, and F. Klimt (eds). *Children and Exercise XII.* Champaign, IL: Human Kinetics, 1986, pp. 67–76.

190. Tanaka, H., and M. Shindo. Running velocity at blood lactate threshold of boys aged 6–15 years compared with untrained and trained young males. *Int. J. Sports Med.* 6:90–94, 1985.

191. Tanner, J. M. Fallacy of per-weight and per-surface area standards and their relation to spurious correlation. *J. Appl. Physiol.* 2:1–15, 1949.

192. Tanner, J. M. *Growth at Adolescence.* (2nd edition). Oxford: Blackwell Scientific, 1962.

193. Tanner, J. M. *The Physique of the Olympic Athlete.* London: George, Allen and Unwin, 1964.

194. Tanner, J. M. *Foetus into Man. Physical Growth from Conception to Maturity.* London: Open Books, 1978.

195. Taylor, H. L., E. R. Buskirk, and A. Henschel. Maximal oxygen intake as an objective measure of cardiorespiratory performance. *J. Appl. Physiol.* 8:73–80, 1955.

196. Tell, G. S. Cardiovascular disease risk factors related to sexual maturation: the Oslo Youth Study. *J. Chron. Dis.* 38:633–642, 1985.

197. Thoden, J. S. Testing aerobic power. J. D. MacDougall, H. A. Wenger, and H. J. Green (eds). *Physiological Testing of the High Performance Athlete.* Champaign, IL: Human Kinetics, 1991, pp. 107–173.

198. Thoden, J. S., B. A. Wilson and J. D. MacDougal. Testing aerobic power, J. D. MacDougal, H. A. Wenger, and H. J. Green (eds). *Physiological Testing of the Elite Athlete.* New York: Mouvement Pubs, 1982, pp. 39–60.

199. Tolfrey, K., and N. Armstrong. The relationship between blood lactate responses to incremental exercise and age. *J. Sports Sci.* 10:563–564, 1992.

200. Vaccaro, P., and A. Mahon. Cardiorespiratory responses to endurance training in children. *Sports Med.* 4:352–363, 1987.

201. Walsh, M. L., and E. W. Bannister. Possible mechanisms of the anaerobic threshold: a review. *Sports Med.* 5:269–302, 1988.

202. Washington, R. L. Anaerobic threshold in children. *Pediatr. Exerc. Sci.* 1:244–256, 1989.
203. Washington, R. L. Anaerobic threshold. T. W. Rowland (ed). *Pediatric Laboratory Exercise Testing.* Champaign, IL: Human Kinetics, 1993, pp. 115–130.
204. Washington, R. L., J. C. van Gundy, C. Cohen, H. M. Sondheimer, and R. R. Wolfe. Normal aerobic and anaerobic exercise data for North American school-age children. *J. Pediatr.* 112:223–233, 1988.
205. Wasserman, K. The anaerobic threshold measurement to evaluate exercise performance. *Am. Rev. Respir. Dis.* 129(Suppl.):S35–S40, 1984.
206. Wasserman, K., B. J. Whipp, S. N. Koyal, and W. L. Beaver. Anaerobic threshold and respiratory gas exchange during exercise. *J. Appl. Physiol.* 35:236–243, 1973.
207. Weaver, M. R., and P. M. Vadgama. An O_2 based enzyme electrode for whole blood lactate measurement under continuous flow conditions. *Clin. Chim. Acta* 155:295–308, 1986.
208. Weil, M. H., J. A. Leavy, E. C. Rackow, and C. J. Halfman. Validation of a semi-automated technique for measuring lactate in whole blood. *Clin. Chem.* 32:2175–2177, 1986.
209. Welsman, J. R., and N. Armstrong. Daily physical activity and blood lactate indices of aerobic fitness in children. *Br. J. Sports Med.* 26:228–232, 1992.
210. Weltman, A., D. Snead, R. Seip, R. Schurrer, S. Levine, et al. Prediction of lactate threshold and fixed blood lactate concentrations from 3200m running performance in male runners. *Int. J. Sports Med.* 8:401–406, 1987.
211. Weymans, M., I. Reybrouck, H. Stijns, and J. Knops. Influence of age and sex on the ventilatory anaerobic threshold in children. R. A. Binkhorst, H. C. G Kemper, and W. H. M. Saris (eds). *Children and Exercise XI.* Champaign, IL: Human Kinetics, 1985, pp. 114–118.
212. Whipp, B. J., and K. Wasserman. Oxygen uptake kinetics for various intensities of constant load work. *J. Appl. Physiol.* 33:351–356, 1972.
213. Williams, J. R., and N. Armstrong. The influence of age and sexual maturation on children's blood lactate responses to exercise. *Pediatr. Exerc. Sci.* 3:111–120, 1991.
214. Williams, J. R., and N. Armstrong. Relationship of maximal lactate steady state to performance at fixed blood lactate reference values in children. *Pediatr. Exerc. Sci.* 3:333–341, 1991.
215. Williams, J. R., N. Armstrong, and B. J. Kirby. The 4mM blood lactate level as an index of exercise performance in 11–13 year old children. *J. Sports Sci.* 8:139–147, 1990.
216. Williams, J. R., N. Armstrong, and B. J. Kirby. The influence of the site of sampling and assay medium upon the interpretation of blood lactate responses to exercise. *J. Sports Sci.* 10:95–107, 1992.
217. Williams, J. R., N. Armstrong, E. M. Winter, and N. Crichton. Changes in peak oxygen uptake with age and sexual maturation in boys: physiological fact or statistical anomaly? J. Coudert and E. Van Praagh (eds). *Children and Exercise XVI.* Paris: Masson, 1992, pp. 35–37.
218. Winter, E. M. Scaling: partitioning out differences in size. *Pediatr. Exerc. Sci.* 4:296–301, 1992.
219. Winter, E. M., F. B. C. Brookes, and E. J. Hamley. Maximal exercise performance and lean leg volume in men and women. *J. Sports Sci.* 9:3–13, 1991.
220. Wirth, A., E. Trager, K. Scheele, D. Mayer, K. Diehm, et al. Cardiopulmonary adjustment and metabolic response to maximal and submaximal physical exercise of boys and girls at different stages of maturity. *Eur. J. Appl. Physiol.* 39:229–240, 1978.
221. Working Party on Ethics of Research in Children. Guidelines to aid ethical committees considering research involving children. *Br. Med. J.* 280:229–231, 1980.
222. Working Party on Research in Children. *The Ethical Conduct of Research in Children.* London: Medical Research Council, 1991.
223. Woynarowska, B. The validity of different estimations of maximal oxygen uptake in children 11–12 years of age. *Eur. J. Appl. Physiol.* 43:19–23, 1980.
224. Yeh, M. P., R. M. Gardner, T. D. Adams, F. G. Yanowitz, and R. O. Crapo. Anaerobic

threshold: problems of determination and validation. *J. Appl. Physiol.* 55:1178–1186, 1983.

225. Yoshida, T. Current topics and concepts of lactate and gas exchange thresholds. *J. Hum. Ergol.* 16:103–121, 1987.

226. Yoshida, T., M. Chida, M. Khioka, and Y. Suda. Blood lactate parameters related to aerobic capacity and endurance performance. *Eur. J. Appl. Physiol.* 56:7–11, 1987.

227. Yoshida, T., N. Takeuchi, and Y. Suda. Arterial versus venous blood lactate increase in the forearm during incremental bicycle exercise. *Eur. J. Appl. Physiol.* 50:87–93, 1982.

228. Yoshizawa, S. A comparative study of aerobic work capacity in urban and rural adolescents. *J. Hum. Ergol.* 1:45–65, 1972.

229. Yoshizawa, S., H. Honda, M. Urushibara, and N. Nakamura. Aerobic-anaerobic energy supply and daily physical activity level in young children. S. Oseid and K-H. Carlsen (eds). *Children and Exercise XIII.* Champaign, IL: Human Kinetics, 1989, pp. 47–56.

230. Yoshizawa, S., T. Ishizaki, and H. Honda. Physical fitness of children aged 5 and 6 years. *J. Hum. Ergol.* 6:41–51, 1977.

15
Effects of Exercise Training on Plasma Lipids and Lipoproteins

J. LARRY DURSTINE, Ph.D.
WILLIAM L. HASKELL, Ph.D.

Major advances have occurred in the understanding of lipoprotein metabolism and its regulation during the last several decades. Although not completely defined, the role of plasma lipids, apolipoproteins, lipoprotein receptors, and lipolytic enzymes in lipoprotein metabolism has become clearer. We have increased our knowledge of lipid function and transport by better understanding intracellular and extracellular movement of lipoproteins. We now better understand many of the interactions between lipoproteins, the lipoprotein metabolic pathways, factors that influence synthesis and catabolism rates, and how lipoproteins exert their physiologic and pathologic effects. Part of this expanded knowledge surrounding lipoprotein metabolism has come from a better understanding of the various genetic and environmental factors that influence the lipoprotein metabolic pathways and ultimately lipoprotein composition. These environmental factors include gender; age; body composition and body fat distribution; dietary intake of various constituents including fats, cholesterol, carbohydrates, fiber, and alcohol; cigarette smoking; medication use; a single session of exercise; and regular participation in exercise activity.

Comprehensive reviews of the effects of endurance [61] and resistance exercise [84] have been published. Since publication of these reviews, a number of reports addressing these topics have been produced. The purpose of this chapter is to appraise the existing knowledge relating both regularly practiced exercise and a single exercise session to lipoprotein composition and metabolism.

LIPOPROTEIN COMPOSITION AND METABOLIC PATHWAYS IN HEALTHY ADULTS

Plasma lipoproteins are the prominent constituent of a complex transport system that provides for the movement of exogenous and endogenous lipid between the liver, the intestine, and peripheral tissues. Since lipids are not water soluble, they must combine with apolipoproteins to form micelle lipid-protein complexes or lipoproteins. These water-soluble macromolecules are spherical, have finite dimensions, and contain cholesterol (both free and esterified), triglyceride, phospholipid, and various apolipoproteins. Four basic classes of lipoproteins have been categorized according to their gravitational density: chylomicron, derived from intestinal absorption of triglyceride (or triacylglycerol); very-low-density lipoprotein (VLDL, or pre-β-lipoprotein), derived from the liver for the export of triglyceride; low-density lipoprotein (LDL, or β-lipoprotein), representing a final stage in the catabolism of VLDL; and high-density lipoprotein (HDL, or α-lipoprotein), involved in the reverse transport of cholesterol. However, other lipoprotein subfractions exist and include intermediate-density lipoprotein (IDL), an intermediate step in VLDL catabolism, found in a density range of 1.006 to 1.019 g/ml; lipoprotein(a) [Lp(a)] with a density range of 1.055 to 1.120 g/ml; and HDL that is typically studied as two separate subfractions: HDL_2 and the more dense HDL_3 (see Table 15.1 for a more detailed description of these lipoprotein classes).

Lipids have important beneficial biologic functions that include the use of triglyceride for energy production or as stored fat in adipose tissue and the use of cholesterol as a component, in conjunction with phospholipids, of cellular membranes or in the synthesis of steroid hormones. However, it is the apolipoprotein portion of the particle that enhances the lipid's aqueous solubility as well as regulates the interaction of the lipoprotein complexes with tissue receptors and lipolytic enzymes. As many as 17 or more apolipoproteins have been identified, with one or more apolipoproteins associated with each lipoprotein complex [16, 17]. In some cases these apolipoproteins exist as isoproteins (e.g., apo B, designated apo B-48 and apo B-100). Though most apolipoproteins are synthesized by the liver or intestine, some such as apo B-100 and apo A-I originate at both sites. Apolipoproteins also direct and regulate enzymatic function (e.g., apo C-II serves as an enzyme cofactor in the activation of lipoprotein lipase [LPL], while apo A-I is a cofactor for the lecithin:cholesterol acyltransferase [LCAT] reaction), serve as lipid transfer proteins (e.g., apo D: a surface component of HDL) [155], and are the binding molecules (ligand) for interaction with lipoprotein receptors (e.g., apo B-100's interaction with extrahepatic LDL receptors) [17]. (For specific apolipoprotein description and function refer to Table 15.2.)

Several enzymes have important roles in the metabolism of plasma lipoproteins. LPL is bound to capillary walls and has been isolated in extracts of many tissues (e.g., heart, adipose tissue, skeletal muscle). LPL is involved in the hydrolysis of the triglyceride core of chylomicrons and VLDL and enhances the uptake of the released fatty acid into extrahepatic tissue. A second enzyme, hepatic lipase (HL), is bound to the liver endothelial capillary lining. This enzyme has different properties than those of LPL and does not react easily with chylomicrons but has several functions. There is evidence that HL participates in the final conversion of chylomicron and VLDL remnants into LDL [121]. In addition, HL works in conjunction with cholesteryl ester transfer protein (CETP) in the degrada-

TABLE 15.1
Composition of Human Plasma Lipoproteins

Fraction	Source	Density (g/ml)	Electroph Motility	Protein (%)	Total Lipid (%)	Composition			
						Percentage of Total Lipid			
						TG	Phos	Chol Ester	Chol (Free)
Chylomicron	Intestine	<0.96	Origin	1–2	98–99	88	8	3	1
VLDL	Liver and intestine	0.96–1.006	Pre β	7–10	90–93	56	20	15	8
IDL	VLDL and chylomicron	1.006–1.019	β	11	89	29	26	34	9
LDL	VLDL and chylomicron	1.019–1.063		21	79	13	28	48	10
Lp(a)	Liver?	1.055–1.120	Pre β	29	69	19	5	37	8
HDL$_2$	Intestine and liver	1.063–1.125	α	33	67	16	43	31	10
HDL$_3$	Intestine and liver	1.125–1.210		57	43	13	46	29	6

Electroph motility = electrophoretic motility; VLDL = very-low-density lipoprotein; LDL = low-density lipoprotein; IDL = intermediate-density lipoprotein; HDL = high-density lipoprotein; TG = triglyceride; Phos = phospholipid; Chol = cholesterol.

TABLE 15.2
Human Apolipoproteins

Apo	Lipoprotein Class				Major Function; Site of Synthesis
	Chylom	VLDL	LDL	HDL	
A-I	Minor	Minor		Major	LCAT activator; synthesized in liver and intestine
A-II	Minor	Minor		Major	LCAT inhibitor and/or activator of heparin releasable hepatic triglyceride hydrolase; synthesized in liver
A-IV	Major			Minor	Synthesized in liver
B-48	Major	Minor			Required for synthesis of chylomicron; synthesized in intestine
B-100	Major	Major	Major		LDL receptor binding; synthesized in liver
Apo(a)			Major		Similar characteristics between Apo(a) and plasminogen, thus may have a prothrombolytic role by interfering with function of plasminogen; site of synthesis not clear
C-I	Minor		Minor	Minor	LCAT activator; synthesized in liver
C-II	Minor	Minor	Minor	Minor	LPL activator; synthesized in liver
C-III	Minor	Major		Minor	LPL inhibitor, several forms depending on content of sialic acids; synthesized in liver
D		Minor		Major	Core lipid transfer protein, possibly identical to the cholesteryl ester transfer protein; site of synthesis not clear
E	Minor	Major		Minor	Remnant receptor binding, present in excess in the beta-VLDL of patients with type III hyperlipoproteinemia and exclusively in HDL-C; synthesized in liver
F				Major	Site of synthesis not clear
G		Major			Site of synthesis not clear
H	Major				Site of synthesis not clear

Apo = apolipoprotein; Chylom = chylomicron.

tion of HDL_2 particles. CETP is associated predominantly with HDL particles and is one of several lipid transfer proteins believed to mediate the transfer of esterified cholesterol from HDL_2 to VLDL and ultimately advances the formation of HDL_3 [156]. LCAT, found in plasma and synthesized by the liver, can bind to HDL_3 and catalyze the esterification of free cholesterol on the HDL surface and promote the movement of esterified cholesterol into the HDL core [173].

A sequence of metabolic steps involved in the delivery of cholesterol to peripheral tissues (referred to as the LDL receptor pathway) has facilitated the overall understanding of cholesterol transport [18]. Though we have increased our knowledge about the transport of cholesterol and triglyceride to the peripheral tissues, less is known about the return of cholesterol from peripheral tissues to the liver: a process referred to as reverse cholesterol transport [48]. Disruption of either of these two processes can cause glaring changes in plasma lipoprotein profiles and result in modified risk for premature coronary artery disease (CAD). Recently, several concise reviews concerning this topic have been published [7, 52, 140, 155].

Exogenous (dietary) triglyceride after intestinal absorption is packaged into large chylomicron particles and secreted into the circulation by means of the lymphatic system. Although some smaller particles resembling VLDL are formed and released from the intestine, their composition is chylomicron [140]. These particles react with LPL, lessen their triglyceride core, form chylomicron remnants, and are catabolized by the liver [140] (Fig. 15.1). On the other hand, most of the triglyceride synthesized by the liver (endogenous) is packaged into the core of VLDL molecules [140]. Since apo B-100 is the primary B protein for the VLDL particle, the metabolic fate is somewhat different from that of chylomicrons with apo B-48 as the principal B apolipoprotein.

When VLDL formed in the liver reacts with LPL, the result is hydrolysis of the triglyceride core and the formation of VLDL remnants and IDL, the precursor to LDL [140]. This catabolism of VLDL into IDL and then into LDL leads to the direct transport of cholesterol by the LDL receptor pathway [18] (Fig. 15.1). Delivery of cholesterol to body cells is mediated by LDL receptors located on the surfaces of almost all cell types [18]. Once LDL is recognized (primarily by its apo B-100) and bound to the cell LDL receptor, it is internalized and exposed to lysosomal enzymes. Cholesterol is released and is used to meet the metabolic needs of that cell. In addition, the release of cholesterol in the cell will result in a reduction of cholesterol synthesis within that cell and promotes storage of excess esterified cholesterol and suppression of LDL receptor synthesis, preventing additional uptake of LDL particles [173].

Reverse cholesterol transport involves the movement of cholesterol by the HDL molecule from peripheral tissues back to the liver, where it is catabolized and excreted into the small intestine as bile (Fig. 1). The reverse transport of cholesterol may incorporate several different pathways for the removal of cholesterol from the circulation [155]. These pathways have the same origin for HDL, but it seems that several different exit points for cholesterol removal may exist [155]. As nascent HDL is secreted from the liver and intestine or is derived from LPL catabolism of chylomicrons and VLDL [140, 173], it quickly reacts with LCAT. LCAT has dual functions. It modifies discoidal HDL particles by transforming cholesterol into cholesteryl ester and shifts the ester to the HDL_3 core [157]. This process enhances a second function: development of a chemical gradient that leads to continual uptake of cholesterol by HDL_2, thereby providing a constant supply of substrate for the LCAT reaction [26]. This constant flow of free cholesterol, succeeded by esterification and movement of the ester into the core, expands the HDL_3 particle and shifts the density range to the less dense HDL_2 particle. As this HDL_2 particle increases in size, two other enzymatic reactions occur. CETP facilitates the transfer of the cholesteryl ester to other lipoproteins (chylomicron and VLDL remnants) in exchange for triglyceride [156]. This allows the movement of cholesteryl ester originating from HDL to the liver by chylomicron and VLDL remnants, where they are catabolized. The resulting increased HDL_2 triglyceride content then provides a good substrate for HL [156]. Thus, the small dense HDL_3 molecule can originate by LPL action; be modified by LCAT, resulting in HDL_2 formation; undergo further processing mediated by CETP and HL; and be transformed into HDL_3 in the liver and released back into the circulatory system to begin the process once again [140, 173]. Additionally, there may be other possible pathways for the removal of HDL-C from the circulation. Since the cholesterol associated with HDL can be quickly transferred to the liver cholesterol pool, one pathway involves the direct action of HL, which results in the uptake of HDL-C and transfer of cholesterol to the liver cholesterol pool [155]. Another pathway includes the hepatic apo E receptor–mediated removal of HDL. Large HDL_2 particles rich with cholesterol ester and containing apo E may be withdrawn from the circulation by receptor–mediated endocytosis by liver LDL receptors [155].

AEROBIC EXERCISE TRAINING EFFECTS ON LIPOPROTEIN CONCENTRATIONS

Early studies evaluating the effects of exercise training on blood lipid parameters only examined triglyceride and cholesterol concentrations.

FIGURE 15.1

Transport of triglyceride and cholesterol between tissues in humans. TG, triglyceride; C, free cholesterol; CE, cholesteryl ester; VLDL, very-low-density lipoprotein; IDL, intermediate-density lipoprotein; LDL, low-density lipoprotein; HDL, high-density lipoprotein; ACAT, acyl-CoA:cholesterol acyltransferase; LCAT, lecithin:cholesterol acyltransferase; LPL, lipoprotein lipase; HL, hepatic lipase; CETP, cholesteryl ester transfer protein; A-I; apolipoprotein A-I; A-II, apolipoprotein A-II; Apo B-100, apolipoprotein B-100; Apo E, apolipoprotein E; heavy dark lines *indicate major pathways,* lighter lines *indicate minor pathways; EX1–4 are points where exercise has a potential impact on lipoprotein metabolism: EX1 is the site for reduced synthesis of triglyceride, EX2 is the site for enhanced activity of LPL, EX3 is the site for enhanced LCAT activity, and EX4 represents enhanced reverse cholesterol transport. Adapted from Mayes, P. A. Cholesterol synthesis, transport, & excretion. R. K. Murray, D. K. Granner, P. A. Mayes, and V. W. Rodwell (eds). Harper's Biochemistry. San Mateo, CA: Appleton & Lange, 1990, p. 255.*

FIGURE 15.1

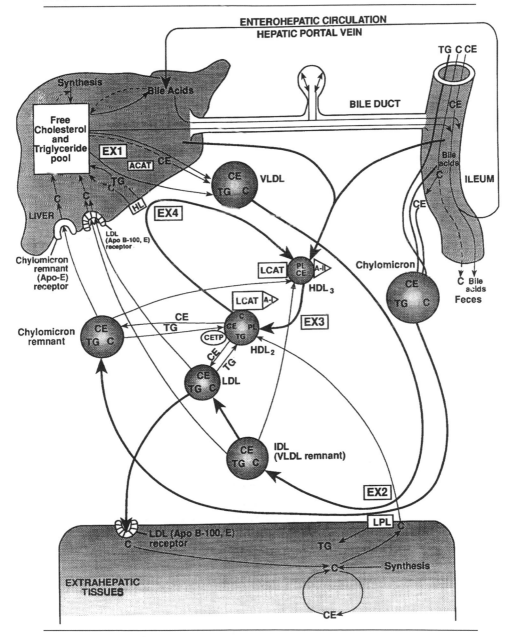

Observations from these early investigations indicated lower triglyceride concentrations in endurance-trained subjects, while total cholesterol was either not changed or only slightly different. However, it became evident that physical activity had an impact on the lipoprotein lipid distribution, and later investigations have focused on the measurement of both the cholesterol and protein content associated with these various lipoproteins. A comprehensive review of these early studies has been presented by Haskell [61]. Since that time, other means of evaluating lipoprotein composition in response to exercise training (to include measurement of apolipoproteins) have been used. Although ultracentrifugation and precipitation procedures remain the principle means for lipoprotein evaluation, measurement of specific flotation intervals for LDL subspecies (small LDL [S_f0-7] and large LDL [S_f7-12]) and the resolution of HDL into a number of subspecies HDL_{2a}, HDL_{2b}, HDL_{3a}, HDL_{3b}, and HDL_{3c}) by gradient gel electrophoresis have been completed. In addition, to understand the mechanisms responsible for these changes, lipolytic enzymes associated with the lipoprotein metabolic pathways have been measured. This information has added greatly to our understanding of the effects of exercise training and change in lipoprotein composition.

Triglyceride

Generally, regular participation in physical activity is associated with lower plasma triglyceride concentrations. Results from cross-sectional studies using endurance athletes [111, 112, 169, 195], cross-country skiers [95], and tennis players [181] indicate lower triglyceride concentrations in active persons than in inactive controls. In some studies subjects who had longer maximal treadmill test times or higher $\dot{V}O_2$max also had lower triglyceride concentrations when adjusted for age, body fat, body weight, and extreme leanness [22, 59, 198]. However, not all reports support these relationships [115, 134]. In some cases where endurance athletes do not have significantly lower triglyceride concentrations than controls (especially in the study of women), the lack of difference was likely due to lower than average values for the inactive controls [34].

Endurance exercise training usually reduces plasma triglyceride concentrations [71, 75, 170, 197] when baseline concentrations are elevated, but not always [97, 105]. The amount of this reduction is related to the pretraining concentration and the volume of exercise completed during the training program [58, 202]. This exercise training reduction in triglyceride is believed to result from both a single exercise session and habitual exercise. After a single session of regular endurance training, plasma triglyceride concentrations are reduced in hypertriglyceridemic subjects [71, 142], whereas individuals who participate regularly in physical activity have lower triglyceride concentrations even though they had not exercised recently [198]. Changes in adiposity or in the composition of dietary intake do not seem to account totally for lower triglyceride concentrations in physically active subjects [30, 82, 135], but in some studies, extreme leanness is related to lower triglyceride concentrations [22, 59, 64, 198].

Presently, few studies have evaluated lipid and lipoprotein differences in physically active older (mean age of 60 years or more) adults. Two cross-sectional studies examining body composition, blood lipoproteins, and physical activity in older adults have recently been published. Reaven et al. [127] observed that older men and women who regularly participate in physical activity had triglyceride concentrations lower than inactive controls. However, the results from Coon et al. [21] would indicate that obesity and the regional distribution of body fat and not physical fitness or age, are major determinants for plasma triglyceride in older men. Longitudinal studies evaluating older men and women after endurance training usually report lower triglyceride concentrations [15, 136, 137, 139]. This is consistent with earlier work by Martin et al. [112], who reported relatively constant mean plasma triglyceride concentrations in male runners from age 20 to 60 years, as compared with a steady increase in triglyceride for inactive males for this age period.

Some attention has been given to blood lipids, lipoproteins, and physical activity levels of children as they advance through developmental stages. Since children generally have low triglyceride concentrations that differ during development periods, and definitions of activity levels differ among studies, one must be cautious when comparing the results from various studies. Two recent reviews concerning this topic have been completed by Després et al. [29] and Armstrong and Simons-Morton [6]. Present results indicate that physically fit and active children tend to have lower triglyceride concentrations than unfit or inactive children [32, 102, 171, 178, 183], but exercise training-induced reductions are not always found [6, 98].

Cholesterol
Although cholesterol is an important component of cell membranes and is needed for the synthesis of steroid hormones, elevated plasma cholesterol concentrations have been implicated in the development of CAD [51]. Some observational studies have reported lower plasma cholesterol concentrations for endurance-trained male [193] and female runners [199], but most studies observe no difference in plasma cholesterol concentrations for male runners [1, 74, 111, 112, 169] female runners [34], cross-country skiers [38], and other endurance-trained athletes [59, 177], compared with inactive counterparts. Similar [10, 11] or higher plasma cholesterol concentrations [41] have been observed for speed-trained and power-trained athletes, compared with inactive controls. Maximal aerobic capacity has been inversely related to cholesterol concentrations [22], but when adjusted for age and body weight, these relationships no longer exist [39, 115]. Accordingly, factors such as body weight, percentage of body fat,

and/or different patterns of dietary intake are important considerations in evaluating the effects of physical activity on plasma cholesterol concentrations. Consequently, the consensus is that physically active individuals do not have significantly lower plasma concentrations than do inactive individuals.

Results from endurance-training studies have not been any more encouraging. Most well-designed and executed studies accounting for gender, dietary intake modifications, changes in plasma volume, body weight change, and altered body composition have not produced significant plasma cholesterol reductions [30, 71, 75, 170, 197]. Some studies have reported reductions in plasma cholesterol after exercise training, but they did not concurrently maintain an inactive control group. Thus, in these investigations seasonal variations and/or interference from other variables may confound interpretation of the results for both men [175] and women [100].

Plasma cholesterol differences for age and gender have been reported. Men have higher total cholesterol concentrations than women between the third and sixth decades of life; after this women have higher concentrations [129]. Reaven et al. [127] completed a cross-sectional study comparing several levels of physical activity in older women and men. Women had higher total cholesterol concentrations than men at all activity levels, but regular exercise had no effect on total cholesterol of women or men. In addition, no exercise training–induced reductions have been reported for older adults [15, 21, 136, 137]. Furthermore, in children, cross-sectional [32, 102, 171, 178, 183] and longitudinal [46, 47, 98] studies generally agree that differences in plasma cholesterol between physically active and inactive children do not exist.

Chylomicrons

Dietary triglyceride is packaged into chylomicrons during absorption from the gastrointestinal tract and transported through the peripheral vascular system where they interact with LPL and are catabolized into fatty acids, glycerol, and chylomicron remnants. These remnants are available to interact with other lipoproteins and enzymes (such as HDL_2 and CETP) to facilitate the exchange of triglyceride for cholesteryl ester and transport back to the liver for metabolism. The cholesterol and cholesteryl ester are metabolized by the liver and either released back into the plasma with other lipoproteins, converted to bile acid and directly secreted in the bile, and/or secreted in bile as a neutral sterol.

Most studies evaluating the effects of regular participation in physical activity on plasma lipoprotein measure these changes in a fasted condition. Since the post-prandial *half-life* of chylomicron triglyceride is less than *five minutes*, few studies have been completed concerning the consequences of endurance exercise training on plasma chylomicron concentration, composition, production, and/or removal rates. Highly trained endurance athletes following a high-fat meal or intravenous lipid load usually remove chylomicrons from plasma faster than inactive controls [13], whereas endurance training has resulted in either no change [116] or an improved triglyceride clearance [3] following a fat load. These inconsistent observations are probably due to differences in the type, amount, and administration of the fat load, in the time after the last exercise session that the load was administered, and/or modifications in diet or body weight during the training program. Weintraub et al. [184] completed a 7-week exercise training study where diet was prescribed to maintain percentage of carbohydrate, fat, and protein, while caloric intake was increased during the training period to prevent weight loss. After endurance training, plasma chylomicron concentrations following a fat load were reduced by 37% and were inversely related to LPL activity. This reduction of postprandial triglyceride-rich lipoprotein was most likely due to an accelerated removal of triglyceride from the circulation by increased LPL activity in adipose tissue, skeletal muscle and cardiac muscle [65, 119].

Very-Low-Density Lipoprotein
Endogenous triglyceride either synthesized by the liver or derived from storage reservoirs is packaged into the VLDL core for transport to peripheral tissues. As a result of the enzyme LPL, the triglyceride core of a VLDL molecule is hydrolyzed and the remnants removed in much the same manner as for chylomicrons. However, unlike the catabolism of chylomicrons, an IDL molecule is formed (the principle protein of this molecule is apo B-100). These IDL molecules undergo further hydrolysis and form LDL molecules. This leads to the transport and direct uptake of cholesterol by the LDL receptor pathway [18]. The VLDL-triglyceride *half-life* in normal lipemic human blood is between *two and four hours.*

Plasma VLDL-triglyceride concentrations are lower following endurance training. This is due either to increased catabolism of triglyceride, decreased hepatic synthesis and secretion, or some combination of both. Evidence favors increased catabolism of VLDL-triglyceride, but some evidence for reduced hepatic synthesis exists. Little is known regarding the mechanism responsible for the reduced synthesis of VLDL-triglyceride following participation in an endurance-exercise training program [54], but much has been learned about the removal of VLDL from the circulation. Both the triglyceride and cholesterol content of the VLDL molecule have been evaluated after endurance-exercise training. Cross-sectional studies of endurance-trained athletes, where lower plasma triglyceride concentrations have been observed, usually also report lower VLDL-triglyceride concentrations [111, 119, 162], and longitudinal training studies that report no changes in plasma triglyceride also report no change in VLDL-triglyceride [122], but not always [28]. In addition, endurance training in hypertriglyceridemic animals [33, 143], involvement in extended periods of vigorous exercise [194], and completing repeated periods of exercise on successive days [20, 58] result in reduced VLDL-triglyceride concentrations. Furthermore, Kiens and Lithell [79] have measured VLDL- triglyceride in blood leaving trained and sedentary muscles under resting conditions and found lower concentrations of VLDL- triglyceride in venous blood leaving the trained muscle.

VLDL-cholesterol (VLDL-C) has been measured directly after ultracentrifugation or estimated [27, 43]. Cross-sectional studies examining VLDL-C concentrations from endurance athletes and sedentary controls have reported lower VLDL-C concentrations in the athletes [34, 111, 112, 177, 193]. Endurance-exercise training usually, but not always [28, 97], results in reductions in VLDL-C [75, 110]. A significant correlation (r = -0.79) between VLDL-C and maximum oxygen consumption has been reported for male athletes [11]. No published results for VLDL-C concentrations in active older adults are available. However, one cross-sectional study observed lower VLDL-C in active black adolescents [32], whereas no endurance-training reductions in VLDL-C have been reported for youth [98].

Low-Density Lipoprotein
Cholesterol is principally carried by low-density lipoprotein (LDL-C) in the blood and has been positively associated with development of premature CAD [51]. LDL is primarily derived from the catabolism of chylomicron and VLDL and has a disappearance *half-time* from the circulation of approximately 2.5 days for LDL containing apo B-100. Several avenues exist for tissues to access cholesterol, including (*a*) uptake of cholesterol by the LDL receptor pathway; (*b*) uptake of free cholesterol from a non-receptor-mediated pathway; (*c*) uptake of free cholesterol from cholesterol-rich lipoproteins to the cell membrane; (*d*) hydrolysis of cholesteryl esters; and (*e*) cell cholesterol synthesis.

Observational studies comparing LDL-C concentrations in men and women athletes from various sports with those of inactive subjects have produced mixed results, with no differences [34, 63, 111, 169, 177] and differences [112, 177, 193] being reported. Athletes participating in power- or speed-related events have LDL-C concentrations either similar to [11] or lower [177] than those of inactive controls. Some, but not all [19, 30, 170], longitudinal endurance-exercise training studies have reported lower LDL-C concentrations for men and women [29, 146, 148, 196] following endurance training. When LDL-C concentrations are lower [19, 28, 148], the change (about 3–8%) has been inversely related to the distance run each week [174, 200]. As was true with total cholesterol, exercise training modifications that result in weight loss, plasma volume expansion, and dietary intake must be considered when reductions in LDL-C occur following exercise training [174, 197]. Cross-sectional studies of active and inactive older adults [70, 127] and youths [6] have observed no differences in LDL-C concentrations. Results from longitudinal exercise-training studies are consistent with cross-sectional results, with no reductions in LDL-C reported for older adults [15, 21, 136, 137] and youth [6, 98].

Since the amount of triglyceride associated with LDL is quite small, it has not often been measured. However, one cross- sectional study of men [111] and another of men and women long-distance runners observed lower LDL-triglyceride concentrations in men but not women, compared with inactive controls [120], whereas Finnish lumberjacks had higher LDL-triglyceride concentrations than sedentary workers [90]. Three longitudinal studies in humans [110, 122, 153] and one in genetically obese rats [33] reported no change in LDL-triglyceride values following exercise training.

Low-Density Lipoprotein Subfractions
Several LDL subspecies exist within its overall flotation interval of S_f0-20. Three general classifications divide the LDL group into small LDL (S_f0–7), large LDL (S_f7–12), and intermediate-density lipoprotein (IDL; S_f12–20). Some evidence indicates that the smaller, apo B–rich LDL and IDL particles are particularly atherogenic [88, 89]. Observational results comparing endurance runners and inactive controls indicate that the smaller LDL mass is significantly lower in runners, with no differences in the mass of the larger LDL and IDL particles [193]. Since the smaller LDL particle mass is reduced in endurance runners, their risk for CAD should also be reduced. However, endurance exercise training of men did not find any changes in these subfractions during a 1-year period, when adjusted for change in body mass index [189, 191]. Presently, no results are available for youth, women, and older adults.

High-Density Lipoprotein
The primary function of HDL has become clearer in recent years. It serves as the cholesterol acceptor in the reverse transport and excretion of cholesterol. Although HDL has several sites of origin, it continually interacts with free cholesterol, cholesteryl ester, and several enzymes within the circulation. The result is a constant flux in HDL composition and a transport mechanism for net movement of cholesterol from the peripheral vascular compartment and tissues to the liver for excretion as bile. The small, dense HDL_3 particle is synthesized either by the liver or by the intestinal epithelial cells or is a product of LPL action (Fig. 15.1). Once in the circulation, HDL_3 is modified by LCAT and transformed into the less dense HDL_2. Continued processing of the HDL_2 molecule is mediated by CETP and HL, resulting in the transformation of the macromolecule into HDL_3. CETP promotes the transfer of cholesteryl ester and triglyceride between HDL_2 and chylomicron and/or VLDL remnants. This allows removal of cholesterol and cholesteryl ester from chylomicron and/or VLDL remnants by the liver, while HL metabolizes the triglyceride portion of the HDL_2 molecule. The newly transformed HDL_3 particle is then released into the circulation and is ready for the process to continue. The *half-life* of HDL in human plasma is approximately five days.

HDL-cholesterol (HDL-C) has been negatively associated with risk for premature development of CAD [128]. Endurance-exercise training has been associated with increased HDL-C concentrations, implying reduced CAD risk. Cross-sectional studies observe a rather consistent elevated HDL-C concentration (typically 20–30%) for endurance-trained athletes, compared with inactive groups [34, 111, 112, 166, 169, 177, 193]. Furthermore, a dose-response relationship between the amount of exercise performed and HDL-C has been suggested [34, 131, 195]. However, longitudinal endurance-training studies have not been as congruent. Some studies have reported a significant difference after an endurance exercise training program [29, 110, 148, 170, 195, 196], while others have not [19, 30, 114, 122, 153, 186]. The reason for this discrepancy is not known, but it is likely related to several factors: the length of the training period, the volume of training completed, changes in body composition, dietary intake, weight loss, and the pretraining HDL-C concentration. Nevertheless, a recently published study that evaluated initially sedentary individuals before and after one year of endurance training found a positive correlation ($r = 0.45$, $P<0.05$) between total distance run and change in HDL-C [196]. In addition, elevated HDL-C concentrations have been reported for women after involvement in a high-volume training program [53] but not for those involved in a low-volume training program [19]. These results provide further support for the dose-response relationship observed in cross-sectional studies between physical activity and HDL-C concentrations.

Results from cross-sectional studies indicate that older physically active men and most older active women, but not all [67, 68], have higher HDL-C concentrations than do inactive controls [69, 70, 127, 138]. Results from longitudinal training studies indicate that HDL-C is elevated after exercise in most, but not all [21], older adults [15, 87, 136, 137]. Although evidence from cross-sectional and longitudinal studies demonstrates that physically active youth may have somewhat higher HDL-C concentrations, these differences are generally not significant [37, 98].

HDL Subfractions
There are two major HDL subfractions: HDL_2 and HDL_3. The specific functions of each are only now being better defined. HDL_3 is most likely the precursor to HDL_2, while HDL_2 serves as the final acceptor of cholesterol in the reverse cholesterol transport process. Higher HDL_2-C and lower HDL_3-C concentrations are observed in comparisons of elite endurance runners and inactive controls [34], with HDL_2-C highly correlated with time spent running each week ($r = 0.673$, $P<0.05$). A recent one-year randomized trial evaluating the changes in lipoprotein subfractions during diet-induced and exercise-induced weight loss in moderately overweight men reported exercise-induced elevated HDL_2-C and HDL_3-C concentrations [196]. However, distance run and $\dot{V}O_2max$ were not associated with

changes in other lipids or lipoprotein subfractions. A follow-up report examining the change in the mass of lipoprotein subfractions found an elevated HDL_2 mass and attributed this increase to an exercise-induced reduction in body mass index [189]. Distance run and $\dot{V}O_2$max were correlated with one-year changes within specific ranges of HDL_2 mass, but these correlations were not significant when adjusted for change in body mass index [189]. In another report, men with known CAD had an increased HDL_2 mass after endurance-exercise training. Increased cholesterol, triglyceride, protein, and phospholipid content were responsible for the increased mass of this subfraction [8]. Recent work indicates that regular exercise can augment the effects of a low-fat diet and result in an improved HDL_2-C concentration in overweight men after one year of diet and exercise intervention [197]. Although similar changes are found in women, the magnitude of change was not as great as observed for men [197]. Presently, little information relative to change in the HDL mass induced by endurance training for youth and the older adults is available.

The two HDL subfractions can also be separated by nondenaturing polyacrylamide gradient gel electrophoresis [14] into three HDL_3 subclasses and two HDL_2 subclasses. These subclasses are defined by their estimated particle diameters: HDL_{3c} (~7.2–7.8 nm), HDL_{3b} (7.8–8.2 nm), HDL_{3a} (8.2–8.8 nm), HDL_{2a} (8.8–9.7 nm) and HDL_{2b} (9.7–12.9 nm) [14]. Williams et al. [192] have described various associations between these HDL subclasses as well as an inverse relationship between HDL_{2a} and HDL_{2b}. Furthermore, the HDL_{3b} was positively related to CAD risk [192]. Presently, only one longitudinal exercise-training study evaluating the effects of weight loss by exercise and by diet on the particle-size distribution of HDL in men has been completed. Williams et al. [190] reported decreased HDL_{3b} and increased HDL_{2b} in both exercisers and dieters. After adjusting for the effects of weight loss, these significant changes (reductions in HDL_{3b} and the increases in HDL_{2b}) for exercisers and dieters were eliminated. However, when adjusted for weight loss, the mean change in the dieter's HDL_{2b} had decreased significantly relative to the means for both exercisers and controls. These results suggest that changes in the HDL subclasses after exercise training may result from metabolic changes secondary to exercise-induced weight loss [190] and that altered caloric balance and/or other factors diminish the rise in HDL_{2b} after weight loss.

Apolipoproteins
Although much remains to be learned about the biologic functions of the various apolipoproteins, clearly they are involved in the transport of lipids, the regulation of enzymes in the lipoprotein metabolic pathway, recognition of specific lipoproteins by cell receptors, and the exchange of lipid among various lipoproteins. Two apolipoproteins have been related to risk for developing CAD: apolipoprotein A-I, the primary protein moiety of the

HDL group, and apolipoprotein B, the principal LDL protein moiety. Angiographic evidence indicates that individuals with elevated concentrations of apolipoprotein A-I have lower incidence of CAD [103]. Apolipoprotein B, on the other hand, has been positively identified with increased risk for CAD [60]. A third protein, apolipoprotein E, is primarily synthesized by the liver and functions in the catabolism of chylomicron, VLDL, and HDL [101]. Apolipoproteins C-I, C-II, and C-III are synthesized in the liver and regulate enzyme activities: C-I is an activator of LCAT, C-II is an activator of LPL, and C-III inhibits LPL activity.

Apolipoprotein A-I activates LCAT. Some cross-sectional studies have reported higher apolipoprotein A-I concentrations in elite women runners [35] and in physically active men [66, 111, 169, 172]. In another respect, forced bed rest as a result of spinal injury in both men and women was associated with lower apolipoprotein A-I concentrations, compared with ambulatory controls [120]. Endurance-training studies have not produced a clear answer relative to exercise-induced change in apolipoprotein A-I. Some investigations have reported an increase in apolipoprotein A-I [81, 135, 190], while others have not [170, 200]. A 10% increase (p = 0.01) in this apolipoprotein was reported for men after a 12-week endurance-training program [81]. In a recent study, Williams et al. [190] found increased apolipoprotein A-I after 12 months of exercise training, likely because of changes associated with exercise-induced weight loss. Nevertheless, Wood et al. [200] observed no change in apolipoprotein A-I concentrations in sedentary men who exercise-trained for 1 year. Furthermore, apolipoprotein A-I did not correlate with miles run (r = 0.16), while significant correlations between miles run, HDL_2 mass, and HDL-C were found. The reason for the difference in these studies is not readily apparent but may be related to change in body weight, calorie intake, and adiposity, and/or a loss of abdominal body fat as a result of increased physical activity. In overweight men, exercise training and a low-fat diet result in an increased apolipoprotein A-I concentration in men but not in women [197]. Few published results for older adults and adolescents are available. Differences in apolipoprotein A-I concentrations have been observed in a cross-sectional study of older active and inactive men [159], but not between active and inactive older women [70]. No differences were reported after exercise training for older adult men [136]. Only small changes have been observed in physically active adolescents [6].

Apolipoprotein A-II is an LCAT inhibitor and/or an HL activator [17]. Most observational exercise studies, but not all [159, 166], have reported no differences in apolipoprotein A-II concentrations [35, 66, 70, 169] between physically active and inactive subjects. Results from longitudinal exercise training studies also support the conclusion that exercise has no effect on apolipoprotein A-II concentrations [170, 200]. However, changes in apolipoprotein A-II have been positively associated with changes in caloric intake (r = 0.39) [200]. Therefore, some of the elevation in apolipoprotein A-II found by Thompson et al. [166] could be explained by the greater caloric intake of elite athletes.

Apolipoprotein B consists of two distinct isoproteins: apo B- 48, primarily found with chylomicrons, and apo B-100, primarily associated with VLDL and LDL. Although most cross-sectional and longitudinal exercise studies evaluating apolipoprotein B have not considered the isoprotein forms, one recently published study by Tamai et al. [158] observed lower plasma apo B-48 ratios in elderly women runners, compared with inactive controls. Observational studies of athletes and sedentary controls do not support any change in apolipoprotein B concentration for women [35] and men [45, 111, 169], nor do most investigations report an exercise training–induced change [30, 110, 200]. However, Després et al. [29] have reported a reduction in apolipoprotein B in concordance with a reduction in plasma LDL-C. In addition, apolipoprotein B has been negatively related (r = 0.29, P<0.05) with distance run each week [200]. A low fat-diet and an exercise program will augment apolipoprotein B reductions in men but not in women [197].

The atherogenic risk index, the ratio of apolipoprotein B to apolipoprotein A-I [118], was favorably influenced by weight loss promoted by a low-fat diet plus exercise training in both men and women, in comparison to a low-fat diet alone group or an inactive control group that did not modify their diet [197]. Observational studies [70, 158, 159] of older active or inactive men and women and longitudinal exercise-training studies of older men [136] have reported no differences for apolipoprotein B concentrations. In the few published studies evaluating apolipoprotein B in adolescence groups either small [102] or no differences [6] have been reported.

Very few studies have been published regarding an exercise-induced effect with either E apolipoprotein or any of the C apolipoproteins. Marti et al. [111] observed no difference in apolipoprotein E concentrations in current and former runners, but both of these groups had significantly lower apolipoprotein E concentrations than a sedentary group. Higher concentrations of apolipoprotein E were reported in young runners, but not in older runners, compared with inactive groups [158]. Endurance-training two hours per week for four months did not alter apolipoprotein E concentrations [110] in older men or women (greater than 60 years of age) [139]. Tamai et al. [159] reported no differences in apolipoproteins C-II and C-III between young and older physically active and inactive men.

Lipoprotein(a)

Lp(a) and LDL are similar in structure and composition with the exception of the apolipoprotein(a) that is bound by covalent disulfide bonds to apo B-100. The amino acid sequence of this apolipoprotein is exceedingly similar to that of human plasminogen. This likeliness has led to the hypothesis that Lp(a) may mimic plasminogen and interfere with the fibrinolytic functions of plasminogen and/or plasmin and promote thrombotic effects. Thus, elevated concentrations of Lp(a) have been associated with an increased risk of CAD [113]. Present information indicates that Lp(a) is a heritable trait [92] and is not linked metabolically with LDL [24]. Therefore, intervention programs that alter plasma concentrations of LDL may have little effect on Lp(a) concentrations [2, 180]. Observational exercise studies support this contention by reporting no relationship between Lp(a) and lowest versus highest fitness quartiles, body composition, and other factors known to influence risk of CAD in adults [93, 149, 158] and in adolescents [152]. Presently, few longitudinal training studies have been published relative to the effects of exercise on Lp(a). Lobo et al. [99] and Seip et al. [139] report no exercise effect on Lp(a) after endurance-exercise training, whereas Mankowitz et al. [104] report no effect on Lp(a) after 14 or more days of detraining.

RESISTANCE EXERCISE TRAINING EFFECTS ON LIPOPROTEIN CONCENTRATIONS

Resistance-exercise training in recent years has become popular, and the benefits of these programs have been reviewed [49, 84, 179]. However, results from cross-sectional and longitudinal studies regarding specific lipid and lipoprotein change have provided inconsistent information. Many early studies did not use a proper experimental design to account for factors known to affect lipoprotein metabolism. These limitations have recently been reviewed by Kokkinos and Hurley [84] and include differences in day-to-day lipid and lipoprotein variations, dietary composition, body composition, plasma volume, the use of small sample sizes, no distinction between a single exercise session and regular practiced exercise, anabolic steroid use, and lack of or improperly selected inactive control groups. Since these factors have confounding influences on plasma lipoproteins, little conclusive information can be gained from these reports. In addition, some confusion has occurred because of the different types of resistance training that exist. Essentially, three different methods of resistance-training programs are used: powerlifting, Olympic weight lifting, and bodybuilding. Powerlifters and Olympic weight lifters primarily use exercise-training regimens that consist of heavy resistance and low number of repetitions with long rest intervals between exercise stations, whereas exercise-training programs used by bodybuilders employ moderate resistance and high number of repetitions with short rest intervals between exercise stations. Generally, bodybuilders and runners have similar lipoprotein profiles, and these profiles are associated with less CAD risk than those of power lifters. Recently published studies have used more appropriate experimental designs, and as a result have added meaningful information about the relationship between resistance-exercise training programs and plasma lipoproteins.

Triglyceride
Cross-sectional studies examining regular participation in resistance exercise training have observed no differences in plasma triglyceride concentrations for male [41] and female [117] bodybuilders, compared with inactive groups. However, Kohl et al. [83] found a direct association between upper and lower body strength and triglyceride concentrations in men, but not in women. Most longitudinal studies have not reported triglyceride changes after resistance exercise training in male [73, 85, 86, 145], female [106], and prepubertal male [185] participants. Conversely, when pretraining plasma triglyceride concentrations were elevated, significantly lower triglyceride concentrations were observed after training in bodybuilders, compared with inactive controls [201], and in females after 16 weeks of resistive exercise training [50].

Cholesterol
Regular participation in resistance-exercise training appears to have little effect on plasma total cholesterol concentrations. Cross-sectional observations indicate that total cholesterol concentrations in male [37] and female [37, 117] bodybuilders do not differ from those of distance runners. Furthermore, Kohl et al. [83] after adjusting for age, body composition, and cardiovascular fitness, observed no association between muscular strength and serum total cholesterol concentrations for men and women. Recent longitudinal studies for men [73, 85, 86, 145] and women [106] report no differences in total cholesterol concentrations after resistance training. In some cases, decreased cholesterol concentrations have been reported [50, 76]. However, this decrease may have been the result of a hemodilution effect occurring as a consequence of exercise training. Fripp and Hodgson [44] evaluated adolescent males after a 9-week resistance-exercise training program and reported no change in total cholesterol concentrations. However, Weltman et al. [185] found a 16% reduction in total cholesterol for prepubertal males after a 14-week resistance-training program.

Lipoproteins
VERY-LOW-DENSITY LIPOPROTEIN AND LOW-DENSITY LIPOPROTEIN. Few studies have evaluated VLDL change relative to resistance training. Studies that observed triglyceride reductions in bodybuilders have also observed reductions in VLDL triglyceride [201] as well as VLDL-C [11]. Some interest has been given to LDL cholesterol. Cross-sectional reports observe lower LDL-C in bodybuilders and runners than in inactive controls and powerlifters [72]. No relationship was observed between muscular strength and serum LDL-C for men and women [83]. Several longitudinal resistance exercise training studies have found reductions in LDL-C for males [73], females [50], and young male adolescents [44]. Nevertheless, most recent studies have found no change in LDL-C concentrations for men [85, 86, 145] and women [106] after resistance exercise training.

HIGH-DENSITY LIPOPROTEIN AND SUBFRACTIONS. Cross-sectional observations indicate that HDL-C concentrations are not elevated in bodybuilders, compared with endurance athletes, and are similar to those of inactive controls for both males and females [37, 117]. Hurley et al. [72] observed significantly lower HDL-C in powerlifters and higher concentrations in bodybuilders than in runners and inactive controls, whereas Farrell et al. [41] found no difference in HDL-C for power lifters and an inactive group. Kohl et al [83] found a significant inverse association between muscular strength and HDL-C concentrations in men but not women. One longitudinal resistance-training study has reported increased HDL-C concentrations [73] after training, but most have found no changes for men [50, 85, 86, 145] and women [50, 106]. Concerning youth, Weltman et al. [185] reported no differences in HDL-C concentrations after resistance training of prepubertal males. On the other hand, Fripp and Hodgson [44] found a 22% increase in HDL-C after 9 weeks of resistance training in male adolescents. Hurley et al. [72] in a cross-sectional study observed lower HDL_2-C concentrations in power lifters than in bodybuilders and runners. From a longitudinal perspective, HDL_2-C was either reduced [73] or not changed [86] after resistance training.

LIPOPROTEIN RATIOS. Various lipid and lipoprotein ratios have also been evaluated in response to resistance-exercise training. Hurley et al [72] observed a smaller ratio of LDL-C to HDL-C in bodybuilders and runners than in power lifters and inactive controls. Elliot et al. [37] evaluated the ratio of total cholesterol to HDL-C and found no differences between bodybuilders and runners. Although Goldberg et al. [50] and Hurley et al. [73] have found significantly decreased total cholesterol to HDL-C ratios after resistance-exercise training, Kokkinos et al. [85] and Manning et al. [106] did not. These changes in lipoprotein ratios, when found, are regarded as favorable relative to CAD risk.

APOLIPOPROTEINS. Few studies have evaluated apolipoproteins changes in response to resistance-exercise training. Manning et al. [106] reported significant changes in apo A-I after 12 weeks of resistance training for women. However, this change did not remain 4 days after the last exercise session. Fripp and Hodgson [44] found no change in apo B, and Manning et al. [106] reported no change in apo B-100 after a resistance-training program.

SINGLE SESSION OF EXERCISE AND ITS EFFECT ON LIPOPROTEIN CONCENTRATIONS

Since some of the modifications ascribed to regular participation in physical activity may be induced partially by a single exercise period, considerable attention has been given to the effects of one physical activity session on plasma lipids and lipoproteins. Currently, over 70 published journal manuscripts and abstracts are available regarding a single period of exercise completed by men and women, which encompass both short and prolonged periods of varying exercise modes and intensities. Since many factors influence lipoprotein metabolism, accounting for these factors is important in evaluating results from these studies. Factors that influence lipoprotein metabolism during and after exercise include volume of work completed (the amount of work should be quantified so that various activities may be compared, i.e., kcal), preexercise lipoprotein concentrations (for change to occur, persons with initially high HDL-C or low total cholesterol concentrations may have to complete a larger volume of work), timing of blood samples, length of postexercise follow-up periods (changes that occur in lipoprotein metabolism many times develop within the 72-hour postexercise period and not necessarily during exertion), change in dietary composition (if an experimental protocol involves several exercise treatments and/or lasts for an extended period of time, then dietary composition must be held constant), lack of and/or incomplete estimation of plasma volume change (plasma volume can contract during an exercise session or expand in the days after exercise by 10% or more: an appropriate estimate of this change would incorporate measurement of both hemoglobin and hematocrit [55] and/or measurement of total plasma proteins), and training state of test subjects (an inactive person may require a smaller absolute volume of exercise to elicit change than an active person). Women present several additional complications that affect the lipid and lipoprotein profile. These factors must be considered when interpreting results from studies using women subjects and include the use of oral contraceptives as well as their position in the menstrual cycle. Selected studies evaluating the effects of a single session of physical activity and their results are summarized and presented in Table 15.3. The studies cited in Table 15.3 and in the following sections are those that have made some adjustment for plasma volume change.

Triglyceride
Triglyceride concentrations are not usually altered immediately following or in the days after an exercise period of short duration and low intensity [4, 25]. However, exercise studies that required subjects to expend large quantities of energy (i.e., marathon running) have found no change immediately after the session [5, 23, 36, 78, 167], but did observe decreased triglyceride concentrations 24 hours after exercise [5, 23, 38, 77, 167]. In some cases, increased triglyceride concentrations have been reported immediately after exercise in women [52, 154] and men [31], but these elevated triglyceride values returned to the preexercise concentrations or were lower than the preexercise concentrations 24 hours after the exercise session. When lower triglyceride concentrations were observed following the exercise period, they slowly returned to preexercise levels during the succeeding days. Following a single session of resistance exercise

TABLE 15.3
Selected Studies of a Single Session of Exercise

Citation	Study Design	Variables Measured	Time Periods for Variable Measurement	Changes
Aerobic exercise sessions with male and female subjects				
Angelopoulos et al., 1993	9 sedentary males completed 3 treadmill protocols: 1) 1 30-min session at 65% $\dot{V}O_2$max 2) 2 30-min sessions at 65% $\dot{V}O_2$max 3) 3 30-min sessions at 65% $\dot{V}O_2$max	TC, TG, HDL-C, HDL_2-C, HDL_3-C	imm. pre, 5 min post, 24 hr post, 48 hr post	Changes found for all 3 protocols: At 5 min post ↑ HDL-C, ↑ HDL_3-C. At 24 hr post ↑ HDL-C. At 48 hr post ↓ HDL_2-C and ↓ HDL_3-C.
Davis et al., 1992	10 trained males completed 2 treadmill protocols: 1) 75% $\dot{V}O_2$max 60 min 2) 50% $\dot{V}O_2$max 90 min	TC, TG, HDL-C, HDL_2-C, HDL_3-C, LDL-C, VLDL-C, apo A-I, apo A-II, apo B	24 hr pre, imm. pre, 18 hr post, 1 hr post, 24 hr post, 48 hr post, 72 hr post	No changes were found at any time point.
Griffin et al., 1988	6 trained males completed 3 different diets and over a 4 day period walked 148 km: 1) normal diet 2) high carbohydrate diet 3) high fat diet	TC, TG, HDL-C, HDL-TG, HDL-protein, HDL_{2a+3a}, HDL_{2b}, HDL_{3b+3c}, LDL-C, VLDL-C, VLDL-TG, LCAT	24 hr pre, imm. pre, 18 hr post, 42 hr post, 90 hr post	At 18 hr post: Normal diet ↑HDL-C, ↓ VLDL-C, ↓ LCAT. High-carbohydrate diet ↓ HDL-C, ↓ HDL-protein, ↑ HDL_{3b+3c}, ↓ LDL-C, ↑ VLDL-C, ↑ VLDL-TG. High-fat diet ↑ HDL-C, ↑ HDL-protein, ↓ HDL_{2a+3a}, ↑ HDL_{2b}, ↓ VLDL-C, ↓ VLDL-TG, ↓ LCAT.
Annuzzi et al., 1987	10 active males completed 2 bicycle protocols: 1) 60 min cycling at 50% max work rate and 30 min treadmill work at 85% max HR 2) Subjects completed 2 of protocol 1	TC, TG, HDL-C, HDL-TG, LDL-C, LDL-TG, VLDL-C, VLDL-TG, apo C-I, apo C-II, apo C-III	24 hr pre, imm. pre, imm. post, 24 hr post, 48 hr post, 72 hr post	At 24 hr post: for protocol 1 ↓ VLDL-TG, ↓ LDL-TG, ↓ VLDL-C, ↓ LDL-C; for protocol 2 ↓ TG, ↓ apo C-I. At 48 hr post: for protocol 2 ↓ TG.

Study	Subjects/Protocol	Variables	Time Points	Results
Kantor et al., 1987	21 males (11 trained and 10 inactive) cycled at 80% $\dot{V}O_2$max Trained completed 120 min, inactive completed 60 min of work	TC, TG, HDL-C, HDL$_2$-C, HDL$_3$-C, LDL-C, LPL, HL	24 hr pre, 10 min post, 24 hr post, 48 hr post, 72 hr post	At 10 min post: Trained subjects ↓ LDL-C, ↑ HDL-C, ↓ LPL; Inactive subjects ↓ TC, ↓ LDL-C, ↓ LPL. At 24 hr post: Trained subjects ↑ HDL-C, ↑ LPL; Inactive subjects ↑ HDL-C, ↑ LPL. At 48 hr post: Trained subjects ↑ TC, ↑ HDL-C, ↑ HDL$_2$-C; Inactive subjects ↑ TC, ↑ HDL-C, ↑ HDL$_3$-C. At 72 hr post: Trained subjects ↑ TC, ↑ HDL-C, ↑ HDL$_2$-C, ↑ HL; Inactive subjects ↑ TC, ↑ HDL-C, ↑ HDL$_3$-C.
Dufaux et al., 1986	14 trained males completed a 3-hr treadmill run at 75% of lactate threshold (4 mmol)	TC, TG, HDL-C, HDL$_2$-C, HDL$_3$-C, Lp(a), apo A-I, apo A-II, apo B, LCAT	24 hr pre, imm. pre, imm. post, 1 hr post, 3 hr post, 24 hr post, 48 hr post, 96 hr post	At imm. post ↑TC, ↑ TG, ↑ HDL-C, ↑ HDL$_3$-C, ↑ apo A-II, ↑ apo A-II, ↑ apo B. At 1 hr post ↑ TG, ↑ HDL-C, ↑ HDL$_3$-C. At 3 hr post ↑ LCAT. At 24 hr post ↓ TC, ↓ TG, ↑ HDL-C, ↑ HDL$_3$-C. At 48 hr post ↓ TC, ↓ TG, ↑ HDL$_2$-C, ↑ LPL, ↑ Lp(a), ↓ LCAT. At 96 hr post ↓ apo A-II.
Sady et al., 1986	10 trained males ran a marathon	TC, TG, HDL-C, HDL$_2$-C, HDL$_3$-C, LDL-C, apo A-I, apo A-II, LPL, HL	24 hr pre, 18 hr post	At 18 hr post ↓ TG, ↓ LDL-C, ↑ HDL-C, ↑ HDL$_2$-C, ↑ LPL.
Kantor et al., 1984	10 trained males ran a marathon	TC, TG, HDL-C, HDL$_2$-C, HDL$_3$-C, LDL-C, apo A-I, apo A-II, HL, LPL	24 hr pre, 18 hr post, 42 hr post	At 18 hr post ↓TG, ↓ LDL-C, ↑ HDL-C, ↑ HDL$_2$-C, ↑ HDL$_3$-C, and ↑ LPL. At 42 hr post ↓ TG, ↑ HDL-C, and ↑ HDL$_2$-C.

TABLE 15.3
Selected Studies of a Single Session of Exercise—continued

Citation	Study Design	Variables Measured	Time Periods for Variable Measurement	Changes
Durstine et al., 1983	10 active males walked on treadmills to exhaustion at 45% V̇O₂max	TC, TG, HDL-C, LDL-C, VLDL-C	imm. pre, 30 min post	At 2 hours of exercise ↑ HDL-C. At 30 min post ↑ TC, ↑HDL-C, ↓ HDL-C/LDL-C ratio.
Cullinane et al., 1982	19 men (10 inactive and 9 trained cyclists) cycled at anaerobic threshold; inactive subjects completed 60 min of work and trained completed 2 protocols; 1) 60 min 2) 120 min	TC, TG, HDL-C, LDL-C	imm. pre, imm. post, 1 hr post, 4 hr post, 24 hr post, 48 hr post, 72 hr post	At imm. post trained subject completing 60 min of work ↑ LDL-C and after 120 min of work ↑ TC, ↑ LDL-C, ↑ HDL-C. At 24 hr post and after the 120 min protocol ↓ TG.
Thompson et al., 1980	12 trained males ran a marathon	TC, TG, LDL-C, HDL-C, apo A-I	24 hr pre, 1 hr pre, 5 min post, 1 hr post, 4 hr post, 18 hr post, 42 hr post, 66 hr post	At 5 min post ↑ HDL-C, ↑ apo A-I. At 1 hr post ↓ apo A-I. At 4 hr post ↓ TC, ↓ LDL-C, ↓ apo A-I. At 18 hr post ↓ TG, ↓ TC, ↓ LDL-C, ↑ HDL-C, ↓ apo A-I. At 42 hr post ↓ TG, ↓ TC, ↓ LDL-C, ↓ apo A-I. At 66 hr post ↓ TG, ↓ TC, ↓ LDL-C, ↓ apo A-I.

Goodyear et al., 1990	12 trained females completed a marathon	TC, TG, HDL, LDL	24 hr pre, 10 min post, 24 hr post, 72 hr post, 120 hr post	At 10 min post ↑ TG and ↓ LDL-C. At 24 hr post ↓ TC, ↑ HDL-C and ↓ LDL-C. At 72 hr post ↓ TC. At 120 hr post ↓ TC.
Skinner et al., 1987	12 trained females completed a marathon	TC, HDL-C, HDL-cholesteryl ester, LDL-C, VLDL-C, apo A-I, apo A-II, apo C, apo E	1 hr pre, imm. post	At imm. post ↑ TC, ↑ HDL-C and ↑ HDL-cholesteryl ester.
Swank et al., 1987	9 healthy females completed a treadmill run for 40 min at 70% $\dot{V}O_2$max	TC, TG, HDL-C, HDL$_2$-C, HDL$_3$-C	imm. pre, 5 min post, 24 hr post, 48 hr post, 96 hr post	At 5 min post ↑ HDL-C and ↑ HDL$_3$-C.
Resistance exercise session with male subjects				
Shoup et al., in review	10 inactive males completed 40 min of circuit-weight training	TC, TG, HDL-C, HDL$_2$-C, HDL$_3$-C, LDL-C, VLDL-C, LPL activity, HL activity	24 hr pre, imm. pre, imm. post, 24 hr post, 48 hr post	At 24 hr post ↑ LPL. At 48 hr post ↑ LPL.
Wallace et al., 1991	10 healthy weight-trained males completed 2 protocols: high-volume weight training and a low-volume weight training	TC, TG, HDL-C, HDL$_2$-C, HDL$_3$-C, LCAT	10 min pre, 5 min post, 24 hr post, 48 hr post, 72 hr post	At 24 hr post the high-volume protocol had ↓ TG, ↑ HDL-C, ↑ HDL$_3$-C, and ↑ LCAT.

TG = triglyceride; TC = total cholesterol; VLDL = very low density lipoprotein; LDL = low-density lipoprotein; HDL = high-density lipoprotein; LCAT = lecithin:cholesterol acyltransferase; LPL = lipoprotein lipase; HL = hepatic lipase; apo = apolipoprotein; $\dot{V}O_2$max = maximal oxygen consumption; pre= before exercise; imm. = immediately; post = after exercise.

triglyceride concentrations have been reported unchanged when the volume of the completed work was low [141], or reduced [182] if the volume of work completed was high. Generally, if an exercise session is prolonged and has a large energy requirement, triglyceride concentrations will be lower immediately afterwards and/or during the days following a single exercise session.

Cholesterol

Studies evaluating exercise periods of short duration have reported no change in total plasma cholesterol concentrations immediately after and in the days following a single exercise session for men [4, 25] and women [94]. A variety of responses have been reported for prolonged exercise periods as characterized by long-distance running and cross-country skiing. Measures of total cholesterol immediately after prolonged exercise include no change for male {23, 38, 77, 124, 167] and female [52] subjects as well as reductions [5] and increases [31, 36]. During the days after a prolonged exercise session, varying responses for total cholesterol concentrations have been reported and include reductions [5, 31, 38, 167], increases [78], and no change [23, 77]. Studies evaluating resistance exercise have reported no change in total cholesterol immediately after and in the days following a single exercise session [141, 182]. In summary, if a single exercise session is to have an impact on total cholesterol concentrations, the exercise must be prolonged and require a large amount of energy expenditure. Even then any effect will most likely not be seen until 24 hours after the end of the exercise session.

Lipoproteins

VERY-LOW-DENSITY LIPOPROTEIN AND LOW-DENSITY LIPOPROTEIN. Exercise periods of short duration using men [25] and women [94] have little impact on VLDL and LDL moieties immediately after and/or in the days following an exercise session. Although not often reported, VLDL-C concentrations immediately after prolonged exercise are lower [5, 56]. In addition, LDL-C concentrations have been reported to be lower in men [5, 77, 78, 167] and women [52] or unchanged [23, 36, 38, 144] immediately after prolonged exercise. Investigations evaluating a single session of resistance exercise do not report any changes in VLDL-C or LDL-C concentrations [141, 182]. Thus, if a single session of exercise is to affect VLDL-C or LDL-C concentrations, the activity should be prolonged and have a large energy requirement.

HIGH-DENSITY LIPOPROTEINS. Since HDL-C is inversely related to risk for developing CAD, this lipoprotein has received considerable attention relative to a single exercise session. Some studies using short-duration and low-intensity exercise designs have reported increased HDL-C immediately after the exercise episode [4, 94]. Durstine et al. [36] have evaluated HDL-C response to low-intensity exhaustive walking (45% of $\dot{V}O_2max$) and found increased HDL-C concentrations after 2 hours of exercise that persisted through exhaustion (exhaustion was reached after 4.5 hours) and into the postexercise period. Davis et al. [25] compared two exercise intensities, 50 and 75% of $\dot{V}O_2$max (energy expenditure for the two activities was held constant at 950 kcal; exercise time was 60 and 90 minutes, respectively) and found no change in HDL-C concentrations or any of the subfractions immediately after or in the days following the exercise episode. Annuzzi et al. [5] found no change in HDL-C after 1.5 hours of exercise requiring about 77% of maximal heart rate. On the other hand, prolonged exercise (more than 1.5 hours) will usually elevate HDL-C concentrations immediately after exercise in men [31, 36, 38, 56, 167] and women [52, 144] as well as in the days following the exercise episode [31, 38, 52, 56, 77, 167]. Thus, although not completely defined, there may be a threshold for the volume of work completed that is necessary to induce consistent increases in HDL-C. In addition, training state of the subject must be considered. In some cases, trained and sedentary have not always responded in the same fashion to a single exercise session. Kantor et al. [78] reported elevated HDL-C concentrations immediately after and in the days following an exercise session in trained subjects, whereas, sedentary subjects did not have elevated HDL-C concentrations immediately after an exercise period, but did have elevated HDL-C concentrations 24, 48, and 72 hours following the exercise session. Investigations evaluating a single session of resistance exercise have observed elevated HDL-C concentrations after a high-volume exercise session [182], but not after a low-volume exercise session [141, 182]. Consequently, to induce HDL-C change immediately after and in the days following a single exercise session, there appears to be a threshold of energy expenditure that has to be reached during the exercise session. The precise energy requirement is not known, but most likely time is a factor (a period of over 1.5 hours) [36] with an energy expenditure of more than 1000 kcal [25].

HDL$_2$ AND HDL$_3$ SUBFRACTIONS. Investigations evaluating the HDL subfractions relative to short-duration activities have found either no change [25] or only modest changes [4, 94] immediately after and in the days following the exercise episode. Studies examining prolonged exercise responses have reported elevations in HDL$_3$-C with no change in HDL$_2$-C immediately after the exercise period, but elevations in both HDL$_3$-C and HDL$_2$-C were found during the days following the exercise period [31, 77]. State of training also seems to be an important consideration when evaluating factors that affect the HDL subfractions. Kantor et al. [78] reported elevations in HDL-C 24, 48, and 72 hours after exercise for both trained and sedentary subjects. However, trained subjects had elevated HDL$_2$-C and unchanged HDL$_3$-C concentrations in the days following the exercise session, whereas, the sedentary subjects had no change in HDL$_2$-C but elevated HDL$_3$-C concentrations during the same follow-up period.

Another important observation was recently made by Kiens and Lithell

[79] in subjects completing a single exercise session after 8 weeks of one-leg training. They found that trained muscle developed more HDL_2-C than nontrained muscle. In addition, diet and exercise responses may have interactive effects upon the subfractions. The consumption of a high-fat diet (75% of the calories were fat) in conjunction with exercise increased HDL-C and HDL_2-C, while a high-carbohydrate diet (85% of the calories were carbohydrate) in combination with exercise decreased HDL-C and HDL_3-C [56]. Furthermore, the consumption of a high-fat diet and exercise involvement resulted in an increase in the HDL_{2b} concentration and a decrease in the HDL_{2a+3a} concentration. No consistent changes were evident while exercising and consuming a high-carbohydrate diet [56]. Finally, a study examining a single session of high-volume resistance exercise reported increased HDL-C and HDL_3-C concentrations in the days following an exercise episode, while HDL_2-C did not change [182]. At the same time a single low- volume resistance-exercise episode had no impact on either HDL_2-C or HDL_3-C concentrations [141, 182].

APOLIPOPROTEINS. Most studies have observed no change in apo A-I and A-II immediately after or in the days following a single exercise episode [25, 31, 77, 133]. In addition, no changes in apo B concentrations have been reported after exercise [25, 31]. Annuzzi et al. [5] found no change in apo C-I, C-II, and C-III 24 hours after a 1.5-hour exercise period (requiring 77% of the person's maximal heart rate). However, 24 hours after a 3-hour exercise period (requiring 77% of the person's maximal heart rate), apo C-I was reduced [5]. Few published results are available concerning changes in Lp(a) and apo E concentrations after a single exercise episode, but modest elevations have been reported in Lp(a) during the days after exercise [31, 56], whereas apo E concentrations after exercise were not changed [56]. Additional studies are required before conclusive comments can be made regarding a single exercise session and change in these apolipoproteins.

POTENTIAL MECHANISMS INVOLVED IN EXERCISE-ALTERED LIPOPROTEIN METABOLISM

Routine participation in physical activity and a single exercise session can alter lipoprotein metabolism, plasma lipid and lipoprotein concentrations, and lipid transport. Our understanding of the precise mechanisms responsible for these modifications is not complete, but present evidence indicates that other factors including diet composition, adiposity, weight loss, plasma volume change, and hormone and enzyme activity interact with exercise to alter the rates of synthesis, transport, and clearance of lipid and lipoproteins from the blood. Clearly, exercise has an impact on triglyceride synthesis (*EX1*, Fig. 15.1), LPL action (*EX2*, Fig. 15.1), LCAT, and CETP regulation (*EX3*, Fig. 15.1) that result in enhanced reverse cholesterol transport (*EX4*, Fig. 15.1). Although numerous investigations have focused on the changes in the lipid and lipoprotein concentrations that occur with exercise, the mechanisms responsible for many of these modifications in synthesis, clearance, and survival remain unclear (e.g., the reduction of triglyceride synthesis after exercise training [54]). Presently, altered lipoprotein enzyme activity has been observed in response to routine participation as well as a single session of exercise. From these observations we have gained valuable insight regarding potential mechanisms responsible for the change in lipoprotein metabolism, composition, and lipid transport.

Lipoprotein Lipase
LPL is responsible for delipidation of chylomicron and VLDL molecules and promotes the clearance of fatty acids and glycerol from the vascular compartment for either storage or use as substrate in energy metabolism. Cross-sectional studies indicate that endurance-trained runners at rest have higher plasma concentrations of heparin-releasable LPL than less active controls [119, 169], but not always [132]. However, no differences were reported between bodybuilders, weight-matched controls, and normal-weight controls for muscle or adipose tissue LPL activity [201]. Inactive men after having undergone endurance-exercise training usually have significantly higher adipose tissue and postheparin LPL activity than before training [126, 170]. Peltonen et al. [126] observed that much of the increase in LPL activity was found after the first week of training and suggested that this higher LPL activity after training was, in part, a response to a single session of exercise.

Information from studies evaluating a single exercise session indicates that energy demand by physical activity increases LPL activity. Depletion of intramuscular triglyceride stores by endurance exercise may promote secretion and/or synthesis of LPL by muscle cells [123]. After sedentary and trained subjects performed a single prolonged session of endurance cycling exercise [78], both groups had higher postheparin LPL activity. Furthermore, the running of a marathon increased both postheparin LPL activity and the clearance rate of an artificial triglyceride emulsion [133]. Although higher postheparin plasma LPL activity may not be evident until 4–18 hours after exercise, augmented LPL activity results in increased chylomicron and VLDL hydrolysis and reductions in plasma triglyceride concentrations [78, 79]. Increased remnants are a consequence of increased catabolism of chylomicron and VLDL (Fig. 1). These remnants in conjunction with HDL$_3$ (as the primary substrate) may combine in a series of reactions that yield HDL$_2$ [165]. This increased HDL$_2$ synthesis appears to be a major contributor to the higher HDL mass resulting from endurance exercise and may occur in the vascular compartment of both muscle [79] and adipose tissue [189]. Kiens and Lithell [79] had subjects complete 8 weeks of one-leg cycle training. At the conclusion of the training period the subjects performed two hours of knee extension. A significant increase in arterial-venous HDL_2-C concentrations across trained skeletal muscle, but not across the nontrained muscle from the same individual, was observed. Further, estimates of total triglyceride degradation and total HDL formation from both trained and nontrained legs were highly correlated (r = 0.91). Although muscle biopsies taken at rest after 8 weeks of exercise training indicated differences in resting muscle LPL activity for trained and nontrained muscle groups, two hours of exercise did not change LPL activity immediately postexercise in either muscle group. However, muscle LPL activity was higher four hours after exercise in only trained muscle [79]. These results suggest that changes in lipoprotein profiles induced by endurance training, in part, are explained by skeletal muscle adaptations that impact LPL activity after exercise.

A different approach has been taken by Williams et al. [189]. This approach was based on the observation that LPL activity is greatest in adipose tissue. Thus, chylomicron and VLDL catabolism is more likely to occur in adipose tissue rather than in muscle tissue [189]. Therefore, depletion of adipocyte triglyceride stores as a result of endurance training–induced weight loss could cause increased adipocyte LPL activity and, in turn, affect lipoprotein concentrations [189]. Regardless of which tissue has the more prominent role, skeletal muscle, heart, and adipose tissue are possible sites for endurance training–induced LPL activity modifications that can result in lipoprotein profile change.

Since increased LPL activity results in increased HDL synthesis, increased synthesis has received much of the credit for the elevated HDL mass associated with endurance exercise. However, present knowledge indicates that exercise training also prolongs the survival of HDL apolipoproteins. The synthesis rates of HDL proteins for competitive runners and sedentary subjects are alike [66] with no change in HDL protein synthesis after endurance training [170]. Additionally, the survival time of HDL protein was 27% longer in the circulation of physically active men, compared with inactive men [66], and endurance training increased the half-lives of apolipoproteins A-I and A-II in formerly inactive men [170]. Both LPL activity and fat clearance were increased in conjunction with the increased HDL survival, but postheparin LPL activity was lower than expected [170] and could reflect qualitative as well as quantitative changes in LPL [165]. Most likely the increased HDL mass associated with endurance training is a result of both increased synthesis and survival.

Hepatic Lipase

HL is bound to the endothelial surface of hepatic tissue and has a primary function in the reverse transport of cholesterol. Cross-sectional studies have observed that HL activity did not differ between active and inactive groups [169] or was lower in active groups [108]. HL was reduced in middle-aged men after 15 weeks of endurance training [126] and after one year of weight loss by exercise and/or dieting [147] and not different after 14 or 32 weeks of endurance training when adjusted for plasma volume change [170]. A single session of endurance exercise [77, 78] and resistive exercise [141] had little or no effect on HL activity. In addition, a significant inverse relationship has been reported between HDL-C and HL in active military academy students [91], negatively correlated with HDL_2-C, but positively correlated with HDL_3-C [160]. Since HL is involved in the process of converting HDL_2 to HDL_3 and since HL activity is either lower or not changed in response to exercise, the higher HDL_2 concentrations and lower HDL_3 reported after endurance exercise training are not unexpected.

Lecithin:Cholesterol Acyltransferase

LCAT resides on the surface of lipoprotein particles in plasma and catalyzes the transfer of plasma fatty acids from lecithin to cholesterol. The esterified cholesterol can then move into the hydrophobic core of the preferred substrate HDL_3, creating a gradient that favors the net transfer of cholesterol from cell membranes onto the lipoprotein surface [187]. Higher LCAT activity has been reported for endurance-trained sportsmen [57, 109, 176] and after endurance training of young men [109] and middle-aged men [107] and is thought to contribute to increased synthesis of HDL_2-C. Increased LCAT activity was correlated with an increase in HDL-C (r = 0.49, P<0.01) [109]. However, Thomas et al. [163] found no change in LCAT activity in men that completed an 11-week interval training program. Nor did Williams et al. [187] observe any change in LCAT mass of men undergoing a 1-year exercise-induced weight-loss program. Thompson et al. [164] withdrew any routine exercise for 6 weeks from physically active men who were expending about 1000 kcal per week in an exercise program and found no change in LCAT activity. The reason for this discrepancy between studies is not readily apparent, but the inconsistency may be related to the volume of training completed and/or the technologic differences used to measure LCAT. The athletes in the study of Marniemi et al. [109] completed approximately 10 hours per week of aerobic activity, while the young military cadets completed over 20 hours per week of combat training that included 4 hours of aerobic training. In this case, $\dot{V}O_2$max was correlated with LCAT activity (r = 0.399, P<0.01), whereas Williams et al. [187] had their subjects exercise 12.7 km per week, and $\dot{V}O_2$max was not significantly related to LCAT activity (r = 0.23). If LCAT activity is modified as a result of endurance training, a threshold above 12.7 km per week appears to be necessary.

A single session of endurance activity may increase LCAT activity [31, 42], but not always [12, 56]. Wallace et al. [182] observed increased LCAT activity in young weightlifters immediately after a 90-minute high-volume weightlifting period, but no change was found after a 90-minute low-volume weight-lifting session with less work completed. Thus, this supports the concept that a threshold of energy expenditure must be reached before physical activity will induce change in LCAT activity and change lipoprotein concentrations.

Cholesteryl Ester Transfer Protein

CETP promotes the transfer of cholesteryl ester from the HDL_2 particle to chylomicron and VLDL remnants in exchange for triglyceride. Once accepted by these lipoproteins, this cholesterol has several fates: it could undergo hepatic degradation and/or it could be a source for tissue deposition. Only recently has information become available regarding an exercise effect on CETP. One recent cross-sectional study observed higher CETP activity in endurance-trained athletes than in inactive controls [57]. In addition, CETP activity was inversely correlated with lipoprotein ratios considered at risk for CAD (i.e., total cholesterol/HDL-C). However, another recent report found lower CETP activity after 9–12 months of endurance-exercise training [139]. Positive associations were found between plasma CETP and LDL-C and between plasma CETP and total cholesterol before and after the exercise training period. Further, Seip et al. [139] reported a positive correlation between body fat and CETP concentrations. This may be evidence in humans for adipose tissue as an important source of CETP. Results from these studies are important because they provide insight into possible explanations regarding previous exercise training observations of lipoprotein profiles after training. For example, increased CETP activity could explain enhanced reverse cholesterol transport despite a coinciding decrease or no change in HDL-C concentration, whereas a decrease in CETP could result in an increased HDL-C.

Reverse Cholesterol Transport

Raising HDL-C concentrations may provide protection from CAD, based on epidemiologic observations, but evidence for increased cholesterol extraction from peripheral tissues of persons regularly involved in physical activity is only now becoming available. To understand the transport of cholesterol from peripheral tissues, the movement both into and out of peripheral cells must be considered. Gupta et al. [57] measured cholesterol movement into and out of cultured fibroblast cells from athletes and inactive controls. The net mass of free cholesterol transported from cultured fibroblast cells into the athletes' serum was greater than that for controls, and net transport of cholesterol mass was positively correlated with CETP and LCAT activities. The outflow of cholesterol from the cultured fibroblasts correlated with HDL-C ($r = 0.26$) and apo A-I ($r = 0.36$) concentrations. Since CETP and LCAT activity were increased and because of the positive correlations with HDL-C and apo A-I, these findings suggest a reduced movement of cholesterol into fibroblasts and support the antiatherogenic role of physical activity [57].

Although this explanation seems plausible, Seip et al. [139] recently reported decreased CETP activity after regular participation in physical activity. These results are contrary to those of Gupta et al. [57], who reported increased CETP activity in athletes. The information from Seip et al. [139] suggest that the exercise-increased HDL-C might be a consequence of reduced transfer of cholysteryl esters from HDL to chylomicron and VLDL remnants for removal from the circulation. Although present information supports an enhanced reverse transport of cholesterol, the precise mechanism for removal of cholesterol from the circulation remains unclear. Therefore, other pathways for the removal of cholesterol must exist and include the direct action of HL that results in transfer of cholesterol from HDL to the liver cholesterol pool, and the hepatic apo E receptor- mediated removal of HDL [155].

Other Factors and Their Interactions With Lipoproteins
Other factors should be considered when evaluating the impact of a single session of exercise or exercise training on lipoprotein metabolism. Increased dietary carbohydrate can reduce HDL-C and increase triglyceride concentrations, but physical activity will diminish this response [168, 170]. At the same time, skeletal muscle and adipose tissue LPL activity is reduced after a diet of complex carbohydrates but not after a simple carbohydrate diet [130]. Weight loss is positively associated with HDL-C and HDL$_2$-C concentrations and negatively with HL activity and total cholesterol and LDL-C concentrations [195]. Caloric restriction will reduce HDL-C concentrations in obese women [161] but increase HDL-C in distance runners [168]. Reduced body fat and increased leanness are important outcomes of exercise training. Leanness has been associated with lower HL activity in physically active people [195].

Adipose distribution, as indexed by the waist-to-hip girth ratio (WHR), is associated with altered lipoprotein patterns. Abdominal adiposity (WHR greater than 1.0) in nonobese males is associated with lower HDL-C and apolipoprotein AI concentrations [9]. Plasma LDL characteristics from subjects with abdominal adiposity closely resemble the attributes of LDLs from patients with CAD [125]. Endurance training may influence lipoprotein concentrations by enhancing beta-receptors' sensitivity to norepinephrine, causing amplified lipolysis. Since abdominal adipocytes are more responsive to catecholamine-induced lipolysis than are femoral adipocytes [96], this suggests, as a result of endurance training, a selective loss of abdominal fat versus femoral and gluteal fat, a reduction in the WHR [195], and perhaps reduced CAD risk [125].

Plasma volume expands with endurance-exercise training [66, 170]. Therefore, blood samples taken after endurance training must be corrected for this change or one may underestimate an exercise effect on plasma HDL concentrations and overestimate the effect on other lipoproteins. The reported endurance training–induced reductions in total cholesterol and LDL-C by some studies could be accounted for by a larger plasma volume [165].

An issue that often arises pertains to the volume of exercise necessary to induce change in lipid and lipoprotein profiles [150]. Since many factors affect lipoprotein metabolism, this issue is complex. Many of these factors have been addressed earlier, but one important consideration is the volume of exercise performed. Presently, many published reports (including a single exercise session and routine participation in an exercise program) do not adequately quantify their exercise protocols. Although some studies report mode, intensity, distance, and duration of the activity, this information does not always allow comparison between studies. Exercise is best quantified by the amount of energy expended and is reported in kcal or joules (1 kcal = 4.184 joules). Results from endurance exercise training studies indicate that plasma HDL-C concentrations are frequently increased by an exercise regimen that requires 1000–1200 kcal, or 4.2–5 megajoules, of energy expenditure [150, 188] per week and appears to have a dose-response relationship. This amount may be less for bed-rested patients[8] or more for active persons who increase their endurance-exercise training [80]. This level of energy expenditure may be necessary to effect changes in lipid and lipoprotein profiles immediately after and/or during the days following a single session of exercise [25, 36]. The relationship between lipid and lipoprotein responses after a single session of exercise and the responses from repeated sessions of exercise has not been completely defined.

HEALTH IMPLICATIONS

Physical activity has a positive effect on the lipid and lipoprotein profile. In normolipemic men and women, increased physical activity is associated with lower plasma triglyceride concentrations, whereas plasma total cholesterol is not altered. Although the triglyceride portion of the VLDL molecule is reduced after endurance-exercise training, the prominent changes in lipoprotein composition associated with endurance training are increased HDL-C, HDL_2-C, and apolipoprotein A-I concentrations. Exercise-induced modifications in LDL-C, its subfractions and apolipoproteins, are only minor without change in adiposity or dietary fat and cholesterol intake. The mechanisms responsible for these modifications are related to increases in LPL and LCAT enzyme activity. These enzymes enhance the reverse transport of cholesterol. The precise process for the removal of cholesterol from HDL is not clear, but it is most likely related to altered CETP and HL enzyme activity and/or an increased hepatic apo E receptor–mediated pathway. Regardless of the pathway for cholesterol removal, the described exercise- induced responses occur in both men and women of all ages and are associated with reduced CAD risk. Although a causal relationship between these two observations has not been established, abundant evidence supports consideration of increased physical activity patterns of previously inactive persons.

Clinical management of hyperlipoproteinemic subjects provides beneficial cardiovascular effects by reducing CAD morbidity and mortality. Although exercise could be considered as a primary therapeutic method of intervention for hyperlipoproteinemia, most professionals consider the role of endurance exercise training as secondary or supportive to dietary intervention or lipid-lowering medications. Few randomized controlled studies evaluating the effects of exercise training on patients with dyslipoproteinemia have been reported other than in hypertriglyceridemic men [58]. Many of these patients have lipoprotein deficiencies that result in abnormal lipid and/or lipoprotein concentrations. Consequently, the effect of exercise on these patients may be substantially different from the effect in patients free of these afflictions. Review of the exercise effect on some of these conditions have been published [151], including the effects of exercise on lipoprotein metabolism in patients with diabetes [62]. Generally, endurance exercise training for patients who are hypertriglyceridemic will result in a reduction of triglyceride concentrations. On the other hand, the precise effects of endurance-exercise training on total plasma cholesterol concentrations of hypercholesterolemic (total cholesterol concentrations above 240 mg/dl) patients have not been completely defined. Nevertheless, intervention programs that emphasize reductions in dietary intake of fat that result in reductions of body fat and body weight and are accompanied by an exercise program will result in reductions of total cholesterol and LDL-C concentrations, while HDL-C concentrations either stay the same or increase [197]. Without exercise there is a less consistent reduction in triglyceride concentration, while HDL-C tends to decrease.

The recent National Cholesterol Education Program Guidelines [40] state that exercise along with diet, weight loss, and medications should be included in the management of dyslipoproteinemias. It is important to know not only the interactive effect of exercise and diet on lipoprotein metabolism, but also the interactions between exercise and various classes of lipid medications now in use. However, studies of such interactions have not been published. The optimal management of these patients will in part depend on understanding these interactions.

REFERENCES

1. Adner, M. M., and W. P. Castelli. Elevated high-density lipoprotein levels in marathon runners. *JAMA* 243(6):534–536, 1980.
2. Albers, J. J., H. M. Taggart, D. Applebaum-Bowden, S. Haffner, C. H. Chestnut III, and W. R. Hazzard. Reduction of lecithin:cholesterol acyltransferase, apolipoprotein D, and the Lp(a) lipoprotein with the anabolic steroid stanozolol. *Biochim. Biophys. Acta* 795:293–296, 1984.

3. Altekruse, E. B., and J. H. Wilmore. Changes in blood chemistries following a controlled exercise program. *J. Occup. Med.* 15(2):110–113, 1973.

4. Angelopoulos, T. J., R. J. Robertson, F. L. Goss, K. F. Metz, and R. E. Laporte. Effect of repeated exercise bouts on high density lipoprotein-cholesterol and its subfractions HDL_2-C and HDL_3-C. *Int. J. Sports Med.* 14(4):196–201, 1993.

5. Annuzzi, G., E. Jansson, L. Kaijser, L. Holmquist, and L. A. Carlson. Increased removal rate of exogenous triglycerides after prolonged exercise in man: time course and effects of exercise duration. *Metabolism.* 36(5):438–443, 1987.

6. Armstrong, N., and B. Simons-Morton. Physical activity and blood lipids in adolescents. Invited presentation to the *International Consensus Conference on Physical Activity Guidelines for Adolescents.* La Jolla, CA, June 11–12, 1993.

7. Assmann, G., and H. Funke. HDL metabolism and atherosclerosis. *J. Cardiovasc. Pharmacol.* 16:(suppl 9):S15–S20, 1993.

8. Ballantyne, F. C., R. S. Clark, H. S. Simpson, and D. Ballantyne. The effect of moderate physical exercise on the plasma lipoprotein subfractions of male survivors of myocardial infarction. *Circulation* 65(5):913–918, 1982.

9. Barakat, H. A., D. S. Burton, J. W. Carpenter, D. Holbert, and R. G. Israel. Body fat distribution, plasma lipoproteins and the risk for coronary heart disease of male subjects. *Int. J. Obes.* 12:423–430, 1988.

10. Berg, A., G. Ringwald, and J. Keul. Lipoprotein cholesterol in well-trained athletes. *Int. J. Sports Med.* 1:137–138, 1980.

11. Berg, A., J. Keul, G. Ringwald, B. Deus, and K. Wybitul. Physical performance and serum cholesterol fractions in healthy young men. *Clin. Chim. Acta* 106:325–330, 1980.

12. Berger, G. M. B., and M. P. Griffiths. Acute effects of moderate exercise on plasma lipoprotein parameters. *Int. J. Sports Med.* 8(5):336–341, 1987.

13. Björntorp, P., P. Berchtold, G. Grimby, B. Lindholm, H. Sanne, et al. Effects of physical training on glucose tolerance, plasma insulin and lipids and on body composition in men after myocardial infarction. *Acta. Med. Scand.* 192:439–443, 1972.

14. Blanche, P. J., E. L. Gong, T. M. Forte, and A. V. Nichols. Characterization of human high-density lipoproteins by gradient gel electrophoresis. *Biochim. Biophys. Acta* 665:408–419, 1981.

15. Blumenthal, J. A., C. F. Emery, D. J. Madden, R. E. Coleman, M. W. Riddle, et al. Effects of exercise training on cardiorespiratory function in men and women > 60 years of age. *Am. J. Cardiol.* 67:633–639, 1991.

16. Breslow, J. L. Genetics of lipoprotein disorders. *Circulation.* 87(suppl III):III16–III21, 1993.

17. Brewer, H. B., R. E. Greg, J. M. Hoeg, and S. S. Fojo. Apolipoproteins and lipoproteins in human plasma: an overview. *Clin. Chem.* 34(8):(suppl B):B4–B8, 1988.

18. Brown, M. S., and J. L. Goldstein. A receptor-mediated pathway for cholesterol homeostasis. *Science* 232:34–47, 1986.

19. Brownell, K. D., P. S. Bachorik, and R. S. Ayerle. Changes in plasma lipid and lipoprotein levels in men and women after a program of moderate exercise. *Circulation* 65(3):477–484, 1982.

20. Carlson, L., and S. O. Fröberg. Blood lipid and glucose levels during a ten-day period of low-calorie intake and exercise in man. *Metabolism* 16(7):624–634, 1967.

21. Coon, P. J., E. R. Bleecker, D. T. Drinkwater, D. A. Meyers, and A. P. Goldberg. Effects of body composition and exercise capacity on glucose tolerance, insulin, and lipoprotein lipids in healthy older men: a cross-sectional and longitudinal intervention study. *Metabolism* 38(12):1201–1209, 1990.

22. Cooper, K. H., M. L. Pollock, R. P. Martin, S. R. White, A. C. Linnerud, and A. Jackson. Physical fitness levels vs. selected coronary risk factors: a cross-sectional study. *JAMA* 236(2):166–169, 1976.

23. Cullinane, E., S. Siconolfi, A. Saritelli, and P. D. Thompson. Acute decrease in serum

triglycerides with exercise: is there a threshold for an exercise effect. *Metabolism* 31(8):844–847, 1982.

24. Dahlen, G. H., J. R. Guyton, M. Attar, J. A. Farmer, J. A. Kautz, and A. M. Gotto. Association of levels of lipoprotein Lp(a), plasma lipids, and other lipoproteins with coronary artery disease documented by angiography. *Circulation* 74(4):758–765, 1986.

25. Davis, P. G., W. P. Bartoli, and J. L. Durstine. Effects of acute exercise intensity on plasma lipids and apolipoproteins in trained runners. *J. Appl. Physiol.* 72(3):914–919, 1992.

26. Deckelbaum, R. J., T. Olivecrona, and S. Eisenberg. Plasma lipoproteins in hyperlipidemia: roles of neutral lipid exchange and lipase. L. A. Carlson and A. G. Olsson (eds). *Treatment of Hyperlipoproteinemia*. New York: Raven Press, 1984, pp. 85–93.

27. DeLong, D. M., E. R. DeLong, P. D. Wood, K. Lippel, and B. M. Rifkind. A comparison of methods for the estimation of plasma low- and very low-density lipoprotein cholesterol: the Lipid Research Clinics Prevalence Study. *JAMA* 256(17):2372–2377, 1986.

28. Després, J. P., A. Tremblay, S. Moorjani, P. J. Lupien, G. Thériault, et al. Long-term exercise training with constant energy intake 3: Effects on plasma lipoprotein levels. *Int. J. Obes.* 14:85–94, 1990.

29. Després, J. P., C. Bouchard, and R. M. Malina. Physical activity and coronary heart disease risk factors during childhood and adolescence. K. B. Pandolf and J. O. Holloszy (eds). *Exercise and Sport Sciences Reviews*. Baltimore: Williams & Wilkins, 1990, pp. 243–261.

30. Després, J. P., S. Moorjani, A. Tremblay, E. T. Poehlman, P. J. Lupien, et al. Heredity and changes in plasma lipids and lipoproteins after short-term exercise training in men. *Arteriosclerosis* 8(4):402–409, 1988.

31. Dufaux, B., U. Order, R. Müller, and W. Hollman. Delayed effects of prolonged exercise on serum lipoproteins. *Metabolism* 35(2):105–109, 1986.

32. DuRant, R. H., C. W. Linder, S. Jay, J. W. Harkness, and R. G. Gray. The influence of a family history of CHD risk factors on serum lipoproteins in black children and adolescents. *J. Adolesc. Health Care* 3:75–81, 1982.

33. Durstine, J. L., K. A. Kenno, and R. E. Shepherd. Serum lipoproteins of the Zucker rat in response to an endurance running program. *Med. Sci. Sports Exerc.* 17(4):567–573, 1985.

34. Durstine, J. L., R. R. Pate, P. B. Sparling, G. E. Wilson, M. D. Senn, and W. P. Bartoli. Lipid, lipoprotein, and iron status of elite women distance runners. *Int. J. Sports Med.* 8:119–123, 1987.

35. Durstine, J. L., R. R. Pate, W. P. Bartoli, E. E. Shoup, L. A. Klingshirn, et al. Apolipoproteins AI and B in elite women runners. *Med. Sci. Sport Exerc.* 21(2):S113, 1989.

36. Durstine, J. L., W. Miller, S. Farrell, W. M. Sherman, and J. L. Ivy. Increases in HDL-cholesterol and the HDL/LDL cholesterol ratio during prolonged endurance exercise. *Metabolism* 32(10):993–997, 1983.

37. Elliot, D. L., L. Goldberg, K. S. Keuhl, and D. H. Catlin. Characteristics of anabolic-androgenic steroid-free competitive male and female bodybuilders. *Physician Sportsmed.* 15(6):169–179, 1987.

38. Enger, S. C., S. B. Strømme, and H. E. Refsum. High-density lipoprotein cholesterol, total cholesterol and triglycerides in serum after a single exposure to prolonged heavy exercise. *Scand. J. Clin. Lab. Invest.* 40:341–345, 1980.

39. Erikksen, J., K. Forfang, and J. Jervell. Coronary risk factors and physical fitness in healthy middle-aged men. *Acta Med. Scand.* 645(suppl):57–64, 1981.

40. Expert panel on detection, evaluation, and treatment of high blood cholesterol in adults. Summary of the second report of the National Cholesterol Education Program (NCEP) Expert panel on detection, evaluation, and treatment of high blood cholesterol in adults (Adult Treatment Panel II). *JAMA* 269(23):3015–3023, 1993.

41. Farrell, P. A., M. G. Maksud, M. L. Pollock, C. Foster, J. Anholm, et al. A comparison of plasma cholesterol, triglycerides, and high-density lipoprotein cholesterol in speed skaters, weight lifters, and nonathletes. *Eur. J. Appl. Physiol.* 48:77–82, 1982.

42. Frey, I., M. W. Baumstark, A. Berg, and J. Keul. Influence of acute maximal exercise on

lecithin:cholesterol acyltransferase activity in healthy adults of differing aerobic performance. *Eur. J. Appl. Physiol.* 62:31–35, 1991.

43. Friedewald, W. T., R. I. Levy, and D. S. Fredrickson. Estimation of the concentration of low density lipoprotein cholesterol in plasma without the use of the preparative ultracentrifuge. *Clin. Chem.* 18(6):499–502, 1972.

44. Fripp, R. R., and J. L. Hodgson. Effect of resistive training on plasma lipid and lipoprotein levels in male adolescents. *J. Pediatr.* 111:926–931, 1987.

45. Giada, F., G. Baldo-Ensi, M. R. Baiocchi, G. Zuliani, E. Vitale, and R. Fellin. Specialized physical training programs: effects on serum lipoprotein cholesterol, apoproteins A-I and B and lipolytic enzyme activities. *J. Sports Med. Phys. Fitness* 31:196–203, 1991.

46. Gilliam, T. B., and M. B. Burke. Effects of exercise on serum lipids and lipoproteins in girls, aged 8 to 10 years. *Artery* 4(3):203–213, 1978.

47. Gilliam, T. B., and P. S. Freedson. Effects of a 12- week school physical fitness program on peak VO_2max, body composition and blood lipids in 7 to 9 year-old children. *Int. J. Sports Med.* 1(2):73–78, 1980.

48. Glomset, J. A. The plasma lecithin:cholesterol acyltransferase reaction. *J. Lipid Res.* 9:155–167, 1968.

49. Goldberg, A. P. Aerobic and resistive exercise modify risk factors for coronary heart disease. *Med. Sci. Sports Exerc.* 21(6):669–674, 1989.

50. Goldberg, L., D. L. Elliot, R. W. Schutz, and F. E. Kloster. Changes in lipid and lipoprotein levels after weight training. *JAMA* 252(4):504–506, 1984.

51. Goodman, D. S. Report of the National Cholesterol Education Program Expert Panel on detection, evaluation, and treatment of high blood cholesterol in adults. *Arch. Intern. Med.* 148:36–69, 1988.

52. Goodyear, L. J., D. R. Van Houten, M. S. Fronsoe, M. L. Rocchio, E. V. Dover, and J. L. Durstine. Immediate and delayed effects of marathon running on lipids and lipoproteins in women. *Med. Sci. Sports Exerc.* 22(5):588–592, 1990.

53. Goodyear, L. J., M. S. Fronsoe, D. R. Van Houten, E. V. Dover, and J. L. Durstine. Increased HDL-cholesterol following eight weeks of progressive endurance training in female runners. *Ann. Sport Med.* 3(1):33–38, 1986.

54. Gorski, J., L. B. Oscai, and W. K. Palmer. Hepatic lipid metabolism in exercise and training. *Med. Sci. Sports Exerc.* 22(2):213–221, 1990.

55. Greenleaf, J. E., V. A. Convertino, and G. R. Mangseth. Plasma volume during stress in man: osmolality and red cell volume. *J. Appl. Physiol.* 47(5):1031–1038, 1979.

56. Griffin, B. A., E. R. Skinner, and R. J. Maughan. The acute effect of prolonged walking and dietary changes on plasma lipoprotein concentrations and high-density lipoprotein subfractions. *Metabolism* 37(6):535–541, 1988.

57. Gupta, A. K., E. A. Ross, J. N. Myers, and M. L. Kashyap. Increased reverse cholesterol transport in athletes. *Metabolism* 42(6):684–690, 1993.

58. Gyntelberg, F., R. Brennan, J. Holloszy, G. Schonfeld, M. Rennie, and S. W. Weidman. Plasma triglyceride lowering by exercise despite increased food intake in patients with type-IV hyperlipoproteinemia. *Am. J. Clin. Nutr.* 30:716–720, 1977.

59. Hagen, R. D., and L. R. Gettman. Maximal aerobic power, body fat, and serum lipoproteins in male distance runners. *J. Cardiac Rehabil.* 3(5):331–337, 1983.

60. Hamsten, A., G. Walldius, A. Szamosi, G. Dahlen, and U. de Faire. Relationship of angiographically defined coronary disease to serum lipoproteins and apolipoproteins in young survivors of myocardial infarction. *Circulation* 73(6):1097–1110, 1986.

61. Haskell, W. L. The influence of exercise on the concentrations of triglyceride and cholesterol in human plasma. R. L. Terjung (ed). *Exercise and Sport Sciences Reviews.* Lexington, MA: Collamore Press, 1984, pp. 205–244.

62. Haskell, W. L., and J. L. Durstine. Impact of exercise training on lipoprotein metabolism. J. Devlin, E. S. Horton, and M. Vranic (eds). *Diabetes Mellitus and Exercise.* Great Britain: Smith-Gordon, 1992, pp. 205–216.

63. Haskell, W. L., H. L. Taylor, P. D. Wood, H. Schrott, and G. Heiss. Strenuous physical

activity, treadmill exercise test performance and plasma high-density lipoprotein cholesterol: the Lipid Research Clinic Program Prevalence Study. *Circulation* 62(suppl IV):53–61, 1980.

64. Haskell, W. L., M. L. Stefanick, and R. Superko. Influence of exercise on plasma lipids and lipoproteins. E. S. Horton, R. L. Terjung (eds). *Exercise, Nutrition, and Energy Metabolism.* New York: Macmillan, 1988, pp. 213–227.

65. Herbert, J. A., L. Kerkhoff, L. Bell, and A. Lopez-S. Effect of exercise on lipid metabolism of rats fed high carbohydrate diet. *J. Nutr.* 105:718–725, 1975.

66. Herbert, P. N., D. N. Bernier, E. M. Cullinane, L. Edelstein, M. A. Kantor, and P. D. Thompson. High-density lipoprotein metabolism in runners and sedentary men. *JAMA* 252(8):1034–1037, 1984.

67. Higuchi, M., K. Iwaoka, K. Ishii, S. Matsuo, S. Kobayashi, et al. Plasma lipid and lipoprotein profiles in pre- and post-menopausal middle-aged runners. *Clin. Physiol.* 10:69–76, 1990.

68. Higuchi, M., K. Oishi, K. Ishii, K. Iwaoka, S. Matsuo, et al. Plasma lipid and lipoprotein profile in elderly female runners. *Clin. Physiol.* 11:545–552, 1991.

69. Higuchi, M., T. Fuchi, K. Iwaoka, K. Yamakawa, S. Kobayashi, et al. Plasma lipid and lipoprotein profile in elderly male long- distance runners. *Clin. Physiol.* 8:137–145, 1988.

70. Higuchi, M., T. Tamai, S. Kobayashi, and T. Nakai. Plasma lipoprotein and apolipoprotein profiles in aged Japanese athletes. Y. Sato, J. Poortmans, I. Hashimoto, and Y. Oshida (eds). *Integration of Medical and Sports Sciences.* Basel:Karger, 1992, pp. 126–136.

71. Holloszy, J. O., J. S. Skinner, G. Toro, and T. K. Cureton. Effects of a six month program of endurance exercise on lipids of middle-aged men. *Am. J. Cardiol.* 14:753–760, 1964.

72. Hurley, B. F., D. S. Seals, J. M. Hagberg, A. C. Goldberg, S. M. Ostrove, et al. High-density-lipoprotein cholesterol in bodybuilders v powerlifters: negative effects of androgen use. *JAMA* 252(4):507–513, 1984.

73. Hurley, B. F., J. M. Hagberg, A. P. Goldberg, D. R. Seals, A. A. Ehsani, et al. Resistive training can reduce coronary risk factors without altering VO₂max or perent body fat. *Med. Sci. Sports Exerc.* 20(2):150–154, 1988.

74. Hurter, R., J. Swale, M. A. Peyman, and C. W. H. Barnett. Some immediate and long term effects of exercise on the plasma lipids. *Lancet* 2:671–675, 1975.

75. Huttunen, J. K., E. Länsimies, E. Voutilainen, C. Ehnholm, E. Hietanen, et al. Effect of moderate physical exercise on serum lipoproteins: a controlled clinical trial with special reference to serum high-density lipoproteins. *Circulation* 60(6):1220–1229, 1979.

76. Johnson, C. C., M. H. Stone, A. Lopez-S, J. A. Hebert, L. T. Kilgore, and R. J. Byrd. Diet and exercise in middle-aged men. *J. Am. Diet. Assoc.* 81:695–701, 1982.

77. Kantor, M. A., E. M. Cullinane, P. N. Herbert, and P. D. Thompson. Acute increase in lipoprotein lipase following prolonged exercise. *Metabolism* 33(5):454–457, 1984.

78. Kantor, M. A., E. M. Cullinane, S. P. Sady, P. N. Herbert, and P. D. Thompson. Exercise acutely increases high density lipoprotein-cholesterol and lipoprotein lipase activity in trained and untrained men. *Metabolism* 36(2):188–192, 1987.

79. Kiens, B., and H. Lithell. Lipoprotein metabolism influenced by training-induced changes in human skeletal muscle. *J. Clin. Invest.* 83:558–564, 1989.

80. Kiens, B., H. Lithell, and B. Vessby. Further increase in high density lipoprotein in trained males after enhanced training. *Eur. J. Appl. Physiol.* 52:425–430, 1984.

81. Kiens, B., I. Jörgenson, S. Lewis, G. Jensen, H. Lithell, et al. Increased plasma HDL-cholesterol and Apo A-I in sedentary middle-aged men after physical conditioning. *Eur. J. Clin. Invest.* 10:203–209, 1980.

82. Kiens, B., P. Gad, H. Lithell, and B. Vessby. Minor dietary effects on HDL in physically active men. *Eur. J. Clin. Invest.* 11:265–271, 1981.

83. Kohl, H. W., N. F. Gordon, C. B. Scott, H. Vaandrager, and S. N. Blair. Musculoskeletal strength and serum lipid levels in men and women. *Med. Sci. Sports Exerc.* 24(10):1080–1087, 1992.

84. Kokkinos, P. F., and B. F. Hurley. Strength training and lipoprotein-lipid profiles: a critical analysis and recommendations for further study. *Sports Med.* 9(5):266–272, 1990.

85. Kokkinos, P. F., B. F. Hurley, M. A. Smutok, C. Farmer, C. Reece, et al. Strength training does not improve lipoprotein-lipid profiles in men at risk for CHD. *Med. Sci. Sports Exerc.* 23(10):1134–1139, 1991.

86. Kokkinos, P. F., B. F. Hurley, P. Vaccaro, J. C. Patterson, L. B. Gardner, et al. Effects of low- and high-repetition resistive training on lipoprotein-lipid profiles. *Med. Sci. Sports Exerc.* 20(1):50–54, 1988.

87. Koro, T. Physical training in the aged person. *Jpn. Circ. J.* 54:1465–1470, 1990.

88. Krauss, R. M., Relationship of intermediate and low- density lipoprotein subspecies to risk of coronary artery disease. *Am. Heart J.* 113:578–582, 1987.

89. Krauss, R. M., F. T. Lindgren, P. T. Williams, S. F. Kelsey, J. Brensike, et al. Intermediate-density lipoproteins and progression of coronary artery disease in hypercholesterolaemic men. *Lancet* ii:62–68, 1987.

90. Kuusela, P. J., E. Voutilainen, K. Kukkonen, and R. Rauramaa. Lipoprotein patterns in lumberjacks. *Scand. J. Sports Sci.* 2(1):13–16, 1980.

91. Kuusi, T., E. A. Nikkilä, P. Saarinen, P. Varjo, and L. A. Laitinen. Plasma high density lipoproteins HDL_2, HDL_3 and postheparin plasma lipase in relation to parameters of physical fitness. *Atherosclerosis* 41:209–219, 1982.

92. Lamon-Fava, S., D. Jimenez, J. C. Christian, R. R. Fabsitz, T. Reed, et al. The NHLBI twin study: heritability of apolipoprotein A-I, B, and low density lipoprotein subclasses and concordance for lipoprotein(a). *Atherosclerosis* 91:97–106, 1991.

93. Lamon-Fava, S., E. C. Fisher, M. E. Nelson, W. J. Evans, J. S. Millar, et al. Effect of exercise and menstrual cycle status on plasma lipids, low density lipoprotein particle size, and apolipoproteins. *J. Clin. Endocrinol. Metab.* 68(1):17–21, 1989.

94. Lee, R., D. Nieman, R. Raval, J. Blankenship, and J. Lee. The effects of acute moderate exercise on serum lipids and lipoproteins in mildly obese women. *Int. J. Sports Med.* 12(6):537–542, 1991.

95. Lehtonen, A., and J. Viikari. Serum triglycerides and cholesterol and serum high-density lipoprotein cholesterol in highly physical active men. *Acta Med. Scand.* 204:111–114, 1978.

96. Leibel, R. L., and J. Hirsch. Site- and sex-related difference in adrenoceptor status of human adipose tissue. *J. Clin. Endocrinol. Metab.* 64(6):1205–1210, 1987.

97. Leon, A. S., J. Conrad, D. B. Hunninghake, and R. Serfass. Effects of a vigorous walking program on body composition, and carbohydrate and lipid metabolism of obese young men. *Am. J. Clin. Nutr.* 32:1776–1787, 1979.

98. Linder, C. W., R. H. DuRant, and O. M. Mahoney. The effect of physical conditioning on serum lipids and lipoproteins in white male adolescents. *Med. Sci. Sports Exerc.* 15(3):232–236, 1983.

99. Lobo, R. A., M. Notelovitz, L. Bernstein, F. Y. Khan, R. K. Ross, and W. L. Paul. Lp(a) lipoprotein: relationship to cardiovascular disease risk factors, exercise and estrogen. *Am. J. Obstet. Gynecol.* 166(4):1182–1190, 1992.

100. Lokey, E. A., and Z. V. Tran. Effects of exercise training on serum lipid and lipoprotein concentrations in women: a meta-analysis. *Int. J. Sports Med.* 10(6):424–429, 1989.

101. Lusis, A. J. Genetic factors affecting blood lipoproteins: the candidate gene approach. *J. Lipid Res.* 29:397–429, 1988.

102. Máček, M., D. Bell, J. Rutenfranz, J. Vavra, J. Masopust, et al. A comparison of coronary risk factors in groups of trained and untrained adolescents. *Eur. J. Appl. Physiol.* 58:577–582, 1989.

103. Maciejko, J. J., D. R. Holmes, B. A. Kottke, A. R. Zinsmeister, D. M. Dinh, and S. J. T. Mao. Apolipoprotein A-I as a marker for angiographically assessed coronary-artery disease. *N. Engl. J. Med.* 309(7):385–389, 1983.

104. Mankowitz, K., R. Seip, C. F. Semenkovich, and G. Schonfeld. Short term interruption of training affects both fasting and post-prandial lipemia. *Atherosclerosis* 95:181–189, 1992.

105. Mann, G. V., H. L. Garrett, A. Farhi, H. Murray, and F. T. Billings. Exercise to prevent coronary heart disease: an experimental study of the effects of training on risk factors for coronary disease in men. *Am. J. Med.* 46:12–27, 1969.

106. Manning, J. M., C. R. Dooly-Manning, K. White, I. Kampa, S. Silas, et al. Effects of a resistive training program on lipoprotein-lipid levels in obese women. *Med. Sci. Sports Exerc.* 23(11):1222–1226, 1991.
107. Marniemi, J., and E. Hietanen. Response of serum lecithin:cholesterol acyltransferase activity to exercise training. E. Hietanen (ed). *Regulation of Serum Lipids by Physical Exercise.* Boca Raton, FL: CRC Press, 1982, pp. 116–118.
108. Marniemi, J., P. Peltonen, I. Vuori, and E. Heitanen. Lipoprotein lipase of human postheparin plasma and adipose tissue in relation to physical training. *Acta Physiol. Scand.* 110:131–135, 1980.
109. Marniemi, J., S. Dahlstrom, M. Kvist, A. Seppänen, and E. Hietanen. Dependence of serum lipid and lecithin:cholesterol acyltransferase levels on physical training in young men. *Eur J. Appl. Physiol.* 49:25–35, 1982.
110. Marti, B., E. Suter, W. F. Riesen, A. Tschopp, H. Wanner, and F. Gutzwiller. Effects of long-term, self-monitored exercise on the serum lipoprotein and apolipoprotein profile in middle-aged men. *Athersclerosis* 81:19–31, 1990.
111. Marti, B., M. Knobloch, W. F. Riesen, and H. Howald. Fifteen year changes in exercise, aerobic power, abdominal fat, and serum lipids in runners and controls. *Med. Sci. Sports Exerc.* 23(1):115–122, 1991.
112. Martin, R. P., W. L. Haskell, and P. D. Wood. Blood chemistry and lipid profiles of elite distance runners. *Ann. NY Acad. Sci.* 301:346–360, 1977.
113. Miles, L. A., and E. F. Plow. Lp(a): An interloper into the fibrinolytic system. *Thromb. Haemost.* 63(3):331–335, 1990.
114. Moll, M. E., R. S. Williams, R. M. Lester, S. H. Quarfordt, and A. G. Wallace. Cholesterol metabolism in non-obese women: failure of physical conditioning to alter levels of high density lipoprotein cholesterol. *Atherosclerosis* 34:159–166, 1979.
115. Montoye, H. J., W. D. Block, and R. Gayle. Maximal oxygen intake and blood lipids. *J. Chronic Dis.* 31:111–118, 1978.
116. Moore, R. A., W. A. F. Penfold, R. D. Simpson, R. W. Simpson, J. I. Mann, and R. S. Turner. High-density lipoprotein, lipid, and carbohydrate metabolism during increasing fitness. *Ann. Clin. Biochem.* 16:76–80, 1979.
117. Morgan, D. W., R. J. Cruise, B. W. Girardin, V. Lutz- Schneider, D. H. Morgan, and W. M. Qi. HDL-C concentrations in weight-trained, endurance-trained, and sedentary females. *Physician Sportsmed.* 14(3):166–181, 1986.
118. Naito, H. K. The association of serum lipids, lipoproteins, and apolipoproteins with coronary artery disease assessed by coronary arteriography. *Ann. NY Acad. Sci.* 454:230–238, 1985.
119. Nikkilä, E. A., M.-R. Taskinen, S. Rehunen, and M. Härkönen. Lipoprotein lipase activity in adipose tissue and skeletal muscle of runners: relation to serum lipoproteins. *Metabolism* 27(11):1661–1671, 1978.
120. Nikkilä, E. A., T. Kuusi, and P. Myllynen. High-density lipoprotein and apolipoprotein A-I during physical inactivity. *Atherosclerosis* 37:457–462, 1980.
121. Nozaki, S., M. Kubo, H. Sudo, Y. Matsuzawa, and S. Tarui. The role of hepatic triglyceride lipase in the metabolism of intermediate-density lipoprotein-postheparin lipolytic activities determined by a sensitive, nonradioisotopic method in hyperlipidemic patients and normals. *Metabolism* 35(1):53–58, 1986.
122. Nye, E. R., K. Carlson, P. Kirstein, and S. Rössner. Changes in high density lipoprotein subfractions and other lipoproteins induced by exercise. *Clin. Chim. Acta* 113:51–57, 1981.
123. Oscai, L. B., D. A. Essig, and W. K. Palmer. Lipase regulation of muscle triglyceride hydrolysis. *J. Appl. Physiol.* 69(5):1571–1577, 1990.
124. Pay, H. E., A. E. Hardman, G. J. W. Jones, and A. Hudson. The acute effects of low-intensity exercise on plasma lipids in endurance-trained and untrained young adults. *Eur. J. Appl. Physiol.* 64:182–186, 1992.
125. Peeples, L. H., J. W. Carpenter, R. G. Israel, and H. A. Barakat. Alterations in low-density lipoproteins in subjects with abdominal adiposity. *Metabolism* 38(10):1029–1036, 1989.

126. Peltonen, P., J. Marniemi, E. Hietanen, I. Vuori, and C. Ehnholm. Changes in serum lipids, lipoproteins and heparin releasable lipolytic enzymes during moderate physical training in man: a longitudinal study. *Metabolism* 30(5):518–526, 1981.

127. Reaven, P. D., J. B. McPhillips, E. L. Barrett-Conner, and M. H. Criqui. Leisure time exercise and lipid and lipoprotein levels in an older population. *J. Am. Geriatr. Soc.* 38(8):847–854, 1990.

128. Rhoads, G. C., C. Gulbrandsen, and A. Kagan. Serum lipoproteins and coronary heart disease in a population study of Hawaii Japanese men. *N.Engl. J. Med.* 294(6):293–298, 1976.

129. Rifkind, B. M., I. Tamir, G. Heiss, R. B. Wallace, and H. A. Tyroler. Distribution of high density and other lipoproteins in selected LRC prevalence study populations: a brief survey. *Lipids* 14(1):105–112, 1979.

130. Roberts, K. M., E. G. Noble, D. B. Hayden, and A. W. Taylor. Lipoprotein lipase activity in skeletal muscle and adipose tissue of marathon runners after simple and complex carbohydrate-rich diets. *Eur. J. Appl. Physiol.* 57:75–80, 1988.

131. Rotkis, T. C., R. Cote, E. Coyle, and J. H. Wilmore, Relationship between high density lipoprotein cholesterol and weekly running mileage. *J. Cardiac Rehabil.* 2(2):109–112, 1982.

132. Sady, S. P., E. M. Cullinane, A. Saritelli, D. Bernier, and P. D. Thompson. Elevated high-density lipoprotein cholesterol in endurance athletes is related to enhanced plasma triglyceride clearance. *Metabolism* 37(6):568–572, 1988.

133. Sady, S. P., P. D. Thompson, E. M. Cullinane, M. A. Kantor, E. Domagala, and P. N. Herbert. Prolonged exercise augments plasma triglyceride clearance. *JAMA* 256(18):2552–2555, 1986.

134. Schwane, J. A., and D. E. Cundiff. Relationships among cardiorespiratory fitness, regular physical activity and plasma lipids in young adults. *Metabolism* 28(7):771–776, 1979.

135. Schwartz, R. S. Effects of exercise training on high density lipoproteins and apolipoprotein A-I in old and young men. *Metabolism* 37(2):1128–1133, 1988.

136. Schwartz, R. S., D. C. Cain, W. P. Shuman, V. Larson, J. R. Stratton et al. Effects of intensive endurance training on lipoprotein profiles in young and older men. *Metabolism* 41(6):649–654, 1992.

137. Seals, D. R., J. M. Hagberg, B. F. Hurley, A. A. Ehsani, and J. O. Holloszy. Effects of endurance training on glucose tolerance and plasma lipid levels in older men and women. *JAMA* 252(5):645–649, 1984.

138. Seals, D. R., W. K. Allen, B. F. Hurley, G. P. Dalsky, A. A. Ehsani, and J. M. Hagberg. Elevated high-density lipoprotein cholesterol levels in older endurance athletes. *Am . J. Cardiol.* 54:390–393, 1984.

139. Seip, R. L., P. Moulin, T. Cocke, A. Tall, W. M. Kohrt, et al. Exercise training decreases plasma cholesteryl ester transfer protein. *Arterioscler. Thromb.* 13:1359–1367, 1993.

140. Shepherd, J. Lipoprotein metabolism: an overview. *Ann. Acad. Med.* 21(1):106–113, 1992.

141. Shoup, E. E., J. L. Durstine, J. M. Davis, R. R. Pate, and W. P. Bartoli. Effects of a single session of resistance exercise on plasma lipoproteins and postheparin lipase activity. *in review.*

142. Siegel, W., G. Blomqvist, and J. H. Mitchell. Effects of a quantitated physical training program on middle-aged sedentary men. *Circulation* 41:19–29, 1970.

143. Simonelli, C., and R. P. Eaton. Reduced triglyceride secretion: a metabolic consequence of chronic exercise. *Am J. Physiol.* 234(3):E221–E227, 1978.

144. Skinner, E. R., C. Watt, and R. J. Maughan. The acute effect of marathon running on plasma lipoproteins in female subjects. *Eur. J. Appl. Physiol.* 56:451–456, 1987.

145. Smutok, M. A., C. Reece, P. F. Kokkinos, C. Farmer, P. Sawson, et al. Aerobic versus strength training for risk factor intervention in middle-aged men at high risk for coronary heart disease. *Metabolism* 42(2):177–184, 1993.

146. Sopko, G., A. S. Leon, D. R. Jacobs, N. Foster, J. Moy et al. The effects of exercise and weight loss on plasma lipids in young obese men. *Metabolism* 34(3):227–236, 1985.

147. Stefanick, M. L., R. B. Terry, W. L. Haskell, and P. D. Wood. Relationships of changes in

postheparin hepatic and lipoprotein lipase activity to HDL-cholesterol changes following weight loss achieved by dieting versus exercise. L. Gallo (ed). *Cardiovascular Disease: Molecular and Cellular Mechanisms, Prevention, and Treatment.* New York: Plenum Press, 1984, pp. 61–68.

148. Stein, R. A., D. W. Michielli, M. D. Glantz, H. Sardy, A. Cohen, et al. Effects of different exercise training intensities on lipoprotein cholesterol fractions in healthy middle-aged men. *Am. Heart J.* 119(2):277–283, 1990.

149. Sullivan, M. H., R. G. Israel, R. Cayton, and R. H. Marks. Relationship between cardiorespiratory fitness and plasma lipoprotein (a) in men. *Med. Sci. Sports Exerc.* 25(5):S204, 1993.

150. Superko, H. R. Exercise training, serum lipids, and lipoprotein particles: is there a change threshold. *Med. Sci. Sports Exerc.* 23(6):677–685, 1991.

151. Superko, H. R., and W. L. Haskell. The role of exercise training in the therapy of hyperlipoproteinemia. *Cardiol. Clin.* 5(2):285–310, 1987.

152. Suter, E., and M. R. Hawes. Relationship of physical activity, body fat, diet, and blood lipid profile in youths 10–15 yr. *Med. Sci. Sports Exerc.* 25(6):748–754, 1993.

153. Sutherland, W. H. F., S. P. Woodhouse, S. Williamson, and B. Smith. Decreased and continued physical activity and plasma lipoprotein lipids in previously trained men. *Atherosclerosis* 39:307–311, 1981.

154. Swank, A. M., R. J. Robertson, R. W. Deitrich, and M. Bates. The effect of acute exercise on high density lipoprotein-cholesterol and the subfractions in females. *Artherosclerosis* 63:187–192, 1987.

155. Tall, A. R. Plasma high density lipoproteins: metabolism and relationship to atherogenesis. *J. Clin. Invest.* 86:379–384, 1990.

156. Tall, A. R. Plasma lipid transfer proteins. *J. Lipid Res.* 27:361–367, 1986.

157. Tall, A. R., and D. S. Small. Plasma high-density lipoproteins. *N. Engl. J. Med.* 299:1232–1236, 1978.

158. Tamai, T., M. Higuchi, K. Oida, T. Nakai, S. Miyabo, and S. Kobayashi. Effects of exercise on plasma lipoprotein metabolism. Y. Sato, J. Pourtmans, I. Hashimoto, Y. Oshida (eds). *Integration of Medical and Sports Sciences.* Basel:Karger, 1992, pp. 430–438.

159. Tamai, T., T. Nakai, H. Takai, R. Fujiwara, S. Miyabo, et al. The effects of physical exercise on plasma lipoprotein and apolipoprotein metabolism in elderly men. *J. Gerontol.* 43(4):M75–79, 1988.

160. Taskinen, M. -R., and E. A. Nikkila. High-density lipoprotein subfractions in relation to lipoprotein lipase activity of tissues in man—evidence for reciprocal regulation of HDL_2 and HDL_3 levels by lipoprotein lipase. *Clin. Chim. Acta.* 112:325–332, 1981.

161. Taskinen, M. -R., and E. A. Nikkilä. Effects of caloric restriction on lipid metabolism in man. *Atherosclerosis* 32:289–299, 1979.

162. Taskinen, M. -R., E. A. Nikkilä, S. Rehunen, and A. Gordin. Effect of acute vigorous exercise on lipoprotein lipase activity of adipose tissue and skeletal muscle in physically active men. *Artery* 6(6):471–483, 1980.

163. Thomas, T. R., S. B. Adeniran, P. W. Iltis, C. A. Aquiar, and J. J. Albers. Effects of interval and continuous running on HDL-cholesterol, apoproteins, A-I and B, and LACT. *Can. J. Appl. Sport Sci.* 10(1):52–59, 1985.

164. Thompson, E. C., T. R. Thomas, J. Araujo, J. J. Albers, and C. J. Decedue. Response of HDL cholesterol, apoprotein A-I, and LCAT to exercise withdrawal. *Atherosclerosis* 54:65–73, 1985.

165. Thompson, P. D. What do muscles have to do with lipoproteins. *Circulation* 81(4):1428–1430, 1990.

166. Thompson, P. D., B. Lazarus, E. Cullinane, L. O. Henderson, T. Musliner, et al. Exercise, diet, or physical characteristics as determinants of HDL-levels in endurance athletes. *Atherosclerosis* 46(3):333–339, 1983.

167. Thompson, P. D., E. Cullinane, L. O. Henderson, and P. N. Herbert, Acute effects of prolonged exercise on serum lipids. *Metabolism* 29(7):662–665, 1980.

168. Thompson, P. D., E. M. Cullinane, R. Eshleman, S. Sady, and P. N. Herbert. The effects of caloric restriction or exercise cessation on the serum lipid and lipoprotein concentrations of endurance athletes. *Metabolism* 33(10):943–950, 1984.

169. Thompson, P. D., E. M. Cullinane, S. P. Sady, M. M. Glynn, C. B. Chenevert, and P. N. Herbert. High density lipoprotein metabolism in endurance athletes and sedentary men. *Circulation* 84(1):140–152, 1991.

170. Thompson, P. D., E. M. Cullinane, S. P. Sady, M. M. Flynn, D. N. Bernier, et al. Modest changes in high-density lipoprotein concentrations and metabolism with prolonged exercise training. *Circulation* 78(1):25–34, 1988.

171. Thorland, W. G., and T. B. Gilliam. Comparison of serum lipids between habitually high and low active pre-adolescent males.*Med Sci. Sports Exerc.* 13(5):316–321, 1981.

172. Tikkanen, H. O., M. Härkönen, H. Näveri, E. Hämäläinen, T. Elovaninio, et al. Relationship of skeletal muscle fiber type to serum high density lipoprotein cholesterol and apolipoprotein A-I levels. *Atherosclerosis* 90:49–57, 1991.

173. Tikkanen, M. J. Plasma lipoproteins and atherosclerosis. *J. Diabetes Complications* 4(2):35–38, 1990.

174. Tran, Z. V., A. Weltman, G. V. Glass, and D. P. Mood. The effects of exercise on blood lipids and lipoproteins: a meta- analysis of studies. *Med. Sci. Sports Exerc.* 15(5):393–402, 1983.

175. Tran, Z. V., and A. Weltman. Differential effects of exercise on serum lipid and lipoprotein levels seen with changes in body weight: a meta analysis. *JAMA* 254(7):919–924, 1985.

176. Tsopanakis, C., D. Kotsarellis, and A. Tsopanakis. Plasma lecithin:cholesterol acyltransferase activity in elite athletes from selected sports. *Eur. J. Appl. Physiol.* 58:262–265, 1988.

177. Tsopanakis, C., D. Kotsarellis, and A. D. Tsopanakis. Lipoprotein and lipid profiles of elite athletes in Olympic sports. *Int. J. Sports Med.* 7(6):316–321, 1986.

178. Välimäki, I., M. L. Hursti, L. Pihlaskoski, and J. Viikari. Exercise performance and serum lipids in relation to physical activity in school children. *Int. J. Sports Med.* 1(3):132–136, 1980.

179. Verrill, D., E. Shoup, G. McElveen, K. Witt, and D. Bergey. Resistive exercise training in cardiac patients. *Sports Med.* 13(3):171–193, 1992.

180. Vessby, B., G. Kostner, H. Lithell, and J. Thomis. Diverging effects of cholestyramine on apolipoprotein B and lipoprotein Lp(a). *Atherosclerosis* 44:61–71, 1982.

181. Vodak, P. A., P. D. Wood, W. L. Haskell, and P. T. Williams. HDL-cholesterol and other plasma lipid and lipoprotein concentrations in middle-aged male and female tennis players. *Metabolism* 29(8):745–752, 1980.

182. Wallace, M. B., R. J. Moffatt, E. M. Haymes, and N. R. Green. Acute effects of resistance exercise on parameters of lipoprotein metabolism. *Med. Sci. Sports Exerc.* 23(2):199–204, 1991.

183. Wanne, O., J. Viikari, and I. Välimäki. Physical performance and serum lipids in 14-16-year-old trained, normally active, and inactive children . J. Ilmarinen and I. Välimäki (eds). *Children and Sport.* Berlin, Springer-Verlag, 1984, pp. 241–246.

184. Weintraub, M. S., Y. Rosen, R. Otto, S. Eisenberg, and J. L. Breslow. Physical exercise conditioning in the absence of weight loss reduces fasting and postprandial triglyceride-rich lipoprotein levels. *Circulation* 79(5):1007–1014, 1989.

185. Weltman, A., C. Janney, C. B. Rains, K. Strand, and F. I. Katch. The effects of hydraulic-resistance strength training on serum lipid levels in prepubertal boys. *Am. J. Dis. Child.* 141:777–780, 1987.

186. Weltman, A., S. Matter, and B. A. Stamford. Caloric restriction and/or mild exercise: effects on serum lipids and body composition. *Am. J. Clin. Nutr.* 33:1002–1009, 1980.

187. Williams, P. T., J. J. Albers, R. M. Krauss, and P. D. S. Wood. Associations of lecithin:cholesterol acyltransferase (LCAT) mass concentrations with exercise, weight loss, and plasma lipoprotein subfraction concentrations in men. *Atherosclerosis* 82:53–58, 1990.

188. Williams, P. T., P. D. Wood, W. L. Haskell, and M. A. Vranizan. The effects of running milage and duration on plasma lipoprotein levels. *JAMA* 247(19):2674–2679, 1982.
189. Williams, P. T., R. M. Krauss, K. M. Vranizan, and P. D. S. Wood. Changes in lipoprotein subfractions during diet-induced and exercise-induced weight loss in moderately overweight men. *Circulation* 81(4):1293–1304, 1990.
190. Williams, P. T., R. M. Krauss, K. M. Vranizan, J. J. Albers, and P. D. S. Wood. Effects of weight-loss by exercise and by diet on apolipoproteins A-I and A-II and the particle-size distribution of high-density lipoproteins in men. *Metabolism* 41(4):441–449, 1992.
191. Williams, P. T., R. M. Krauss, K. M. Vranizan, J. J. Albers, R. B. Terry, and P. D. S. Wood. Effects of exercise-induced weight loss on low density lipoprotein subfractions in healthy men. *Arteriosclerosis* 9(5):623–632, 1989.
192. Williams, P. T., R. M. Krauss, K. M. Vranizan, M. L. Stefanick, P. D. S. Wood, and F. T. Lindgren. Associations of lipoproteins and apolipoproteins with gradient gel electrophoresis estimates of high-density lipoprotein subfractions in men and women. *Arterioscler. Thromb.* 12(3):332–340, 1992.
193. Williams, P. T., R. M. Krauss, P. D. Wood, F. T. Lindgren, C. Giotas, and K. M. Vranizan. Lipoprotein subfractions of runners and sedentary men. *Metabolism* 35(1):45–52, 1986.
194. Wirth, A., C. Diehm, M. Kohlmeier, C. C. Heuck, and I. Vogel. Effect of prolonged exercise on serum lipids and lipoproteins. *Metabolism* 32(7):669–672, 1983.
195. Wood, P. D., and M. L. Stefanick. Exercise, fitness, and atherosclerosis. C. Bouchard, R. J. Shephard, T. Stephens, J. R. Sutton, and B. D. McPherson. (eds). *Exercise, Fitness, and Health.* Champaign, IL: Human Kinetics Books, 1990, pp. 409–423.
196. Wood, P. D., M. L. Stefanick, D. M. Dreon, B. Frey-Hewitt, S. C. Garay, et al. Changes in plasma lipids and lipoproteins in overweight men during weight loss through dieting as compared with exercise. *N. Engl. J. Med.* 319(18):1173–1179, 1988.
197. Wood, P. D., M. L. Stefanick, P. T. Williams, and W. L. Haskell. The effects on plasma lipoproteins of a prudent weight-reducing diet, with or without exercise, in overweight men and women. *N. Engl. J. Med.* 325(7):461–466, 1991.
198. Wood, P. D., W. L. Haskell, H. Klein, S. Lewis, M. P. Stern, and J. W. Farquhar. The distribution of plasma lipoproteins in middle-aged male runners. *Metabolism* 25(11):1249–1257, 1976.
199. Wood, P. D., W. L. Haskell, M. P. Stern, S. Lewis, and C. Perry. Plasma lipoprotein distributions in male and female runners. *Ann. NY Acad. Sci.* 301:748–763, 1977.
200. Wood, P. D., W. L. Haskell, S. N. Blair, P. T. Williams, R. M. Krauss, et al. Increased exercise level and plasma lipoprotein concentrations: a one-year randomized, controlled study in sedentary middle-aged men. *Metabolism* 32(1):31–39, 1983.
201. Yki-Järvinen, H., V. A. Koivisto, M.-R. Taskinen, and E. A. Nikkilä. Glucose tolerance, plasma lipoproteins and tissue lipoprotein lipase activities in body builders. *Eur. J. Appl. Physiol.* 53:253–259, 1984.
202. Zavaroni, I., Y. I. Chen, C. E. Mondon, and G. M. Reaven. Ability of exercise to inhibit carbohydrate-induced hypertriglyceridemia in rats. *Metabolism* 30(5):476–480, 1981.

Index

*Numbers followed by the letter t indicate tables; numbers followed by the letter f indicate figures.